THE PATHOLOGY OF THE
AGING HUMAN NERVOUS SYSTEM

THE PATHOLOGY OF THE AGING HUMAN NERVOUS SYSTEM

Serge Duckett, M.D. *(Université de Paris);* Ph.D.
*(Royal Postgraduate Medical School, University of
London);* Dr. es Sc. *(Université de Paris).*

*Director and Professor, Bernard J. Alpers Neuropathology
Laboratory, Department of Neurology, Jefferson Medical
College of the Thomas Jefferson University, Philadelphia,
Pennsylvania.*
*Professeur Associé, Département de Biophysique, Faculté
de Médecine de Paris XII, CHU Henri Mondor (Créteil),
France.*
*Visiting Professor, Department of Pathology,
Massachusetts General Hospital, Boston, Massachusetts.*

Lea & Febiger • *Philadelphia* • *London* • *1991*

Lea & Febiger
200 Chester Field Parkway
Malvern, PA 19355-9725
U.S.A.
(215) 251-2230

Library of Congress Cataloging-in-Publication Data

The Pathology of the aging human nervous system / edited by Serge
    Duckett.
        p.   cm.
    ISBN 0-8121-1355-1
        1. Geriatric neurology. . 2. Nervous system—Diseases—Age factors.
    3. Aged—Diseases.   I. Duckett, Serge.
        [DNLM: 1. Aging.   2. Nervous System—pathology.   3. Nervous
    System Diseases—in old age.   WL 102 P297]
    RC346.P34   1991
    618.97′8—dc20
    DNLM/DLC   90-6638
    for Library of Congress   CIP

PRINTED IN THE UNITED STATES OF AMERICA

Print number: 3   2   1

Reprints of chapters may be purchased from Lea & Febiger in quantities of 100 or more.

Dedication

This book is dedicated to the memory of William H. McMenemey (1905–1977).

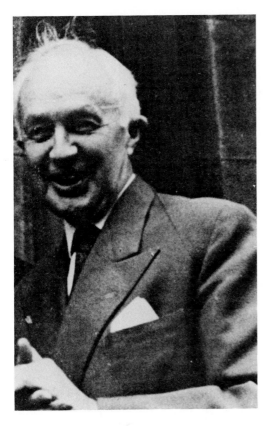

William Henry McMenemey died on November 24, 1977, at the age of 72. He retired from active participation in neuropathology in 1970, to the tranquility of his home in Morden, Surrey, where in the company of his wife, Dr. Robina Insker McMenemey (Rubie), he pursued his "other" career as a medical historian.

Professor McMenemey was emeritus Professor of Pathology at the Institute of Neurology (London). He was a fellow of three Royal Colleges—those of the Pathologists, Psychiatrists and Physicians of London. He was at one time or other president of the Association of Clinical Pathologists (1958), the British Neurological Society (1957–60), the British Neuropathological Society (1957–60), the section of Neurology (1960–61), the section of History of Medicine (1962–64) of the Royal Society of Medicine, and the International Society of Clinical Pathology (1966–69). He held numerous other posts in national and international medical organizations.

He was educated at Merton College, Oxford, and received his medical training at St. Bartholomew's Hospital. He trained in psychiatry and pathology at the Napsbury and Shenley hospitals and at Maida Vale Hospital. He was appointed assistant pathologist to the West End Hospital for Nervous Diseases in 1934, assistant pathologist to the Radcliffe Infirmary in 1937, pathologist to the Royal Infirmary, Worcester in 1940, pathologist to the Maida Vale Hospital in 1949, where he remained until his retirement.

His areas of interest in neuropathology were dementia, senility, brain tumors and demyelinating diseases to which he contributed classic descriptions and studies. He wrote the chapter on dementia in Greenfield's Neuropathology (1955, 1963) and contributed the section on diseases of the nervous system in Systemic Pathology by Payling-Wright and Symmers (1966).

He introduced the use of electron micros-copy, CSF electrophoresis and histochemistry in the diagnosis of disease at Maida Vale Hospital in the late fifties and early sixties, some-times in the face of not only disinterest but of active opposition. He was always ready to keep and support people whose ideas did not fit in with the preconceived notions of the mandarins of neuropathology and neurology of the times, and he was also an internation-alist and thus, in Britain, he was popular with some and unpopular with others. There was unanimity in other lands where he was just popular.

His "other" career was a medical historian. His first contribution was "A History of the Worcester Royal Infirmary" published in 1947, which is much more interesting than the title suggests, because it deals with development of the care of patients in a provincial English hos-pital, set against the background of the evolu-tion of scientific and medical thinking, and the change from superstition to a rational ap-proach to diagnosis and treatment. The de-tailed information available in this book sug-gests many hours poring over ancient catalogues and musty registers in many vil-lages throughout Worcestershire. Here, as in other writings on Sir James Parkinson (1955), Sir Charles Hasting, founder of the British Medical Association (1959), Thomas Wakley, founder of The Lancet (1962), the style is clear and concise, the phrases short and the atmo-sphere usually positive—the bottle is not half empty it is half full. William McMenemey pos-sibly felt a kinship with Parkinson, Hasting and Wakley who were revolutionaries working within the system.

He awakened and stimulated an interest in medical history in those around him. Thus to celebrate his nomination as president of the section of history of medicine of the RSM, his assistants Robin Barnard (his successor at Maida Vale), Richard Bergland (Associate Pro-fessor Neurosurgery, Harvard Medical Col-lege) and I, delighted the master by surprising him with a presentation of biographical stud-ies of John Hunter's Irish Giant and Pourfour du Petit the father of experimental neurology. In accordance with the lack of ceremony de ri-gueur at Maida Vale, the "meeting" took place at tea-time and began as soon as the four of us

met. These studies were subsequently pub-lished, after considerable editing by Professor McMenemey. History, for him, was not a col-lection of data to titillate the elderly members of a historical society, but the analysis of data useful to guide modern medicine.

Tea-time at Maida Vale will be remembered by many neuropathologists, neurologists, and neurosurgeons throughout the world as a unique event. It took place Monday to Friday, barring holidays and catastrophes, at 3:30 p.m. in the so-called microscopy room, a small room which served as the permanent work area for visiting students. There was a long desk covered with microscopes, journals, trays of celloidin and paraffin sections where tea and biscuits were deposited. Professor Mc-Menemey, assisted by Mrs. Hall, presided at tea-time with humor, calm and gentility. In regular attendance were the staff, residents and visiting foreign students—a crew of strong-willed individuals from many lands, who for these occasions, managed to calm their scientific passions and engage in courte-ous discourse. During my time as registrar, the regulars included Wendy Grant, Robin Bar-nard, Michael Kidd, P.K. Thomas, Madame Gravilescu (Roumania), John Prineas (Austra-lia), Thaddeus Mandybar (Poland), Richard Bergland (USA), Forbes Norris (USA), Georges Bischoff (Switzerland) and many others, all of whom went on to successful careers and con-tributed to neurological knowledge. Some were not so lucky, among them two neurosur-geons from Haiti who were eventually shot by firing squads in that country and others jailed for political views. Then there were the occa-sional visiting neurologists and neurosurgeons, Sam Nevin, Lord Brain, Ronald Henson, Ger-ald Kelly, Valentine Logue, R.T.C. Pratt, Sir Francis Walsh, Sir Charles Symonds and oth-ers. The foreign visitors at one time or other included Ludo van Bogaert (Belgium), Webb Haymaker (USA), Robert Terry (USA), Ells-worth Alvord (USA), Orville Bailey (USA), Mde. Osetowska (Poland), Wolfgang Zeman (USA), Serge Brion (France), Moise Pollak (Ar-gentina) and others. There were his two spe-cial friends and co-conspirators R.O. Norman and W. Payling-Wright, who visited from time to time. These meetings were highly educa-tional for the trainees who learned about recent neuropathological and neurological studies, the fine art of academic politics and plain gossip.

Professor McMenemey's manner of teaching was Socratic. He never said we were wrong, rather he would state his views as questions: "I wonder what that is?" he would say adjusting the pointer to an obvious mitotic cell or a few epithelial cells in a smear of brain tissue, after he had been told that the tissue looked normal. For a laboratory with few autopsies, there was more material than we could cope with, sent to us from all over the British Isles, the Commonwealth and other countries. His final diagnosis was always right and sometimes it took months of observation and meditation.

This gentle and unassuming man could not digest pomposity, and he certainly came in contact with it in his milieu. He would take delight in telling us of some cinematic episode where ostentation had again been triumphantly deflated by the Marx brothers or W.C. Fields.

He fitted in better with the consultant crew of Maida Vale than elsewhere, possibly because it was less formal, younger and it included other reformists such as Lord Brain and Sam Nevin. This tandem helped direct the destiny of BRAIN; from 1961 to 1966 Lord Brain was editor, Dr. Nevin was secretary and treasurer, and Professor McMenemey was part of "the help." They certainly did not agree in all subjects but they were conservative, committed to medical reform and creative. Each materialized his need for reform by action in his own way, thus McMenemey's way was in organization—to join persons of similar interest for their common interest. This talent for organization was first manifested when he went to the Worcester Royal Infirmary mentioned above; he founded the Virgonian Society for the purpose of arranging clinico-pathological conferences for local physicians and medical members of allied forces stationed locally. He was one of the organizers of the Association of Clinical Pathologists, a body representing the interests of provincial pathologists. In Britain, this work is considered by some to be his major contribution to pathology. We, who live beyond those shores, consider the next display of his organizational capabilities to be his major contribution—the International Association of Neuropathologists.

As one of the senior members of the international neuropathology community, he was highly qualified to unionize its members. He shared this difficult task with Ludo van Bogaert. Difficult because there was reticence and bitterness in the postwar period between members of opposite warring nations and a lack of communication between neuropathologists of both sides of the so-called Iron Curtain. McMenemey was the diplomatic envoy who travelled extensively all over Europe and the Americas and with the help of sympathetic and understanding colleagues everywhere, built bridges between the neuropathologists of the world. The organization of the 1955 International Congress in London depended largely upon his organization. This work was recognized and honored during his lifetime by learned societies in Australia, USA, France, Germany, Roumania, Spain and other countries.

Many of us will remember this remarkable Renaissance man who pursued so successfully different careers and arranged to bring together men and women of good will of different outlook and culture.

(Reproduced with permission from Duckett, S.: William Henry McMenemey (1905–1977). In Memoriam. J. Neuropathol. Exp. Neurol., 37(4):452–455, 1978.)

Foreword

In the most developed parts of the planet, population growth has ceased and the median age has risen dramatically in recent decades. Average length of life in the United States has increased from slightly over 47 years in 1900 to almost 75 years now, an increase of almost 60%. The causes of illness and death have shifted strikingly from infectious disorders to the vascular, degenerative, and neoplastic diseases encountered in later life. This astonishing change has taken place within so brief a span of time as to be encompassed by living memory. Coupled with and causatively linked to the demographic changes just mentioned is the knowledge explosion in biology and medicine. The implications of these trends for diseases of the nervous system and our understanding of them are far-reaching to say the least.

In this broadly conceived monograph on disorders of the aging nervous system, Professor Duckett and his collaborators address the neuropathologic consequences of the recent revolution in human biology. At the outset Professor Duckett cogently reminds us that pathology is the study of disease, and that such study may be undertaken by any means that come to hand. Said in another way, pathology is not simply an exercise in examining congealed tissues infiltrated with paraffin and stained with aniline dyes. Approaches to disorders of the aging nervous system used in this monograph include immunologic, molecular, pharmacologic and imaging techniques.

The choice of such a broad approach to the neurologic concurrents of aging was a wise one, because purely morphologic study of the brain has been disappointing in some respects. For example, using standard morphologic techniques, it may not be possible to distinguish the brain of a profoundly retarded person requiring institutionalization from the brain of a highly accomplished member of our society. The most likely explanation for this state of affairs is that present morphologic methods provide almost no measure of connectivity in the brain. The crucial details of neuron-to-neuron connections and how they work, and further, how they cumulatively translate into learning, memory, and human experience remain obscure. Standard morphologic methods as applied to the brain offer little insight into this key problem. But this is a shortcoming of a particular field of research, and not of the monograph so skillfully assembled by Professor Duckett. We can hope that future editions will be able to address more directly the issues of neural connectivity in the brain and the effects thereon of aging and disease.

Arthur K. Asbury, M.D.
Van Meter Professor of Neurology
University of Pennsylvania
School of Medicine
Philadelphia, Pennsylvania

Preface

Once upon a time, the study of the pathology of the nervous system was the exclusive domain of the histologist who monopolized the title of neuropathologist. There were chemists and cytologists who examined cells and measured the chemical constituents of CSF, blood, and urine; microbiologists who identified and grew bugs, and diagnosed neurologic diseases; but they were not considered to be real neuropathologists. Real neuropathologists in Europe were supposed to be—and sometimes were—monocled eccentric elitists who spent afternoons examining gorgeous multicolored miniature paintings on histologic slides with a microscope or viewing projection slides of silver and gold engravings by the Italian school (Golgi), the Spanish school (Cajal), and the aniline blue abstractions of the German school. Tea was served in mid-afternoon in the company of other neuropathologists engaging in erudite fluid conversations on Proust, Kraepelin, de Stael, and Jung. Neurologists were avoided as voluble, therapeutically powerless, eponym-conscious creatures. Neurosurgeons were considered quaint and Nordic. General pathologists were characterized as a cupiditous lot, whose cultural horizons were limited to numbers. These fraternal sentiments were reciprocated. So much for a fair and objective professional assessment. It was said by unkind tongues that, in the United States, the real neuropathologists were hastily recruited appendices of pathology departments without neurologic knowledge or experience, qualified not necessarily by training but by a sentence of years of hard labor in a general pathology lab, followed by a union certification referred to as "the boards." Their eventual activity was essentially restricted to tumor diagnosis. This is, of course, a simplified caricature because the great mass of neuropathologists were thoughtful and hard-working physicians, who often made diagnoses under limiting and difficult circumstances, namely, an absence of clinical information. There were genial neuropathologists in many countries who laid down the morphologic foundations upon which was built the future multidisciplined neuropathology that we have now. That future began to emerge in the 1970s and 1980s when basic scientists, neuropathologists, neurologists, neurosurgeons, neuroradiologists, and members of allied disciplines slowly joined forces in the pursuit of the correct diagnosis. This is where we are today.

The discipline of neuropathology includes histology, radiology, genetics, microbiology, immunology, chemistry, physics, and epidemiology. My colleagues and I have attempted in this textbook to reflect this multidisciplinary approach. The authors were urged to write their contribution in simple language in the light of their experience and knowledge, because our book is meant to be read by anyone who has the responsibility of the care of the aged. There was little editorial interference. Authors from the United States, Canada, France, Sweden, and England have contributed different views concerning diseases that can afflict humans.

As I write, important legislation is being presented in the United States Congress concerning the cost and financial support for the care of the aged faced with catastrophic illness. Frequently now, new and important discoveries concerning the pathogenesis of neurologic diseases are reported. This text has been revised to keep up with this new information, but now, let us publish.

Philadelphia, Pennsylvania   Serge Duckett

Acknowledgments

I am grateful to the large and varied group of friends and colleagues who have helped in the production of this book. I thank Robert J. Schwartzman, M.D., Chairman of the Department of Neurology, who gave his unreserved and wholehearted support to this enterprise, without which it would not have come to fruition; Shirley Sadak, B.S., our chief editorial and administrative officer, who organized this complicated international effort very efficiently and diplomatically to improve the content and quality of the many manuscripts, and graciously relinquished many leisure hours; Dr. David Macfadyen, now of the World Health Organization, then Associate Dean of Health Policy at the Jefferson Medical College, whose humane and international outlook on medicine was helpful and inspirational in the writing of the introductory chapter; the illustrators, Diane Armao, M.D., of Albuquerque, New Mexico, and Jean-Francois Duckett of the Charlotte Observer, Charlotte, North Carolina; Dr. Thaddeus Mandybur (Cincinnati, Ohio), Dr. Richard M. Torack (St. Louis, Missouri), and Dr. Donald B. Calne (Vancouver, BC, Canada), who very graciously read and commented on many contributions; the multitude of students, interns, and residents who read and corrected the text and verified the references—Greg di Russo, Mark Bej, M.D., Neil Culligan, M.D., and Chris Huntington, M.D.; Mr. Dan Williams, Assistant Director of Human Resources, Thomas Jefferson University, who provided the data concerning the cost and legislation of the care of the aged; Mr. John de Carville, friend and agent, who organized the publication of this book with Ken Bussy, friend and editor; Ms. Leslie Davis, Neurosensory Care Program Manager, for her gracious support and advice; Mrs. Lee Vespi, Mrs. Joanne Hall, and Mr. Joseph Severdia of the Bernard J. Alpers Neuropathology Laboratory who contributed photographic and histologic preparations to many chapters; friends who did bibliographic searches on varied subjects—Claude and Claire Barnwell, Jean and Rollande Rodier, Jean and Danielle Schere, Michel and Martine Souillac, Jean-Claude and Annick Baclet, Pat and Carol Foley; Danielle Giuliano and Gertrude Rapaport for patiently typing and retyping manuscripts; Loraine Emanuel for her preparation of Chapter 18; J. Dellanave, I. Coquart, and V. Deprat for preparation of Chapter 3; Edward F. Mannino, Peter Eck, Bruce Sheffler, Jack Land, and Richard L. Gerson for wise counsel and moral support; Paula Bavasso Duckett for her bibliographic research for Chapter 1, her patience, and understanding; and finally, the many other associates who helped in this undertaking in many ways.

S.D.

Contributors

O.F. Agee, M.D.
Professor
Department of Radiology
University of Florida College of Medicine
Gainesville, Florida

Christer Alling, M.D., Ph.D.
Professor in Medical Neurochemistry
Department of Psychiatry & Neurochemistry
Lund University
Lund, Sweden

Ellsworth C. Alvord, Jr., M.D.
Professor of Pathology (Neuropathology)
Department of Pathology
University of Washington School of Medicine
Seattle, Washington

Everett J. Austin, M.D.
Department of Neurology
Kaiser Permanente Medical Center
San Francisco, California

Anca Bereanu, M.D.
Neuropathology Fellow
Bernard J. Alpers Neuropathology Laboratory
Department of Neurology, Jefferson Medical College
of the Thomas Jefferson University
Philadelphia, Pennsylvania

Timothy Block, Ph.D.
Assistant Professor
Department of Microbiology, Jefferson Medical College
of the Thomas Jefferson University
Philadelphia, Pennsylvania

Serge Brion, M.D.
Professeur de Psychiatrie
Laboratoire Universitaire de Neuropathologie
Hôpital Sainte Anne
Paris, France

Pia Delaere, Ph.D.
Laboratoire de Neuropathologie R. Escourolle
Hôpital de la Salpetrière
Paris, France

Serge Duckett, M.D., Ph.D., D.Sc.
Director and Professor
Bernard J. Alpers Neuropathology Laboratory
Department of Neurology, Jefferson Medical College
of the Thomas Jefferson University
Philadelphia, Pennsylvania

Charles Duyckaerts, M.D., Ph.D.
Assistant Professeur
Laboratoire de Neuropathologie R. Escourolle
Hôpital de la Salpetrière
Paris, France

Michael Gordon, M.D., FRCP(C)
Medical Director
Baycrest Center for Geriatric Care
North York, Ontario, Canada

Francoise Gray, M.D.
Maître de Conférence des Universités
Département de Neuropathologie
Faculté de Médicine de l'Université de Paris XII
CHU Henri Mondor
Créteil, France

Jean-Jacques Hauw, M.D.
Professeur de Pathologie (Neuropathologie)
Laboratoire de Neuropathologie R. Escourolle
Hôpital de la Salpetrière
Paris, France

Ronald C. Kim, M.D.
Staff Neuropathologist
Department of Veterans Affairs Medical Center
Long Beach, California

Robert L. Knobler, M.D.
Associate Professor
Department of Neurology, Jefferson Medical College
of the Thomas Jefferson University
Philadelphia, Pennsylvania

Vei H. Mah, M.D.
Assistant Professor
Bernard J. Alpers Neuropathology Laboratory
Department of Neurology, Jefferson Medical College
of the Thomas Jefferson University
Philadelphia, Pennsylvania

Samuel H. Markind, M.D.
Neuropathology Fellow
Bernard J. Alpers Neuropathology Laboratory
Department of Neurology, Jefferson Medical College
of the Thomas Jefferson University
Philadelphia, Pennsylvania

Jacqueline Mikol, M.D.
Professeur des Universités
Faculté Lariboisière-St. Louis, Université Paris 7
Paris, France

Joel Plas, M.D.
Psychiatre des Hôpitaux
Centre Hospitalier
Versailles, France

Jacques Poirier, M.D.
Professeur de Pathologie (Neuropathologie)
Département de Neuropathologie
Faculté de Médecine de l'Université de Paris XII
CHU Henri Mondor
Créteil, France

Harold G. Preiksaitis, M.D., Ph.D., C.M., FRCP(C)
Research Fellow
Department of Medicine
Toronto Western Hospital
Toronto, Ontario, Canada

David Roeltgen, M.D.
Associate Professor
Department of Neurology
Hahnemann University School of Medicine
Philadelphia, Pennsylvania

Francesco Scaravilli, M.D.
Department of Neuropathology
Institute of Neurology
The National Hospital Queen Square
London, England

Robert E. Schmidt, M.D.
Associate Professor
Department of Pathology/Neuropathology
Washington University
St. Louis, Missouri

Scott Schoedler, M.D.
Neuropathology Fellow
Bernard J. Alpers Neuropathology Laboratory
Department of Neurology, Jefferson Medical College
of the Thomas Jefferson University
Philadelphia, Pennsylvania

Cheng-Mei Shaw, M.D.
Professor of Pathology (Neuropathology)
Department of Pathology
University of Washington School of Medicine
Seattle, Washington

Michael E. Shy, M.D.
Associate Professor
Bernard J. Alpers Neuropathology Laboratory
Department of Neurology, Jefferson Medical College
of the Thomas Jefferson University
Philadelphia, Pennsylvania

J. Bruce Smith, M.D.
Professor of Medicine, Microbiology, and Immunology
Department of Rheumatology, Jefferson Medical
College of the Thomas Jefferson University
Philadelphia, Pennsylvania

Mark Stacy, M.D.
Fellow, Parkinson Disease Center and Movement
Disorder Clinic
Department of Neurology
Baylor College of Medicine
Houston, Texas

Joo Ho Sung, M.D.
Professor in Laboratory Medicine and Pathology
Department of Laboratory Medicine and Pathology
University of Minnesota School of Medicine
Minneapolis, Minnesota

Rudolph E. Tanzi, M.D.
Department of Neurogenetics
Massachusetts General Hospital
Boston, Massachusetts

Harry V. Vinters, M.D., FRCP (C)
Associate Professor
Department of Neuropathology
UCLA School of Medicine
Los Angeles, California

Anne Vital, M.D.
Maître de Conférences en Anatomie Pathologique
Université Bordeaux II
Bordeaux, France

Claude Vital, M.D.
Professeur d'Anatomie Pathologique
Université Bordeaux II
Bordeaux, France

Contents

CHAPTER 1

The Normal Aging Human Brain

SERGE DUCKETT

The purpose of this chapter is to provide general information concerning the morphology and behavior of the normal aging human brain. We will also examine the population numbers and the geographic distribution of humans over the age of 65 years (65+).

The terms "aging" and "old" imply mental and physical decline. Shakespeare said it pithily; "When the age is in, the wit is out."[1] Such generalizations are entertaining but simplistic. The indiscriminate use of the plural is a demonstration of ignorance. Literature, cinema, and television, the world's most popular sources of information—the university-without-walls—have traditionally portrayed elderly citizens in simplistic terms as nasty, nasty and rich, submissively kind, demented, benevolent, amusing and/or amnesic individuals gravitating inevitably down the gentle slope of mental decline. This popular view was accepted scientifically until the early 70s because of inadequate psychologic and morphologic research. Sadly enough, too many older persons have had their self-image hurt by negative external views even though they realized that their own experience and self-analysis contradicted the outside image.[2,3] Worse still, they accepted it.[4] Many have resented the consequent injustices, particularly in the job market. Others have not paid attention, particularly politicians and artists. The average age of the leaders of the 12 European Common Market nations is 67 (1989), George Bush is 67 and Gorbachev at age 59 is considered to be a youngster. Picasso, Titian, Cezanne, and Michaelangelo were producing masterpieces in their 80s and 90s. Goethe finished Faust at 82 and Cervantes finished Don Quixote at 72. The list is long.

Although there are many productive women and men over the age of 65 and a newly defined aggressive and positive gerontologic attitude, numerous elderly citizens accept passively their presumed fate and wait for death in an armchair. This attitude may be justified for health reasons but in too many cases it is

1

unjustified. The role of gerontologists and geriatricians is to define the limits of the possible for aged citizens.

The ability to grow old contentedly is limited to a small portion of our society, often financially secure and always mentally trained and equipped to rely upon cerebral rather than physical activities. The vast majority of our elderly citizens are poor, uneducated, and most often depressed; they form the hidden majority who subsist solely on their meager earnings or on Social Security checks. In 1987 there were 6,772,000 men and women 65 years of age and older living on a yearly income of $5,000 or less in the United States with a medical aid program worse than any in the Western or Communist world.[5]

AGING AND BEHAVIOR

It was the classical view of anatomists and psychologists that the normal aging human brain atrophies and loses cells, that its ventricular system enlarges, and that behavior and mentation gradually regress. This was voluminously documented in the literature mostly on the basis of cross-sectional studies. However, we now know that the morphologic and psychologic methods used to reach these conclusions were grossly inadequate and that these resulted in negative generalizations which affected human lives.

The reassessment of the hypothesis that the normal aging brain is a "normally" degenerating organ began in the late 1960s when respected and authoritative voices in psychology and gerontology criticized traditional research methods in aging and consequently the conclusions. In 1974 Schaie[6] wrote "The presumed universal decline in adult intelligence is at best a methodological artifact and at worst a popular misunderstanding of the relation between individual development and sociocultural change" and "the major finding produced in the gerontology laboratory in the area of intellectual functioning is the demolishing (of the idea) of serious intellectual decrement in the aged." Some of Schaie's more traditional colleagues differed with this view and their responses were rather direct. In a personal reference to Schaie concerning the views

expressed above Horn and Donaldson[7] wrote "Humans have a well-developed ability for wishful thinking, and most humans who derive their livelihood and status from exercise of their intellectual abilities have a strong wish that these abilities not wane." Nevertheless, the majority of psychologists were clearly in agreement with Schaie, which meant that the time had come to review the methods and possibly reinterpret or at least re-evaluate conclusions.

There were two traditional previous methods of studying human aging—cross-sectional and longitudinal studies. A cross-sectional study compared the performance of various age groups but did not take into account the differences in health care, education, and nutritional habits of each group. For example, a group of octogenarians would contain immigrants and natives brought up in a period less conscious of proper nutrition and exercise than a group of trigenerians of the vegetarian jogging generation. The longitudinal study compared the activities of individuals over a long period of time—say 10 years, but did not take into account the dropout rate, the physical and mental conditions of the individual during this period, and it ended with a small group of relatively well-preserved citizens. Individuals were compared to one another but the changes within an individual were not taken into account. In view of the limitations of these two methods, Schaie and his associates[8] devised a method which permitted a comparison of the cross-sectional and longitudinal data from the same study populations. Thus, they noted significantly low scores for a multitude of cognitive capacities in the older groups in 1963—a conclusion that was in agreement with contemporary psychologic thinking. However, in 1970 these same subjects were retested and the age-related cognitive declines predicted earlier had disappeared. This longitudinal study suggested that the ability to adapt intellectually and emotionally as measured by reasoning and spatial tests and the retainment of acquired knowledge as measured with verbal tests occurred at significantly later ages than indicated by the 1963 cross-sectional studies. Schaie and his colleagues deduced that these differences could not be explained simply by the human aging process as indicated by the study of cohorts (groups of individuals) but rather by the differences between individuals within a cohort. Thus, they felt each human being was different because of education, genes, nutrition, employment, geography of activities, response to life's vicissitudes, physical ills, and intelligence (however defined). Kenyon[2] has proposed the term "personal existence" to underline the importance of studying not only the physical and behavioral characteristics of each individual, but other parameters of life such as the ability to benefit themselves or others from their life experience and their wisdom. Wisdom is defined as an "ability to exercise good judgement about important but uncertain matters in life."[9]

Support for Schaie's revolutionary view was clearly demonstrated by the analysis of scores of the Wechsler Adult Intelligence Scale. Comparison of groups of mixed educational background indicated decrements associated with age but comparisons of groups of individuals of equal education showed no such age decrement. These studies indicated that cognitive losses in late middle life may be caused in part by extrinsic factors and therefore can be prevented and even reversed.[10-12]

The immediate benefit of the academic dispute between the traditional and revolutionary psychologists was the enhancement of the ongoing explosion of research into aging manifested by the exponential growth of publications, research programs, and by the creation of centers for the care or the counseling of the aged. Other major forces which contributed to this interest were the 65+ population explosion and its costs to society. Governmental legislators were quick to realize it was cheaper to keep the 65+ in the working force than pay them for "doing nothing" (i.e. retirement), so that in 1985 in the United States the Pepper Act was passed which pushed the retirement age to 70. Thus, the pragmatism of our money oriented society has been beneficial to the self respect of older citizens.

Recently, psychologists and gerontologists have concluded that the research in aging during these past two decades has been "data-rich but theory-poor."[13] "The paucity of theory in social gerontology is an embarrassment to academic students of human aging."[14] Research in aging has emphasized average age-related losses and neglected the substantial heterogeneity of older persons. The effects of the aging process itself have been exaggerated and the modifying effects of diet, exercise, personal habits and psychosocial factors underestimated, according to Rowe and Kahn.[15]

CREATIVITY AND AGING

Creativity is proportional to the ability and ambition of the individual and can vary from gardening to the production of Don Quixote. Individuals 65 years old and older have problems, tasks, issues, and motivations different from younger folk, which influence their sense of creativity. There may be a reduction in the intensity of striving and ambition may be diminished by experience. Older people may feel that they have less time left and may develop an urge to accomplish some last goal or dream. Some individuals, such as Grandma Moses, may have a sudden surge of late life creativity which expresses or reaffirms past creative work or tendencies. Having established a difference between what is important to them and what are distractions, the 65+ may approach their last years with a special sense of vocation. Older citizens may develop a sense of spiritual sufficiency that makes them less dependent than young people on external stimulation. Such introspection can lead to meditation and reflectiveness, or contented solitude and in gifted individuals can result in creative masterpieces.[16-21]

The list of major accomplishments by women and men 65+ is long and the following few names illustrate this point:

Adams, John (1735 to 1826): Second president of the United States from ages 62 to 66.

Adams, John Quincy (1767 to 1848): Sixth president of the United States from ages 58 to 62, politically active until age of 81.

Anthony, Susan B. (1820 to 1906): London International Council of Women delegate at age 79, National American Woman Suffrage Association president until age 80.

Barton, Clara (1821 to 1912): Founder at age 80 and director of the National Association of First Aid until her death at 91.

Bellini, Giovanni (1430 to 1516): At age 75 painted the portrait of the "doge Loredano".

Bernhardt, Sarah (1844 to 1923): Acted in "Daniel" in London at age 75, starred in Rostand's "La Gloire" at 75, in Verneull's "Regine Armand" at 76, and final performance in "Daniel" at 78.

Boyd, William (1885 to 1979): Trained as a psychiatrist, Boyd established his reputation as a writer of pathology texts. William Boyd wrote his last edition of *Introduction to the Study of Disease* at the age of 86. He personally went out of print in his 94th year, lucid (and a lover of Scotch whiskey) to the end.

Buffon, G.L. (1707 to 1788): At 80 was hard at work on the 14th volume of Natural History, at 72 published the Epochs of Nature volume on birds, and at 76 to 81 published 5 volumes on minerals.

Clemenceau, Georges (1841 to 1929): Prime minister of France during WWI at ages 76 to 79.

Cervantes, Saavedra Miguel De (1547 to 1616): Completed "Don Quixote" in his 70s.

Churchill, Winston (1874 to 1965): Became wartime prime minister at 65, finished six volume history of the war at 70, prime minister for second time at 77 to 81.

Corot, J.B. (1796 to 1875): Painted "Doual Belfry", "Head of an Italian Girl", and "The Blue Lady" at age 74.

Disraeli, Benjamin (1801 to 1881): Statesman participating in the conclusion of the Treaty of Versailles at 71, premier and leader of his party at 76.

Edison, Thomas A. (1847 to 1931): Conducted experiments and improvements in his existing inventions until his last years.

Franklin, Benjamin (1706 to 1790): Represented his country in France at ages 76 to 79, member of Constitutional Convention at 81, President of Pennsylvania from 79 to 82.

Galileo (1564 to 1642): Physicist and astronomer engaged in the study of mechanics and projection, published his dialogues on mechanics at age 74.

Gladstone, William Evart (1809 to 1898): British statesman, orator, and author at age 80, began his Midlothian campaign overthrowing the Conservative Government and put himself and his party in power, premier for the fourth time from 83 to 85.

Goethe, Wolfgang von (1749 to 1832): Completed "Faust" at 82.

Hals, Franz (1584 to 1666): Painted "The Old Toper of Haarlem", and after 74 painted "The Young Man in the Flop Hat" and "Guardians of the Poorhouse."

Hardy, Thomas (1840 to 1928): English poet and novelist, married at age 74 and wrote "Late Lyrics" at 82, "Queen in Cornwall" (play) at 83, "Human Shows" at 85, and "Christmas in the Elgin Room" at 87.

Holmes, Oliver Wendell (1809 to 1891): American poet, essayist, and physician. Published his "Medical Essays" and "Pages from an Old Volume of Life" at 71, "Over the Teacups" at 75, and other works between 75 to 80.

Hugo, Victor (1802 to 1885): French poet and novelist. At 75 published the second series of "Legende des Siecles" followed by "The Art of Being a Grandfather", also wrote poems at ages 69 to 75 and produced his most famous novels in his 70s, still vigorous at 80.

Ingres, Jean Auguste Dominque (1780 to 1867): Painted "La Source" at age 76.

Jefferson, Thomas (1743 to 1826): Third United States president at age 58 to 66, founded University of Virginia at 76 and devoted himself to his plans for the school until his death at 83.

Mantegna, Andrea (1431 to 1506): Painted "The Madonna of Victory" at 65 and "Parnassus" at 70.

Madison, James (1751 to 1836): Fourth president of the United States at age 58 to 66, rector of the University of Virginia at 76, participated in Virginia Constitutional Convention at 79 and wrote on political subjects until his death.

Michaelangelo (1475 to 1564): Painter, sculptor, and architect. Chief architect of St. Peter's from 72 to 89, sculpted until his death.

Newton, Sir Isaac (1642 to 1727): English mathematician and philosopher working productively until the age of 83.

Rossini, Gioacchino Antonio (1792 to 1868): Produced a musical masterpiece named "Petite Messe Solennelle" at age 72.

Saint Saens, Charles Camille (1835 to 1921): French pianist, organist, conductor, composer and author, wrote an opera, an oratorio and other compositions after 76.

Shaw, George Bernard (1856 to 1950): Dramatist and critic, published after age 74 "What I Really Wrote About the War", "Adventures of the Black Girl in Her Search for God", "The Future of Political Science in America" and more, heard over international radio programs in 1934 and mentally alert until his death at 93.

Sophocles (495 to 406 B.C.): Greek dramatist and tragic poet, produced "Philoctetus" and "Oedipus at Colonus" after 74. and in his ninetieth year wrote a striking play.

Tennyson, Alfred (1809 to 1892): English poet at 71 years old produced "Ballads and Poems", at age 75 took his seat in the House of Lords and published "Becket", at age 80 "Demeter" and other notable poetry at 83.

Titian (1477 to 1576): Italian artist painting several portraits after 80, at 90 years painted "Transfiguration" and "Annunciation", between 94 and 98 painted "Battle of Lepanto" and at 99 was working on the "Pieta" at the time of his death.

Verdi, Guiseppe (1813 to 1901): Composed at age 74 "Othello", "Falstaff" at 80 and produced four sacred works at 85.

Voltaire, J.F.A. (1694 to 1778): Author and free-thinker who at 80 was an active farmer and manufacturer, published "Irene" at age 83 and remained active until his death at 84.

THE MORPHOLOGY OF THE NORMAL AGING BRAIN (See Chap. 5)

Until recently there were no longitudinal studies of the morphology of an aging human brain. The advent of modern radiologic techniques now permits comparisons of the brain and ventricles of one human at various times during life and after death. However, there are no methods available at present which permit histologic comparisons before and/or after death in a human except for the theoretic possibility of the comparison of a fortuitous brain biopsy (i.e. tumor diagnosis) with cerebral tissue obtained at post mortem. The information concerning the morphology of the human brain such as loss of cells and atrophy was based on cross-sectional studies and therefore tentative. There were legitimate criticisms concerning reference to a loss of neurons in a human whose brain was examined once, usually after death, or to brain atrophy without neuropathologic changes. These and other criticisms concerning the relationship and therefore the obvious necessity of the examination of the morphology and the function of a human brain have been expressed in recent years and this has resulted in the amelioration of methods of study of the brain.[22,23]

BRAIN SIZE

Tomlinson in 1972 wrote on the subject of morphologic brain changes in non-demented old people.[24] He was dissatisfied with previous studies[25-27] because he felt that the identification of normal and abnormal brains was unclear due to a lack of precise premortem information and consequently a lack of proper identification of normal and demented patients. Together with Blessed and Roth, a joint study was devised consisting of a full physical and psychologic examination and eventual postmortem examinations of the brains of 28 "non-demented" individuals, 16 women and

12 men, ages 65 to 92.[28] There was no histologic evidence of dementia in these brains. Neurofibrillary changes, senile plaques, and granulovacuolar changes were found in a small number of cases but never significantly. There were few instances of cerebral softening. Evidence of cerebral atrophy was slight or absent in the majority and their brain weights and ventricular size did not differ greatly from those of younger subjects. The brain weights of males were 1170 to 1430 g (mean of 1320 g; SD 77.9) and in females, 1080 to 1390 g (mean of 1213 g; SD 91.8). These figures are similar to those noted in normal aging adults.

The mean weight for the brain of normal young adult males varies from 1304 to 1380 g.[29-31] The mean brain weight for females under 50 years of age in Tomlinson's series was 1268 g (SD 158) which is not significantly heavier than the mean of 1213 g of the brains of intellectually well-preserved old females, 65+.[24] This relatively close approximation of the brains from these intellectually well-preserved old people to those of younger subjects presents a somewhat different picture than that given by many other authors in relation to the brain in old age. Hoch-Ligeti gives 1160 g as the average male brain weight at 90 years and Korenchevski[32] reviewing the studies of several authors besides his own cases gives a mean brain weight in males over the age of 70 years as 1274 g. In Tomlinson's series of 246 cases there was nothing to suggest that the brain weight diminished markedly after the age of 65 years.

Terry and his colleagues[33] compared the brain weights, cortical thickness, and cell counts in the midfrontal region and superior temporal gyrus of 18 patients with senile dementia of the Alzheimer type (SDAT) and 12 age-matched normal specimens between the ages of 70 and 89 years. There was a full examination of the well-documented physical and psychologic examinations of all these patients. The brain weights for the normal group were 930 to 1350 g (mean 1152 ± 45 g), and of the SDAT group were 918 to 1150 g (1055 ± 20 g), which indicates that there was no significant statistical difference. There was no statistical difference in the size of the cortical thickness, the packing density, or number of the cortical cells of both groups, as studied with a Quantimet image analyzer, except for the number of large neurons (larger than 90 μm^2) which was 40% fewer in SDAT brains. There were more plaques in the SDAT brains.

Terry and Hanson[34] studied morphologic parameters of the brains of patients with Alzheimer's disease and of the brains of normal humans. Their conclusion was that the neuronal loss per unit volume in the normal brain was much less than previously reported and that the findings in patients with Alzheimer's disease at any age were clearly different from those of normal controls.

CELL NUMBERS

According to past medical literature, there is a loss of neurons in the normal aging brain. This conclusion is based on the examination of histologic slides of the cerebral grey matter after death and comparison with similar material from younger adults.[34-44]

Normal cerebral aging is associated with the loss of neurons, dendrites, and dendritic spines in various areas of the brain cortex but apparently not in the temporal lobe.[45-47] It has been recently proposed that the loss of neurons in the frontal cortex is the result rather than the cause of a diminution of the total size of this area. No changes in total volume or in the number or size of the neurons could be observed in areas 7 and 17. This is in agreement with the observation that a decrease of muscarinic cholinergic receptor binding sites in the frontal cerebral cortex increases with age in people without any morphologic evidence of senile degeneration. In non-demented brains there were only minimal non-specific finds of cerebral degeneration.

VENTRICULAR SIZE

The lateral ventricles were normal in 7 of the 28 cases studied by Tomlinson and slightly or moderately dilated in the rest.[24] The mean ventricular volume in 19 measured cases in that series was 26.6 ml and up. This does not differ significantly from the mean of 22/ml in a series of Last and Thompset[48] which included only 3 patients above the age of 65 years. These two series provide little support for the idea that the cerebral ventricles are larger in non-demented old people than in young adults.

Davis and Wright[44] developed a technique which allows the examiner at autopsy to measure the ratio of the volume of the brain and that of the cranial vault. They examined 63 individuals, ages 7 to 82, and noted that the ratio was constant at about 0.92 until age 55, and then declined to 0.83 at age 90.

NEURORADIOLOGY AND THE AGING BRAIN

Neuroradiology was revolutionized by computed tomographic reconstruction techniques, one of which is based on the use of x rays (x ray CT), the other dependent on proton-molecule or proton-proton interactions, magnetic resonance imaging (MRI). X ray CT and/or MRI permit the visualization of various tissues such as blood, blood vessels, fat, water, the identification of organs or structures in the living brain such as gray and white matter, globus pallidus, thalamus, red nucleus and of pathological processes, such as edema, demyelination, dilatation of ventricles, and cerebral atrophy. These techniques which permit the study of changes in living tissue at different stages of disease have vastly extended our understanding of the pathology of the nervous system.

Soon after the introduction of the CT scanning technique, radiologists started to study the normal and pathologic aging brain.[50-64] These early studies were cross-sectional and confirmed previous studies. This topic is reviewed in Chapter 1.

BIOCHEMISTRY

The brain is the most actively metabolizing organ in the body but it has no energy reserves. It is dependent on a constant supply of energy furnished primarily by the oxidative breakdown of glucose. Part of the glucose taken up by the brain is not oxidized, but after glycolytic breakdown it is disposed of into the venous blood in the form of lactic acid.

Bernsmeier and Gottstein[65] measured the cerebral circulation in relation to aging and showed that circulation decreased as the vascular resistance increased after the age of 50. They concluded that in older people circulation is impaired and the utilization of oxygen is diminished by vascular pathologic conditions.

In 1956, Kety[66] concluded that there was a remarkable decline in both cerebral blood flow and oxygen uptake from childhood through adolescence followed by a more gradual but progressive reduction through the third decade of life onward through middle and old age. Fazekas et al.[67] found no variation in these biologic values in individuals younger than 40 years of age, but noted that in individuals over the age of 50 there was significant reduction both in brain blood flow and oxygen consumption. The individual data of these cerebral values show great variation with age. Scheinburg et al.[68,69] obtained a significantly lower cerebral blood flow in two age groups (mean age 50 and 63) with normal brain function as compared to a young healthy adult control group aged 25 years. However, cerebral metabolic rate (CMR) of oxygen did not vary between the age groups. No differences were found by Schieve and Wilson[70] in brain blood flow and oxygen consumption within different age groups of healthy people. The contradiction in these findings might be due to the fact that the young and elderly individuals investigated were volunteers living in the community and hospitalized patients. They were designated as normal by exclusion of mental and vascular disease. In well-documented mentally and physically intact elderly individuals, Lassen et al.[71] found no age related change in cerebral blood flow but CMR oxygen decreased significantly by 6% with age. Dastur et al.[72] and Sokoloff[73] described no significant variation in blood flow in healthy individuals age 71 years old on the average as compared to healthy young controls; CMR oxygen dropped insignificantly by 6% but CMR glucose was found to be significantly diminished by 23%.

As far as cerebral glucose consumption is concerned, Alavi et al.[74] found a 26% reduction in psychometrically normal elderly subjects age 72 years as compared to 22-year-old controls. Kuhl et al.[75] measured exactly the same degree of reduction by comparing normal elderly subjects age 78 years with normal

18-year-old controls. These findings are in agreement with those of Dastur[72] so that a reduction in CMR glucose of about 25% may in fact occur with normal cerebral aging. CMR glucose does evidently diminish with normal aging. Hoyer[76] studied cerebral glucose and energy metabolism in Wistar rats and found that there was diminution with time. His findings support the assumption that oxidative and energy metabolism of the brain may decrease with normal cerebral aging. Thus, Patel[77] reported diminished oxidation of glucose by about 40% in cerebral cortical slices of 2-year-old rats and Gibson and Peterson demonstrated 20 to 40% in 3-year-old mice.[78]

POPULATION [1979–1983]

The world is aging [Figs. 1–1 to 1–4] and the proportion of the population 65 and over is ex-

pected to double during the next 40 years. The average American is growing older [Table 1–1; Figs. 1–4 to 1–7]. Since the mid 70s the U.S., as a society, has been getting older. The number of humans 65 and older is growing more rapidly than the rest of the population [Fig. 1–5 and Table 1–1].

According to the U.S. Census Bureau, the country's median age in 1950 was 30.2 years. It was 29.4 in 1960 and it reached a low of 27.9 in 1970 when the bulk of the baby boomers were in their early to mid 20s. From that point on, as the boomers became full-fledged adults, the median age began to rise. It was 30.0 in 1980 and according to Census Bureau projections will be 33.0 in 1990, 36.3 in the year 2000, 38.4 in 2010 and 39.3 in 2020. In 1950, 12 million Americans or 8% of the population were 65 or older. By 1987 that number had doubled to almost 30 million people or more

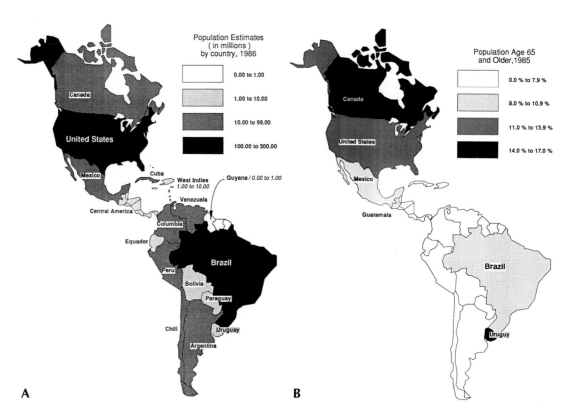

Fig. 1–1. A. Geographic distribution of humans, in millions, in the Americas, 1986. B. Distribution of humans, age 65+, in the Americas, 1985. From Statistical Abstract of the United States, 1987, 107th Edition, U.S. Bureau of Census, Washington, D.C., and from Bureau of Census, Center for International Research, International Database on Aging: International Population Reports Series P-95, No. 78, September, 1987, Washington, D.C.

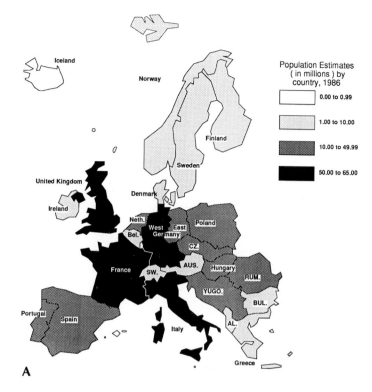

Fig. 1–2.   A. Geographic distribution of humans, in millions, in Europe, 1986. From Statistical Abstract of the United States, 1987, 107th Edition, U.S. Bureau of Census, Washington, D.C.

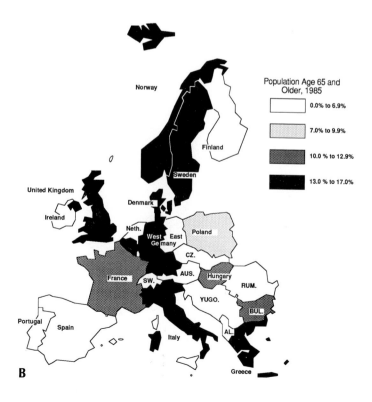

Fig. 1–2. (Continued)   B. Distribution of humans, age 65+, in Europe, 1985. From Bureau of Census, Center for International Research, International Database on Aging: International Population Reports Series P-95, No. 78, September, 1987, Washington, D.C.

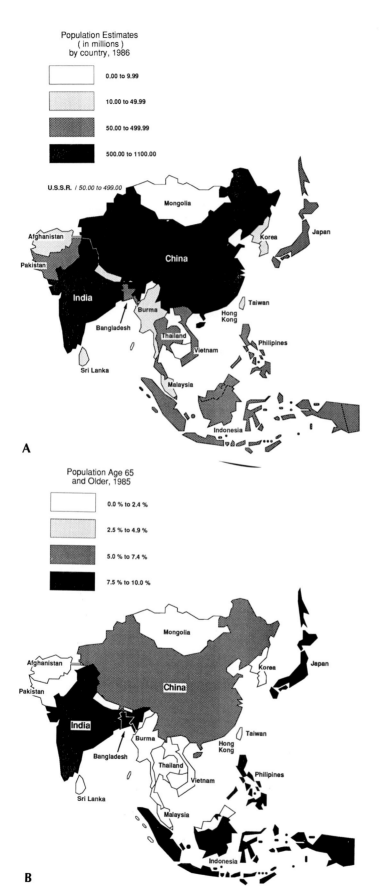

Fig. 1–3. A. Distribution of the human population in millions, in Asia, 1986. From Statistical Abstract of the United States, 1987, 107th Edition, U.S. Bureau of Census, Washington, D.C.

Fig. 1–3 *(Continued)* B. Distribution of humans, age 65+, in millions, in Asia, 1985. From Bureau of Census, Center for International Research, International Database on Aging: International Population Reports Series P-95, No. 78, September, 1987, Washington, D.C.

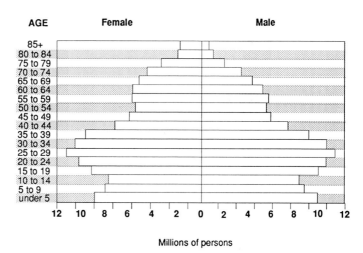

Fig. 1–4. Distribution of the U.S. population, in millions, by age and sex, 1986. From U.S. Bureau of the Census. "Estimates of the Population of the United States by Age, Sex, and Race: 1980–1986" Current Population Reports Series P-25, No. 1000 (February 1987).

than 12% of the population. The population of the United States today is approximately 249,657,000 of which 31,697,000 are 65+, including 3,313,000 85+. In the year 2000 the population will be 267,955,000 (an increase of 7.3%) and 34,697,000 humans will be 65+ (an increase of 9.5%) and 4,926,000 age 85+ (an increase of 49%). In 2020, that is 30 years from now, the biggest population group will be over the age of 60. The Census Bureau predicts that by 2040 the 65 over population will be 67 million people—that is 1 in every 5 Americans.

In 1990 there were 3.3 million people 85 and older. That number is expected to increase to more than 4-fold by 2040 [Fig. 1–5 and Table 1–1]. At that point 1 in every 25 Americans will be "old-old." The number of people over 85 will total 12 million in 50 years and the number of baby boomers over 65 will be 67 million, a quarter of the population.

According to the Census Bureau in 1990, those of the age of 65 have nearly doubled since the 1950s. By 1980 there were 14,200 people 100 years or older, and in 1986, 25,000; by 2000, 108,000 people will be 100+ years or older [Fig. 1–8]. The U.S. has the third largest elderly population (age 65+) and the largest "old-old" population (age 80+) in the world.

TABLE 1–1. Past, Present, and Future Growth of the Population 65+ and over. 1900–2050

		(Numbers in thousands)								
	Total population all ages	55 to 64 Years		65 to 74 years		75 to 84 years		85 years and over		65 years and over	
Year		Number	Percent	Number	Percent	Number	Percent	Number	Percent	Number	Percent
1900	76,303	4,009	5.3	2,189	2.9	772	1.0	123	0.2	3.064	4.0
1910	91,972	5,054	5.5	2,793	3.0	989	1.1	167	0.2	3,950	4.3
1920	105,711	6,532	6.2	3,464	3.3	1,259	1.2	210	0.2	4,933	4.7
1930	122,775	8,397	6.8	4,721	3.8	1,641	1.3	272	0.2	6,634	5.4
1940	131,669	10,572	8.0	6,375	4.8	2,278	1.7	365	0.3	9,019	6.8
1950	150,967	13,295	8.8	8,415	5.6	3,278	2.2	577	0.4	12,270	8.1
1960	179,323	15,572	8.7	10,997	6.1	4,633	2.6	929	0.5	16,560	9.2
1970	203,302	18,608	9.2	12,447	6.1	6,124	3.0	1,409	0.7	19,980	9.8
1980	226,505	21,700	9.6	15,578	6.9	7,727	3.4	2,240	1.0	25,544	11.3
1990	249,657	21,051	8.4	18,035	7.2	10,349	4.1	3,313	1.3	31,697	12.7
2000	267,955	23,767	8.9	17,677	6.6	12,318	4.6	4,926	1.8	34,921	13.0
2010	283,238	34,848	12.3	20,318	7.2	12,326	4.4	6,551	2.3	39,195	13.8
2020	296,597	40,298	13.6	29,855	10.1	14,486	4.9	7,081	2.4	51,422	17.3
2030	304,807	34,025	11.2	34,535	11.3	21,434	7.0	8,612	2.8	64,581	21.2
2040	308,559	34,717	11.3	29,272	9.5	24,882	8.1	12,834	4.2	66,988	21.7
2050	309,488	37,327	12.1	30,114	9.7	21,263	6.9	16,034	5.2	67,411	21.8

From Spencer, Gregory. US Bureau of Census. "Projections of the United States, by Age, Sex and Race 1900–2050" Current Population Reports Series P-25 No. 862 (May 1984).

Population

(Numbers in the thousands)

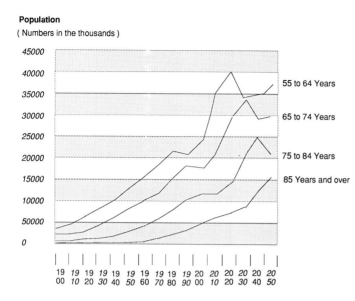

Fig. 1–5. Actual and projected growth of the population of humans 55 and older in the United States, 1987. From Statistical Abstract of the United States, 1987, 107th Edition, U.S. Bureau of Census, Washington, D.C.

This increase in the population of the world is due to decreased infant mortality and advances of medical science and social welfare. The trend is apparent not only in Western Europe, the Soviet Union, and North America, but in the under-developed countries as well. If present trends continue, those age 60 years or older will account for about 10% of the world's population in 20 years. The declining birthrate in industrialized countries has further augmented the aging of populations. For example, at the present time about 20% of the inhabitants of West Germany are older than 60 years. In the year 2000 it will be 23% and

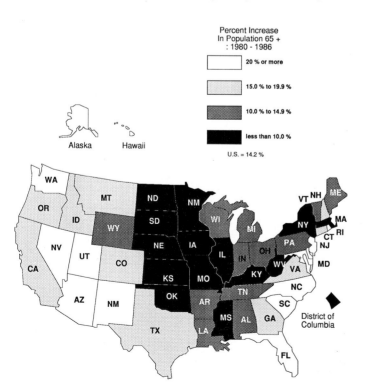

Fig. 1–6. Geographic distribution of the increase in the human population in the United States between 1980 and 1986. From U.S. Bureau of the Census. "State Population and Household Estimates With Age, Sex, and Components of Change: 1981 to 1985." Current Population report Series P-25, No. 1010 (September 1987).

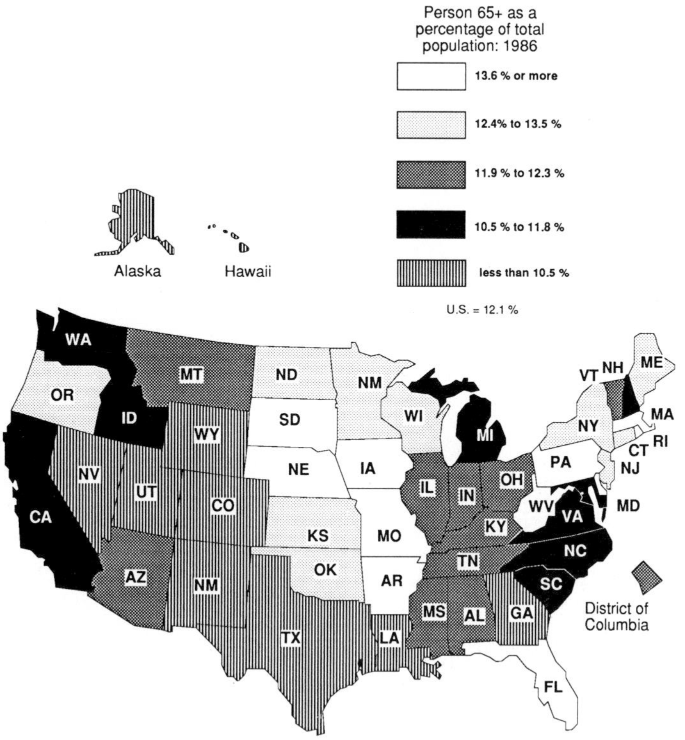

Person 65+ as a
percentage of total
population: 1986

	13.6 % or more
	12.4% to 13.5 %
	11.9 % to 12.3 %
	10.5 % to 11.8 %
	less than 10.5 %

U.S. = 12.1 %

Fig. 1–7. Humans age 65+, as a percentage of the total population of the United States, 1986. From U.S. Bureau of the Census. "State Population and Household Estimates With Age, Sex and Components of Change: 1981 to 1985." Current Population report Series P-25, No. 1010 (September 1987).

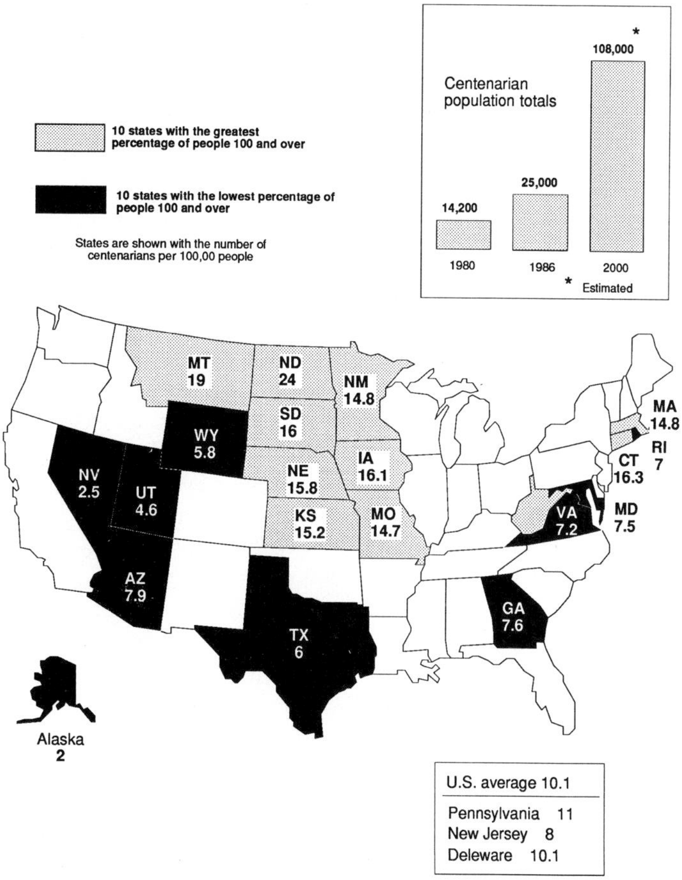

Centenarian
population totals

108,000 *
25,000
14,200

1980   1986   2000
* Estimated

| | 10 states with the greatest percentage of people 100 and over |
| | 10 states with the lowest percentage of people 100 and over |

States are shown with the number of
centenarians per 100,00 people

Fig. 1–8. Distribution of the centenarian population in the United States. From Social Security Administration, U.S. Bureau of Census. The Philadelphia Inquirer/David Pierce.

U.S. average 10.1

Pennsylvania   11
New Jersey   8
Deleware   10.1

in the year 2030 about 33% over the age of 60. It appears likely that in West Germany, between 1975 and 1990, the age group from 75 to 90 will increase by 17%, those from 80 to 85 by 51%, and those over the age of 90 years by 42%.

GEOGRAPHIC DISTRIBUTION

In the United States more than half of the elderly live in just 8 states: California, New York, Florida, Pennsylvania, Texas, Illinois, Ohio and Michigan [Table 1–2]. Each of these states had over one million persons age 65 + in 1985. Alaska had the smallest number of elderly (18,000), 3% of its total population. But Alaska and Nevada also experienced the largest percentage increases (50%) in their elderly population between 1980–1986. Sixteen of 21 northern states had percentages of elderly above the national average, while 9 out of 30 southern and western states including Washington, D.C. were above the national level. Today, persons 65 + constitute 13.6% of the total population in 10 states: Florida, Pennsylvania, Rhode Island, Iowa, Arkansas, South Dakota, Missouri, West Virginia, Nebraska, and Massachusetts. Florida has the largest proportion of residents 65 +. The proportion of elderly in Florida, 17.7%, is close to the proportion expected nationally in 2020. Florida is the "oldest" state (median age 36.0), and Utah is the "youngest state" (median age 25.5). Houston, Texas had the smallest percentage of elderly in 1980 (7%) for a major metropolitan area. New York had over one million elderly residents in the 1980 census.

Older persons tend to remain where they have spent much of their adult lives. Rates of moving decline with increasing age. With younger people leaving and older people staying, some areas of the country are becoming grayer. Most of the areas of the country that are becoming grayer are in the nation's heartland (agricultural areas) due to a lower birth rate and heavy out-migration by the young. There is a high proportion of elderly in: Iowa, Kansas, Missouri, Nebraska, South Dakota, Arkansas, Maine, Massachusetts, Rhode Island, and Pennsylvania. There is an older population in Florida and in the Ozark Plateau in Arkansas and the Texas hill country because

there are large retirement centers. In 1980, for the first time, more elderly persons lived in the suburban areas than in central cities. Older persons are found disproportionately in suburbs which were established before World War II. These older suburbs have lower average resident income levels, more rental housing, lower home values, and higher population densities.

Sunbelt states are experiencing an aging of their population due to the migration of older persons during their early retirement years.

MIGRATION

Between 1980–1986 the elderly population grew in the South and West. The growth of the elderly population in the Northeast and Midwest was and is less than the national average. Of the nearly 1.7 million Americans over age 60 who moved out of state between 1975–1980, half went to five states: Florida, California, Arizona, Texas, or New Jersey. Three states had large increases in older immigrants: Arizona, Texas, and Florida. One quarter of all older immigrants moved to Florida. States where people are moving from are: (1) New York, (2) California, (3) Illinois, (4) Florida, (5) New Jersey. Older persons who move are affluent, well-educated and are frequently accompanied by their spouses. People move to nonmetropolitan areas because of family, friends, property, or positive images of rural or small town life.

COUNTERMIGRATION

During the past decade there has been a statistically significant and increasing phenomenon—namely the countermigration of retired persons back to their original home base for psychologic and/or financial reasons. The term countermigration in this context means migration away from the warm to the cold climates. An important reason for this type of countermigration has been loneliness for family and familiar surroundings. There has also been a migration of retired citizens from the south to states with better benefit and health systems such as Michigan, New York, Ohio and Pennsylvania. These countermigrants usually have incomes below the poverty level, many are disabled or are living in institutions

TABLE 1–2.   Distribution of the 65+ Population in the United States

Number of persons 65+			Persons 65+ as percent of state's population			Percent change in number of persons 65+, 1980–1986		
Rank		State	Number (000s)	Rank	State	Percent	Rank	State	Percent

Rank		State	Number (000s)	Rank	State	Percent	Rank	State	Percent
1	(1)	California	2,848	1	Florida	17.7	1	Alaska	55.3
2	(2)	New York	2,283	2	Pennsylvania	14.6	2	Nevada	51.3
3	(5)	Florida	2,071	3	Rhode Island	14.6	3	Hawaii	35.8
4	(4)	Pennsylvania	1,736	4	Iowa	14.5	4	Arizona	33.2
5	(3)	Texas	1,583	5	Arkansas	14.5	5	New Mexico	24.5
6	(6)	Illinois	1,386	6	South Dakota	13.9	6	South Carolina	23.6
7	(7)	Ohio	1,320	7	Missouri	13.7	7	Florida	22.7
8	(8)	Michigan	1,039	8	West Virginia	13.6	8	Delaware	22.3
9	(9)	New Jersey	981	9	Nebraska	13.6	9	Utah	22.2
10	(12)	Massachusetts	794	10	Massachusetts	13.6	10	North Carolina	21.1
11	(10)	North Carolina	731	11	Oregon	13.4	11	Washington	20.5
12	(15)	Missouri	694	12	Kansas	13.4	12	Virginia	19.9
13	(14)	Indiana	657	13	Maine	13.3	13	Idaho	19.7
14	(17)	Wisconsin	624	14	Connecticut	13.3	14	Maryland	19.6
15	(11)	Georgia	608	15	Wisconsin	13.0	15	Oregon	19.3
16	(13)	Virginia	606	16	North Dakota	13.0	16	Colorado	18.9
17	(16)	Tennessee	590	17	New Jersey	12.9	17	California	18.0
18	(21)	Minnesota	526	18	New York	12.8	18	Georgia	17.7
19	(20)	Washington	520	19	Minnesota	12.5	19	Montana	17.3
20	(22)	Alabama	496	20	Oklahoma	12.4	20	Connecticut	15.8
21	(19)	Maryland	473	21	Arizona	12.3	21	Texas	15.5
22	(18)	Louisiana	454	22	Ohio	12.3	22	New Hampshire	15.2
23	(23)	Kentucky	449	23	Tennessee	12.3	23	Wyoming	14.5
24	(28)	Connecticut	423	24	Alabama	12.2	24	New Jersey	14.1
25	(29)	Iowa	414	25	Dist. of Col.	12.2	25	Tennessee	13.9
26	(26)	Oklahoma	411	26	Montana	12.1	26	Michigan	13.9
27	(25)	Arizona	409	27	Kentucky	12.0	27	Pennsylvania	13.4
28	(30)	Oregon	362	28	Illinois	12.0	28	Ohio	12.9
29	(24)	South Carolina	355	29	Mississippi	12.0	29	Alabama	12.8
30	(33)	Arkansas	344	30	Indiana	11.9	30	Louisiana	12.3
31	(32)	Kansas	330	31	Vermont	11.9	31	Indiana	12.1
32	(31)	Mississippi	314	32	Washington	11.7	32	Rhode Island	11.8
33	(27)	Colorado	294	33	New Hampshire	11.6	33	Maine	10.8
34	(34)	West Virginia	261	34	North Carolina	11.5	34	Wisconsin	10.7
35	(36)	Nebraska	217	35	Delaware	11.4	35	Vermont	10.6
36	(38)	Maine	156	36	Michigan	11.4	36	Arkansas	10.0
37	(37)	New Mexico	144	37	Idaho	11.2	37	Illinois	9.8
38	(42)	Rhode Island	142	38	Maryland	10.6	38	West Virginia	9.8
39	(35)	Utah	133	39	California	10.6	39	Minnesota	9.7
40	(40)	New Hampshire	119	40	South Carolina	10.5	40	North Dakota	9.6
41	(41)	Idaho	112	41	Virginia	10.5	41	Kentucky	9.5
42	(39)	Hawaii	103	42	Nevada	10.3	42	Oklahoma	9.3
43	(43)	Nevada	99	43	Louisiana	10.1	43	Massachusetts	9.2
44	(44)	Montana	99	44	Georgia	10.0	44	Mississippi	8.7
45	(45)	South Dakota	99	45	New Mexico	9.8	45	South Dakota	8.4
46	(46)	North Dakota	88	46	Hawaii	9.7	46	Kansas	7.7
47	(48)	Dist. of Col.	77	47	Texas	9.5	47	Missouri	7.0
48	(47)	Delaware	72	48	Colorado	9.0	48	Iowa	6.9
49	(49)	Vermont	64	49	Wyoming	8.4	49	Nebraska	5.7
50	(51)	Wyoming	43	50	Utah	8.0	50	New York	5.7
51	(50)	Alaska	18	51	Alaska	3.4	51	Dist. of Col.	3.1

From U.S. Bureau of the Census. "State Population and Household Estimates. With Age, Sex, and Components of Change: 1981 to 1986." *Current Population Reports* Series P.25, No. 1010 (September 1987). Rankings compiled by the U.S. Administration on Aging.

or homes for the aged. Small numbers of older people who move to another state at retirement are moving back home or to a state where family members live. This trend is relatively small in absolute numbers, though still statistically significant. People are leaving the Sunbelt area for: Michigan, New York, Ohio, and Pennsylvania—all these states also send migrants to Florida. Fifty-six percent of 9000 elderly Florida residents who moved to New York between 1975 to 1980 were born in New York; the average age was 73 years. This was more than double the number who moved to New York from Florida between 1965 to 1970. Another Sunbelt state—California—lost older migrants to other areas, but not to states that generally lose large numbers to California.

COST OF CARE [Fig. 1–9]

As noted above, the 65+ population is rising faster than any other age group. The cost of health care is also rising rapidly. The 65+ population needs long-term health care. Long-term care consists of medical and support services which include nursing care at home or in institutions and custodial care at home. In 1985, 12% of the American population over 65 accounted for 30% of hospital and medical bills. Over 6.6 million Americans, age 65+,

needed long-term care, that is, health and social services; in 1990, the number is 8.6 million and in 2000 it will be 9.3 million. At age 65 there is a 43% chance of needing nursing home care, 50% of which is financed directly by patients and their families. The House Select Committee on Aging has determined that $\frac{2}{3}$ of elderly people living alone would be impoverished after 13 weeks in a nursing home, where the average yearly cost is $25,000 and rising. Medicare covers only short-term convalescent care after illness, it does not pay for long-term care. Medicaid, a federal-state insurance program, covers long-term care of the poor aged—poverty being defined as below $5,000. Some people with income over $5,000 are forced to give away their money in order to qualify for Medicaid. Medicaid finances 41.5% and Medicare 2.1% of all nursing home care.

THE COST OF CARE OF SENILITY

In 1985 in the United States there were 4.28 million demented elderly patients, which is about 15% of the total 65+ population. Alzheimer's disease and multi-infarct dementia represent 85% of all dementia cases according to an older British study. The cost of senile dementia was $13.26 billion, which includes

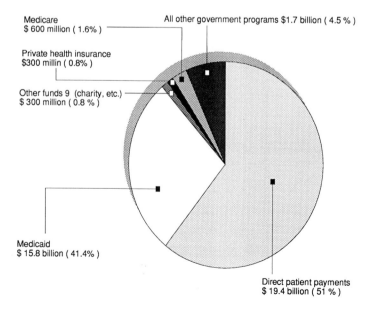

Medicare
$ 600 million (1.6%)

All other government programs $1.7 billion (4.5 %)

Private health insurance
$300 millin (0.8%)

Other funds 9 (charity, etc.)
$ 300 million (0.8 %)

Medicaid
$ 15.8 billion (41.4%)

Direct patient payments
$ 19.4 billion (51 %)

Fig. 1–9. The payers of nursing care. From Department of Health and Human Services. Based on a chart in the New York Times, November 26, 1987.

$6.36 billion for medical care, $2.56 billion for nursing care and $4.34 billion for social service agency costs. The indirect cost for community home care was $31.46 billion. The cost of premature death and loss of productivity was about $43.17 billion.[85]

THE PREVENTION AND REVERSAL OF MENTAL DECLINE

In recent years it has been suggested that parameters of mental performance of some elderly subjects—such as inductive reasoning, cognitive problem solving, memory span— could be improved by training. Since many of these and previous studies were cross-sectional in design, Schaie and Willis[11] felt that it was not possible to determine whether the improvement represented an amelioration of a prior cognitive decline or the acquisition of new performance levels. They felt that cognitive rehabilitation required a long-term longitudinal study in which training improvement could be assessed by comparison of the individual's prior level of cognitive functioning. There were 229 participants in this study, age 65 to 95 years, examined repeatedly over a 14 year span on their abilities for inductive reasoning and spatial orientation as a result of training. They reported that in a substantial number of the participants there was reversal of decline for these two cognitive parameters and an enhancement of performance for the stable participants.

Another interesting study was that of Avorn and Langer[86]; participants with average age of 78 years were rated for proficiency and speed in problem solving, and were randomly placed in 3 groups and asked to do a simple jigsaw puzzle individually. The first group were verbally encouraged; the second group were assisted and the third group were neither encouraged nor assisted. The first group did well, the second group did badly, and the third group did what their pre-experimental test suggested—no better, no worse. These authors suggested that direct assistance cultivated the mental inertia of the second group. Rowe and Kahn reviewing this and other studies suggested that encouraged or denied assistance of

personal self-esteem could be a major factor in the determination of usual and successful aging.[15]

REFERENCES

1. Shakespeare: Much Ado About Nothing. Act III, Scene 5, L 33, 1572.
2. Kenyon, G.: Basic Assumptions in Theories of Human Aging. In: *Emergent Theories of Aging*. Edited by J.E. Birren, Vern L. Bengtson, New York, Springer Publishing Company, 1988.
3. De Beauvoir, S.: *The Coming of Age*. New York, Warner, 1973.
4. Philibert, M.: The phenomenological approach to images of aging. In: *Philosophical Foundations of Gerontology*. Edited by P. McKee. New York, Human Sciences Press, 1982.
5. U.S. Bureau of Census. Money Income of Households, Families, and Persons in the United States: 1987. Current Populations Reports, Consumer Income, Series P-60, No. 162, pp. 154, 1987.
6. Schaie, K.W.: Translations in gerontology from lab to life: Intellectual functioning. Am. Psychol., *29*:802, 1974.
7. Horn, J.L., and Donaldson, G.: On the myth of intellectual decline in adulthood. Am. Psychol., *Oct*:701, 1976.
8. Schaie, K.W., and Labouvie-Vief, G.: Generational versus ontogenetic components of change in adult cognitive behavior: A fourteen-year cross-sequential study. Dev. Psychol., *10*:105, 1974.
9. Dittman-Kohli, and Baltes, P.: Toward a neofunctionalist conception of adult intellectual development: Wisdom as a prototypical case of intellectual growth OSC p1–30. In: *Beyond Formal Operations: Alternative Endpoints to Human Development*. Edited by C. Alexander, E. Langer, New York, Cambridge University Press (in press).
10. Green, R.F.: Age-intelligence-relationship between ages 16 and 64: A rising trend. Dev. Psychol., *1*:618, 1969.
11. Schaie, K.W., and Willis, S.L.: Can Decline in Adult Intellectual Functioning Be Reversed? Dev. Psychol., *22(2)*:223, 1986.
12. Labouvie-Vief, G.: In: *Handbook of the Psychology of Aging*. Edited by J.E. Birren, and K.W. Schaie. New York, Van Nostrand Reinhold, 1985.
13. Preface.: In: *Emergent Theories of Aging*. Edited by J.E. Birren, and V.L. Bengtson. New York, Springer Publishing Co., 1988.
14. Moody, H.R.: Toward a Critical Gerontology. In: *Emergent Theories of Aging*. Edited by J.E. Birren, and Vern L. Bengtson. New York, Springer Publishing Co., 1988.
15. Rowe, J.W., and Kahn, R.L.: Human Aging: Usual and Successful. Science, *237*:143, 1988.
16. Stern, F.H.: Creative Aging Is Within the Reach of All. Psychosomatics, *7(20)*:59, 1967.
17. Dawson, A.M., and Baller, W.R.: Relationship Between Creative Activity and the Health of Elderly Persons. J. Psychol., *82*:49, 1972.
18. Simonton, D.K.: Creative Productivity, Age, and Stress: A Biological Time-Series Analysis of 10 Classical Composers. J. Personal. Soc. Psychol., *25(11)*:791, 1977.

19. Hayslip, Jr., B., and Sterns, H.L.: Age Differences in Relationships Between Crystallized and Fluid Intelligences and Problem Solving. J. Geron., *34(3):*404, 1979.

20. Ager, C.L., et al.: Creative Aging. Intern. J. Aging Hum. Develop., *14(1):*67, 1982.

21. Pruyser, P.W.: Creativity in Aging Persons. Bull Menninger Clinic, *51:*425, 1987.

22. Mc Menemey, W.H.: Degenerations. In: *Pathology of the Nervous System,* Vol. 2, pp. 1372. Edited by J. Minckler. New York, McGraw-Hill, 1971.

23. Reier-Ruge, W.: Morphometric Methods and Their Potential Value for Gerontological Brain Research. In: *Histology and Histopathology of the Aging Brain.* Edited by H.P. von Hahn. Basel, Karger, 1988.

24. Tomlinson, B.E.: Morphological brain changes in non-demented old people. In: *Aging of the Central Nervous System.* Edited by H.M. Van Progg, and H.F. Kalverboer. De Erven F. Bohn, Haarlem, 1972.

25. Gellerstedt, N.: Upsala Lak.—Foren Forh. *38:*193, 1933.

26. Hirano, A., and Zimmerman, H.M.: Alzheimer's Neurofibrillary Changes. Arch. Neurol. (Chic.), *7:*227, 1963.

27. Corsellis, J.A.N.: In: *Mental Illness and the Aging Brain.* London, Oxford University Press, 1962.

28. Blessed, G., Tomlinson, B.E., and Roth, M.: The association between quantitive measures of dementia and of senile change in the cerebral grey matter of elderly subjects. Br. J. Psych., *114:*797, 1968.

29. Hoch Ligeti, C.: Effect of Aging on the Central Nervous System. J. Amer. Geriat. Soc., *II:*403, 1963.

30. Davies, D.V., and Davies, F.: *Gray's Anatomy.* 33rd Ed. London, Longmans, Green, 1962.

31. Ranson, S.W.: *The Anatomy of the Nervous System.* 8th Ed. Revised by S.L. Clark, Philadelphia, Saunders, 1951.

32. Korenchevsky, V.: *Physiological and Pathological Aging.* Edited by G.H. Bourne. New York, Karger, 1961.

33. Terry, R., et al.: Some morphometric aspects of the brain in senile dementia of the Alzheimer type. Ann. Neurol, *10(2):*184, 1981.

34. Terry, R.D., Hansen, L.A.: Some Morphometric Aspects of Alzheimer Disease and of Normal Aging. In: *Aging and the Brain.* Edited by R.D. Terry. New York, Raven Press, 1988.

35. Mc Menemey, W.H.: Degenerations. In: *Pathology of the Nervous System,* Vol 2, pp. 1373. Edited by J. Minckler. New York, McGraw-Hill, 1971.

36. Braak, H., and Braak, E.: Morphology of the Human Isocortex in Young and Aged Individuals: Qualitative and Quantitative Findings. In: *Histology and Histopathology of the Aging Brain.* Edited by H.P. von Hahn. Basel, Karger, 1988.

37. Brody, H.: Organization of cerebral cortex, III. A study of aging in human cerebral cortex. J. Comp. Neurol., *102:*511, 1955.

38. Konigsmark, B.W., and Murphy, E.A.: Volume of ventral cochlear nucleus in man: Its relationship to neuronal population and age. J. Neuropathol. Exp. Neurol., *31:*304, 1972.

39. Shefer, V.F.: Absolute number of neurons and thickness of the cerebral cortex during aging, senile and vascular dementia, and Pick's and Alzheimer's disease. Neurosci. Behav. Physio., *6:*319, 1973.

40. Monagle, R.D., and Brody, H.: The effects of age upon main nucleus of inferior olive in the human. J. Comp. Neurol., *155:*61, 1974.

41. Ball, M.J.: Neuronal loss, neurofibrillary tangles and granulovacuolar degeneration in the hippocampus with aging and dementia. Acta Neuropath., *37:*11, 1977.

42. Brody, H.: Cell counts in cerebral cortex and brainstem. In: *Alzheimer's Disease: Senile Dementia and Related Disorders* (aging vol. 7). Edited by R.D. Terry, K. Bick. New York, Raven Press, 1978.

43. Henderson, G., Tomlinson, B.E., and Gibson, P.H.: Cell counts in human cerebral cortex in normal adults throughout life using an image analyzing computer. J. Neurol. Sci., *46:*113, 1980.

44. Bowen, D.M., et al.: Accelerated aging or selective neuronal loss as an important cause of dementia? Lancet, *1:*11, 1979.

45. Scheibel, M.E., et al.: Progressive dendritic changes in aging human cortex. Exp. Neurol., *47:*392, 1975.

46. Scheibel, A.B.: Structural aspects of the aging brain: spine systems and dendritic arbor. In: *Alzheimer's Disease: Senile Dementia and Related Disorders* (Aging Vol. 7), Edited by R. Katzman, R.D. Terry, and K.L. Bick. New York, Raven, 1978.

47. Huttenlocher, P.R.: Synaptic density in human frontal cortex: developmental changes and effects of aging. Brain Res. *163:*195, 1979.

48. Last, R.J., and Tompsett, D.H.: Casts of the Cerebral Ventricles. Br. J. Surg., *40:*525, 1953.

49. Davis, P.J.M., and Wright, E.A.: New method for measuring cranial cavity volume and its application to the assessment of cerebral atrophy at autopsy. Neuropath. App. Neurobio., *3:*341, 1977.

50. Barron, S.A., Jacobs, L. and Kinkel, W.R.: Change in size of normal lateral ventricles during aging determined by computed tomography. Neurol., *26:*1101, 1976.

51. Gonzalez, C.F., Lantieri, R.L., and Nathan, R.J.: The CT scan appearance of the brain in the normal elderly population: A correlative study. Neuroradiology, *16:*120, 1978.

52. Gyldensted, C.: Measurements of the normal ventricular system and hemispheric sulci of 100 adults with computed tomography. Neurorad., *14:*183, 1977.

53. Haug, G.: Age and sex dependence of the size of normal ventricles on computed tomography. Neurorad., *14:*201, 1977.

54. Yamaura, H., et al.: Brain atrophy during aging: a quantitative study with computed tomography. J. Geront. Aging, *35:*492, 1980

55. Jacoby, R.J., Levy, R., and Dawson, J.M.: Computed tomography in the elderly. I. The normal population. Br. J. Psych., *136:*249, 1980.

56. Hughes, C.O., and Gado, M.: Computed tomography and aging of the brain. Radiology, *139:*291, 1981.

57. Cala, L.A., et al.: Brain density and cerebrospinal fluid space size: CT of normal volunteers. Am. J. Neuroradiol., *2:*41, 1981.

58. Brinkman, S.D., et al.: Quantitative indexes of computed tomography in dementia and normal aging. Radiology, *138:*89, 1981.

59. Gado, M., et al.: Volumetric measurements of the cerebrospinal fluid spaces in demented subjects and controls. Radiology, *144:*535, 1982.

60. Damasio, H., et al.: Quantitative computed tomographic analysis in the diagnosis of dementia. Arch. Neurol., *40:*715, 1983.

61. Laffey, P.A., et al.: Computed tomography in aging: results in a normal elderly population. Neuroradiol., *26:*273, 1984.

62. LeMay, M.: Radiologic changes of the aging brain and skull. AJR, *143*:383, 1984.

63. Schwartz, M., et al.: Computed tomographic analysis of brain morphometrics in 30 healthy men, aged 21 to 81 years. Ann. Neurol., *17(2)*:146, 1985.

64. Nagata, K., et al.: A quantitative study of physiological cerebral atrophy with aging: a statistical analysis of the normal range. Neuroradiol., *29*:327, 1987.

65. Bernsmeier, A., and Gottstein, H.: Hirndurchblutung und Alter. Verh. dtsch. Ges. Dreisl.-Forsch., *24*:248, 1958.

66. Kety, S.S.: Human cerebral blood flow and oxygen consumption as related to aging. J. Chron. Dis., *3*:478, 1956.

67. Fazekas, J.F., Alivan, R.W., and Bessman, A.N.: Cerebral physiology of the aged. Am. J. Med. Sci., *223*:245, 1952.

68. Scheinberg, P., Blackburn, I., Rich, M., et al.: Effects of aging on cerebral circulation and metabolism. Arch. Neurol. Psychiat., *70*:77, 1953.

69. Scheinberg, P., and Stead, Jr., E.A.: The cerebral blood flow in male subjects as measured by the nitrous oxide technique: normal values for blood flow, oxygen utilization, glucose utilization and peripheral resistance with observations on the effect of tilting and anxiety. J. Clin. Invest., *28*:1163, 1949.

70. Schieve, J.F., and Wilson, W.P.: The influence of age, anesthesia, and cerebral arteriosclerosis on cerebral vascular activity to CO_2. Am. J. Med., *15*:171, 1953.

71. Lassen, N.A., Feinberg, I., and Lane, M.H.: Bilateral studies of cerebral oxygen uptake in young and aged normal subjects and in patients with organic dementia. J. Clin. Invest., *39*:491, 1960.

72. Dastur, D.K., et al.: Effects of aging on cerebral circulation and metabolism in man. In: *Human Aging. A Biological and Behavioral Study.* Edited by J.E. Birren, R.N. Butler, S.W. Greenhouse, et al.: Washington D.C., U.S. Gov. Print. Off., 1963.

73. Sokoloff, L.: Cerebral circulatory and metabolic changes associated with aging. Res. Pub. Ass. Nerv. Ment. Dis., *41*:237, 1966.

74. Alavi, A., et al.: Regional cerebral glucose metabolism in aging and senile dementias as determined by 18-F-deoxyglucose and positron emission tomography. Exp. Brain Res. Suppl. 5. Hoyer, S. (ed.), Berlin, Heidelberg, New York: Springer, 1982, pp. 187–195.

75. Kuhl, D.E., et al.: Effects of human aging on patterns of local cerebral glucose utilization determined by the 18F fluorodeoxyglucose method. J. Cereb. Blood Flow Metabol., *2*:163, 1982.

76. Hoyer, S.: Plasticity of the Brain in Old Age. Advances in Neuropathology. In: *Advances in Neurosurgery.* Edited by W. Piotrowski, M. Brock, and M. Klinger. Berlin, Springer-Verlag, 1984.

77. Patel, M.S.: Age-dependent changes in the oxidative metabolism in rat brain. J. Geront., *32*:643, 1977.

78. Gibson, G.E., and Peterson, C.: Neurotransmitter and carbohydrate metabolism during senescence. In: *The Aging Brain. Physiological and Pathophysiological Aspects.* Exp. Brain Res. Suppl. 5. Hoyer, S. (ed.), New York, Springer, 1982, pp. 113–139.

79. Normal Human Aging: The Baltimore Longitudinal Study of Aging. NIH Publication No. 84-2450, Nov., 1984.

80. Aging America: Trends and Projections. Prepared by the U.S. Senate Special Committee on Aging in conjunction with the American Association of Retired Persons, the Federal Council on the Aging, and the U.S. Administration on Aging, 1987–88 Edition.

81. U.S. Bureau of the Census. Estimates of the Population of the United States by Age, Sex, and Race: 1980–86. Current Population Reports Series P-25, No. 1000 (February 1987).

82. Spencer, G.: U.S. Bureau of the Census. Projections of the Population of the United States by Age, Sex, and Race: 1983–2080. Current Population Reports Series P-25, No. 952 (May 1984).

83. U.S. Bureau of the Census. State Population and Household Estimates With Age, Sex, and Components of Change: 1981–1986. Current Population Reports Series P-25, No. 1010 (September 1987).

84. Wang, H.S.: In: *Aging and Dementia.* Edited by W.L. Smith, and M. Kinsbourne. New York, Spectrum Pub. Inc., 1977.

85. Rivlin, A.M., Wiener, J.M., Hanley, R.J., et al.: Who Will Pay? Washington, D.C., Brookings Institution, XVIII, 1988.

86. Avorn, J., and Langer, E.: Induced disability in nursing home patients. Control trial. J. Am. Ger. Soc., *30(6)*:397, 1982

CHAPTER 2

Vascular Diseases*

HARRY V. VINTERS
and VEI H. MAH

This chapter discusses cerebral vascular diseases, particularly cerebrovascular diseases that are prone to cause morbidity and mortality in the geriatric population. Many forms of "stroke" and cerebrovascular disease do not respect age boundaries, although certain patterns of disease are more common in young and middle aged patients, whereas others are more prevalent in the elderly. As well, some principles of anoxic-ischemic brain injury can be applied to many situations that affect the adult brain, regardless of age (the pediatric age group of course deserves special consideration in this regard). Thus, common underlying mechanisms of anoxic-ischemic brain damage will be discussed without regard to patient age.

We have arbitrarily divided the chapter into three main sections, namely: (1) cerebral in-

farcts and ischemic lesions, (2) encephalic hemorrhage, and (3) multi-infarct or vascular dementia. These divisions are arbitrary and will overlap with issues (e.g. dementia) discussed in other chapters. Throughout, we shall attempt to emphasize cerebrovascular problems that are particularly common in elderly individuals with an appropriately expanded discussion, whereas disease entities that are less important in the geriatric age group will be de-emphasized, perhaps disproportionately. For example, vascular disease affecting the spinal cord will not be discussed. We accept responsibility for this sense of perspective. We also wish to emphasize that any extensive work on cerebrovascular disease owes a huge debt to the monograph of W.E. Stehbens[1] which, though it was published in 1972, must remain the authoritative text on cerebrovascular neuropathology. Numerous citations to it throughout this chapter will attest to this. Other recent important volumes and reviews on clinicopathologic aspects of stroke and ce-

---

*Dedicated to Professor *John C.E. Kaufmann,* Professor of Pathology and Clinical Neurological Sciences, University of Western Ontario, on the occasion of his retirement.

rebrovascular disease[2-6] must also serve as reference works for the interested reader.

CEREBRAL INFARCTS AND ISCHEMIC LESIONS

ANOXIA/ISCHEMIA AND THE BRAIN

Cerebral infarction has been defined as an area of necrosis with irreversible damage to all cell types within a specific vascular territory of the brain. The transition zone between an infarcted area and normal brain often contains partial changes such as neuronal necrosis with surviving astrocytes. In the brain, neurons are the cells most sensitive to ischemic insults, followed by oligodendroglia, astrocytes and endothelial cells. Among neuronal populations, the CA1 pyramidal cells of the hippocampus and cerebellar Purkinje cells appear most vulnerable, followed by medium-sized neurons within striatum and neocortical neurons in layers 3, 5 and 6.[7,8]

The pathophysiology of cerebral ischemia is influenced by factors both extrinsic and intrinsic to brain. Hypoperfusion initiates cellular changes which lead to irreversible damage if flow is not restored rapidly. Even with recirculation restored following transient ischemia, there may be secondary impairments to blood flow that contribute to pathologic changes.

Studies have been performed to try to elucidate the molecular mechanisms of ischemic injury in discrete regions of the brain. In rats examined after severe transient ischemia, damage to neurons was seen to increase progressively 24 to 72 hours after cerebral reperfusion. Measurements of regional cerebral blood flow and glucose metabolism in the rat following forebrain ischemia showed that abnormalities of these functions could not explain delayed onset and progression of neuronal injury in hippocampal neuronal populations.[7] Measurements of brain phosphocreatine, adenosine triphosphate (ATP) and lactate concentrations showed near complete recovery of energy reserves followed by secondary decline in the hippocampus and striatum.[7]

In experiments where the Schaffer collateral input to CA1 pyramidal cells was interrupted, the CA1 pyramidal cells in the ipsilateral hippocampus showed apparent protection from ischemic injury compared to the contralateral hippocampus, suggesting that neurotransmitter input may have been a factor in selective ischemic injury to neurons.[7]

In early experiments and clinical observations of the brain after cardiac arrest, cerebral ischemia of more than 4 to 5 minutes duration appeared to result in irreversible brain damage. Post-ischemic recirculation was a limiting factor of cerebral recovery.

After circulation is reinitiated after ischemia, there is a period of reactive hyperemia. Disturbances in recirculation include the "no reflow" phenomenon and delayed postischemic hypoperfusion. The "no reflow" phenomenon may be due to a combination of increased blood viscosity, microvascular compression by adjacent swollen glial cells, increased intracranial pressure, disseminated intravascular coagulation or hypotension. There appears to be close correlation of the "no reflow" phenomenon with the appearance of histologic lesions in primates. Postischemic hypoperfusion develops after the reactive hyperemic phase has subsided and is characterized by disrupted autoregulation with vascular constriction and uncoupling of blood flow and metabolic activity.[8]

After prolonged ischemia, other delayed postischemic disturbances—such as permeability changes of the blood-brain barrier, alteration of calcium-mediated processes and secondary depression of previously recovered metabolic activity—have been noted.

Measurements of blood flow show that it is lower in normal white matter than grey matter, as is the metabolic rate. In ischemia, metabolic changes in white matter are greater than within cortical areas. Since the white matter is supplied by smaller caliber penetrating arteries and intercapillary distances are greater, a compromised blood flow may have greater effects on it.[9]

Calcium. An influx of calcium into the cell is associated with significant ischemia. Several processes are enhanced by increased intracellular calcium, including lipolysis through phospholipase A2 and phospholipase C activities, disaggregation of microtubules into tubulin subunits,[10,11] degradation of neurofilaments and other cytoskeletal components by neutral calcium dependent proteases, and protein phosphorylation.[10] Activation of these processes could lead to damage of cell membranes and disruption of transport mechanisms. Calcium entry blockers have shown beneficial effects in models of complete and incomplete ischemia.[10] Although a temporal association between calcium accumulation and ischemic brain injury has been noted,[10] there is no definite proof that cell death is a consequence of the calcium influx itself. For illustrative purposes, an early ischemic brain lesion (from an experimental animal) is shown in Figure 2–1.

Glutamate. Glutamate, a nonessential amino acid and the most abundant free amino acid in the central nervous system (CNS), is a putative excitatory neurotransmitter in several pathways including cortical association fibers, corticofugal, hippocampal, cerebellar and spinal cord pathways. Glutamate has neurotoxic properties and enhanced glutamatergic neu-

rotransmission may cause cell damage and lead to neuronal death.[12,13]

Glutamate receptors have been categorized with respect to their most specific agonist (N-methyl-D-aspartate (NMDA), quisqualate and kainate), or antagonist (L-2-amino-4-phosphonobutyrate (AP4)). The NMDA receptor is involved in excitatory neurotransmission and is felt to be important in long term potentiation,[12] which is theoretically involved in learning and memory.

In cerebral ischemia there is an increase in extracellular glutamate levels and decreased high affinity glutamate uptake, thereby possibly increasing its neurotoxicity. The cerebral cortex and hippocampus, areas susceptible to ischemic insult in adults, contain high concentrations of glutamate receptors. Pharmacologic blocking of glutamate receptors by antagonists or disruption of glutamatergic innervation to the hippocampus has resulted in reduction of

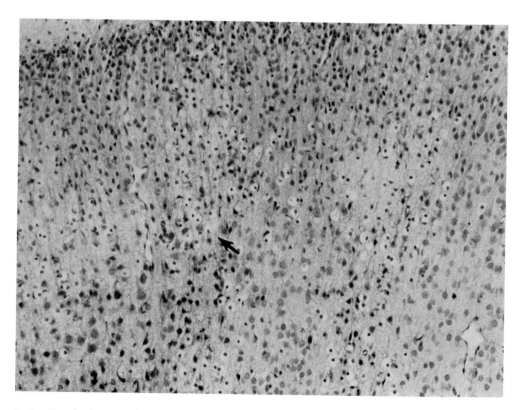

Fig. 2–1. Cerebral cortex from a rat examined several days after induction of ischemia by ligation of internal carotid arteries. Note patchy areas of vacuolization of the neuropil, pyknotic neurons at the centers of enlarged perineuronal spaces (arrow), and many regions in which the neurons appear healthy. (hematoxylin and eosin, ×190).

neuronal damage and neurologic deficits in appropriately treated experimental animals.[12,14]

HYPOGLYCEMIA

Histologically, the neuronal appearances in ischemia and hypoglycemia are similar.[15] However, other significant differences have been noted.[16,17] (1) Cellular redox systems are reduced in ischemia and oxidized in hypoglycemia. (2) pH is decreased in ischemia due to lactic acid formation and pH is increased in hypoglycemia. Lactic acid formation is not a component of hypoglycemia. (3) Energy failure is less severe in hypoglycemia than ischemia. (4) Hypotension in hypoglycemia does not lead to increased neuronal necrosis.[18]

Recent morphologic studies of the distribution of hypoglycemic brain injury in rats have shown a selective neuronal necrosis related to the distance of the site from the subarachnoid spaces.[17] The cerebral cortex shows a decreasing gradient of neuronal necrosis from superficial to deep layers. Both small and large neurons are affected. The location of the neuronal dendritic tree with respect to the subarachnoid space also appears to be an important factor, in addition to the location of the cell body. Astrocytes, oligodendrocytes and other cell types are preserved. Occasionally only unilateral damage was observed. Electron microscopic studies[16,19] have shown swollen dendrites with swollen mitochondria as the earliest changes, followed by changes in the cell body, and then neuronal necrosis. The pathologic process appears to spare axons.

In hypoglycemic tissue, there is a 3- to 4-fold increase in levels of aspartate, an excitatory amino acid.[16,17,20] Glutamate levels are decreased. From this and other data pertaining to cerebrospinal fluid (CSF) and tissue fluid dynamics, an excitotoxic mechanism of neuronal death in hypoglycemia has been hypothesized.[16,17,20]

ATHEROSCLEROSIS

Atherosclerosis is the principal cause of and contributes significantly to mortality from myocardial and cerebral infarcts. To some extent, the lesions of atherosclerosis are age-related, although important metabolic factors also come into play.[21-25]

The earliest atherosclerotic lesions are the fatty streaks commonly found in large arteries of young adults and children. These lesions contain macrophages and some smooth muscle cells. Recent animal studies have demonstrated the importance of monocyte interactions with possibly altered endothelium as an early event in the pathogenesis of atherosclerosis. The monocytes appear to migrate between endothelial cells and accumulate lipid, becoming foam cells. Progression of this process occurs with continuing attachment and migration of monocytes and gradual migration from the media of smooth muscle cells that also accumulate lipid.[21] After prolonged insult, the endothelial cells retract such that the macrophages and underlying connective tissues are exposed to the circulation. This allows for platelet adherence and the formation of mural thrombi.

The fibrous plaque representing more advanced atherosclerosis consists of excessive intimal smooth muscle cells, connective tissue matrix and variable amounts of lipid. These are generally covered with a dense fibrous cap of smooth muscle and connective tissues. Beneath this is a cellular zone containing smooth muscle and macrophages with lipid droplets, connective tissue and sometimes other leukocytes. Beneath this cellular region there may be necrotic debris, cholesterol crystals, and calcium.[21] "Complicated" atheroma, which is often symptomatic, contains the latter structures, and there is usually resultant ulceration of the plaque, with or without mural thrombus formation. Examples of thrombosed segments of the carotid artery are illustrated in Figure 2–2.

Endothelial cells can produce various vasoactive agents, growth factors and inhibitors which can affect both monocytes and smooth muscle cells. One of these is a mitogen resembling platelet derived growth factor (PDGF). Endothelial cells also form antithrombotic substances such as prostacyclin and heparin. Smooth muscle cells can produce large amounts of connective tissue matrix, accumulate lipid and can migrate in response to chemotactic factors. They have receptors for low density lipoprotein (LDL) and growth factors such as PDGF.

The platelets which interact with subendo-

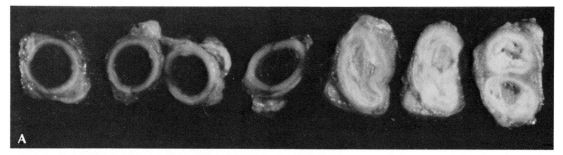

Fig. 2–2. A. Serial sections of common carotid artery and carotid bifurcation examined at autopsy. Both internal carotid and external carotid branches show old thrombus within severely atherosclerotic vessels. The four sections at left show more recent thrombus.

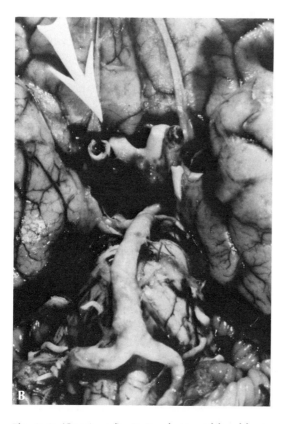

Fig. 2–2. *(Continued)* B. Basal view of fixed brain from patient with ICA occlusion (arrow). Note that vertebrobasilar system also shows severe atheromatous change. Left ICA also appears to demonstrate significant complicated atheromatous change.

of substances—including interleukin-1, which induces increased adherence of leukocytes to endothelium; leukotriene B4, which is a strong chemoattractant; and fibroblast growth factor, which is a potent mitogen for endothelial cells and fibroblasts.

Fisher et al.[26] defined the morbid anatomy of atherosclerosis of the intra- and extracranial carotid and vertebral arteries in an exhaustive autopsy study of 178 patients. The conclusion from this illuminating work was that atherosclerosis within the carotid arteries was less than that observed in the aorta, but greater than that of the vertebral and cerebral arteries. In relation to patient age, the discrepancy between aortic and carotid atherosclerosis became particularly prominent in both normotensive and hypertensive males after the age of 50 years (aortic lesions being more severe), and in normotensive and hypertensive females after the age of 60. Almost 10% of patients showed one or more *total* vascular occlusions within the neck and 6 patients had them intracranially. Of remaining patients, 40% had some degree of vascular stenosis. When symptomatic, carotid occlusion tended to be extracranial while vertebral occlusion was intracranial. The study highlighted the frequency of asymptomatic stenosis and occlusion of vertebral and carotid arteries, and the often highly *focal* nature of carotid (as opposed to vertebral) atherosclerosis. Hypertension was found to be an aggravating factor for cerebral atherosclerosis overall, and especially basilar atherosclerosis and stenosis. Finally, severity of atherosclerosis was usually about the same in the anterior and posterior regions of the circle of Willis. Among other things, this important

thelial connective tissues are stimulated to release their granule contents. PDGF is both chemotactic and mitogenic and therefore can induce smooth muscle cell migration and proliferation. Macrophages can produce a number paper highlighted the importance of carefully examining the neck vessels in any patient who comes to autopsy following a "stroke".

CEREBRAL INFARCTS—GROSS AND MICROSCOPIC FEATURES

Infarcts can be classified as hemorrhagic or anemic. The clinical importance of cerebral infarcts can be judged by the results of one autopsy study, in which 320 cases of ischemic cerebrovascular disease were found among 944 consecutive necropsies. Their importance in the *geriatric* age group was highlighted by the median age of patients in whom ischemic cerebrovascular disease was present: 73.2 years in men, 75.6 years in women.[27] Anemic (or bland) infarcts contain little or no hemorrhage because, in theory, the circulation to them is completely blocked. They generally, though not always, result from *in situ* thrombosis of a severely atherosclerotic vessel.[1,2] It is important to realize, however, that occlusion of a vessel feeding the cerebral circulation need not produce tissue necrosis, and that 'late' or delayed cerebral ischemic events distal to occluded arterial segments have been described.[28] The probable mechanism involved in a hemorrhagic infarct is reperfusion of the infarcted area after vascular endothelial damage has occurred, thus allowing for extravasation of red blood cells. Hemorrhagic infarcts (Fig. 2–3) more commonly result from vascular emboli, originating in the heart or elsewhere. In addition, post-anoxic swelling of tissues may lead to venous compression and elevated intravascular pressures, exacerbating the process of hemorrhage into necrotic tissue.

After irreversible anoxic damage to the CNS, visible changes occur following a sequence which correlates to a large extent with the time interval between the insult and the point at which the brain is examined.

Gross Appearances. The early changes of coagulative necrosis occur between approximately 8 and 48 hours. There is swelling of cortex and white matter and blurring of the cortex-white matter junction. The affected cortex becomes slightly hyperemic and darker in appearance due to vascular dilatation (Fig. 2–4).[1] Between 48 and 96 hours the swelling reaches a maximum (Fig. 2–5), and during this time the greatest risk of fatal brain herniation occurs. The infarcted area becomes clearly delineated and a separation of the necrotic tissues from the relatively unaffected tissues can be observed (sometimes designated "cracking artifact"). Between 7 days and 3 weeks the

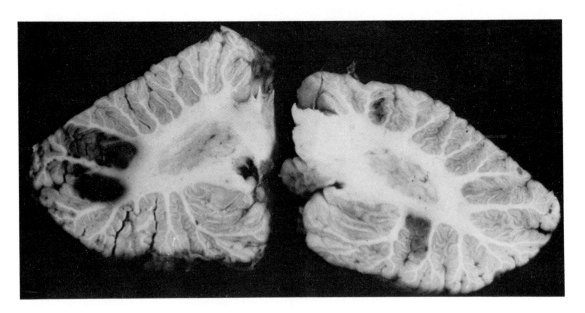

Fig. 2–3. Patchy areas of recent infarction within both cerebellar hemispheres. Infarcts on the left appear more hemorrhagic than those on the right.

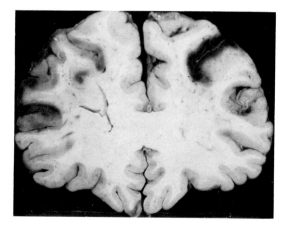

Fig. 2–4. Coronal section through fixed cerebral hemispheres near genu of corpus callosum. Recent infarcts are identified in both cerebral hemispheres. Infarct in left hemisphere occupies most of the territory of the left MCA, while the rather more hemorrhagic infarct in the right hemisphere is approximately at the watershed between right MCA and ACA vessels. Note fracture of white matter, partly artifactual, in left centrum semiovale.

process of liquefactive necrosis occurs. The swelling resolves and the affected tissues become soft and friable.

After approximately 3 weeks, cavitation of the brain substance begins to occur, as there is little fibroblastic activity or collagen deposition to replace the infarcted tissues, which are resorbed by macrophages. The lesion is replaced by an irregular fluid-filled cystic cavity traversed by variable numbers of blood vessels and gliotic trabeculae (Fig. 2–6), regardless of whether the infarct is large or small (Fig. 2–7).[1] When the overlying leptomeninges are involved, they become thickened and opaque. There is usually preservation of an intensely gliotic molecular layer of cortex overlying the infarct. Extensive infarcts may fail to resorb completely. Eventual resolution of the infarct results in contraction and collapse of remaining tissues (Fig. 2–6B).

Microscopic Features. Between 6 and 24 hours after irreversible ischemia, neurons may become (1) shrunken and angulated with in-

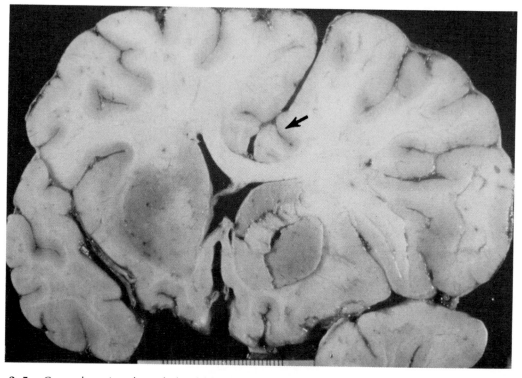

Fig. 2–5. Coronal section through fixed brain demonstrates right MCA territory infarct associated with ICA occlusion, approximately 2 to 3 days old. Extensive cracking artifact is noted at cortex-white matter junction in right MCA territory, as well as in the junction between the basal ganglia and internal capsule. Infarct has caused significant edema, manifested by right to left of midline structures, including marked subfalcine herniation of the cingulate gyrus (arrow). Left cerebral hemisphere appears relatively normal.

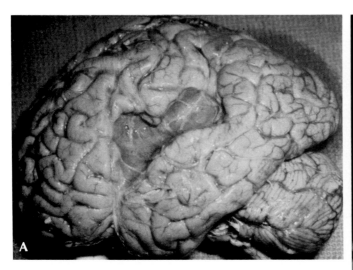

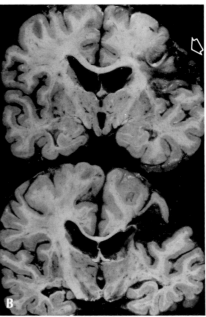

Fig. 2–6.   A. Fixed brain, left lateral view. Note large cystic cavity in left lateral frontoparietal cortex and subcortical white matter, representative of an old infarct. Portions of the MCA territory are, however, spared. B. Coronal sections from another brain containing an old cystic infarct in right MCA territory (arrowhead). Note relative preservation of surrounding brain, but collapse of brain parenchyma into the cyst. The cyst cavity is filled with gliotic material and blood vessels. There is compensatory enlargement of the right lateral ventricle. The internal capsule on the right is also thin and shrunken, probably secondary to Wallerian degeneration.

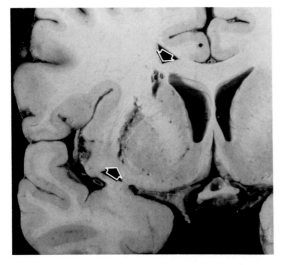

Fig. 2–7.   Coronal section of fixed brain. Arrowheads indicate a relatively small old cystic infarct in territory of distal penetrating branches of the left MCA.

tensely eosinophilic homogeneous cytoplasm and pyknotic basophilic nuclei or (2) swollen and pale staining. The axons become swollen and fragmented and myelin sheaths disintegrate (Fig. 2–8).[1] Oligodendrocytes swell and show enlarged perinuclear halos. Astrocytes and endothelial cells also become swollen. Microvacuolation of the neuropil may occur and become visible at the light microscopic level (Fig. 2–9). With disintegration of myelinated axons, oligodendrocytes and astrocytes, the neuropil takes on a granular appearance. Polymorphonuclear leukocytes may migrate into the region of the infarct within 1 to 3 days after its occurrence, though in our experience the severity of this inflammation is extremely unpredictable from case to case.

By electron microscopy, at 5 hours after ischemia there is microvacuolation of mitochondria and at 24 hours, swelling of the Golgi complex and endoplasmic reticulum and accumulation of ribosomal rosettes.[15] Between 24 and 48 hours after an infarct, neutrophils mar-

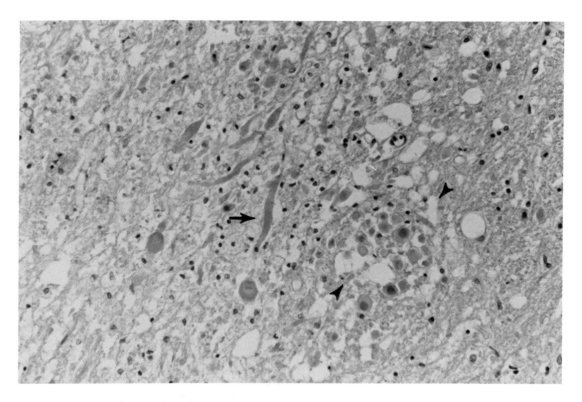

Fig. 2–8. Section shows edge of a recent infarct. Tissue at right is relatively preserved. However, left two thirds of the micrograph show vacuolization of the tissue, as well as enlarged (ischemic) axons, some of which are cut in longitudinal section (arrow), while others are cut in cross section (arrowheads). (hematoxylin and eosin, ×190).

ginate along blood vessel walls and migrate into brain substance. After 48 hours, macrophages appear in increasing numbers and phagocytose myelin breakdown products, thus acquiring their foamy appearance. They initially aggregate around capillary walls and are most prominent at the edges of infarcted zones. At approximately 2 to 3 weeks, the number of macrophages tends to reach a maximum.[1] Thereafter, they gradually disappear, although some may persist for many years. Whether the macrophages derive from microglia or monocytes of hematogenous origin is still debated.[29]

Between 2 and 4 weeks, there is endothelial cell proliferation with formation of new capillaries (Fig. 2–10), and reactive astrocytic proliferation and hypertrophy followed by formation and deposition of glial fibers (astrocytic gliosis, Fig. 2–11).[1] Astrocytic activity is maximal at approximately 6 weeks. The changes

are most prominent along the borders of the infarct. After 4 weeks there is a decrease in prominence of the capillaries, gradual disappearance of the necrotic tissue and macrophages and eventual glial scar formation (Fig. 2–12).

Watershed Infarcts. Watershed or border-zone infarcts are those which occur along the boundaries between two arterial territories, generally the major cerebral arteries such as the anterior and middle or the middle and posterior cerebral arteries (Fig. 2–13). They have also been documented between cerebellar artery territories and in the basal ganglia. Watershed infarcts account for approximately 10% of all brain infarcts.[30] They have been the subject of meticulous clinicopathologic human autopsy and experimental studies.[31,32] There are several hypotheses as to the mechanisms involved in their development. These include hypotension, microemboli, carotid artery occlusion, and cerebral thromboangiitis obliterans.[30,33]

Watershed infarcts are most commonly associated with a sharp drop in systemic blood pressure. Clinically, this is a particular problem in elderly individuals with atherosclerotic cerebral blood vessels undergoing major general or cardiovascular surgery. Their most frequent location is the territory between the anterior and middle cerebral arteries. It is hypothesized that the decrease in blood flow in such circumstances may be more severely decreased in the arterial endfields. There may be diffuse nerve cell loss in the cortex in addition to localized frank infarcts. Emboli consisting of cholesterol crystals or atheromatous debris (Fig. 2–14) from a more proximally situated plaque can block vessels within watershed zones. In general, these tend to pass distally from their site of origin until the arterial lumen becomes too narrow or tortuous for their further passage.

Carotid artery occlusions are associated with watershed infarcts.[30,34] The occurrence of platelet aggregates in overlying leptomeningeal vessels has been noted.[35] The watershed infarcts in this setting were thought to be due to decreased blood flow, i.e. mechanisms similar to those involved in hypotension. Alternatively, they may have resulted from microemboli, e.g. from mural thrombi within the carotid artery.[36]

Lacunar Infarcts. These are small infarcts occurring in deep brain structures, most often in association with hypertension.[37] They accounted for approximately 19% of cerebral infarcts in one study.[38] The majority of these infarcts measure from 2 to 15 mm in greatest dimension. Commonly affected sites are the basal ganglia, thalamus, internal capsule or basis pontis (Fig. 2–15). These structures are in the territories of the lenticulostriate or thalamoperforant arteries, or paramedian branches of the basilar artery. Such vessels have in common their small size, a tendency to arise di-

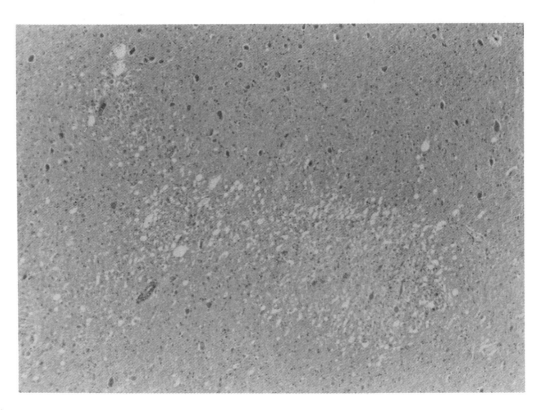

Fig. 2–9. Recent micro-infarct shows pale central staining of neuroglial tissue, and surrounding vacuolization, possibly representing edema. Preserved neurons are seen at top of micrograph. (hematoxylin and eosin, ×50).

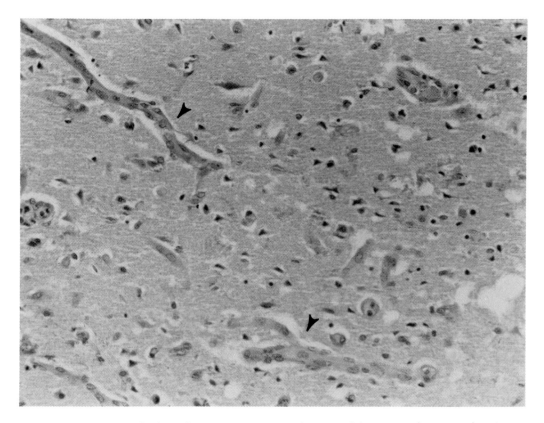

Fig. 2–10.   Recent cortical infarct shows extensive vacuolization of the neuropil, many pyknotic neurons (right of field), and prominent capillaries (arrowheads). Patient had a long history of peripheral vascular disease including carotid endarterectomy performed 3 years before death. Extensive cerebral infarcts occurred during a prolonged cardiovascular surgical procedure, from which the patient did not awaken. Clinically, infarcts were at least 3 to 4 days old. Vascular endothelial proliferation such as this suggests they may have been even older. (hematoxylin and eosin, ×190).

rectly from large arteries, and an unbranching end artery configuration. Generally, lacunar infarcts are not frequently found in cerebral neocortex, subcortical white matter, corpus callosum, or spinal cord. The fact that similar small blood vessels supply these areas argues against a generalized small vessel disease as the underlying etiology of lacunes. Lacunes usually have the histologic features of small infarcts (Figs. 2–16 and 2–17). However, several French studies have suggested that the term 'lacune' encompass a more broadly de-

fined group of lesions, including dilated perivascular spaces, the walls of which show no gliosis or other destructive/reactive changes, and microhemorrhages. Rarely 'expanding' cerebral lacunae in hypertensives may behave as space occupying lesions.[39,40]

Several forms or components of arterial and arteriolar lesion have been described in association with lacunar infarcts, including fibrinoid necrosis, hyalinosis, lipohyalinosis and microatheroma (Fig. 2–18). Vascular hyalinosis and fibrinoid necrosis both occur in the

⟶

Fig. 2–12.   Micrograph from edge from an old cystic infarct, comparable to that shown in Figure 2–11 (both sections are from the same patient). Preserved, severely gliotic rim of molecular layer (arrowheads) is seen immediately deep to the leptomeninges. Lower portion of micrograph shows many histiocytes, and a cystic cavity traversed by glial fibers and microvessels. Histology is characteristic of an old cystic infarct, the precise dating of which is problematic. (hematoxylin and eosin, ×76).

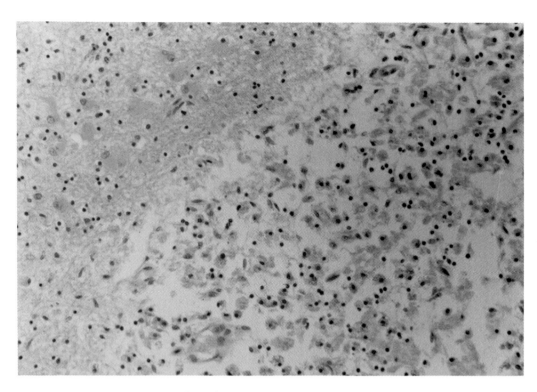

Fig. 2–11. Edge of an old cystic infarct shows numerous gemistocytic astrocytes in preserved neuroglial tissue at upper left. By contrast, right half of micrograph shows numerous foamy macrophages (compound granular corpuscles, gitter cells). Gitter cells contain hemosiderin, even in an otherwise anemic infarct. (hematoxylin and eosin, ×190).

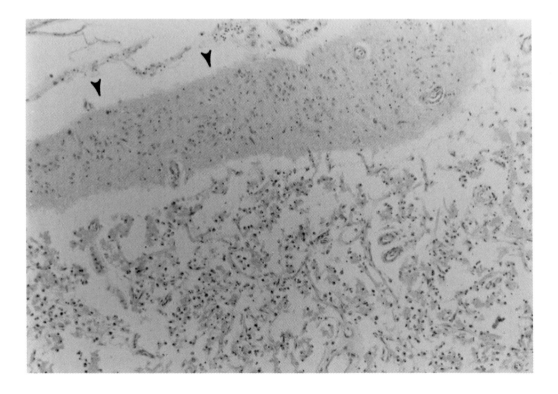

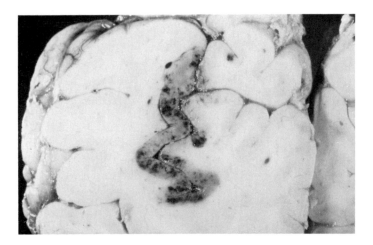

Fig. 2–13. Coronal section of fixed brain through parietal lobes. Typical hemorrhagic watershed infarct in brain parenchyma between territories of supply of ACA (to right of infarct) and MCA (to left). Patient was an elderly female who suffered profound hypotension during a cardiac surgical procedure.

brain in the context of hypertension, and occur segmentally along arteries. Hyalinosis, medial hypertrophy and atherosclerotic change are commonly found in association with chronic long-standing hypertension.[41] Fibrinoid necrosis occurs with extreme elevations of blood pressure (i.e. malignant hypertension, eclampsia) and similar changes may be seen in arterioles and capillaries of the kidneys and retina as well as brain.[42] The change has also been noted in cerebral blood vessels in cases of benign hypertension and with no history of hypertension.[43,44] In these cases, fibrinoid necrosis was not seen in visceral blood vessels. Histologically, fibrinoid degeneration/necrosis consists of alterations in blood vessel walls with replacement of normal mural components by homogeneous or finely granular dark eosinophilic material resembling fibrin.

Atheromatous disease involving small penetrating arteries in cases of capsular infarcts has been described by Fisher.[41] The change consisted mostly of masses of lipid-filled macrophages in affected blood vessel walls (lipohyalinosis). In this study, the arterial lesions were associated with relatively larger infarcts in a greater percentage of the cases.

Fisher and others have described various clinical syndromes referred to as lacunar syndromes, although they are not invariably associated with lacunar infarcts. The most common is pure motor hemiplegia.[45] The classical presentation includes unilateral paresis or paralysis of the face and upper and lower extremities with general sparing of sensation, vision, language, and behavior. The severity of

impairment is variable. Dysarthria is often present, and some patients have sensory complaints. This syndrome has been described in association with capsular and pontine infarcts.

A second syndrome consists of isolated unilateral sensory symptoms.[46,47] Paresthesias involve the arm, leg, usually the face and sometimes axial structures. Partial syndromes with focally affected areas have been reported. Pathologic studies have shown infarcts most commonly in the ventroposterior thalamic nucleus. Symptoms tend to improve, often within weeks.

A third syndrome, ataxic hemiparesis,[47] consists of gait difficulties, incoordination and sometimes paresthesias. Hemiparesis is more severe in the lower extremity. Studies have shown variable localization of infarcts to the contralateral basis pontis and contralateral thalamocapsular area. Other syndromes encompassing sensorimotor stroke, dysarthria-clumsy hand syndrome, hemichorea-hemiballismus, pure dysarthria, and other permutations and combinations of brainstem or vertebral artery territory signs and symptoms (such as internuclear opthalmoplegia, cerebellar ataxia, gaze palsies) have been described.[47–49]

Infarcts in Specific Vascular Territories.

Anterior Choroidal Artery. The anterior choroidal artery (AChA) measures approximately 7 to 20 mm in diameter at its origin, usually from the internal carotid artery 2 to 4 mm distal to the origin of the posterior communicating artery.[50] It supplies portions of the

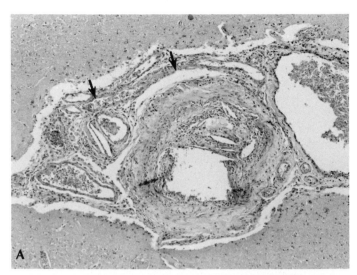

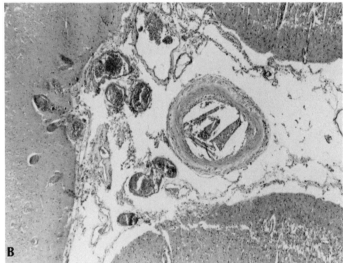

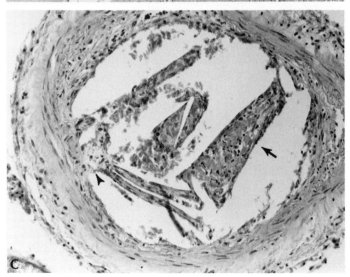

Fig. 2-14. Atheroembolic material within leptomeningeal arteries from a patient who died following multiple watershed cerebral infarcts. A. Two arteries of variable size (arrows) show occlusion of lumina by atheroembolic material that must have included cholesterol, i.e. note residual cholesterol clefts in both lumina. A portion of the occlusive material in the larger vessel has fallen away during tissue processing. Note that adjacent veins have patent lumina. B. A small leptomeningeal artery adjacent to three infarcted gyri (note prominent vacuolization of neuropil) shows plugging of lumen by atheromatous material. C. Magnified view of section of vessel illustrated in B shows prominent acicular clefts representing cholesterol material within remaining portion of the embolic material. Cells within more solid portions of the occlusive substance (arrow) probably represent histiocytes. Note point of attachment of atheroembolic material to the vessel wall (arrowhead). (all sections hematoxylin and eosin; A ×76, B ×50, C ×190).

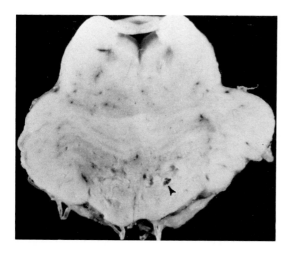

Fig. 2–15. Horizontal section through pons. Multiple lacunar infarcts are present in the basis pontis, including infarcts in both corticospinal tracts (arrowhead).

posterior limb of the internal capsule, lateral geniculate nucleus, anterior hippocampus, optic tract, amygdala, optic radiations, rostral portions of the cerebral peduncles, inner portion of the globus pallidus, body and tail of the caudate nucleus and choroid plexus of the inferior horn of the lateral ventricle.[51] The clinical picture of an infarct from complete AChA occlusion includes contralateral hemiplegia, hemianesthesia and homonymous hemianopia.[51,52] Bilateral AChA infarcts are rare and clinical presentations are variable. Some patients with right sided AChA infarcts show spatial hemineglect similar to that seen with parietal lobe lesions.[51,52] Language disorders are variable and minor, most often consisting of a mild dysarthria.[52]

AChA infarcts have been noted in association with cardiogenic embolism, arterial aneurysm and conditions which predispose to small

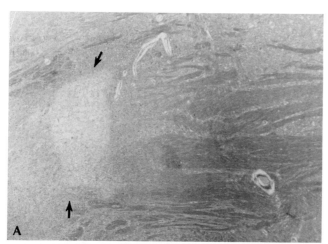

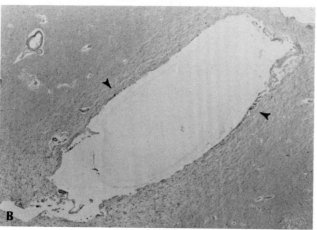

Fig. 2–16. A. Section of basis pontis shows old cystic lacunar infarct (arrows), which has interrupted pontocerebellar fibers. Neurons of pontine nuclei are also affected. B. Relatively large lacunar infarct in deep central grey matter shows intense astrocytic gliosis around its margins. In one or two foci, small peripheral aggregates of hemosiderin-laden macrophages (arrowheads) can also be identified. The occluded vessel responsible for the infarct cannot be seen in this section. (both sections hematoxylin and eosin; A ×24, B ×24).

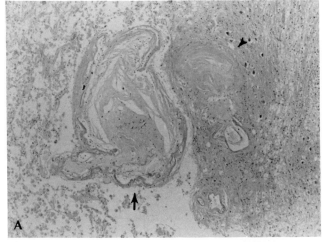

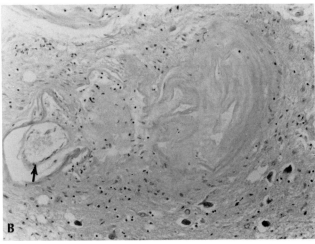

Fig. 2–17. A. Edge of a lacunar infarct in the basis pontis. Numerous lipid-laden histiocytes are seen at left, whereas scattered preserved neurons are seen in right of field. Note the tortuous, apparently thrombosed microvessel in the center (arrow). Grazing section of a microvessel on the right (arrowhead) shows apparent hyaline thickening of the wall, but preserved lumen. B. Magnified view of microvessel indicated by arrowhead in A. Note small patent lumen (arrow). (hematoxylin and eosin; A ×76, B ×190).

vessel disease (i.e. hypertension and diabetes). In one study 2 patients developed infarcts after temporal lobe resection for intractable epilepsy.[50]

Vertebrobasilar Arteries. The vertebral arteries arise from the subclavian arteries, course upwards through the cervical spine, enter the subarachnoid space at the level of the atlantooccipital interspace, run adjacent to the medulla and join to form the basilar artery at approximately the pontomedullary junction. The basilar artery supplies the pons and the superior and anterior portions of cerebellum. The vertebral arteries supply the medulla and inferior cerebellum.[2]

In a series studied by Castaigne et al.,[53] occlusion in the vertebrobasilar system was caused by atherosclerosis in approximately 80% of cases, cardiogenic embolism in approx-

imately 9% and was of undetermined cause in 11%. The risk of thrombotic occlusion in the context of atherosclerosis appeared to correlate with the degree of stenosis. Of vertebral artery occlusions, 88% were due to atherosclerosis, with most of these due to superimposed thrombosis. Most of the thromboses occurred in the distal portion of the vertebral artery, in contrast to the findings of several other studies showing an increased incidence of occlusion and stenosis in its more proximal portions. Anterograde thrombosis from proximal vertebral artery occlusions was a rare event.

In 50% of cases of vertebral artery occlusion, no infarction of either medulla or cerebellum was seen. Where either was present, occlusion of the origin of the posterior inferior cerebellar artery (PICA) was observed in most cases. Fisher et al. noted that 75% of patients with

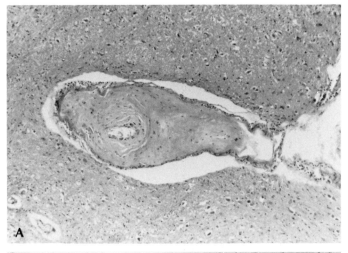

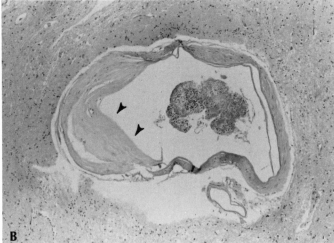

Fig. 2–18. A. Pronounced hyaline thickening of a parenchymal microvessel from a patient who had multiple lacunar infarcts elsewhere within the brain. B. A parenchymal artery (section taken from basal ganglia) shows eccentric hyaline thickening of the vessel wall (arrowheads). (hematoxylin and eosin; A ×76, B ×76).

lateral medullary infarcts had occlusion of the vertebral artery.[54]

Of 18 basilar artery occlusions, the vast majority were the result of atherosclerosis, 77.8% resulting from thrombosis superimposed on stenosis. Of these, 50% had anterograde thrombus and 28.5% had retrograde thrombus. Of those with anterograde thrombosis, posterior cerebral artery territory infarcts were relatively common.[53] No correlation between severity of atherosclerosis in the vertebrobasilar system and the carotid arteries was seen. The variable clinicopathologic consequences of basilar artery occlusion had previously been described by Kubik and Adams.[55] Patients (8 of 18 were 60 years old or older) were described as having a change in their state of consciousness together with signs and symptoms indic-

ative of brainstem dysfunction. The extent of brainstem infarcts was variable from patient to patient.

Cerebellar Infarction. In cases of acute cerebellar infarction, atherosclerosis and occlusion of the vertebral artery are common etiologies often associated with hypertension, diabetes or generalized cardiovascular disease.[56] Clinically, onset tended to be sudden with symptoms including vomiting, dizziness, vertigo and ataxia. Some patients had intermittent symptoms in the preceding days or weeks consisting of dizziness, vertigo, ataxia, dysarthria, confusion or blurred vision. On admission, most patients showed some combination of impaired consciousness, cerebellar signs, ocular movement abnormalities, cranial nerve dysfunction and motor system involvement.[56]

Motor system involvement, usually spastic quadriparesis and decerebrate posturing, and disturbances of respiration appeared late in the course of disease, usually in association with the onset of coma.

Cerebellar edema resulting from necrosis may lead to brainstem compression, with respiratory failure and hydrocephalus. The mortality rate for acute cerebellar infarction is relatively high, between 20 and 50%.[56,57] Surgical decompression by removal of infarcted tissue may be beneficial in some cases.[57]

Posterior Cerebral Artery. The majority of posterior cerebral artery (PCA) occlusions can be attributed to atherosclerosis—either from stenosis or embolism of atheromatous material.[53] Most PCA occlusions are associated with concomitant vertebral artery or basilar artery atherosclerotic disease. Another significant cause of PCA occlusion is anterograde thrombosis from basilar artery occlusion.

The PCA territory includes the occipital pole, inferior temporal lobe and posteromedial portions of the cerebral hemispheres (Fig. 2–19).[2] Various penetrating branches supply the midbrain tegmentum, subthalamus, portions of the thalamus, mammillary bodies and adjacent hypothalamus. Superficial PCA branches supply the hippocampus, inferior

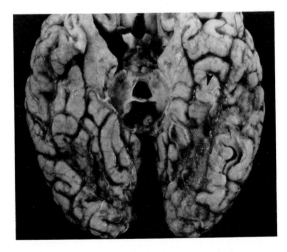

Fig. 2–19. Basal view of fixed brain. Note motheaten appearance on the undersurfaces of both temporal lobes. These represent old cystic infarcts in the PCA territories bilaterally. Note that even leptomeningeal vessels show atherosclerotic change (arrowhead).

surface of the temporal lobe, medial surface of the posterior parietal and occipital lobes, visual cortex and posterior one-sixth of the corpus callosum.[2]

Among patients with PCA territory infarcts associated with vertebral artery disease, two main categories of clinical presentation were noted by Koroshetz and Ropper.[58] Half of patients had a major brainstem syndrome with medullary symptoms, and visual field abnormalities ensued. The other half had minor single brainstem symptoms, with visual field abnormalities being the most prominent presenting feature. Acute confusional states have been documented in some patients with bilateral or dominant PCA territory infarcts.[59] In a study of 35 patients with occipital infarction from a PCA lesion,[60] embolism (diagnosed by angiographic and clinical features) was the most common etiologic mechanism. Five patients had a history of migraine headaches and no other risk factors. Neurologic deficits were maximal at onset in most patients. Symptoms commonly included headache and visual field defects, sensory loss, dyslexia, memory disturbance, nystagmus, unsteady gait and hemiparesis.

Posterior Inferior Cerebellar Artery. The posterior inferior cerebellar artery (PICA) supplies portions of the lateral medulla, including the nucleus ambiguus, lateral spinothalamic tract, inferior cerebellar peduncle, descending tracts and nucleus of the 5th cranial nerve, descending sympathetic tract, vestibular nuclei, and the dorsal motor nucleus of the vagus nerve. It also supplies the inferior portions of cerebellum, including the dentate nucleus.[2] However, there is considerable variation in its territory of supply.

Occlusion of the PICA or vertebral artery can result in the lateral medullary syndrome (Wallenberg's syndrome).[54] Clinical features include ipsilateral facial pain or numbness, vertigo, nausea, vomiting, dysphagia, hoarseness, dysarthria, diplopia, gait ataxia, Horner's syndrome, facial weakness, and contralateral sensory loss. With involvement of spinocerebellar tracts or the inferior cerebellar peduncle, there may be nystagmus, intention tremor, and falling toward the side of the lesion.

Internal Carotid Artery. Thromboembolic occlusion of the internal carotid artery (ICA) results in infarcts in approximately 80% of cases,[35] according to one autopsy study. These vary from small white matter lesions to those involving most of a hemisphere, depending on the pattern of patent and anastomosing arteries. The extent of actual tissue infarction is dependent on the efficiency of collateral circulation, particularly from the circle of Willis and anterior communicating artery, connections between the external carotid and ophthalmic arteries, anastomoses of major cerebral arteries in the leptomeninges, and blood supply by the vertebrobasilar system through the posterior communicating artery.[35]

Clinical presentations are variable. Onset of symptoms is often abrupt with impaired consciousness, flaccid hemiparesis, decreased deep tendon reflexes, and contralateral homonymous hemianopia. Many patients have prodromal symptoms. Transient ischemic episodes due to carotid insufficiency may produce loss of vision (amaurosis fugax), dysphasia, or dyslexia.[61] A few patients remain asymptomatic and others have a slowly progressive course.

In general, infarcts with occlusions of extracranial segments of the ICA are smaller than those associated with occlusion of intracranial segments. Intracranial carotid occlusions often extend into the circle of Willis. These patients may have a sudden onset of symptoms and entire middle cerebral artery territory involvement or entire hemispheric involvement.[35] Edema (Fig. 2–5) is a frequent complication leading to raised intracranial pressure, uncal herniation, and fatal brainstem hemorrhage. Other patterns seen include boundary zone infarcts, capsular infarcts, isolated PCA or anterior cerebral artery (ACA) territory infarcts, or partial middle cerebral artery (MCA) territory infarcts.[15,62]

Middle Cerebral Artery. The middle cerebral artery (MCA) supplies the lateral orbitofrontal cortical surface, and most of the lateral surface of the cerebral hemispheres except the area along the superior and inferolateral borders of the temporal lobe.[2] It also supplies subjacent white matter, putamen, outer globus pallidus, posterior limb of the internal capsule, portions of the anterior limb of the internal capsule and the caudate nucleus. The MCA is the most common major vessel to be involved

by occlusive cerebrovascular disease. Lhermitte et al.[63] found associated ICA occlusion in two-thirds of their patients. Embolism (see below) was an important etiologic factor.

Differentiating between ICA and MCA occlusion by clinical symptoms may be difficult. Most commonly, a completed deficit occurs at onset,[64] but some patients have progressive or fluctuating courses. Symptoms can include headache and decreased level of consciousness. A pure motor hemiplegia similar to that seen in lacunar infarcts can occur with occlusion of deep penetrating branches from the MCA. Seizures at onset have been described in as many as 12% of patients.[64]

Anterior Cerebral Artery. Deep penetrating branches from the anterior cerebral artery (ACA) supply portions of the anterior limb of the internal capsule, head of the caudate nucleus, putamen, external segment of globus pallidus, anterior commissure and anterior fornix. Superficial branches supply the anterior five-sixths of the corpus callosum, medial half of the orbital frontal lobe and medial surface of the frontal lobe and most of the parietal lobe.[2]

Isolated ACA infarcts are rare, constituting 3% of ischemic infarcts seen by CT scan in one study.[65] It has been hypothesized that anatomic and hemodynamic factors may account for this low occurrence rate. In some patients, ACA occlusion is associated with ICA occlusion. Local thrombosis is rare. Clinical symptoms associated with ACA territory infarcts include contralateral mono- or hemiplegia with sensory loss (if the postcentral gyrus is affected). If the dominant hemisphere is involved, there may be variable degrees of dyspraxia or motor dysphasia. In one study, transcortical motor aphasia was associated with involvement of the supplementary motor area and involvement of the cingulate area alone resulted in alterations in verbal memory.[66]

CEREBRAL EMBOLISM

The incidence of strokes of embolic origin is variable.[2] Possible sources of cerebral emboli are listed in Table 2–1. With respect to cerebrovascular disease, most emboli consist of fibrin-platelet aggregates, thrombus or ather-

TABLE 2–1.   Possible Causes of Cerebral Embolism

A. Cardiac origin:
   1. atrial fibrillation and other arrhythmias
   2. rheumatic heart disease
   3. myocardial infarction with mural thrombus
   4. congenital heart disease with right to left shunt (paradoxical embolism)
   5. bacterial or non-bacterial thrombotic (marantic) endocarditis
   6. following cardiac surgery
   7. cardiac valve prosthesis
   8. atrial myxoma
B. Local embolism:
   1. atherosclerosis/thrombosis from the internal carotid artery, vertebrobasilar, subclavian, innominate arteries and aorta
   2. trauma to neck vessels
   3. complications of neck and thoracic surgery
C. complications of arteriographic studies
D. septic emboli
E. metastatic tumor
F. fat embolism
G. air embolism
H. ova or parasites
I. pulmonary vein thrombus

Adapted and modified from C.M. Fisher.[2]

oma.[2] The majority of cerebral emboli originate from the heart or locally from carotid, basilar, vertebral, or subclavian arteries. Emboli from a cardiac source are especially problematic in the geriatric population, members of which are likely to have atherosclerotic coronary artery disease (leading to myocardial infarcts), or arrhythmias (e.g. atrial fibrillation) that may produce mural thrombi within the cardiac chambers.

Emboli characteristically lodge at arterial bifurcations and points of narrowing.[2] The arterial wall at the embolic site is generally free of reactive change. Definite pathologic documentation of embolic material can be difficult, since emboli tend to migrate or lyse with time. Often the diagnosis is made on circumstantial evidence such as a ready source, absence of atherosclerosis or other arteriopathy in the occluded vessel, embolic occlusion with infarction in other organs, multiple scattered brain infarcts in several vascular territories, or embolic fragments in distal branches of the artery under suspicion. Hemorrhagic infarcts are often attributed to embolic phenomena and, at least on gross inspection, tend to involve grey matter and spare white matter.[2] Usually the hemorrhage is petechial but it may become confluent. Blood in subarachnoid spaces or

ventricles, however, is not common. As a crude generalization, occlusions of the MCA and PCA often tend to be embolic, while occlusions of the ICA and vertebral arteries often tend to be from atherosclerosis and in situ thrombosis.

The term "local embolism" or athero-embolism has been used to refer to emboli arising at atherosclerotic sites within arteries, that then migrate distally to smaller branches of the artery. Most consist of fibrin and platelets or aggregates of cholesterol and atheromatous material. Sometimes foreign body giant cell reactions (to cholesterol) and organization are present. Local embolism is common in the carotid artery system, and may also be a complication of carotid sinus pressure.[67]

Intravascular fat embolism to the brain is rare and is associated with limb and limb girdle fractures.[15,68,69] It has also been reported to occur after open heart surgery. Both clinical scenarios are common for elderly patients. At 3 to 4 days, the white matter shows diffuse pericapillary petechial hemorrhages—ring and ball type.

Sometimes there is necrosis of capillary walls and fat globules are visible on appropriate stains of frozen sections. Hemorrhage does not occur in the grey matter. With longer time intervals, foci of necrosis in deeper layers of cortex, cerebellum and brainstem have been noted. In patients who survive for several months, gross atrophy of the white matter has been noted.[15]

VENOUS SINUS THROMBOSIS

Thrombosis of dural venous sinuses occurs as a rare complication of various infectious and noninfectious processes. Noninfectious conditions reported in association with dural venous sinus thrombosis include polycythemia, sickle cell anemia or trait, paroxysmal nocturnal hemoglobinuria, arteriovenous malformation, trauma, vasculitis, pregnancy, oral contraceptive use, congenital heart disease, dehydration, marasmus, hyperlipidemia and compression by mass lesions such as tumor or aneurysm.[70] Clearly, only a small number of these is of import for elderly patients.

The cavernous sinuses, located at the base of the skull superior and lateral to the sphenoid sinuses, are the most commonly involved by septic thrombosis. The most common primary site of infection associated with cavernous sinus thrombosis was the medial third of the face.[70] The usual pathogens included gram positive bacteria, especially *Staphylococcus aureus*. More recently, the frequency of association with infection of the sphenoid and ethmoid air sinuses has increased. Dental infections, usually involving maxillary teeth have occurred in nearly 10% of cases of septic cavernous thrombosis. Before the availability of antibiotics, otitis media was often an associated entity. Orbital infection is rarely complicated by cavernous sinus thrombosis.

Common clinical symptoms are headache, periorbital edema, fever, extraocular muscle weakness, proptosis, chemosis, ptosis and mental status changes. Lethargy, diplopia, and photophobia are not common as early complaints.[70] An early neurologic finding may be lateral gaze palsy, as the abducens nerve traverses the cavernous sinus medially, near the carotid artery, whereas the third and fourth cranial nerves pass along the lateral aspects of the cavernous sinus and are surrounded by thick fibrous sheaths. The ophthalmic and maxillary branches of the trigeminal nerve also traverse the lateral aspect of the cavernous sinus. Involvement of these nerves can lead to hypo- or hyperesthesias within the appropriate dermatomes.

Thrombosis in the cavernous sinus can extend to involve other dural sinuses, such as the petrosal, sigmoid, lateral and inferior.[71] Spread of infection to the pituitary gland and resultant necrosis have been noted. Other associated findings have included leptomeningitis, brain abscess and cortical vein thrombosis with hemorrhagic or nonhemorrhagic infarction.[71] Mortality rate is approximately 30%, and less than 40% of patients survived without serious impairments.[70]

Septic lateral sinus thrombosis is nearly always associated with spread of infection from the mastoid air cells, following acute or chronic otitis media.[70,71] It is generally a subacute illness with symptoms persisting for several weeks prior to hospital admission. Headache and earache are the most frequent symptoms. Other complaints may include nausea, vomiting and vertigo. Fever and bilat-

eral papilledema were relatively common. Less common findings were nuchal rigidity, change in mental status, decreased visual acuity or hemiparesis. The pathogens usually associated with otitis media or mastoiditis are *Proteus* species, *Staphylococcus aureus,* anaerobes or *E. coli.* Complications noted have included meningitis, cerebellar abscess, septic pulmonary embolism, cavernous sinus thrombosis, and cortical vein thrombosis with associated cerebral infarct and sepsis.

Septic superior sagittal sinus thrombosis is less common than cavernous or lateral sinus thrombosis. The most common predisposing condition is bacterial meningitis, with probable spread along the diploic veins. Air sinus infection has been the second most commonly associated entity.

Onset of symptoms is relatively rapid and may include severe headache, nausea, and vomiting, followed by confusion which progresses to coma. Focal or grand mal seizures refractory to anticonvulsant therapy may occur following the onset of confusion. High fever and altered mental status are frequent findings. Cortical vein thrombosis, associated cerebral infarcts and subsequent hemiparesis were also relatively frequent. A lesser percentage of patients showed signs of brainstem compression or papilledema. CSF pressure was often elevated due to impaired resorption by arachnoid villi in the occluded sinus. Mortality rate has approached 80%. In autopsy studies, 92% showed thrombosis of the entire superior sagittal sinus and 41% also showed occlusion of other dural sinuses. Cortical vein thrombosis with hemorrhagic cerebral infarcts was noted in 50% of the patients, while pulmonary emboli were seen in 33% of patients. Pathologic findings often include granulation tissue or a frank abscess overlying the thrombosed sinus, and thrombi may extend into the jugular veins.[71]

VASCULITIS

The reader is referred to several excellent reviews for current concepts on the nature of systemic vasculitides that affect the CNS, as well as vasculitides that are confined to the nervous system.[72-75] A recent classification is presented in Table 2–2. Many of these are rare,

TABLE 2–2.   Vasculitides That Affect the Nervous System:

1. Polyarteritis nodosa group—systemic necrotizing (includes allergic angiitis).
2. Hypersensitivity vasculitis (includes Henoch-Schönlein purpura, cutaneous hypersensitivity vasculitis, etc.).
3. Wegener's granulomatosis.
4. Lymphomatoid granulomatosis.
5. Giant cell arteritis (includes temporal arteritis, Takayasu's).
6. Behçet's disease.
7. Isolated CNS angiitis.
8. Nervous system vasculitis secondary to other disease.

Adapted and modified from P.M. Moore and T.R. Cupps, Neurological complications of vasculitis. Ann. Neurol., *14*:155, 1983.

if even reported, in the elderly (e.g. Henoch-Schönlein purpura, Takayasu's arteritis, Behçet's disease), whereas others are a major problem. Pathologically, the lesions are classified depending on (1) the size and type of blood vessel affected, and (2) the histologic nature of the inflammatory infiltrate. The frequency of neurologic abnormality also varies with the type of vasculitis,[72] e.g. neurologic involvement occurs in 20–40% of patients with polyarteritis nodosa, but only 10% of patients with temporal arteritis.

The most "age-related" vasculitis of the group may well be giant cell or temporal arteritis, an eminently treatable entity.[76] Its incidence in patients over the age of 50 years was found to increase significantly (in one study) between the years 1950 and 1975.[76] In the period 1970 to 1974, the average annual incidence per 100,000 people over age 50 years was 17.4. The disease presents with a fairly characteristic clinical picture of headache, visual complaints, weight loss, and the syndrome of polymyalgia rheumatica. The temporal artery biopsy shows a characteristic picture of transmural lympho-histiocytic infiltration (Fig. 2–20), within which giant cells *may* be present,[76,77] though their presence within the biopsy has no apparent influence on the patient's clinical course. "Skip" areas may also be seen on the biopsy, so special care must be taken in its detailed examination, often using subserial sections. The vasculitis responds to steroid therapy.

A detailed postmortem study has shown that in patients dying during the active phase of giant cell arteritis, there was a high incidence of involvement of the superficial temporal, vertebral, ophthalmic, and posterior ciliary arteries, with less common severe inflammation of the internal carotid, external carotid and central retinal arteries.[78] Furthermore, there appeared to be a significant correlation between the susceptibility to giant cell arteritis and the amount of elastic tissue within the adventitia and media of the arteries in the head and neck.

Isolated angiitis of the CNS, though of considerable biologic interest,[74,75] is only rarely identified in patients above the age of 60 years. Lymphomatoid granulomatosis (LG) is defined by an atypical (? pre-neoplastic) infiltrate of blood vessel walls, especially within the lung, CNS and skin, with attendant angionecrosis.[79–81] It is perhaps more appropriately discussed together with malignant lymphoproliferative lesions than angiitides, since it is now considered an angiocentric T-cell lymphoma.[82] LG may occur in the geriatric age group, though it has no predilection for doing so.

MISCELLANEOUS MICROANGIOPATHIES

Rarely, microangiopathies of unknown etiology may produce cerebral necrosis. One of these is thrombotic thrombocytopenic purpura (TTP).[1,83] Thrombosis of small blood vessels (in the brain and viscera) is seen in association with "microangiopathic" hemolytic anemia. The clinical presentation of TTP may mimic that of disseminated intravascular coagulation (DIC). In one review,[83] 3 of 11 patients were beyond the age of 60 years. Histologic findings in the brain include microscopic platelet thrombi within the lumina of microvessels, hyaline subendothelial deposits, and marked endothelial proliferation (Fig. 2–21).

Some forms of microvascular "disease" in the brain are asymptomatic. Mineralization of small blood vessels (Fig. 2–22) is commonly noted in the globus pallidus of elderly patients.[84] The affected vessel walls (primarily the media) show variable amounts of basophilic material which, on appropriate study, has the staining characteristics of iron and calcium. There is no good evidence that mineral-

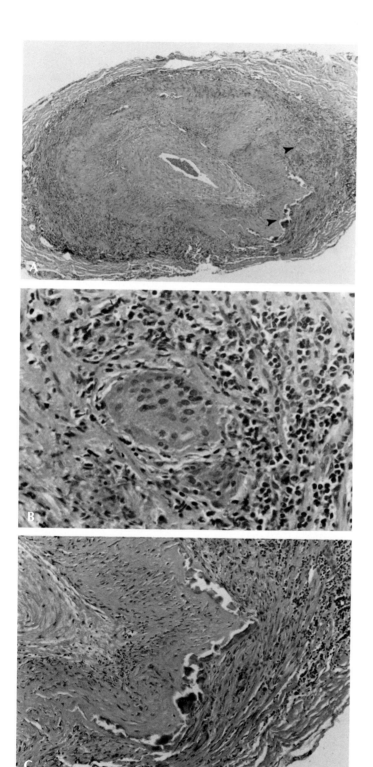

Fig. 2–20. Temporal artery biopsy, giant cell arteritis. A. Cross section of entire vessel shows compromise of vascular lumen. The most striking abnormality, however, is transmural inflammation around the entire circumference of the vessel. Inflammation is most prominent in the media and adventitia. Upper arrowhead indicates a single multinucleated giant cell, while lower arrowhead indicates an area of calcification and fragmentation of the elastica. These regions are shown at higher magnifications in B and C. B. Magnified view of multinucleated giant cell indicated by arrowhead in panel A. Numerous mononuclear inflammatory cells, mainly lymphocytes and histiocytes, surround the giant cell. C. Fragmented and calcified internal elastic lamina is seen. Note mononuclear inflammatory cells in upper right of the panel. At left, pronounced fibrous intimal hyperplasia is noted. (hematoxylin and eosin; A ×76, B ×495, C ×190).

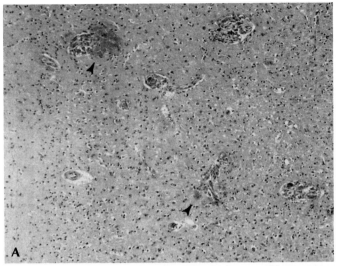

Fig. 2–21. Section of cortex from patient with thrombotic thrombocytopenic purpura (TTP). A. Petechial hemorrhages surround many microvessels (arrowheads). Cellular thickening of the vascular lumina is also identified. B. Magnified view of one of the hyperplastic microvessels shows proliferated cells which, on immunocytochemical staining, had the features of endothelial cells. The patient was a 67-year-old Oriental male. (both sections hematoxylin and eosin; A ×76, B ×495).

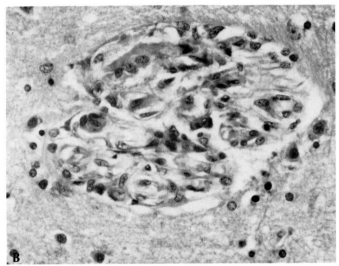

ized vessels cause brain ischemia or hemorrhage. Slager and Wagner[84] found, in an autopsy study, that mineralized ganglionic microvessels occur over the age range 15 to 103 years, while 43% of patients with the lesion were over 60 years old and 20% were over 70. There was no association of vascular mineralization with any specific systemic disorder.

INTRACRANIAL HEMORRHAGE

Hemorrhage into the various cranial compartments will be considered separately, beginning with the most superficial, i.e. hematomas of the epidural or extradural space. To some extent, this is an arbitrary division, since some of the etiological mechanisms operative in (for example) subarachnoid hemorrhage are also important in the genesis of intraparenchymal hemorrhage. Nevertheless, it seems to allow for a logical clinicopathologic subdivision of syndromes.

EXTRADURAL OR EPIDURAL HEMORRHAGE

Epidural hemorrhage (EDH) is more properly discussed in relation to craniocerebral trauma,[85] since spontaneous epidural hematomas almost never occur. EDH after closed head injury presents as a rapidly evolving neurologic deficit because the bleeding is usually

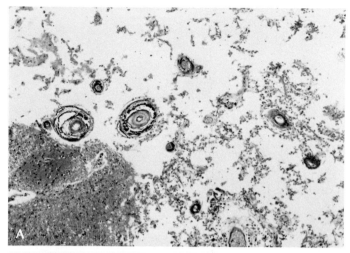

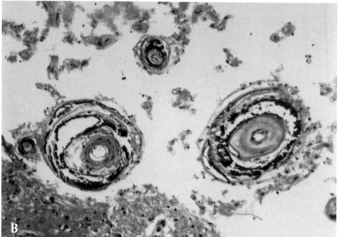

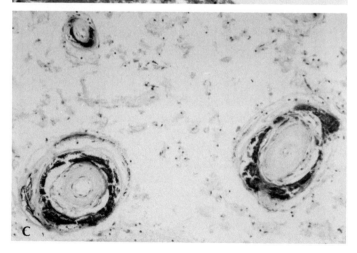

Fig. 2–22. Mineralization (ferruginization, siderocalcinosis) of small arteries within the globus pallidus. A. Note many vessels with mineralized walls, especially media. The vessels are at the center of an area of cystic necrosis, which was unrelated to the mineralized vasculature. B. Magnified view of the two most prominently calcified vessels seen in panel A. Localization of the material (which had staining properties of both iron and calcium) is apparent. C. Iron stain of parallel section shows reactivity of material in the microvessel walls. (A, B, hematoxylin and eosin; C, Perl's Prussian blue stain for iron; A ×76, B ×190, C ×190).

from an arterial source (e.g. the middle meningeal artery) secondary to a skull fracture. It constitutes a neurosurgical emergency.[86,87] Mortality from the condition irrespective of age group is high, usually 10 to 20%, but for the geriatric population this figure is much higher.[87] An ominous sign suggestive of evolving EDH in a patient brought to the emergency room after a closed head injury is clouding of consciousness or deepening of the degree of unconsciousness,[86] and the diagnosis should be apparent on computerized tomographic (CT) scan studies. If treated early by drainage of the clotted blood, the patient may make an uneventful recovery although usually the context of EDH—i.e. severe head trauma with or without subdural hematoma and encephalic contusion or hemorrhage—makes the prognosis less favorable.

Elderly patients in particular are more likely to succumb to the sequelae of head injury than are the resilient young[85] and, as implied above, postoperative mortality with EDH correlates with the level of consciousness at the time of operation.[87] EDH is much less common in the geriatric population than among those in the first two decades of life overall.[86] EDHs may be bilateral and in various locations within the cranial cavity, though posterior fossa EDHs are common in the elderly as they are at the other extreme of life,[86] perhaps because both groups tend to experience falls onto the back of the head. Posterior fossa EDH also carries the highest mortality rate.[86]

The documentation of a fatal EDH must be made at the time of necropsy, since if this is not done upon unroofing of the calvarium, another opportunity will not in all likelihood arise. Since most cases of EDH will have medico-legal implications, postmortem photographs are valuable and the amount of clotted extradural blood can be either weighed or measured by volumetric displacement to give an objective assessment of the space it has occupied in the cranial cavity. This must be done immediately after the skull is unroofed, since the blood has a tendency to slip from the dura and become "lost," particularly if the hemorrhage is reasonably fresh. Further evidence of its effects on the brain will become obvious when herniation of the appropriate brain structures is subsequently documented or demonstrated at the time of brain cutting after formalin fixation.

SUBDURAL HEMORRHAGE

Subdural hematomas (SDHs), described historically by Virchow as "pachymeningitis hemorrhagica interna," of both the acute and chronic variety are a much greater problem in the geriatric population than in the young, in large part because of their protean clinical manifestations and insidious evolution and presentation. Unlike epidural hematomas, they are not always associated with trauma or at least clinically perceived, documented or reported trauma. There clinical evolution occurs with a more sedate tempo because the bleeding is usually from a venous source, i.e. the bridging veins between the dura mater and the leptomeninges and brain surface, especially parasagittal bridging veins. As will be discussed below, however, it must be remembered that SDH may, in a small number of patients, represent dissection of blood from the subarachnoid space—where it originates from an arterial source such as a berry aneurysm or arteriovenous malformation—into the subdural compartment. The investigational and therapeutic implications of this are obvious.

Elderly patients are also at greater risk for developing SDH because age- (or dementia-) related brain atrophy increases the space between the dura mater and the brain surface, i.e. the distance over which bridging veins must course. They are thus more prone to rupture as a result of minimal trauma that causes movement of the brain with respect to its coverings.[88] Furthermore, a mildly demented or simply forgetful geriatric patient may fail to recall or report the "guilty" traumatic episode that has precipitated an SDH. The hematoma may, in turn, worsen a relatively subtle cognitive deficit. All of these considerations mean that a clinician faced with an elderly patient who has a slowly evolving neurologic deficit must always consider SDH in the differential diagnosis, whether or not a clear history of head trauma is given by the patient or his/her family.

The broad etiologic differential diagnosis of chronic SDH[88] includes (1) trauma, as a result of direct or indirect cranial trauma that may produce rupture of the parasagittal bridging veins, or (less commonly) skull fractures that lacerate the venous sinuses—a concomitant brain contusion may or may not be present, (2) arteriovenous malformations or aneurysms that rupture into the subdural space as well as the subarachnoid space or directly into brain parenchyma, (3) infections, (4) brain tumors (e.g. convexity meningiomas), (5) meningeal carcinomatosis/sarcomatosis, and (6) hemorrhagic diathesis or coagulopathies, either secondary to hemophilia or hepatic disease, or iatrogenic anticoagulant therapy (a major problem in the geriatric age group). As regards the latter issue, a large epidemiologic study from the Netherlands[89] has shown the occurrence of SDH in patients receiving anticoagulant therapy to be 7 times as high in males and 26 times as high in females, as that in the non-anticoagulated population. As well, the elderly were more likely to be on anticoagulant therapy than the young. Elderly patients who are more likely to have significant cerebral atrophy or a cerebrospinal fluid (CSF) shunt (placed for the treatment of normal pressure hydrocephalus) and thus lowered intracranial pressure

are especially prone to SDH, because the minor subdural bleeding that would normally stop because of counter-pressure of the cerebral hemispheric parenchyma continues relatively unchecked.

As a SDH organizes, its innermost portion (i.e. that closest to brain) comes to be composed of granulation tissue, which is identical to the granulation tissue that would form around foci of bleeding elsewhere within the body (Fig. 2–23). The richly vascular outer SDH membrane, initially containing fibrin and fibrin degradation products, may become completely organized with resorption of the subdural membrane[88] or, alternatively, serve as the locus from which a gradually enlarging hematoma may emerge. Local "hyperfibrinolysis", which results in liquefaction of the clotted subdural blood, may also lead to continuing hemorrhage from the thin-walled and tortuous microvessels of the inner neomembrane, with enlargement of a chronic SDH. Another theory to explain the continuing enlargement of a chronic SDH was based on the assumption that the osmotic pressure resulting from the breakdown of cellular con-

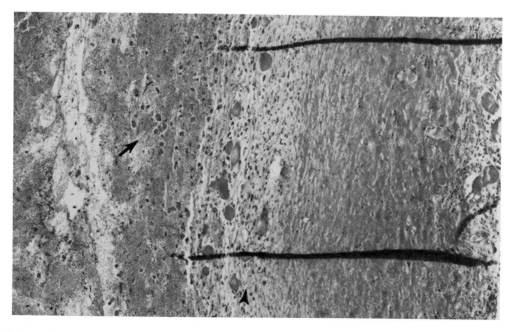

Fig. 2–23. Dura mater (right of field) with subdural membrane. Dark streaks represent artifactual folds in tissue section. Dura mater is at right of field. Old blood, including hemosiderin-laden macrophages (arrow) is seen at left of field. Center of section is occupied by thin-walled vascular channels in loose fibrotic tissue, i.e. granulation tissue (arrowhead). (hematoxylin and eosin, ×76).

stituents within the hematoma cavity would lead to massive movement of CSF into the subdural sac.[90] This theory has been questioned on several grounds.[88]

When the pathologist examines a SDH of "clinically" uncertain age, the degree of organization of the subdural membranes can be used to date the hematoma. The inner capsule of a SDH is generally less vascular than its richly vascularized outer capsule. Different types of neomembranes which form whenever the inner dural layer comes into contact with blood, fibrin, or fibrin degradation products, have been distinguished.[91] Not unexpectedly, similar membranes are observed in induced subdural hematomas in mongrel dogs.[92] Ultrastructurally, the capsules of chronic SDHs have been noted to contain capillary endothelial cells with prominent cytoplasmic protrusions and fenestrations, with incomplete envelopment by basement membrane, and focally degenerate endothelial cells, suggesting a high degree of vessel wall permeability.[88,93] SDHs treated by osmotherapy had prominent collagen fibrils apparently emanating from fibroblasts, and endothelial cells appeared less permeable. Subdural neomembranes indicative of asymptomatic remote subdural hemorrhage are a relatively common autopsy finding,[91] even in elderly patients who have no history of clinical features that might predispose them to develop such hematomas.

An important study from Finland[94] examined the influence of patient age on symptoms, signs and thickness of chronic SDHs. It concluded that: (1) younger patients clinically had more evidence of increased intracranial pressure with this lesion, whereas older patients had greater evidence of mental deterioration and signs and symptoms of lesions of the corticospinal tracts; (2) the interval from trauma to surgical intervention was briefer among younger patients; and (3) thickness of the SDH itself (as measured by angiograms, since the paper was published in the early CT scan era) increased directly with age of the patient. The latter two findings were attributed to the natural age-related decrease in brain weight and corresponding increase in the size of the space between the brain and skull. The latter increase was stated by the authors to change from 6 to 11% of total intracranial space during the age interval 50 to 80 years. Thus, an evolving hematoma in the elderly has greater room to expand before causing a rise in intracranial pressure or, for that matter, any other signs or symptoms.

Debates that have occupied neurosurgeons as to the optimal way to make the diagnosis of acute, subacute and chronic SDH, and subsequently to treat it,[95–98] are now somewhat redundant, given the effectiveness of CT scans in verifying the clinical diagnosis.[88] Nevertheless, isodense (on CT scan) SDHs, particularly when bilateral, are occasionally found.[88] Contrast-enhanced CT scans improve the diagnostic accuracy. Radionuclide brain scanning is also an excellent confirmatory neurodiagnostic tool. Angiography may be indicated in some patients, especially those in whom the SDH is strongly suspected to have arisen from a ruptured berry aneurysm or, less likely, an intraparenchymal arteriovenous malformation. The latter would be more likely to show up on a CT scan.

The treatment of choice appears to be drainage of the hematoma, though there is debate as to whether this ought to be done by twist-drill or burr-hole trephination, or craniotomy to remove the membranes[88,98] which, as discussed above, may be the source of recurrent or repetitive subdural bleeds. In the elderly, particularly those patients in whom a dementing illness has caused loss of brain parenchyma, re-accumulation of subdural blood is always a risk[99] and such individuals are more likely to have complicating medical disorders than are younger patients. One group[100] has advocated conservative (nonsurgical) treatment of SDHs by a combination of bedrest, corticosteroids, and/or mannitol. A large proportion of patients experienced a favorable outcome with this non-interventional regimen.

SUBARACHNOID HEMORRHAGE

Hemorrhage into the subarachnoid space is a major cause of morbidity and mortality for the elderly, as it is in younger age groups.[1] Its less conspicuous profile in the elderly may simply reflect the fact that other types of intracranial "cerebrovascular accident", usually related to atherosclerosis, microangiopathy, etc., are more common in the geriatric age group than in the young. Subarachnoid hemorrhage (SAH) may be secondary to intraparenchymal brain hemorrhage, i.e. caused by dissection of clot into the subarachnoid space, or it may be the primary result of rupture of an aneurysm on the circle of Willis or one of its branches, a vascular malformation within brain parenchyma (usually an arteriovenous malformation) or systemic causes. Each of these etiologic mechanisms will be considered separately.

Berry or Saccular Aneurysms. Stehbens[1] has defined an aneurysm as "a localized and persistent [pathologic] dilatation [of the heart or a blood vessel] that results from the yielding of components of the wall". Aneurysms usually occur within arteries. Berry aneurysms, often also referred to as "congenital" or saccular, usually occur at the major bifurcation points of the circle of Willis (Fig. 2–24). Over half occur on the anterior portions of the circle, usually at the following vascular bifurcation

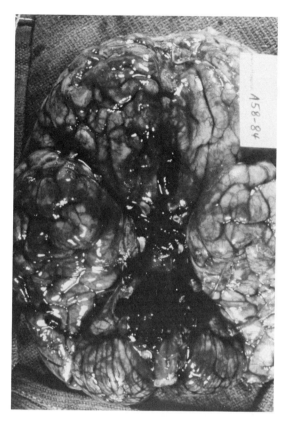

Fig. 2–25. Patient who suffered fatal subarachnoid hemorrhage from an anterior cerebral artery-anterior communicating artery junction berry aneurysm. The brain is diffusely congested, edematous, and shows extensive subarachnoid blood, particularly on the undersurface of the right frontal lobe and right temporal lobe. As well, the basal cisterns are filled with fresh clotted blood, which effectively obscures the cranial nerve exit regions and the circle of Willis itself. It is important to remove all clotted blood and to identify the berry aneurysm(s) at the time of autopsy in such a patient.

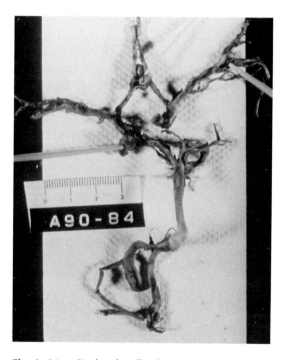

Fig. 2–24. Circle of Willis dissected free from the base of the brain. Multiple berry aneurysms are identified at the ends of pointers. Biloculated aneurysms present on anterior cerebral-anterior communicating artery junction (top of field), right ICA-posterior communicating artery junction, and left MCA bifurcation (right of field). Berry aneurysms may be multiple, as in this case.

points: internal carotid artery—posterior communicating artery or anterior choroidal artery, middle cerebral artery bi/trifurcation within the Sylvian fissure, and anterior cerebral artery—anterior communicating artery junctions. Of patients with berry aneurysms, most who are below the age of 40 years are males, whereas those who are over that age are females. Most berry aneurysms present between the ages of 40 and 70 years, so they are a more important clinical problem in middle-aged than geriatric patients. One third of patients have multiple berry aneurysms (Fig. 2–24), sometimes as many as 8 or 9. The aneurysm, since it expands gradually into the subarachnoid space (or sometimes displaces brain parenchyma) rarely produces symptoms prior to rupture. The rupture may present as a small bleed ("warning leak") or a large, potentially life-threatening hemorrhage (Fig. 2–25).[101]

Though referred to as "congenital", berry aneurysms are almost never found in the pediatric age group, though this does *not* rule out the possibility that the mature berry aneurysm found in later life represents growth of a focus of mechanical 'weakening' in the younger vessel. This theory, however, has been disputed.[1] Alternatively, berry aneurysms may result from degenerative change within cerebral blood vessels, possibly secondary to loss of tensile strength due to weakening of connective tissues within the vessel walls. Theories as to the cause of berry aneurysms and the precipitating factors leading to their rupture have been discussed at length by Stehbens and others[1,101] and a detailed discussion of such is beyond the scope of this chapter. Cerebral berry aneurysms are associated with polycystic kidney disease and coarctation of the aorta, and familial cases are reported.[1]

The peak incidence of rupture of a berry aneurysm producing an initial subarachnoid hemorrhage (SAH) is at the age of 60 years, with the above noted variable male/female preponderance in different age groups.[1] Subarachnoid hemorrhage from berry aneurysm continues as a significant cause of neurologic morbidity into the 9th and 10th decades of life. Not only can rupture of a berry aneurysm produce SAH, but it can cause bleeding directly into the brain parenchyma (Fig. 2–26) or ventricular system. The precise site of extravasation of blood depends on the location of the aneurysmal dome—i.e. if it points into the brain (as an anterior cerebral artery—anterior communicating artery junction or middle cerebral artery trifurcation aneurysm may well do), rupture can lead to an intraparenchymal blood clot. This is particularly important to remember in the workup of elderly patients, in whom peripherally or "unusually" situated encephalic hematomas may be interpreted to result from age- or Alzheimer disease-related cerebral amyloid angiopathy (see below). Ruptured berry aneurysm must also be considered in the differential diagnosis of such a parenchymal bleed. Rarely, a ruptured berry aneu-

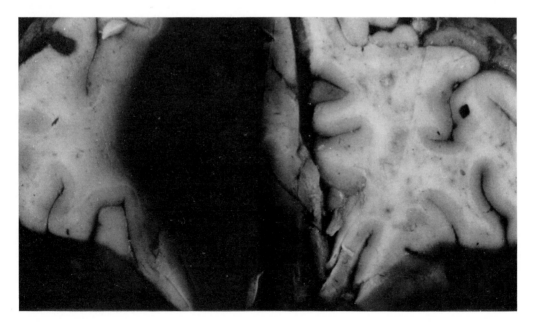

Fig. 2–26. Direct bleeding into the brain parenchyma from a berry aneurysm. A large berry aneurysm located at the internal carotid-ophthalmic artery junction had its dome embedded in the left frontal lobe. Bleeding was thus predominantly into the brain parenchyma rather than the subarachnoid space. A large clot is present in the deep white matter and cortex-white matter junction of the left frontal lobe.

rysm will leak some blood into the subdural space, as described above.

Berry aneurysms are found in necropsy in from 0.2–9% of patients, according to different investigators.[1] A reasonable incidence figure in our experience is 2 to 5%. Only larger aneurysms, those with a diameter of 5 to 10 mm,[102] are considered prone to rupture. Some authors claim that unruptured aneurysms under 1 cm in diameter have a very low probability of subsequent rupture.[103] Aneurysm size as measured at necropsy is, of course, likely to represent an underestimate of the in vivo dimensions.[104] In general, debate persists in the neurosurgical community as to optimal management of patients with one or more berry aneurysms,[105–110] especially if they are discovered prior to having bled, e.g. in the course of cerebral angiogram for some other type of investigation. The treatment of choice for a patient with ruptured berry aneurysm is clipping of the aneurysm. The optimal time of clipping after an aneurysm ruptures is again a subject of considerable controversy. As regards elderly patients (defined as those older than 60 years), the literature suggests that (except for those with aneurysms at the basilar artery bifurcation) older patients tolerate surgical clipping as well as younger individuals, but with a higher risk of subsequent death related to cardiac and vascular disease.[105,111] In general, those who are physically fit benefit from surgical treatment to the same extent as younger patients.

Small aneurysms may produce no mass effect in the cranial cavity, or they may displace and compress a cranial nerve, usually the third, in its extramedullary course. Giant intracranial aneurysms, conversely, are likely to produce a mass effect just as a tumor might. Such aneurysms may show extensive intraluminal organization of thrombus, probably due to platelet-fibrin interaction on the luminal surface, leading to cycles of thrombosis and recanalization.[112] It is not difficult to envision how platelet-fibrin emboli may become dislodged from the cavity of such an aneurysm and float distally in the circulation to produce transient ischemic attacks.

The pathologic anatomy of berry aneurysms is characteristic,[1,113] and is best illustrated using an elastic stain or Movat's pentachrome technique. As one follows the dome of the aneurysm wall from its site of attachment to the parent vessel, the internal elastic lamina becomes fragmented and eventually disappears entirely. The wall of the aneurysm instead shows collagenous connective tissue and smooth muscle cells, in a layer that may be fairly thick but, unfortunately, lacks the tensile strength normally provided by the elastica. In a small aneurysm, particularly in an elderly patient and, in our experience, when it is an incidental finding at autopsy, the aneurysm will often show atherosclerotic change within its dome (Fig. 2–27), though this atherosclerotic change does not apparently play a role in the etiopathogenesis of the aneurysm itself. In aneurysms that have ruptured, the rupture site may fortuitously be identified or it may have

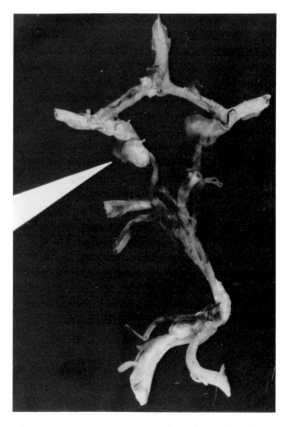

Fig. 2–27. Berry aneurysm found incidentally at autopsy on an 84-year-old female. The circle of Willis itself shows moderate patchy atheromatous disease. Pointer indicates a large berry aneurysm at the right ICA-posterior communicating artery junction. Dome of the aneurysm shows moderately severe atherosclerotic change. There was no evidence that the aneurysm had ruptured during life.

sealed over with thrombus. Evidence of old subarachnoid hemorrhage must be sought, especially if there is a suggestion that the patient may have bled from the aneurysm at a time in the distant past.

Patients who survive rupture of a berry aneurysm are prone to hydrocephalus, secondary to reparative processess induced by hemorrhage in the subarachnoid space and basal cisterns, and delayed cerebral ischemia caused by vasospasm, the exact etiology of which is unknown.[114-116] Vasospasm tends to be more common in *females* who experience subarachnoid hemorrhage, and is difficult to treat by medical or surgical means,[117,118] though interventional neuroradiologic (endovascular) techniques appear to offer some promise (J. Dion, F. Vinuela, personal communication). Although vasospasm is clinically a major problem in the management of aneurysm-related SAH, structural changes found within vasospastic vessels on the circle of Willis and its branches examined at necropsy are relatively non-specific and difficult to find unless a meticulous search is undertaken.[119,120]

Inflammatory Aneurysms. Sometimes also described (somewhat inaccurately) as "mycotic" aneurysms, these are lesions that are almost always associated with either subacute or acute bacterial endocarditis.[121,122] The microorganisms causing the endocarditis may be varied and are often of low virulence. In one series, they included five different bacteria (including enterococcus, *Staphylococcus aureus*, *Streptococcus viridans*) in 5 different patients. Of interest is the fact that the cardiac disease may go clinically unsuspected until rupture from an inflammatory aneurysm occurs.[122] In one series from a major center that specializes in the treatment of cerebrovascular disease including subarachnoid hemorrhage,[122] 2.6% of intracranial aneurysms were judged to be inflammatory in origin, while 4.6% of patients with bacterial endocarditis developed such an aneurysm. These figures, now some 23 years out of date, reflected diagnostic modalities available at the time and probably a different prevalence of endocarditis.

Inflammatory aneurysms, unlike berry aneurysms (see above), are usually situated peripherally in the cerebral circulation. Branches of the middle cerebral artery have been said to be most frequently involved. Rupture of an inflammatory aneurysm may result in subarachnoid or intraparenchymal hemorrhage. The aneurysm, being friable and weakened because of inflammation in the vessel wall, is often resected by the neurosurgeon in the course of removal of an intracerebral clot. It is then incumbent upon the pathologist to do an appropriate examination of any lesions that may look suspicious for an aneurysm, in particular since he/she may be the key individual to make the diagnosis in a patient who has experienced an otherwise mysterious cerebral hemorrhage. The wall of an inflammatory aneurysm will contain abundant acute and chronic inflammatory cells, though not necessarily stainable microorganisms.

The precise pathogenesis of an inflammatory aneurysm due to an infected heart valve is hypothesized to be secondary to a septic embolus that lodges within a branch artery, with extension of microorganisms from the embolus into the vessel wall. Alternatively, passage of infected microemboli into vasa vasorum may occur, with subsequent seeding of the artery wall, weakening and aneurysm formation.[121] Inflammatory or "mycotic" aneurysms are not a disproportionately severe problem in elderly patients.

Dissecting Aneurysms. Dissecting aneurysms are distinctively a problem of younger and middle-aged individuals, and are almost never described in the elderly. Nevertheless, they will briefly be considered here for the sake of completeness. In a recent excellent clinicopathologic study, Farrell et al.[123] described autopsy findings on seven individuals (age range 20 to 63 years) with this syndrome. When dissection had occurred in the anterior circulation, the site of dissection was found between the internal elastic lamina and the media, and had in general produced intravascular thrombosis. When dissection had occurred in the posterior circulation, transmural dissection had frequently resulted in subarachnoid hemorrhage. Variable degrees of acute inflammation were present at the sites of dissection examined histologically, but primary vasculopathies of a degenerative or inflammatory nature could not specifically be identified.

Clincial studies of dissection of the vertebral

arteries confirm that this is a condition of younger patients.[124–126] Nevertheless, one 69-year-old man[127] was reported to have dissection of the basilar artery, and other papers that have reviewed the extensive literature on this entity[128–130] describe reports of occasional patients between the ages of 60 to 70 years who have experienced dissecting aneurysms. Various etiologies[131] for arterial dissection were presented. Clinically, dissection frequently occurs after trauma (including relatively minimal trauma), following exercise, in association with migraine headaches, or after administration of heparin. Pathologic changes in blood vessel walls that have been associated with arterial dissection include syphilitic arteritis, cystic medial degeneration or necrosis, and rather poorly defined "congenital defects" within vessel walls.

Fusiform Aneurysms. Also sometimes referred to as serpentine aneurysms, these are unusual lesions overall but a relatively important clinical problem in elderly patients.[132,133] They tend to be more common in men than in women. In a recent clinicopathologic review, we found 7 patients with this lesion at necropsy, with an age range of 56 to 65 years. In other series,[133] over 80% of patients with fusiform aneurysms were more than 60 years old. Fusiform aneurysms, as the name implies, usually result from enlargement and widening of a vessel along its length (Fig. 2–28). Most often, fusiform aneurysms are found along the length of the basilar artery. They may reach giant proportions, and tend to have laminated thrombi within their walls. The laminated thrombus results from severe complicated atheromatous change, which in turn suggests the pathogenesis of these aneurysms: unlike saccular or berry aneurysms, they are widely supposed to result from severe and complicated atheromatous change within the blood vessel wall.[132] However, acute and chronic inflammatory change has often been found within the walls of fusiform aneurysms, suggesting other possible pathogenetic mechanisms.[132] Naturally, the inflammatory reaction might be in response to the atheromatous change, or related thrombosis or rupture of the aneurysm.

When located on the length of the basilar artery,[134] these aneurysms can enlarge to the point where they cause significant brainstem

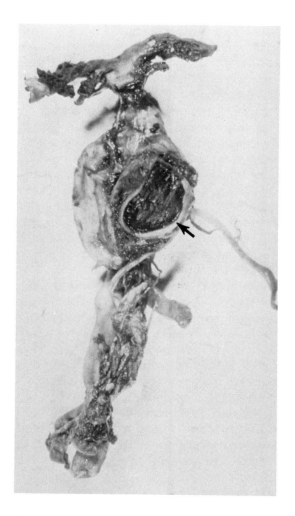

Fig. 2–28. Fusiform aneurysm along the length of the basilar artery. Vertebral arteries are at bottom of figure, and basilar bifurcation is seen at top. Note severe atherosclerosis throughout the entire basilar artery. A large amount of clotted blood is seen adjacent to the rupture site of this fusiform aneurysm (arrow). The pathogenesis of fusiform aneurysms is disputed. However, atherosclerosis within affected vessels is a common finding. The aneurysms may thrombose or rupture.

displacement and compression and may even produce cranial neuropathies. Because laminated thrombus is present within their lumina, platelet fibrin or atheromatous embolic material may embolize distally to produce transient ischemic attacks or permanent infarcts in the distal branches of the vertebrobasilar circulation.[134] However, these aneurysms may also rupture to produce subarachnoid bleeding.[132,133]

Fusiform aneurysms are also seen in the anterior circulation,[135] e.g. the supraclinoid internal carotid artery and the middle cerebral artery. As expected, because they occur along the length of important feeding vessels to the brain, they are extremely difficult to treat. The aim of the treatment is usually obliteration of the aneurysm and yet preservation of adequate blood flow to the brain. Nevertheless, various treatment modalities have been attempted, including entrapment and decompression of the aneurysm, internal carotid artery ligation (when the aneurysm occurs on the anterior circulation), and wrapping of the aneurysms. In addition to the more recent clinicopathologic studies, earlier excellent descriptions of the morbid anatomy of these fusiform or serpentine aneurysms have been published.[136]

Arteriovenous and Other Vascular Malformations. Arteriovenous malformations (AVMs), the clinically most important type of vascular malformation,[1] may cause intraparenchymal intracerebral hemorrhage and/or subarachnoid hemorrhage, but we shall take the prerogative of discussing them in this section, since many authors group them with vascular malformative lesions that include berry aneurysms, discussed above. An exhaustive and superb chapter on vascular malformations was published by Stehbens,[1] and both the quality and quantity of the information presented in that volume cannot be surpassed in terms of its providing an excellent clinicopathologic review of a complex group of entities. Excellent clinical reviews on the controversies involved in management of vascular malformations, in particular AVMs, as well as their natural history, have also been published, e.g. by Drake and by Luessenhop.[137,138]

Vascular malformations of the brain deserve slightly less emphasis in a volume devoted to geriatric neuropathology. Vascular malformations primarily present in young or middle-aged patients. AVMs, for example, have a peak clinical incidence in the age group 20–40 years. They are unusual in patients over the age of 60 years, only approximately 5% of all AVMs are in this age group.[1] AVMs may occur in any portion of the brain. They are usually found in the middle cerebral artery territory, and rarely are present on the circle of Willis itself,[139] in contradistinction to berry aneurysms and fusiform or serpentine aneurysms, discussed above. It is rare for symptoms from an AVM to onset beyond the age of 60 years.

Cerebral AVMs (also sometimes called arteriovenous *aneurysms*) are more likely to be seen by the surgical pathologist than the autopsy pathologist. Their morphology is quite characteristic,[140] and is illustrated in Figs. 2–29 to 2–31. They consist of a collection of vascular channels of varying wall thickness and diameter embedded within extremely abnormal, gliotic and occasionally malformed brain parenchyma.[141] The brain parenchyma may or may not show evidence of old hemorrhage, but the absence of hemosiderin or hematoidin within the neuroglial parenchyma does not rule out the possibility that the AVM has previously bled (T.H. Lanman, N.A. Martin, and H. V. Vinters, unpublished data). It is not uncommon to find thrombosed, and thrombosed and recanalized vascular channels within an

Fig. 2–29. Right mesial temporal arteriovenous malformation. Because of extensive surrounding hemorrhage, the AVM (arrows) is barely visible on a dark background. By comparison to the left temporal lobe and hippocampus, however, one can see extensive hemorrhagic destruction of the right mesial temporal lobe. Blood was seen in the subarachnoid space and extensive intraventricular clot (arrowhead) was also present. The patient had an associated berry aneurysm on the circle of Willis.

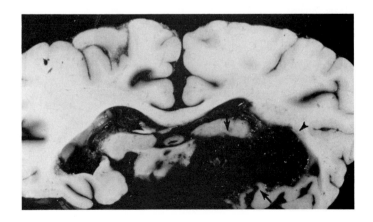

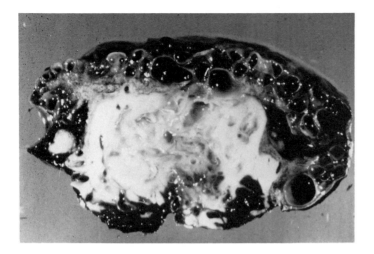

Fig. 2–30. Typical appearance of an arteriovenous malformation received in the Surgical Pathology cutting room. At the center of the specimen is disorganized neuroglial tissue, which has a pale appearance. Surrounding this are ectatic vascular channels of varying wall thickness and diameter. Fresh hemorrhage is seen in and around the AVM.

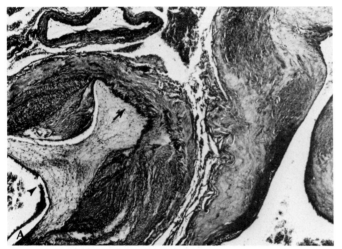

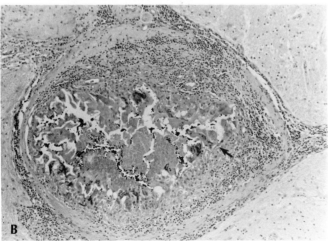

Fig. 2–31. Microscopic features of AVMs. A. Section of AVM stained with elastic van Gieson stain. Note pronounced fibromuscular intimal hyperplasia (arrowhead) of the vascular channel at left. This vessel wall also shows focal reduplication and fragmentation of the elastica, but in some areas the elastica is intact (arrow). By contrast a thickened blood vessel wall at right shows either total absence or sparse amounts of elastica. B. AVM embolized several weeks previously with a mixture of plastic adhesive material and tantalum (black particles within vascular lumen). There is transmural lympho-histiocytic inflammation, and foreign body giant cells are seen around the embolotherapy material (arrow). For details, see reference 149. (B hematoxylin and eosin; magnifications A ×76, B ×130).

AVM. Occasionally, "foreign" paticles, covered by endothelium and associated with a foreign body giant cell reaction, are found within the walls of the vascular channels.[142] Rarely, amyloid is found within the walls of vessels that constitute the AVM, especially in older patients. A recent finding of considerable interest is that the amyloid can be shown to be immunohistochemically similar to the beta-peptide that is present within the walls of amyloidotic vessels found in elderly patients, including elderly patients with Alzheimer's disease (see below).[143]

McCormick[144–146] has published several excellent reviews on the neuropathology of AVMs as well as clinically less important types of vascular malformation (cavernous hemangiomas, venous angiomas, capillary telangiectasia, etc.). The latter (Figs. 2–32 and 2–33) are not a particularly significant clinical problem in elderly patients, and in many cases are not a clinical problem at all, since many forms of vascular malformation exclusive of AVMs virtually never give rise to clinical symptoms. Exceptions to this rule appear to be cavernous hemangiomas and venous angiomas, which may bleed. All of the ways in which AVMs produce clinical symptoms are not clearly understood, although rupture from an AVM often produces obvious bleeding into the sub-

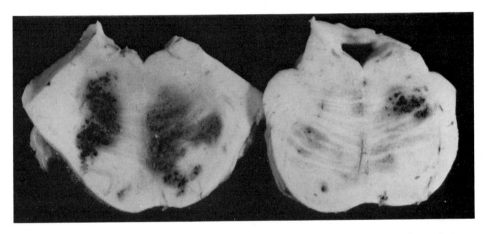

Fig. 2–32. Multiple cavernous hemangiomas present throughout the basis pontis and pontine tegmentum in a patient who died of unrelated causes. There were no documented symptoms related to these lesions during life.

Fig. 2–33. Vascular malformation typical of cavernous hemangioma. Right of field shows many vascular channels of varying wall thickness, some partly thrombosed (arrow). Gliotic brain parenchyma is seen at left. Arrowhead indicates extensive foci of hemosiderin, indicating previous hemorrhage from the malformation. (hematoxylin and eosin, ×76).

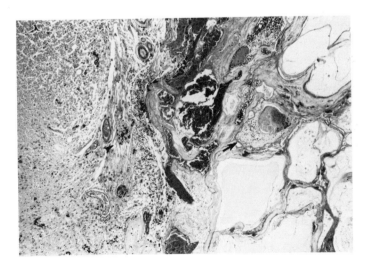

arachnoid space or brain parenchyma. The large blood flow through an AVM may also produce a relative "steal" of blood from the surrounding brain parenchyma with resultant ischemic change in the brain adjacent to an AVM.[147]

The origin of AVMs and other types of vascular malformation is debated, and it is not entirely clear whether these lesions are congenital or acquired (e.g. as a result of repeated subclinical trauma to the head).[1,140] The association between vascular malformations and other brain malformations suggests that at least in some cases there is a dysplastic neurovascular component important in their etiopathogenesis.[141]

Options for the treatment of vascular malformations have been discussed in several excellent reviews.[137,148] From a practical standpoint, it is important to remember that many treatment modalities are being attempted, including the relatively new and innovative interventional neuroradiologic methodology of embolotherapy. This simply means that the vascular malformation is purposefully injected with one or more substances, which may then remain within the vascular malformation and induce a foreign body giant cell reaction or other inflammatory or reactive changes. The examining pathologist must be aware that these materials may be present (Fig. 2–31) and can induce unique tissue reactions.[149,150] Because embolization therapy is increasingly used as a nonsurgical approach to treatment of these lesions, such foreign or iatrogenic materials are increasingly likely to be found within AVMs, especially in older patients who may survive effective treatment in middle age and live for many more years.

Miscellaneous Causes of Subarachnoid Hemorrhage. Patients on anticoagulant therapy, those who have coagulopathies and patients who are thrombocytopenic may experience subarachnoid hemorrhage as a result of these conditions.[151] Several of these will be considered in more detail below as a predisposing factor for intraparenchymal brain hemorrhage. In a large study of patients who experienced subarachnoid hemorrhage of unknown etiology,[152] 8 of 51 patients were over the age of 60 years although the mean age of the individuals affected was substan-

tially lower. In many cases, it was felt that the hemorrhage might be due to a berry aneurysm that was undergoing thrombosis at the time of hemorrhage, making it difficult to detect angiographically. Subsequent recanalization of such a lesion might produce a low incidence of further bleeding. Small (<2 mm greatest dimension) aneurysms might also destroy themselves at the time of the hemorrhage and pose no further risk of subarachnoid bleeding.

A practical clinical point is that subarachnoid hemorrhage may be from a spinal rather than a cranial source.[151,153–155] For example, it may originate from a spinal hemangioma, and blood might subsequently track into the cranial subarachnoid space. An investigation restricted to intracranial vascular abnormalities would thus prove unrewarding, whereas examination of the spinal canal and spinal vasculature might be instructive. Traumatic basal subarachnoid hemorrhage is also seen after relatively trivial trauma to the head.[156]

INTRAPARENCHYMAL HEMORRHAGE

As will be discussed below, it has recently been argued that the etiologic factor considered for many decades to be the most important in the pathogenesis of primary nontraumatic intraparenchymal brain hemorrhage, i.e. hypertension, has decreased as a relatively important consideration, while other etiologic mechanisms (e.g. related to agressive chemotherapeutic treatment of solid tumors, leukemias, and lymphomas) have become more prominent as causes of primary brain hemorrhage. Again, as with the discussion of subarachnoid hemorrhage, the different etiologic mechanisms will be considered separately. For historic reasons, we will begin with a consideration of hypertensive brain hemorrhage.

Large population-based studies, e.g. those from the Mayo Clinic, indicate that primary intraparenchymal brain hemorrhage decreased substantially between the 1940s and 1970s.[157] The annual age-adjusted incidence for spontaneous intracerebral hemorrhage declined significantly when one considered the 8-year intervals from 1945 to 1976. The rate of hemorrhage was always higher in males than females, and the incidence of hypertension diagnosed before the intraparenchymal hematoma had been higher in the earlier years of the study. The median age at onset of the primary intraparenchymal hemorrhage increased from 65 years (for the 8-year span 1945 to 1952) to 71 years of age (for the study period 1969 to 1976). This study eliminated anticoagulant-related hemorrhages from the statistical analysis described above. Of interest was the fact that, after the advent and frequent use of the CT scan as a modality used to assess patients with stroke in the mid 1970s, the relative incidence of intraparenchymal hemorrhage increased again at the Mayo Clinic (i.e. in the years 1975 to 1979). This was felt to be a function of the ability of the CT scan to identify more frequently smaller primary intraparenchymal hemorrhages.[158]

Another large population-based study from Japan has shown a diminution in the annual incidence of intracerebral hemorrhage from the year 1961 to 1983.[159] Among males older than 40 years of age, this figure decreased from 3.1/1000 (in the time period 1961 to 1970) to 1.2/1000 for the time period 1974 to 1983. In autopsy series, the incidence of intracerebral hemorrhage varies from center to center, as would be expected. There are many obvious explanations for this, e.g. the clinical interests of a given center, the population base from which individuals are referred to the center, etc. In general, the incidence of the finding of spontaneous cerebral hemorrhage falls within the range of 2.5 to 10% of autopsies, a figure comparable to the observed incidence of cerebral infarcts.[160] A consideration of etiologic mechanisms, at least in the somewhat older studies, suggests that hypertension is still the commonest single etiologic factor responsible for spontaneous intracerebral bleeding.[160,161] Berry aneurysms (discussed above) cause approximately 20% of hemorrhages,[161] whereas other explanations for the bleeding (e.g. blood dyscrasias and vascular malformations, primary or secondary brain tumors, vascular diseases, anticoagulation) lag behind. This interpretation of the relative incidence of causality of cerebral hemorrhage is strongly questioned in other studies, however.

For example, the significance of hypertension as a cause of primary intraparenchymal hemorrhages has been disputed by McCormick.[162,163] In over two-thirds of patients examined at necropsy, his group found a readily apparent cause of the hemorrhage (e.g. a berry aneurysm, angioma, vasculitis, neoplasm, leukemia, hemophilia, etc.) Hypertensives were in the minority, and roughly a third of the patients who were judged to be hypertensive had another discernible cause of primary intracerebral hemorrhage.[162] Thus hypertension was only implicated as the cause of the intraparenchymal hemorrhage in approximately 25% of the patients. It is possible that the currently aggressive investigation and treatment of all forms of hypertension, including essential hypertension, is gradually leading to a decline in this factor as an important etiologic mechanism in the pathogenesis of intracerebral hemorrhage. The reader is referred to several excellent clinical reviews of spontaneous brain hemorrhage,[163-168] which describe its evolution and clinical diagnosis, the latter frequently performed these days by the CT scan in combination with the evaluation of an astute clinician.

Hypertension. As mentioned, for historic reasons this etiologic mechanism will be considered at the outset. The assignment of the cause of a primary intracerebral hemorrhage to hypertension is usually done by inference, and careful exclusion of other causes. A typical patient has (usually) a deep intraparenchymal hemorrhage and, either during the period of clinical investigation or at autopsy, no obvious etiologic mechanism of the types already described is found by the clinician or pathologist. The examining physician may also be biased by a history of clinically documented, sometimes treated hypertension (though this is not always available), and evidence to support this clinical diagnosis is sought at necropsy. For example, the pathologist seeks evidence of increased heart weight, left ventricular hypertrophy, and evidence of gross and microscopic features of renal disease that may represent the cause or effect of hypertension. For several reasons, this approach is problematic.

The significance of an increased heart weight[169] or left ventricular hypertrophy found at autopsy is often far from clear. Arguably, the most common cause of left ventricular hypertrophy is systemic arterial hypertension.[170] Systemic hypertension also tends to be the cause of the most severe degrees of left ventricular hypertrophy. Yet other causes of cardiomegaly and left ventricular hypertrophy must be considered, including aortic stenosis or regurgitation, ventricular septal defect, chronic adhesive pericarditis, and coronary atherosclerosis with or without an infarct.[170] The latter two conditions are particularly common in the elderly.

Using a rigorous autopsy definition of apparent high blood pressure (i.e. a heart weight greater than the mean heart weight of autopsy controls plus 1.5 standard deviations),[171] one investigator found that only 46% of patients with primary intracerebral hemorrhage had cardiac hypertrophy by this criterion. A sobering finding was that many patients with primary intracerebral intraparenchymal hemor

rhage had been healthy all their lives without evidence of cardiovascular or cerebrovascular disease. Again, the implication is that other causes of primary intraparenchymal hemorrhage must be sought.[172] In some respects, hypertension as a cause of the hemorrhage must be considered a diagnosis of exclusion or of last resort, though perhaps this view is too extreme.

The classic teaching about hypertensive primary intraparenchymal brain hemorrhages is that their most common location is deep within the grey matter (Fig. 2–34), usually in the lateral or medial basal ganglia (e.g. putamen, thalamus).[160,173,174] In many of the older series, approximately one half of such lesions were noted in these locations. 10 to 15% of hy

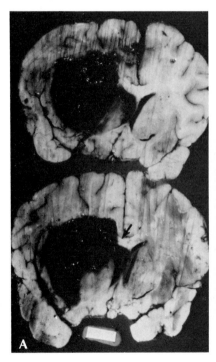
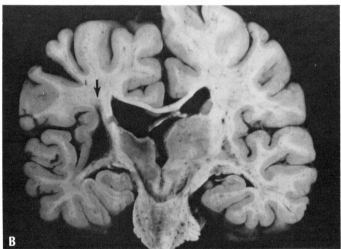

Fig. 2–34. A. Coronal sections of fixed brain reveal typical appearances of a primary hypertensive intracerebral hematoma. The hematoma, which apparently began in the lateral basal ganglia, has dissected extensively into the white matter of the centrum semiovale on the left, and shows intraventricular extension (arrow). There is extensive cerebral edema on the left, with left to right shift of midline structures. B. Coronal section of fixed brain, slice at the level of the hippocampi and lateral geniculate nuclei. A large triangular cystic cavity is present in the region of the left lentiform nucleus (arrow). Microscopic sections showed evidence of hemosiderin laden macrophages within and at the margins of the cavity. Appearances strongly suggest an old hypertensive ganglionic hematoma. Note compensatory dilatation of the left lateral ventricle, and shrinkage of left internal capsule. Wallerian degeneration is evident in the corticospinal tracts of the left basis pontis (bottom of photograph). An old destructive lesion was also seen within the left thalamus.

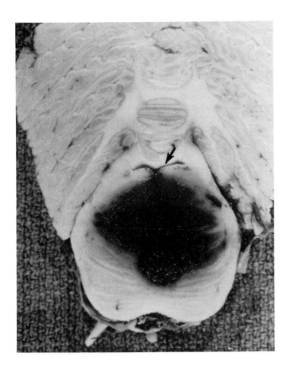

Fig. 2–35. Another common location for primary hypertensive hemorrhages is the basis pontis. This patient survived a pontine hemorrhage for several weeks in a comatose state. Note large amount of clotted blood in pontine tegmentum and basis pontis. A small amount of blood appears to track into the fourth ventricle (arrow). The hematoma has produced distention and enlargement of the pons.

pertensive hemorrhages occur in the cerebral hemispheres, usually the hemispheric white matter. Seven to 15% of hematomas are cerebellar, while 10–15% are pontine (Fig. 2–35). The clinical features of pontine hemorrhages, one-third of which occurred in patients 60 years of age or older, have been reviewed in detail.[175] In one autopsy based study,[173] the age bracket in which hypertension-related intracerebral hemorrhage was most common was that of 50 to 59 years, with a decreasing incidence in each decade thereafter. Primary intraparenchymal hemorrhages caused by hypertension can track into the ventricular cavities, the subarachnoid space and (rarely) even the subdural space.[173]

In addition to extracranial lesions associated with hypertension, the examining pathologist might find microscopic lesions within the brain parenchyma that are said to be associated with long-standing hypertension. These are referred to as hyalinosis, lipohyalinosis or onion-skin thickening, and are found in small arteries and arterioles (see Figs. 2–17 and 2–18). The specific lesions are described above, under a consideration of hypertensive microvascular disease. Fisher,[176] in the course of meticulous serial section studies, was able to find bleeding sites in small parenchymal blood vessels adjacent to intraparenchymal clots. Furthermore, he found small "fibrin globes", consisting of microhemorrhages with central cores of platelets, at the edges of large hematomas.

Another finding freqently sought on routine brain sections from hypertensive patients with parenchymal bleeds, but one uncommonly found, is that of miliary aneurysms (also known as Charcot-Bouchard aneurysms). First described in the late 1800s, these microaneurysms were demonstrated to correlate with clinical or pathologic evidence of hypertension by elegant microinjection studies of postmortem brain specimens.[177–180] They were found in 46% of hypertensive brains, but only 7% of control brains, and the incidence of the microaneurysms increased with age. They were often associated with microhemorrhages, but tended not to be related to microinfarcts. When miliary Charcot-Bouchard aneurysms were seen in relation to cystic lesions, these lesions were usually interpreted as being small old hemorrhages. The examining pathologist must be careful in the morphologic interpretation of miliary aneurysms, particularly on routine hematoxylin and eosin-stained sections. Regions of brain around hematomas can contain blood vessel-related artifacts that may mimic the appearance of microaneurysms. For example, the perivascular space may be distended by blood which tracks from the hematoma.[180]

The pathogenesis of miliary aneurysm formation is unknown, but it may be related to fibrinoid degeneration of microvessel walls. However, fibrinoid degeneration is not always associated with malignant hypertension.[43,44] As well, at least some studies suggest that fibrinoid degeneration is not a requisite for Charcot-Bouchard microaneurysm formation. It is of interest that Charcot-Bouchard type microaneurysms have also been seen in the context of other forms of cerebral microangiopathy, e.g. cerebral amyloid angiopathy, to be discussed below.

Electron microscopic examination of ruptured small arteries in surgical specimens removed from regions of brain adjacent to hypertensive intracerebral hemorrhages[181] has shown that rupture sites of miliary aneurysms are only rarely identified. Degeneration of smooth muscle cells was observed, and was suggestive of prolonged tension or spasm of the blood vessel wall. Obviously, such results based on tissue removed from regions adjacent to severely damaged brain must be interpreted with great caution.

Miscellaneous Causes. Some etiologic mechanisms important in intraparenchymal hemorrhage (e.g. berry aneurysms) have been discussed above under a consideration of subarachnoid hemorrhage. Intraparenchymal hemorrhage is a common cause of death in patients with leukemia, variants of which occur in elderly patients.[182–185] Intraparenchymal hemorrhage as well as subarachnoid hemorrhage are associated with low platelet counts and markedly elevated white blood cell counts. Platelet levels are usually in the range of 5 to 20,000/cu mm, while white blood cell counts (e.g. occurring in the course of blast crisis in leukemic patients) may be in the range of 200 to 300,000/cu mm. In such unfortunate patients, intraparenchymal hemorrhage is usually multifocal and is often associated with bleeding in extracranial sites. Intraspinal and intracranial hematomas may be associated with anticoagulant therapy[186] and are seen in patients with various forms of hemophilia,[187] though the latter is a more significant etiologic consideration in younger patients.[187,188] Spontaneous intraparenchymal brain hemorrhages as the presenting manifestation of CNS vasculitis are unusual but have been described.[189] Chronic, often encapsulated intracerebral hematomas have been observed in younger patients, and sometimes are associated with an underlying occult vascular malformation.[190,191] Both primary and secondary brain tumors (Fig. 2–36) can bleed very extensively,[192] given the high vascularity of malignant primary brain tumors and of many forms of metastatic cancer. The pathologist called to examine brain biopsy tissue removed in the course of a craniotomy for evacuation of a hematoma must thus be particularly vigilant and keep nonvascular causes of bleeding into brain in mind as he/she reads the biopsy. Intracerebral hemorrhage related to alcoholism, often due to the coagulopathy associated with liver damage and low platelet counts, usually occurs in younger patients.[193]

The advent of CT scanning has revolutionized the clinician's ability to assess and plan for long term followup of patients with the diagnosis of primary intraparenchymal brain hemorrhage.[194–199] Many patients with small hematomas do well clinically.[196] The optimal management for some forms of primary intraparenchymal brain hemorrhage—especially *lobar* hematomas—is still the subject of debate between neurologists and neurosurgeons.[200]

Cerebral Amyloid Angiopathy. Cerebral amyloid angiopathy (CAA), defined as a microvascular lesion of the brain parenchyma and subarachnoid space identified by an infiltration of the media and adventitia of small blood vessels by a hyaline eosinophilic material with the staining properties of amyloid, is a particularly important diagnostic consideration in elderly patients with stroke (especially primary intraparenchymal hemorrhage).[201,202] This is because the primary identifiable risk factors for the development of CAA are aging[203,204] and the development of Alzheimer's disease (AD) or senile dementia of Alzheimer type (SDAT).[205] CAA is also identified in the brains of middle-aged patients with Down syndrome.[201]

CAA is a form of microangiopathy that affects the brain in a patchy distribution.[206] Microvessels involved by CAA may be seen in only one or two sections of cerebral cortex and/or overlying leptomeninges, or the entire neocortex may be involved by extensive and severe CAA. Affected microvessels (Fig. 2–37) often run from the subarachnoid space into the cerebral cortical parenchyma, but microvessels of the white matter, deep central grey matter or brainstem are almost never affected by the microangiopathy. Cerebellar vessels (including parenchymal vessels) may be involved in a patchy distribution.[206,207] It seems that only patients with severe, longstanding CAA develop the vascular "substrate" for stroke, in particular cerebral hemorrhage.

Cerebral hemorrhages related to CAA occur

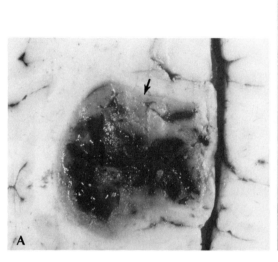
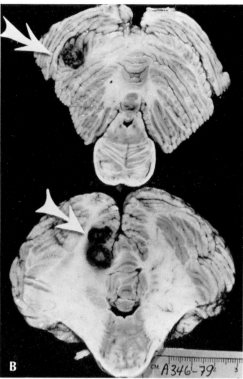

Fig. 2–36. It is important to remember that not all hemorrhagic lesions within the brain are related to vascular disease. A. Frontal lobe oligodendroglioma, with extensive central hemorrhage. Surrounding discolored tissue (arrow) showed typical features of an oligodendroglial neoplasm. B. Various metastatic tumors (e.g. melanoma, hypernephroma, choriocarcinoma) can produce extensive parenchymal brain hemorrhage. In this patient, severely hemorrhagic metastases are seen in the left cerebellum (arrows).

in a fairly stereotyped clinical pattern and physical distribution within the brain.[202,208–211] They usually manifest as hematomas of moderate size within the peripheral (subcortical) brain substance (Fig. 2–38), with frequent dissection directly into the subarachnoid space, a distinctly unusual occurrence in primary hypertensive hemorrhages. This is not surprising, given the topographic localization of the microvascular lesions.[206] Deep ganglionic, brainstem or cerebellar hematomas are thus distinctly unusual in the context of CAA. The hematomas may occur in multiple loci in both cerebral hemispheres over a period of months or years,[212] and many patients have been reported to make surprisingly good recoveries from the stroke-like episodes induced by the occurrence of the hematomas. In a given patient, cerebral function may be compromised

by the co-existent lesions of Alzheimer's disease, however.[205]

Although the most severe and extensive degrees of CAA appear to occur in patients with overt AD/SDAT,[205,206] fairly severe degrees of CAA can be found in patients with relatively normal mentation, and in whom microscopic hallmarks of AD/SDAT are only minimally present or entirely absent at the time of necropsy examination of the brain. CAA is not associated with the deposition of amyloid in other viscera.

The actual pathogenesis of the degenerative changes within the microvessels (Fig. 2-39) that lead to weakening and subsequent rupture (e.g. fibrinoid necrosis, microaneurysm formation) to produce intracerebral hemorrhage are not known.[213,214] Ultrastructural studies of amyloidotic microvessels have been

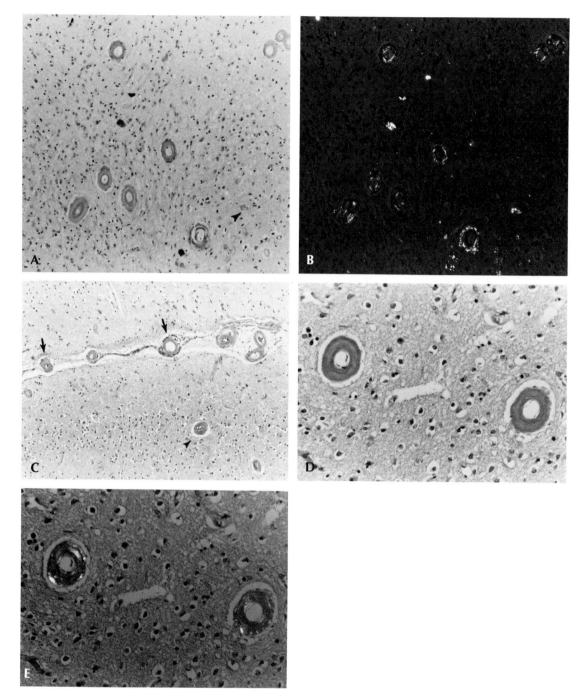

Fig. 2–37.   Cerebral amyloid angiopathy (CAA). A. This panel shows cerebral cortex (with extensive astrocytic gliosis) in which many vessel walls show hyaline thickening. The thickened material has an affinity for Congo red dye, used to stain this section. Section viewed under non-polarized light. B. Identical section viewed under polarized light shows birefringence of the vessel wall material. Birefringence was characteristically apple-green. Parenchymal senile plaques (arrowhead in A) also show birefringence. (A, B ×200). C. Hematoxylin and eosin-stained section shows severe microvascular amyloidosis of leptomeningeal vessels (arrows) and an adjacent parenchymal microvessel of comparable size (arrowhead). (magnification × 200). D. Congo red stained section of brain from patient with severe CAA shows details of hyaline vascular wall thickening. Note that endothelium appears to be relatively intact. E. Identical section viewed under polarized light shows birefringent material in both vessel walls. (magnification ×500).

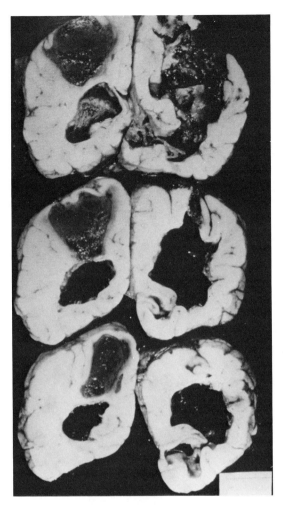

Fig. 2–38. Multiple coronal sections through parietal lobes of brain from a patient with severe CAA and multiple CAA-related brain hematomas. Note that hemorrhage has occurred within the cortex and white matter of both cerebral hemispheres. Hematomas at left communicate directly with the subarachnoid space, while hematoma at right appears to have extended into ventricle. The patient had a long-standing history of multiple stroke episodes and dementia.

few, and those carried out on postmortem specimens are suboptimal in terms of tissue preservation and interpretation of subtle ultrastructural details.[215–217] The rare studies carried out on biopsy material indicate that, *ultrastructurally*, the amyloid is identical to biochemically heterogeneous amyloids deposited in different viscera in a variety of clinical conditions. The material is composed of irregularly arranged skeins of fibrils with a diameter of 7 to 10 nm. It has been observed that intracerebral hemorrhage in patients with CAA may be more likely to occur after relatively minor neurosurgical procedures,[218] suggesting that the amyloidotic microvessels are unable to "handle" the changes in perfusion pressure or blood pressure that might occur in the course of such a procedure. Thus, one could argue that the optimal treatment for a patient with a CAA-related brain hemorrhage is largely supportive. On the other hand, if a peripheral hematoma, particularly from an elderly person, is submitted for histologic examination the examining pathologist must be aware of the possibility of discovering CAA within the biopsy tissue,[219] and thus making an etiologic diagnosis.

The past 3 to 4 years have witnessed an explosion of biochemical and molecular biological information on the nature of brain amyloids in general, in particular amyloid associated with AD/SDAT. Amyloidotic microvessels have been isolated from the meninges or brain cortical parenchyma of patients with AD/SDAT or Down syndrome and subjected to biochemical characterization.[220–222] This has shown that the microvascular amyloid consists of a unique peptide with a molecular weight of approximately 4200 Daltons (the A4 or Alzheimer beta-peptide), and a unique amino acid composition and sequence. The peptide is encoded by a gene on chromosome 21.[223,224] Biochemical and immunocytochemical studies suggest that the peptide is identical to that found in the amyloidotic cores of senile plaques, another important microscopic hallmark of AD/SDAT.[225–227] There has been some debate as to whether the peptide is identical to the amyloid found within the neurofibrillary tangles that are also seen in AD/SDAT cortex.[228,229] Using immunocytochemical techniques, antibodies to portions of the above described 4200 Dalton molecular weight peptide label amyloidotic microvessels, senile plaque cores (Fig. 2-40) and possibly the neuritic component of senile plaques.[226,227,230] Such antibodies do not decorate neurofibrillary tangles. Details as to the microscopic lesions of AD/SDAT are to be found elsewhere in this volume.

Despite its association with brain aging and

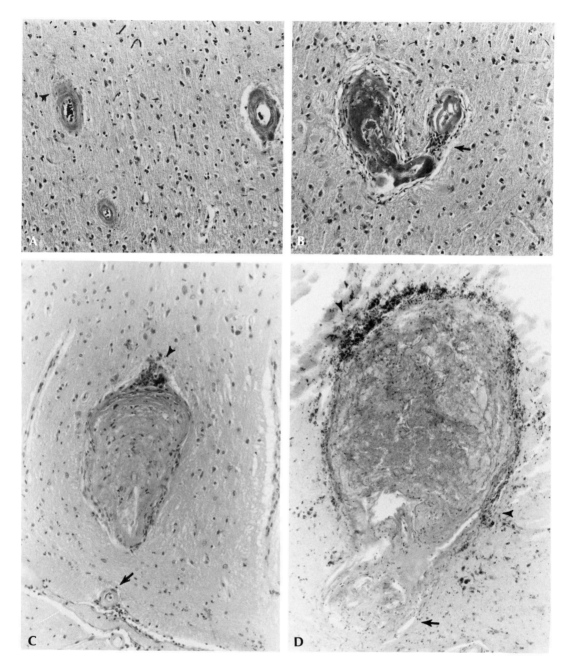

Fig. 2–39. Severe CAA and associated vasculopathies. A. Patient with changes of severe AD/SDAT, with cortical microvessels that show extensive infiltration of vessel walls by amyloid. Amyloid in some areas appears to extend directly into the brain parenchyma (arrowhead). (hematoxylin and eosin, ×190). B. Another section of cerebral cortex from same patient shows less prominent amyloid infiltration of the vessel wall, but hyaline material (which was intensely eosinophilic) on intimal aspect of a tortuous microvessel. Scattered mononuclear inflammatory cells (arrow) are also seen in and around the vessel wall. Surrounding brain shows gemistocytic astrocytes indicative of reactive gliosis. (hematoxylin and eosin, ×190). C and D. Two microaneurysms of the Charcot-Bouchard type in the cerebral cortex of a patient with severe CAA. In C, a leptomeningeal amyloidotic microvessel can be identified (arrow). An adjacent cortical microvessel shows thickening and hyalinosis of its wall, with an apparently preserved lumen. A small cluster of hemosiderin-laden macrophages is seen on the adventitial aspect of the vessel (arrowhead). A larger microaneurysm was seen (D) in cortex a few millimeters from the area illustrated in panel C. The parent

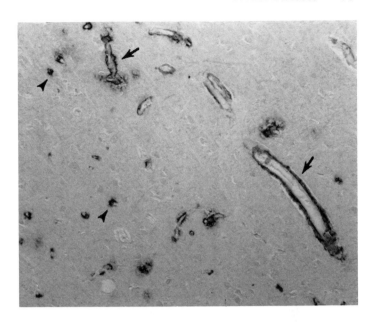

Fig. 2–40. Section of cerebral cortex from a Japanese patient with severe CAA. Staining procedure is an avidin-biotin-peroxidase technique using antiserum to a synthetic 28-amino-acid peptide fragment of the AD A4 or beta-peptide amyloid precursor (see references 226, 227 for details). Amyloidotic microvessels of both the arteriole and capillary size stain intensely (arrows), and senile plaque cores (arrowheads) are also heavily stained. (magnification ×190).

AD/SDAT, the pathogenesis of CAA is currently not understood.[230] It is not even clear whether the abnormal peptide deposited within affected brain blood vessel walls originates from the circulation or directly from the brain cortical parenchyma, and much research is currently devoted to trying to understand this process. It is of interest that another form of CAA found in an isolated area of Iceland, transmitted by autosomal dominant inheritance, and also responsible for the production of intracerebral hemorrhage, results from deposition of an entirely unrelated peptide in microvessel walls within the brain.[231,232] This peptide is related to gamma-trace or cystatin C, a larger molecule than the beta-peptide described above. In the Icelandic patients, cerebral hemorrhages result from CAA, though they occur in much younger patients. As well, the patients do not have other histologic hallmarks or clinical features to suggest the diagnosis of AD/SDAT.

Degenerative microscopic changes described above in the context of hypertensive microvascular disease (e.g. fibrinoid necrosis, microaneurysm formation) have also been observed in association with CAA.[213,214] This suggests that mechanisms such as fibrinoid necrosis and microaneurysm formation are simply a final common pathway of degenerative microangiopathy, rather than being related specifically to hypertensive disease.

Though the association between CAA and primary intraparenchymal brain hemorrhage is well established, the association between CAA and brain infarcts is less clear.[207] Patients with severe CAA may have a superimposed thickening of the amyloidotic vessel wall by non-amyloid materials, and this may eventually lead to complete thrombosis of the vessel.[227] Ischemic lesions are seen in association with CAA, and these may result from such a microangiopathic process.[207] As well, the role (if any) of CAA in the causation of signs and symptoms of Alzheimer's disease must be considered. This opens the broader question of the role of CAA in the etiopathogenesis of vascular dementias (see below).

←———————————————————————

vessel of this microaneurysm is shown at the bottom of the micrograph (arrow). Upper part of micrograph shows ballooning of the vessel wall, and the dome of the microaneurysm appears to be filled by blood and lipid-laden histiocytes. Numerous hemosiderin-laden macrophages are seen immediately outside the aneurysm (arrowheads) and fresh hemorrhage is seen at the top of the field. The parent vessel for the microaneurysm did not itself show extensive amyloid deposition, despite the severe degree of CAA present elsewhere in the brain. (magnifications: C ×200, D ×120).

INTRAVENTRICULAR HEMORRHAGE

Primary intraventricular hemorrhage (IVH) is common in pre-term infants in acute respiratory distress, but extremely rare in adults. There is no particular propensity for primary IVH to occur in the geriatric population, although elderly patients with this condition have been described. It must always be remembered that in a given patient with IVH identified on an imaging modality, the most likely cause is the passage of blood from a primary intraparenchymal lesion or the subarachnoid space into the ventricular cavity. For example, hypertensive bleeds adjacent to the lateral ventricle may easily move *into* the lateral ventricle, as may blood from a ruptured berry aneurysm that sits in close apposition to a ventricular cavity.

Nevertheless, primary IVH in adults has been described. In one series[233] of 5 adults with an age range of 53 to 62 years, all patients had a history of hypertension and all had well documented severe atherosclerotic disease. Three of the individuals had bilateral carotid occlusions, one patient had a unilateral internal carotid artery occlusion and one had a thrombosed middle cerebral artery. Detailed necropsy neuropathologic evaluation of one patient showed several small hemorrhagic lacunar infarcts around the lateral ventricular cavity, one of these showing continuity of hemorrhage between the lacune and a larger intraventricular blood clot. This suggested (but did not prove) that the intraventricular hematoma may have originated from a particularly hemorrhagic lacunar infarct. The most striking point of the study was the high frequency (in patients with primary IVH) of severe occlusive atherosclerotic disease in vessels feeding the brain.

In another study,[234] in which the age range of patients with spontaneous IVH was 21 to 70 years (mean 46 years), two groups of patients were considered. The first of these were individuals in whom intraventricular hemorrhage occurred in the absence of a lesion within the brain parenchyma. The second group was one in which patients experienced the passage of blood from a lesion adjacent to the ventricle, into the ventricular cavity. Patients in the former group in general had a much better prognosis.

Finally, in a third study of primary IVH,[235] 3 patients were found to be over the age of 60 years. Primary IVH constituted 3.1% of all cases of intracerebral hemorrhage in this prospective series of almost 3000 patients with stroke. An underlying vascular malformation was commonly discovered to be the cause of the intraventricular bleed.

MULTI-INFARCT OR VASCULAR DEMENTIA

A consideration of cerebrovascular disease in the elderly without some mention of vascular or multi-infarct dementias, and their relationship to the much maligned and misunderstood entity of Binswanger's subcortical leukoencephalopathy, would be incomplete. We recognize that this entity will be discussed in other chapters throughout this volume, given the importance of dementia as a clinical syndrome in elderly individuals. The many controversies in this field have recently been placed into perspective by a thoughtful review of the subject.[236]

A takeoff point for this discussion might be a mention of two classic articles published by Tomlinson and co-workers in 1968 and 1970.[237,238] These straightforward yet elegant studies examined several gross and microscopic parameters in the brains of "mentally normal" elderly individuals, and compared them with similar parameters in the brains of demented patients of comparable age. In the 50 patients with clinically documented dementia, approximately 50% were felt to have gross and microscopic features of relatively pure AD/SDAT, without a significant ischemic component. Over 10% were thought to have a relatively pure "arteriosclerotic" dementia, and another 5% had "probable" arteriosclerotic dementia. Approximately one tenth of the patients were felt to have mixed dementia, i.e. with histologic and gross features suggestive of AD/SDAT admixed with a component of vascular disease or multifocal brain softening.

The concept of vascular, ischemic or arteriosclerotic or atherosclerotic dementia (multi-infarct dementia, MID) was further refined by Hachinski et al.[239] They concluded that when vascular disease is responsible for dementia, this occurs through the mechanism of multiple small or large infarcts throughout the brain. The corresponding clinical syndrome is a step-wise progression of the dementing illness, i.e. a clinical presentation *unlike* that observed in patients with AD/SDAT.

A consensus appears to be that a minority of patients with the clinical diagnosis of dementia appear to become demented on the basis of step-wise neurologic progression of disease produced by discrete brain infarcts and (probably much less often) hemorrhages, or a combination of the two processes. Large cerebral infarcts have been thought to produce dementia when a certain critical volume of brain (cerebral only ?) tissue was destroyed. The minimal figure of 50 to 100 ml of brain substance loss has been suggested,[238] but there is little doubt that strategically placed lesions of much smaller size can result in a dementia-like condition. Infarcts in the vertebrobasilar territory, for instance, that produce destruction within the inferior and mesial temporal and occipital cortex and white matter, might be expected to more effectively precipitate a dementing syndrome or at least an amnestic syndrome than would lesions of comparable size in the middle cerebral artery or anterior cerebral artery territories. This impinges to some extent on two related questions: 1. What is the anatomic substrate of the global decline in higher intellectual function that we call dementia? and 2. Can lesions of the hippocampal formations *alone* produce dementia?[240,241]

Lacunar infarcts, which have traditionally been attributed to cerebral microvascular disease secondary to hypertension (lipohyalinosis; see consideration of microvascular disease above), do not seem to correlate with the presence of dementia, even when present in substantial numbers in a given brain, though detailed clinicopathologic studies remain to be done in this area. As well, one could envision strategically placed lacunar infarcts that would certainly produce a dementia-like syndrome. Nevertheless, rare syndromes of progressive dementia secondary to widespread cerebral microvascular occlusions have been docu-mented.[242] Thus, most cases of true multi-infarct dementia (MID) are probably secondary to large vessel (atherosclerotic) disease of extracranial vessels or thromboemboli that originate within the heart.[239,243] As has been pointed out,[239] these are important considerations given that some of the risk factors for such forms of vascular disease can be treated, and hence the likelihood of dementia developing in patients at jeopardy can be decreased by more direct medical intervention than is possible in patients with primary parenchymal dementia (e.g. AD/SDAT, Pick's disease). One might even predict that, just as other forms of stroke related to hypertension and atherosclerosis appear to be on the decline, so the diagnosis of pure MID is one likely to become extinct or nearly so, though this view may be overly optimistic.

There seems to be no compelling evidence that the pathogenesis of AD/SDAT is attributable to such risk factors or their related forms of vascular disease. A detailed study of both hippocampal and calcarine macro- and microvasculature in brains from young, normal old, and AD/SDAT patients[244] has recently confirmed that cerebrovascular capacity in AD is at least as good as in the normal old, if not marginally better.

The issue of the role of CAA (see above) in the causation of the parenchymal lesions of AD/SDAT remains unsettled. Some investigators, for example, have claimed that there is a 1:1 correlation between the presence of amyloidotic capillaries within brain parenchyma, and the presence of amyloid-laden senile plaques, important microscopic lesions in the diagnosis of AD/SDAT.[230] Miyakawa et al.[245,246] have suggested that serial sections through all amyloid-laden senile plaques will eventually yield an amyloid-laden capillary or arteriole immediately adjacent to the plaque. Others who have looked at AD/SDAT brains as critically, using non-ultrastructural techniques, do not find the association so compelling (M.A. Bell, M.J. Ball, unpublished observations). One study has shown that the correlation between senile plaque density and capillary density (at least within the confines of the calcarine cortex) was better in normal aged brain than in brain tissue from patients with AD/SDAT.[244] The matter has yet to be resolved.

A further vexing question remains: to what extent does the CAA of AD/SDAT produce or aggravate, on an ischemic basis, neurologic signs and symptoms that contribute to dementia? In a sense, this reopens the additional question: to what extent is AD/SDAT a vascular dementia? In extreme forms, CAA—whether in the context of AD/SDAT or the hereditary Iceland form—causes multiple repeated cerebral parenchymal hemorrhages which have a characteristic distribution, clinical and radiographic presentation. CAA in the context of AD/SDAT also appears to commonly produce cortical microinfarcts. Both of these changes may depend upon CAA-related vessel wall degenerations within affected arteries. These have been discussed above, and include microaneurysm formation, obliterative intimal change (with or without degeneration of the elastica, with or without degeneration of media), transmural inflammation, and fibrinoid necrotizing vascular change.[213,214] As has been described, the pathogenesis of these apparent sequelae of the microangiopathy is now amenable to study using immunohistochemical methods. The importance (if any) of other age-related deformities of the cerebral microvasculature (e.g. "glomerular-loop" formations, vascular bundles and "wickerworks")[247] in the pathogenesis of dementia is also unknown.

The debate as to the existence of the nosologic entity of Binswanger's subcortical leukoencephalopathy, or subcortical arteriosclerotic encephalopathy (SAE), will be raised in this volume by other authors. One accepts the notion that the entity has a rather poorly defined pathologic substrate, even as it was described by Binswanger himself.[248] The current debate hinges on whether Binswanger's disease is a true leukoencephalopathy related purely to long-standing hypertension, or whether it represents the sequelae of multiple lacunar infarcts or other forms of ischemic insult throughout the brain.[249–253] It is particularly intriguing that several elderly patients have recently been described, in whom a fairly severe degree of patchy subcortical leukoencephalopathy was associated with either hemorrhagic or non-hemorrhagic cerebral amyloid angiopathy.[254–256] It was proposed[255] that a common mechanism for leukoencephalopathy on the basis of microangiopathy, whether caused by CAA or another form of microvascular disease, might be hypoperfusion of the distal white matter, with or without alterations of the blood-brain barrier.

The matter has become further complicated by the relatively common finding of white matter lesions (Fig. 2-41) within the brains of patients with AD/SDAT.[257] Histologically, these appear to be relatively bland and can often only be visualized on whole brain sections stained with appropriate methods to show myelin and axons. The latter studies show a diminution in the amount of myelin and the number of oligodendrocytes, together with a decline in the number of axons. There is a subtle astrocytic gliosis and occasional macrophages, presumably digesting axonal or myelin debris, are present. Subcortical U-fibers are often spared. Some have suggested that the lesion represents an "incomplete infarct" within the white matter, one related to either the commonly observed vascular hyaline stenosis of microvessels within the white matter itself or to clinically documented hypotensive episodes experienced by the affected patients.[257]

With the advent of high resolution scanning techniques (CT, MRI), white matter lesions in the brains of normal elderly patients as well as the brains of elderly demented individuals are increasingly identified.[258–261] It is extremely important that the pathologic correlate of these lesions be clearly established. For example, some subcortical white matter lesions identified on MRI scanning were found (on autopsy studies) to be associated with arteriosclerosis, dilated perivascular spaces and vascular ectasia.[262]

A group that has studied a large cohort of "normal elderly" and demented patients with extensive neuropsychologic testing, electroencephalographic and CT and MRI studies[263–266] has found that many normal elderly, and in particular *demented* elderly patients have patchy or diffuse areas of attentuation within the subcortical white matter (on CT scans), without any change in the ventricular size or the overlying sulci. This finding has been given the name "leuko-araiosis" (LA), though

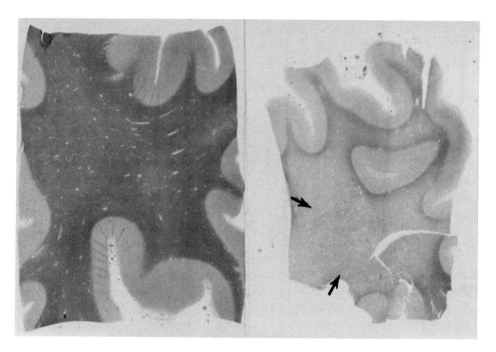

Fig. 2–41. Whole mounts of paraffin sections of comparable thickness taken from same regions of frontal white matter of two demented patients. Both sections stained with Weil stain to demonstrate myelin. Section at left shows relatively normal white matter, while section (from different patient) at right shows severe myelin loss in white matter (arrows), with relative sparing of subcortical U-fibers. (magnification ×3.2). (Reproduced from Vinters, H.V., et al.: Vascular dementia: Immunocytochemical study of brain microvascular and parenchymal lesions associated with Alzheimer's disease. In: *Proceedings of the 16th Princeton Conference on Cerebrovascular Disease.* Edited by M.D. Ginsberg and W.D. Dietrich. New York, Raven Press, 1989. Reproduced with permission).

its pathologic substrate is not yet entirely clear. Cognitive and clinical neurologic correlates of the lesion have been studied, but its pathogenesis is undefined. Given the association of some forms of leukoencephalopathy with overlying meningocortical CAA (described above), it will be of interest to see whether the more commonly observed lesion of LA also correlates with overlying CAA. Clinical studies suggest that LA correlates with risk factors for stroke and cerebrovascular disease.

Excellent clinicopathologic studies of vascular dementia continue to be published, e.g. from large geriatric centers in Japan, where vascular dementias in general appear to be more common than they are in North America.[267,268] Nevertheless, primary parenchymal degenerative dementias (e.g. AD/SDAT) may be difficult to differentiate fully from MID on clinical, and sometimes even on morphologic grounds.[269,270] Some of the reasons for this

have been discussed at length. Even in the current literature, claims are made that vascular dementia is either underdiagnosed[271] or overdiagnosed.[272] Further clinicopathologic studies are thus warranted. A reasonable statement to summarize the 'enigma' of vascular dementias in general is one proposed by Dr. C. Miller Fisher at an NIA-John Douglas French Foundation Symposium on the subject held in June, 1987: "Vascular dementia is a clinical syndrome [of decline in higher intellectual function] in which the underlying chronic brain damage is primarily the result of disturbances of the cerebral circulation—thrombosis, embolism, hemorrhage, systemic hypotension, hypertension, anoxia, abnormalities of the circulating blood, etc. A knowledge of cerebrovascular disease is essential in approaching the subject. The dementia is generally the product of strokes, and since strokes are common, it follows that vascular dementia is also a common condition". An optimistic view is that more effective treatments for cerebrovascular disease[273] will lead to a decline in the incidence of vascular dementias.

ACKNOWLEDGMENTS

The authors gratefully acknowledge the skillful assistance of the following in the final preparation of this ms.: Mr. Roy Bailey, Ms. Laurel Reed and Mrs. Beverly Chandler, Ms. Diana Lenard Secor, Mr. Stephen Kaufman, Ms. Carol Appleton, and Mr. Scott D. Brooks. Ongoing work in Dr. Vinters' laboratory supported by PHS grant #NS 26312

REFERENCES

1. Stehbens, W.E.: *Pathology of the Cerebral Blood Vessels.* St. Louis, C.V. Mosby Co., 1972.
2. Miller Fisher, C.: The anatomy and pathology of the cerebral vasculature. In: *Modern Concepts of Cerebrovascular Disease.* Edited by J.S. Meyer, New York, Spectrum Publications Inc., 1975, pp 1-41.
3. Hachinski, V., and Norris, J.W.: *The Acute Stroke.* Philadelphia, F.A. Davis Co., 1985.
4. Barnett, H.J.M., Mohr, J.P., Stein, B.M., and Yatsu, F.M. (eds.): *Stroke-Pathophysiology, Diagnosis, and Management.* New York, Churchill Livingstone, 1986.
5. Toole, J.F. (ed.): *Cerebrovascular Disorders.* 3d Ed. New York, Raven Press, 1984.
6. Harrison, M.J.G., and Dyken, M.L. (eds.): *Cerebral Vascular Disease.* London, Butterworths, 1983.
7. Pulsinelli, W.A.: Selective neuronal vulnerability: morphological and molecular characteristics. Prog. Brain Res., 63:29, 1985.
8. Hossmann, K.-A.: Post-ischemic resuscitation of the brain: selective vulnerability versus global resistance. Prog. Brain Res., 63:3, 1985.
9. Welsh, F.A.: Role of vascular factors in regional ischemic injury. Prog. Brain Res., 63:19, 1985.
10. Siesjo, B.K.: Calcium and ischemic brain damage. Eur. Neurol., 25 (Suppl. 1):45, 1986.
11. Kakiuchi, S., and Sobue, K.: Ca^{2+} and calmodulin-dependent flip-flop mechanism in microtubule assembly-disassembly. FEBS Lett., 132:141, 1981.
12. Greenamyre, J.T.: The role of glutamate in neurotransmission and in neurologic disease. Arch. Neurol., 43:1058, 1986.
13. Rothman, S.M., and Olney, J.W.: Glutamate and the pathophysiology of hypoxic-ischemic brain damage. Ann. Neurol., 19:105, 1986.
14. Kochhar, A., Zivin, J.A., Lyden, P.D., et al.: Glutamate antagonist therapy reduces neurologic deficits produced by focal central nervous system ischemia. Arch. Neurol., 45:148, 1988.
15. Brierley, J.B., and Graham, D.I.: Hypoxia and vascular disorders of the central nervous system. In *Greenfield's Neuropathology.* 4th Ed. Edited by J.H. Adams, J.A.N. Corsellis, and L.W. Duchen. London, Edward Arnold, 1984, pp. 125-207.
16. Auer, R.N.: Progress review: Hypoclycemic brain damage. Stroke, 17:699, 1986.
17. Siesjö, B.K.: Hypoglycemia, brain metabolism, and brian damage. Diabetes Metab. Rev., 4:113, 1988.
18. Auer, R.N., Hall, P., Ingvar, M., et al.: Hypotension as a complication of hypoglycemia leads to enhanced energy failure but no increase in neuronal necrosis. Stroke, 17:442, 1986.
19. Auer, R.N., Kalimo, H., Olsson, Y., et al.: The temporal evolution of hypoglycemic brain damage. II. Light- and electron-microscopic findings in the hippocampal gyrus and subiculum of the rat. Acta Neuropathol. (Berl.), 67:25, 1985.
20. Auer, R.N., Wieloch, T., Olsson, Y., et al.: The distribution of hypoglycemic brain damage. Acta Neuropathol. (Berl.), 64:177, 1984.
21. Ross, R.: The pathogenesis of atherosclerosis—an update. N. Engl. J. Med., 314:488, 1986.
22. McGill, H.C. Jr.: Persistent problems in the pathogenesis of atherosclerosis. Arteriosclerosis, 4:443, 1984.
23. McGill, H.C. Jr.: The pathogenesis of atherosclerosis. Clin. Chem., 34:B33, 1988.
24. Schaefer, E.J., McNamara, J.R., Genest, J., et al.: Genetics and abnormalities in metabolism of lipoproteins. Clin. Chem., 34:B9, 1988.
25. Tell, G.S., Crouse, J.R., and Furberg, C.D.: Relation between blood lipids, lipoproteins, and cerebrovascular atherosclerosis. A review. Stroke, 19: 423, 1988.
26. Fisher, C.M., Gore, I., Okabe, N., et al.: Atherosclerosis of the carotid and vertebral arteries—extracranial and intracranial. J. Neuropathol. Exp. Neurol., 24:455, 1965.
27. Jorgensen, L., and Torvik, A.: Ischaemic cerebrovascular diseases in an autopsy series. Part 2. Prevalence, location, pathogenesis, and clinical course of cerebral infarcts. J. Neurol. Sci., 9:285, 1969.
28. Barnett, H.J.M.: Delayed cerebral ischemic episodes distal to occlusion of major cerebral arteries. Neurology, 28:769, 1978.
29. Jordan, F.L., and Thomas, W.E.: Brain macrophages: questions of origin and interrelationship. Brain Res. Reviews, 13:165, 1988.
30. Torvik, A.: Editorial. The pathogenesis of watershed infarcts in the brain. Stroke, 15:221, 1984.
31. Adams, J.H., Brierley, J.B., Connor, R.C.R., et al.: The effects of systemic hypotension upon the human brain. Clinical and neuropathological observations in 11 cases. Brain, 89:235, 1966.
32. Brierley, J.B., and Excell, B.J.: The effects of profound systemic hypotension upon the brain of *M. Rhesus:* Physiological and pathological observations. Brain, 89:269, 1966.
33. Romanul, F.C.A., and Abramowicz, A.: Changes in brain and pial vessels in arterial border zones. A study of 13 cases. Arch. Neurol., 11:40, 1964.
34. Bogousslavsky, J., and Regli, F.: Borderzone infarctions distal to internal carotid artery occlusion: Prognostic implications. Ann. Neurol., 20:346, 1986.
35. Torvik, A., and Jörgensen, L.: Thrombotic and embolic occlusions of the carotid arteries in an autopsy series. Part 2. Cerebral lesions and clinical course. J. Neurol. Sci., 3:410, 1966.
36. Torvik, A., and Skullerud, K.: Watershed infarcts in the brain caused by microemboli. Clin. Neuropathol., 1:99, 1982.
37. Miller Fisher, C.: Lacunes: small, deep cerebral infarcts. Neurology, 15:774, 1965.

38. Mohr, J.P., et al.: The Harvard cooperative stroke registry: A prospective registry. Neurology, 28:754, 1978.
39. Poirier, J., Gray F., Gherardi, R., et al.: Cerebral lacunae. A new neuropathological classification. J. Neuropathol. Exp. Neurol., 44:312, 1985.
40. Derouesné, C., Gray, F., Escourolle, R., et al.: 'Expanding cerebral lacunae' in a hypertensive patient with normal pressure hydrocephalus. Neuropathol. Appl. Neurobiol., 13:309, 1987.
41. Miller Fisher, C.: Capsular infarcts. The underlying vascular lesions. Arch. Neurol., 36:65, 1979.
42. Chester, E.M., Agamanolis, D.P., Banker, B.Q., et al.: Hypertensive encephalopathy: A clinicopathologic study of 20 cases. Neurology, 28:928, 1978.
43. Rosenblum, W.I.: Miliary aneurysms and "fibrinoid" degeneration of cerebral blood vessels. Hum. Pathol., 8:133, 1977.
44. Rosenblum, W.I.: Letter to the editor. J. Neuropathol. Exp. Neurol., 44:624, 1985.
45. Mohr, J.P.: Lacunes. Stroke, 13:3, 1982.
46. Fisher, C.M.: Pure sensory stroke involving face, arm, and leg. Neurology, 15:76, 1965.
47. Miller, V.T.: Lacunar stroke. A reassessment. Arch. Neurol., 40:129, 1983.
48. Ropper, A.H., Miller Fisher, C., et al.: Pyramidal infarction in the medulla: A cause of pure motor hemiplegia sparing the face. Neurology, 29:91, 1979.
49. Miller Fisher, C.: Ataxic hemiparesis. A pathologic study. Arch. Neurol., 35:126, 1978.
50. Helgason, C., Caplan, L.R., Goodwin, J., et al.: Anterior choroidal artery-territory infarction. Report of cases and review. Arch. Neurol., 43:681, 1986.
51. Bogousslavsky, J., et al.: Subcortical neglect: Neuropsychological, SPECT, and neuropathological correlations with anterior choroidal artery territory infarction. Ann. Neurol., 23:448, 1988.
52. Decroix, J.P., Graveleau, P., Masson, M., et al.: Infarction in the territory of the anterior choroidal artery. A clinical and computerized tomographic study of 16 cases. Brain, 109:1071, 1986.
53. Castaigne, P., et al.: Arterial occlusions in the vertebro-basilar system. A study of 44 patients with postmortem data. Brain, 96:133, 1973.
54. Fisher, C.M., Karnes, W.E., and Kubik, C.S.: Lateral medullary infarction—the pattern of vascular occlusion. J. Neuropathol. Exp. Neurol., 20:323, 1961.
55. Kubik, C.S., and Adams, R.D.: Occlusion of the basilar artery—a clinical and pathological study. Brain, 69:73, 1946.
56. Sypert, G.W., and Alvord, E.C. Jr.: Cerebellar infarction. A clinicopathological study. Arch. Neurol., 32:357, 1975.
57. Macdonell, R.A.L., Kalnins, R.M., and Donnan, G.A.: Cerebellar infarction: Natural history, prognosis, and pathology. Stroke, 18:849, 1987.
58. Koroshetz, W.J., and Ropper, A.H.: Artery-to-artery embolism causing stroke in the posterior circulation. Neurology, 37:292, 1987.
59. Devinsky, O., Bear, D., and Volpe, B.T.: Confusional states following posterior cerebral artery infarction. Arch. Neurol., 45:160, 1988.
60. Pessin, M.S., et al.: Clinical features and mechanism of occipital infarction. Ann. Neurol., 21:290, 1987.
61. Barnett, H.J.M.: Transient cerebral ischemia. Pathogenesis, prognosis and management. Ann. Royal College Phys. Surg. Canada, 7:153, 1974.
62. Rodda, R.A.: The arterial patterns associated with internal carotid disease and cerebral infarcts. Stroke 17:69, 1986.
63. Lhermitte, F., Gautier, J.C., and Derouesné, C.: Nature of occlusions of the middle cerebral artery. Neurology 20:82, 1970.
64. Bogousslavsky, J., et al.: Atherosclerotic disease of the middle cerebral artery. Stroke, 17:1112, 1986.
65. Gacs, G., Fox, A.J., Barnett, H.J.M., et al.: Occurrence and mechanisms of occlusion of the anterior cerebral artery. Stroke, 14:952, 1983.
66. Bogousslavsky, J., Assal, G., et Regli, F.: Infarctus du territoire de l'artère cérébrale antérieure gauche. II. Troubles du langage. Rev. Neurol. (Paris), 143:121, 1987.
67. Beal, M.F., Park, T.S., and Fisher C.M.: Cerebral atheromatous embolism following carotid sinus pressure. Arch. Neurol., 38:310, 1981.
68. Dines, D.E., Burgher, L.W., and Okazaki, H.: The clinical and pathologic correlation of fat embolism syndrome. Mayo Clin. Proc., 50:407, 1975.
69. Kamenar, E., and Burger, P.C.: Cerebral fat embolism: A neuropathological study of a microembolic state. Stroke, 11:477, 1980.
70. DiNubile, M.J.: Septic thrombosis of the cavernous sinuses. Arch. Neurol., 45:567, 1988.
71. Southwick, F.S., Richardson, E.P., and Swartz, M.N.: Septic thrombosis of the dural venous sinuses. Medicine, 65:82, 1986.
72. Moore, P.M., and Cupps, T.R.: Neurological complications of vasculitis. Ann. Neurol., 14:155, 1983.
73. Moore, P.M., and Fauci, A.S.: Neurologic manifestations of systemic vasculitis. A retrospective and prospective study of the clinicopathologic features and responses to therapy in 25 patients. Am. J. Med., 71:517, 1981.
74. Cupps, T.R., Moore, P.M., and Fauci, A.S.: Isolated angiitis of the central nervous system. Prospective diagnostic and therapeutic experience. Am. J. Med., 74:97, 1983.
75. Calabrese, L.H., and Mallek, J.A.: Primary angiitis of the central nervous system. Report of 8 new cases, review of the literature, and proposal for diagnostic criteria. Medicine, 67:20, 1987.
76. Huston, K.A., et al.: Temporal arteritis. A 25-year epidemiologic, clinical, and pathologic study. Ann. Intern. Med., 88:162, 1978.
77. Barricks, M.E., Traviesa, D.B., Glasser, J.S., et al.: Ophthalmoplegia in cranial arteritis. Brain, 100:209, 1977.
78. Wilkinson, I.M.S., and Russell, R.W.R.: Arteries of the head and neck in giant cell arteritis. A pathological study to show the pattern of arterial involvement. Arch. Neurol., 27:378, 1972.
79. Patton, W.F., and Lynch, J.P. III.: Lymphomatoid granulomatosis. Clinicopathologic study of four cases and literature review. Medicine, 61:1, 1982.
80. Bone, R.C., Vernon, M., Sobonya, R.E., et al.: Lymphomatoid granulomatosis. Report of a case and review of the literature. Am. J. Med., 65:709, 1978.
81. Simon, R.H., et al.: Lymphomatoid granulomatosis with multiple intracranial lesions. Case report. J. Neurosurg., 55:293, 1981.
82. Kadin, M.E., and Said, J.: T-cell lymphomas and leukemias of post-thymic differentiation. Clinics in Laboratory Medicine, 8:135, 1988.
83. Umlas, J., and Kaiser, J.: Thrombohemolytic thrombocytopenic purpura (TTP). A disease or a syndrome? Am. J. Med., 49:723, 1970.

84. Slager, U.T., and Wagner, J.A.: The incidence, com-position, and pathological significance of intracere-bral vascular deposits in the basal ganglia. J. Neuro-pathol. Exp. Neurol., 15:417, 1956.

85. Maloney, A.F.J., and Whatmore, W.J.: Clinical and pathological observations in fatal head injuries. A 5-year survey of 173 cases. Br. J. Surg., 56:23, 1969.

86. Jamieson, K.G., and Yelland, J.D.N.: Extradural he-matoma. Report of 167 cases. J. Neurosurg., 29:13, 1968.

87. McKissock, W., Taylor, J.C., Bloom, W.H., et al.: Ex-tradural haematoma. Observations on 125 cases. Lancet, 2:167, 1960.

88. Markwalder, T.-M.: Chronic subdural hematomas: a review. J. Neurosurg., 54:637, 1981.

89. Wintzen, A.R., and Tijssen, J.G.P.: Subdural hema-toma and oral anticoagulant therapy. Arch. Neurol., 39:69, 1982.

90. Taarnhøj, P.: Chronic subdural hematoma. Historical review and analysis of 60 cases. Cleve. Clin. Q., 22:150, 1955.

91. Friede, R.L.: Incidence and distribution of neomem-branes of dura mater. J. Neurol. Neurosurg. Psychi-atry., 34:439, 1971.

92. Goodell, C.L., and Mealey, J. Jr.: Pathogenesis of chronic subdural hematoma. Experimental studies. Arch. Neurol., 8:99, 1963.

93. Sato, S., and Suzuki, J.: Ultrastructural observations of the capsule of chronic subdural hematoma in var-ious clinical stages. J. Neurosurg., 43:569, 1975.

94. Fogelholm, R., Heiskanen, O., and Waltimo, O.: Chronic subdural hematoma in adults. Influence of patient's age on symptoms, signs, and thickness of hematoma. J. Neurosurg., 42:43, 1975.

95. Echlin, F.A., Sordillo, S.V.R., and Garvey, T.Q. Jr.: Acute, subacute, and chronic subdural hematoma. JAMA, 161:1345, 1956.

96. Rosenbluth, P.R., Arias, B., Quartetti, E.V., et al.: Current management of subdural hematoma. Anal-ysis of 100 consecutive cases. JAMA, 179:759, 1962.

97. Robinson, R.G.: The treatment of subacute and chronic subdural haematomas. Br. Med. J., 1:21, 1955.

98. Heiss, E.: Results of treatment in chronic subdural hematomas. Adv. Neurosurg., 12:192, 1984.

99. Sprung, Ch., Collmann, H., Kazner, E., et al.: Chronic subdural hematoma in geriatric patients—factors affecting prognosis. Adv. Neurosurg., 12:204, 1984.

100. Bender, M.B., and Christoff, N.: Nonsurgical treat-ment of subdural hematomas. Arch. Neurol., 31:73, 1974.

101. Sekhar, L.N., and Heros, R.C.: Origin, growth, and rupture of saccular aneurysms: A review. Neurosur-gery, 8:248, 1981.

102. Kassell, N.F., and Torner, J.C.: Size of intracranial aneurysms. Neurosurgery, 12:291, 1983.

103. Wiebers, D.O., Whisnant, J.P., and O'Fallon, W.M.: The natural history of unruptured intracranial aneu-rysms. N. Engl. J. Med., 304:696, 1981.

104. McCormick, W.F., and Acosta-Rua, G.J.: The size of intracranial saccular naeurysms. An autopsy study. J. Neurosurg., 33:422, 1970.

105. Drake, C.G.: Management of cerebral aneurysm. Stroke, 12:273, 1981.

106. Wilkins, R.H.: Update—Subarachnoid hemorrhage and saccular intracranial aneurysms. Surg. Neurol., 15:92, 1981.

107. Heiskanen, O.: Risk of bleeding from unruptured an-eurysms in cases with multiple intracranial aneu-rysms. J. Neurosurg., 55:524, 1981.

108. Wiebers, D.O., Whisnant, J.P., Sundt, T.M. Jr., et al.: The significance of unruptured intracranial saccular aneurysms. J. Neurosurg., 66:23, 1987.

109. Drake, C.G.: On the surgical treatment of intracranial aneurysms. Annals Royal College Phys. and Surg. Canada, 11:185, 1978.

110. Winn, H.R., et al.: The long-term outcome in patients with multiple aneurysms. Incidence of late hemor-rhage and implications for treatment of incidental aneurysms. J. Neurosurg., 59:642, 1983.

111. Frowein, R.A., and Stammler, A.: Cerebral aneu-rysms in elderly patients. Adv. Neurosurg., 12:180, 1984.

112. Sutherland, G.R., Drake, C.G., and Kaufmann, J.C.E.: Extensive organization in a thrombosed giant intracranial aneurysm: case report. Clin. Neuro-pathol., 4:19, 1985.

113. Sahs, A.L.: Observations on the pathology of saccu-lar aneurysms. J. Neurosurg., 24:792, 1966.

114. Heros, R.C., Zervas, N.T., and Varsos, V.: Cerebral vasospasm after subarachnoid hemorrhage: An up-date. Ann. Neurol., 14:599, 1983.

115. Chyatte, D., and Sundt, T.M. Jr.: Cerebral vasospasm after subarachnoid hemorrhage. Mayo Clin. Proc., 59:498, 1984.

116. Kassell, N.F., Sasaki, T., Colohan, A.R.T., et al.: Ce-rebral vasospasm following aneurysmal subarach-noid hemorrhage. Stroke, 16:562, 1985.

117. George, B., Zerah, M., Dematons, C., et al.: L'anéurysme artériel intra-crânien. Une origine et un pronostic différents chez l'homme et chez la femme. Neurochirurgie, 33:196, 1987.

118. George, B., et al.: Efficacité d'un traitement médical (isoprotérénol + aminophylline) du spasme des rup-tures anéurysmales. Neurochirurgie, 30:273, 1983.

119. Smith, R.R., et al.: Arterial wall changes in early human vasospasm. Neurosurgery, 16:171, 1985.

120. Hughes, J.T., and Schianchi, P.M.: Cerebral artery spasm. A histological study at necropsy of the blood vessels in cases of subarachnoid hemorrhage. J. Neu-rosurg., 48:515, 1978.

121. Molinari, G.F., Smith, L., Goldstein, M.N., et al.: Pathogenesis of cerebral mycotic aneurysm. Neu-rology, 23:325, 1973.

122. Roach, M.R., and Drake, C.G.: Ruptured cerebral an-eurysms caused by micro-organisms. N. Engl. J. Med., 273:240, 1965.

123. Farrell, M.A., Gilbert, J.J., and Kaufmann, J.C.E.: Fatal intracranial arterial dissection: clinical patho-logical correlation. J. Neurol. Neurosurg. Psychiatry, 48:111, 1985.

124. Hart, R.G.: Vertebral artery dissection. Neurology, 38:987, 1988.

125. Mokri, B., Houser, O.W., Sandok, B.A., et al.: Spon-taneous dissections of the vertebral arteries. Neurol-ogy, 38:880, 1988.

126. Caplan, L.R., et al.: Dissection of the intracranial ver-tebral artery. Neurology, 38:868, 1988.

127. Alexander, C.B., Burger, P.C., and Goree, J.A.: Dis-secting aneurysms of the basilar artery in 2 patients. Stroke, 10:294, 1979.

128. Yonas, H., Agamanolis, D., Takaoka, Y., et al.: Dis-secting intracranial aneurysms. Surg. Neurol., 8:407, 1977.

129. Sato, O., Bascom, J.R., and Logothetis, J.: Intracranial dissecting aneurysm. Case report. J. Neurosurg., 35:483, 1971.

130. Friedman, A.H., and Drake, C.G.: Subarachnoid hemorrhage from intracranial dissecting aneurysm. J. Neurosurg., 60:325, 1984.

131. Nedwich, A., Haft, H., Tellem, M., et al.: Dissecting aneurysm of cerebral arteries. Review of the literature and report of a case. Arch. Neurol., 9:477, 1963.

132. Shokunbi, M.T., Vinters, H.V., and Kaufmann, J.C.E.: Fusiform intracranial aneurysms. Clinicopathologic features. Surg. Neurol., 29:263, 1988.

133. Nijensohn, D.E., Saez, R.J., and Reagan, T.J.: Clinical significance of basilar artery aneurysms. Neurology, 24:301, 1974.

134. Steel, J.G., Thomas, H.A., and Strollo, P.J.: Fusiform basilar aneurysm as a cause of embolic stroke. Stroke, 13:712, 1982.

135. Little, J.R., St. Louis, P., Weistein, M., et al.: Giant fusiform aneurysm of the cerebral arteries. Stroke, 12:183, 1981.

136. Courville, C.B.: Arteriosclerotic aneurysms of the circle of Willis. Some notes on their morphology and pathogenesis. Bull. L.A. Neurol. Soc., 27:1, 1962.

137. Drake, C.G.: Cerebral arteriovenous malformations: Considerations for and experience with surgical treatment in 166 cases. Clin. Neurosurg., 26:145, 1979.

138. Luessenhop, A.J.: Natural history of cerebral arteriovenous malformations. In: Intracranial Arteriovenous Malformations. Edited by C.B. Wilson and B.M. Stein. Baltimore, Williams & Wilkins, 1984, pp. 12-23.

139. McArdle, J.E., Dwan, P., Cancilla, P.A., et al.: Arteriovenous malformations and multiple anomalies of the circle of Willis. Bull. Clin. Neurosci., 51:47, 1986.

140. Jellinger, K.: Vascular malformations of the central nervous system: a morphological overview. Neurosurg. Rev., 9:177, 1986.

141. Bailey, O.T.: The vascular component of congenital malformations in the central nervous system. J. Neuropathol. Exp. Neurol., 20:170, 1961.

142. Vinters, H.V., Kaufmann, J.C.E., and Drake, C.G.: 'Foreign' particles in encephalic vascular malformations. Arch. Neurol., 40:221, 1983.

143. Hart, M.N., et al.: Beta-amyloid protein of Alzheimer's disease is found in cerebral and spinal cord vascular malformations. Am. J. Pathol., 132:167, 1988.

144. McCormick, W.F.: The pathology of angiomas. In: Cerebrovascular Surgery. Edited by J.M. Fein and E.S. Flamm. New York, Springer-Verlag, 1985, Volume IV, pp. 1073-1095.

145. McCormick, W.F.: Pathology of vascular malformations of the brain. In: Intracranial Arteriovenous Malformations. Edited by C.B. Wilson and B.M. Stein. Baltimore, Williams & Wilkins, 1984, pp. 44-63.

146. McCormick, W.F.: The pathology of vascular ("arteriovenous") malformations. J. Neurosurg., 24:807, 1966.

147. Costantino, A., and Vinters, H.V.: A pathologic correlate of the 'steal' phenomenon in a patient with cerebral arteriovenous malformation. Stroke, 17:103, 1986.

148. Stein, B.M., and Wolpert, S.M.: Arteriovenous malformations of the brain. I and II. Current concepts and treatment. Arch. Neurol., 37:1,69, 1980.

149. Vinters, H.V., Lundie, M.J., and Kaufmann, J.C.E.: Long-term pathological follow-up of cerebral arteriovenous malformations treated by embolization with bucrylate. N. Engl. J. Med., 314:477, 1986.

150. Lanman, T.H., Martin, N.A., and Vinters, H.V.: The pathology of encephalic arteriovenous malforma-

tions treated by prior embolotherapy. Neuroradiology, 30:1, 1988.

151. Vinters, H.V., Barnett, H.J.M., and Kaufmann, J.C.E.: Subdural hematoma of the spinal cord and widespread subarachnoid hemorrhage complicating anticoagulant therapy. Stroke, 11:459, 1980.

152. Hayward, R.D.: Subarachnoid haemmorhage of unknown aetiology. A clinical and radiological study of 51 cases. J. Neurol. Neurosurg. Psychiatry, 40:926, 1977.

153. Henson, R.A., and Croft, P.B.: Spontaneous spinal subarachnoid haemorrhage. Q. J. Med., 25:53, 1956.

154. Plotkin, R., Ronthal, M., and Froman, C.: Spontaneous spinal subarachnoid haemorrhage. Report of 3 cases. J. Neurosurg., 25:443, 1966.

155. Parkinson, D., and West, M.: Spontaneous subarachnoid hemorrhage first from an intracranial and then from a spinal arteriovenous malformation. Case report. J. Neurosurg., 47:965, 1977.

156. Dowling, G., and Curry, B.: Traumatic basal subarachnoid hemorrhage. Report of six cases and review of the literature. Am. J. Forensic Med. Pathol., 9:23, 1988.

157. Furlan, A.J., Wisnant, J.P., and Elveback, L.R.: The decreasing incidence of primary intracerebral hemorrhage: A population study. Ann. Neurol., 5:367, 1979.

158. Drury, I., Whisnant, J.P., and Garraway, W.M.: Primary intracerebral hemorrhage: Impact of CT on incidence. Neurology, 34:653, 1984.

159. Ueda, K., et al.: Intracerebral hemorrhage in a Japanese community, Hisayama: Incidence, changing pattern during long-term follow-up, and related factors. Stroke, 19:48, 1988.

160. Jellinger, K.: Pathology and aetiology of ICH. In: Spontaneous Intracerebral Haematomas. Advances in Diagnosis and Therapy. Edited by H.W. Pia, C. Langmaid, and J. Zierski. New York, Springer-Verlag, 1980, pp. 13-29.

161. Russell, D.S., Falconer, M.A., Beck, D.J.K., et al.: Discussion: The pathology of spontaneous intracranial haemorrhage. Proc. Royal Soc. Med., 47:689, 1954.

162. McCormick, W.F., and Rosenfield, D.B.: Massive brain hemorrhage: A review of 144 cases and an examination of their causes. Stroke, 4:946, 1973.

163. McCormick, W.F.: Vascular Diseases. In: The Clinical Neurosciences; Neuropathology (Volume 3). Edited by R.N. Rosenberg and S.S. Schochet, Jr. New York, Churchill Livingstone, 1983, pp. 35-83.

164. Ojemann, R.G., and Heros, R.C.: Spontaneous brain hemorrhage. Stroke, 14:468, 1983.

165. Kase, C.S., Williams, J.P., Wyatt, D.A., et al.: Lobar intracerebral hematomas: Clinical and CT analysis of 22 cases. Neurology, 32:1146, 1982.

166. Ransohoff, J., Derby, B., and Kricheff, I.: Spontaneous intracerebral hemorrhage. Clin. Neurosurg., 18:247, 1971.

167. Kase, C.S., and Mohr, J.P.: Supratentorial intracerebral hemorrhage. In: Stroke-Pathophysiology, Diagnosis, and Management, Volume 1. Edited by H.J.M. Barnett, et al. New York, Churchill Livingstone, 1986, pp. 525-547.

168. Kase, C.S., and Mohr, J.P.: General features of intracerebral hemorrhage. In: Stroke-Pathophysiology, Diagnosis, and Management, Volume 1. Edited by H.J.M. Barnett, et al. New York, Churchill Livingstone, 1986, pp. 497-523.

169. Brewer, D.B., Fawcett, F.J., and Horsfield, G.I.: A necropsy series of non-traumatic cerebral haemor-

rhages and softenings, with particular reference to heart weight. J. Pathol. Bacteriol., 96:311, 1968.

170. Batsakis, J.G.: Cardiac Enlargement. In: *Pathology of the Heart and Blood Vessels*. 3d Ed., Edited by S.E. Gould. Springfield. Charles C Thomas, 1968, pp. 532-533.

171. Bahemuka, M.: Primary intracerebral hemorrhage and heart weight: A clinicopathologic case-control review of 218 patients. Stroke, 18:531, 1987.

172. Brott, T., Thalinger, K., and Hertzberg, V.: Hypertension as a risk factor for spontaneous intracerebral hemorrhage. Stroke, 17:1078, 1986.

173. Freytag, E.: Fatal hypertensive intracerebral haematomas: a survey of the pathological anatomy of 393 cases. J. Neurol. Neurosurg. Psychiatry, 31:616, 1968.

174. Ojemann, R.G., and Mohr, J.P.: Hypertensive brain hemorrhage. Clin. Neurosurg., 23:220, 1976.

175. Goto, N., Kaneko, M., Hosaka, Y., et al.: Primary pontine hemorrhage: Clinicopathological correlations. Stroke, 11:84, 1980.

176. Fisher, C.M.: Pathological observations in hypertensive cerebral hemorrhage. J. Neuropathol. Exp. Neurol., 30:536, 1971.

177. Cole, F.M., and Yates, P.: Intracerebral microaneurysms and small cerebrovascular lesions. Brain, 90:759, 1967.

178. Cole, F.M., and Yates, P.O.: Comparative incidence of cerebrovascular lesions in normotensive and hypertensive patients. Neurology, 18:255, 1968.

179. Russell, R.W.R.: Observations on intracerebral aneurysms. Brain, 86:425, 1963.

180. Cole, F.M., and Yates, P.O.: Pseudo-aneurysms in relationship to massive cerebral haemorrhage. J. Neurol. Neurosurg. Psychiatry, 30:61, 1967.

181. Takebayashi, S., and Kaneko, M.: Electron microscopic studies of ruptured arteries in hypertensive intracerebral hemorrhage. Stroke, 14:28, 1983.

182. Law, I.P., and Blom, J.: Adult central nervous system leukemia: Incidence and clinicopathologic features. South. Med. J., 69:1054, 1976.

183. Freireich, E.J., et al.: A distinctive type of intracerebral hemorrhage associated with "blastic crisis" in patients with leukemia. Cancer, 13:146, 1960.

184. Moore, E.W., Thomas, L.B., Shaw, R.K., et al.: The central nervous system in acute leukemia. Arch. Intern. Med., 105:451, 1960.

185. Pochedly, C.: Neurologic manifestations in acute leukemia. N.Y. State J. Med., 75:575, 715, 878, 1975.

186. Lizuka, J.: Intracranial and intraspinal haematomas associated with anticoagulant therapy. Neurochirurgia, 15:15, 1972.

187. Martinowitz, U., et al.: Intracranial hemorrhage in patients with hemophilia. Neurosurgery, 18:538, 1986.

188. Almaani, W.S., and Awidi, A.S.: Spontaneous intracranial bleeding in hemorrhagic diathesis. Surg. Neurol., 17:137, 1982.

189. Biller, J., et al.: Isolated central nervous system angiitis first presenting as spontaneous intracranial hemorrhage. Neurosurgery, 20:310, 1987.

190. Pozzati, E., et al.: Chronic expanding intracerebral hematoma. J. Neurosurg., 65:611, 1986.

191. Masuzawa, T., et al.: Chronic encapsulated hematomas in the brain. Acta Neuropathol. (Berl.), 66:24, 1985.

192. Vinters, H.V.: Cerebral hemorrhage: New ideas about causes and pathology. In: *Pathology Update Series*, Volume 2 (17). Edited by W.R. Platt. Princeton, N.J., Continuing Professional Education Center, Inc., 1985.

193. Weisberg, L.A.: Alcoholic intracerebral hemorrhage. Stroke, 19:1565, 1988.

194. Hayward, R.D., and O'Reilly, G.V.A.: Intracerebral haemorrhage. Accuracy of computerised transverse axial scanning in predicting the underlying aetiology. Lancet, 1:1, 1976.

195. Lipton, R.B., et al.: Lobar vs. thalamic and basal ganglion hemorrhage: clinical and radiographic features. J. Neurol., 234:86, 1987.

196. Scott, W.R., and Miller, B.R.: Intracerebral hemorrhage with rapid recovery. Arch. Neurol., 42:133, 1985.

197. Mosdal, C., Jensen, G., Sommer, W., et al.: Spontaneous intracerebral haematomas. Clinical and computertomographic findings and long-term outcome after surgical treatment. Acta Neurochir. (Wien), 83:92, 1986.

198. Tanaka, Y., et al.: Lobar intracerebral hemorrhage: Etiology and a long-term follow-up study of 32 patients. Stroke, 17:51, 1986.

199. Fieschi, C., et al.: Changing prognosis of primary intracerebral hemorrhage: Results of a clinical and computed tomographic follow-up study of 104 patients. Stroke, 19:192, 1988.

200. Masdeu, J.C., and Rubino, F.A.: Management of lobar intracerebral hemorrhage: Medical or surgical. Neurology, 34:381, 1984.

201. Vinters, H.V.: Cerebral amyloid angiopathy—a critical review. Stroke, 18:311, 1987.

202. Gilbert, J.J., and Vinters, H.V.: Cerebral amyloid angiopathy: Incidence and complications in the aging brain. I. Cerebral hemorrhage. Stroke, 14:915, 1983.

203. Yamada, M., Tsukagoshi, H., Otomo, E., et al.: Cerebral amyloid angiopathy in the aged. J. Neurol., 234:371, 1987.

204. Masuda, J., Tanaka, K., Ueda, K., et al.: Autopsy study of incidence and distribution of cerebral amyloid angiopathy in Hisayama, Japan. Stroke, 19:205, 1988.

205. Glenner, G.G., Henry, J.H., and Fujihara, S.: Congophilic angiopathy in the pathogenesis of Alzheimer's degeneration. Ann. Pathol., 1:120, 1981.

206. Vinters, H.V., and Gilbert, J.J.: Cerebral amyloid angiopathy: Incidence and complications in the aging brain. II. The distribution of amyloid vascular changes. Stroke, 14:924, 1983.

207. Ferreiro, J.A., Ansbacher, L.E., and Vinters, H.V.: Stroke related to cerebral amyloid angiopathy. The significance of systemic vascular disease. J. Neurol. In press.

208. Ishii, N., Nishihara, Y., and Horie, A.: Amyloid angiopathy and lobar cerebral haemorrhage. J. Neurol. Neurosurg. Psychiatry, 47:1203, 1984.

209. Jellinger, K.: Cerebrovascular amyloidosis with cerebral hemorrhage. J. Neurol., 214:195, 1977.

210. Mandybur, T.I., and Bates, S.R.D.: Fatal massive intracerebral hemorrhage complicating cerebral amyloid angiopathy. Arch. Neurol., 35:246, 1978.

211. Kalyan-Raman, U.P., and Kalyan-Raman, K.: Cerebral amyloid angiopathy causing intracranial hemorrhage. Ann. Neurol., 16:321, 1984.

212. Finelli, P.F, Kessimian, N., and Bernstein, P.W.: Cerebral amyloid angiopathy manifesting as recurrent intracerebral hemorrhage. Arch. Neurol., 41:330, 1984.

213. Okazaki, H., Reagan, T.J., and Campbell, R.J.: Clini-

copathologic studies of primary cerebral amyloid angiopathy. Mayo Clin. Proc., *54*:22, 1979.

214. Mandybur, T.I.: Cerebral amyloid angiopathy: The vascular pathology and complications. J. Neuropathol. Exp. Neurol., *45*:79, 1986.

215. Vanley, C.T., Aguilar, M.J., Kleinhenz, R.J., et al.: Cerebral amyloid angiopathy. Hum. Pathol., *12*:609, 1981.

216. Regli, F., Vonssattel, J.-P., Perentes, E., et al.: L'angiopathie amyloïde cérébrale. Rev. Neurol. (Paris), *137*:181, 1981.

217. Okoye, M.I., and Watanabe, I.: Ultrastructural features of cerebral amyloid angiopathy. Hum. Pathol., *13*:1127, 1982.

218. Torack, R.M.: Congophilic angiopathy complicated by surgery and massive hemorrhage. A light and electron microscopic study. Am. J. Pathol., *81*:349, 1975.

219. Hinton, D.R., Dolan, E., and Sima, A.A.F.: The value of histopathological examination of surgically removed blood clot in determining the etiology of spontaneous intracerebral hemorrhage. Stroke, *15*:517, 1984.

220. Glenner, G.G., and Wong, C.W.: Alzheimer's disease: Initial report of the purification and characterization of a novel cerebrovascular amyloid protein. Biochem. Biophys. Res. Commun., *120*:885, 1984.

221. Glenner, G.G., and Wong, C.W.: Alzheimer's disease and Down's syndrome: Sharing of a unique cerebrovascular amyloid fibril protein. Biochem. Biophys. Res. Commun., *122*:1131, 1984.

222. Pardridge, W.M., et al.: Amyloid angiopathy of Alzheimer's disease: Amino acid composition and partial sequence of a 4,200-Dalton peptide isolated from cortical microvessels. J. Neurochem., *49*:1394, 1987.

223. Kang, J., et al.: The precursor of Alzheimer's disease amyloid A4 protein resembles a cell-surface receptor. Nature, *325*:733, 1987.

224. Tanzi, R.E., et al.: Amyloid beta protein gene: cDNA, mRNA distribution, and genetic linkage near the Alzheimer locus. Science, *235*:880, 1987.

225. Wong, C.W., Quaranta, V., and Glenner, G.G.: Neuritic plaques and cerebrovascular amyloid in Alzheimer disease are antigenically related. Proc. Natl. Acad. Sci. U.S.A., *82*:8729, 1985.

226. Vinters, H.V., Pardridge, W.M., and Yang, J.: Immunohistochemical study of cerebral amyloid angiopathy: Use of an antiserum to a synthetic 28-amino-acid peptide fragment of the Alzheimer's disease amyloid precursor. Hum. Pathol., *19*:214, 1988.

227. Vinters, H.V., Pardridge, W.M., Secor, D.L., et al.: Immunohistochemical study of cerebral amyloid angiopathy. II. Enhancement of immunostaining using formic acid pretreatment of tissue sections. Am. J. Pathol., *133*:150, 1988.

228. Masters, C.L., et al.: Neuronal origin of a cerebral amyloid: Neurofibrillary tangles of Alzheimer's disease contain the same protein as the amyloid of plaque cores and blood vessels. EMBO J., *4*:2757, 1985.

229. Guiroy, D.C., et al.: Amyloid of neurofibrillary tangles of Guamanian parkinsonism-dementia and Alzheimer disease share identical amino acid sequence. Proc. Natl. Acad. Sci. U.S.A., *84*:2073, 1987.

230. Vinters, H.V., Miller, B.L., and Pardridge, W.M.: Brain amyloid and Alzheimer disease. Ann. Intern. Med., *109*:41, 1988.

231. Jensson, O., et al.: Hereditary central nervous system gamma-trace amyloid angiopathy and stroke in Icelandic families. In: *Amyloidosis.* Edited by G.G. Glenner, et al. New York, Plenum Pub. Corp., 1986, pp. 789-801.

232. Jensson, O., et al.: Hereditary cystatin C (gamma trace) amyloid angiopathy of the CNS causing cerebral hemorrhage. Acta. Neurol. Scand., *76*:102, 1987.

233. Gates, P.C., et al.: Primary intraventricular hemorrhage in adults. Stroke, *17*:872, 1986.

234. Verma A., Maheshwari, M.C., and Bhargava, S.: Spontaneous intraventricular haemorrhage. J. Neurol., *234*:233, 1987.

235. Darby, D.G., et al.: Primary intraventricular hemorrhage: Clinical and neuropsychological findings in a prospective stroke series. Neurology, *38*:68, 1988.

236. Scheinberg, P.: Dementia due to vascular disease—a multifactorial disorder. Stroke, *19*:1291, 1988.

237. Tomlinson, B.E., Blessed, G., and Roth, M.: Observations on the brains of non-demented old people. J. Neurol. Sci., *7*:331, 1968.

238. Tomlinson, B.E., Blessed, G., and Roth, M.: Observations on the brains of demented old people. J. Neurol. Sci., *11*:205, 1970.

239. Hachinski, V.C., Lassen, N.A., and Marshall, J.: Multi-infarct dementia. A cause of mental deterioration in the elderly. Lancet, *2*:207, 1974.

240. Hyman, B.T., Van Hoesen, G.W., Damasio, A.R., et al.: Alzheimer's disease: Cell-specified pathology isolates the hippocampal formation. Science, *225*:1168, 1984.

241. Ball, M.J., et al.: A new definition of Alzheimer's disease: A hippocampal dementia. Lancet, *1*:14, 1985.

242. Torvik, A., Endresen, G.K.M., Abrahamsen, A.F., et al.: Progressive dementia caused by an unusual type of generalized small vessel thrombosis. Acta Neurol. Scand., *47*:137, 1971.

243. Fields, W.S.: Multi-infarct dementia. Neurol. Clin., *4*:405, 1986.

244. Bell, M.A., and Ball, M.J.: The correlation of vascular capacity with the parenchymal lesions of Alzheimer's disease. Can. J. Neurol. Sci., *13*:456, 1986.

245. Miyakawa, T., Shimoji, A., Kuramoto, R., et al.: The relationship between senile plaques and cerebral blood vessels in Alzheimer's disease and senile dementia. Virchows Arch. [Cell Pathol.], *40*:121, 1982.

246. Miyakawa, T., and Uehara, Y.: Observations of amyloid angiopathy and senile plaques by the scanning electron microscope. Acta Neuropathol. (Berl.), *48*:153, 1979.

247. Hassler, O.: Arterial deformities in senile brains. The occurrence of the deformities in a large autopsy series and some aspects of their functional significance. Acta Neuropathol. (Berl.), *8*:219, 1967.

248. Olszewski, J.: Subcortical arteriosclerotic encephalopathy. Review of the literature on the socalled Binswanger's disease and presentation of two cases. World Neurology, *3*:359, 1962.

249. Burger, P.C., Burch, J.G., and Kunze, U.: Subcortical arteriosclerotic encephalopathy (Binswanger's disease). A vascular etiology of dementia. Stroke, *7*:626, 1976.

250. Huang, K., Wu, L., and Luo, Y.: Binswanger's disease: Progressive subcortical encephalopathy or multi-infarct dementia? Can. J. Neurol. Sci., *12*:88, 1985.

251. Babikian, V., and Ropper, A.H.: Binswanger's disease: A review. Stroke, *18*:2, 1987.

252. Lotz, P.R., Ballinger, W.E. Jr., and Quisling, R.G.: Subcortical arteriosclerotic encephalopathy: CT spec-

trum and pathologic correlation. A.J.N.R., 7:817, 1986.

253. Goto, K., Ishii, N., and Fukasawa, H.: Diffuse white-matter disease in the geriatric population. A clinical, neuropathological, and CT study. Radiology, 141:687, 1981.

254. Salama, J., et al.: Post-anoxic delayed encephalopathy with leukoencephalopathy and non-hemorrhagic cerebral amyloid angiopathy. Clin. Neuropathol., 5:153, 1986.

255. Dubas, F., Gray, F., Roullet, E., et al.: Leucoencéphalopathies artériopathiques (17 cas anatomo-cliniques). Rev. Neurol. (Paris), 14:93, 1985.

256. Gray, F., Dubas, F., Roullet, E., et al.: Leukoencephalopathy in diffuse hemorrhagic cerebral amyloid angiopathy. Ann. Neurol., 18:54, 1985.

257. Brun, A., and Englund, E.: A white matter disorder in dementia of the Alzheimer type: A pathoanatomical study. Ann. Neurol., 19:253, 1986.

258. Drayer, B.P.: Imaging of the aging brain. Part I. Normal findings. Radiology, 166:785, 1988.

259. Drayer, B.P.: Imaging of the aging brain. Part II. Pathologic conditions. Radiology, 166:797, 1988.

260. Awad, I.A., et al.: Incidental subcortical lesions identified on magnetic resonance imaging in the elderly. I. Correlation with age and cerebrovascular risk factors. Stroke, 17:1084, 1986.

261. McQuinn, B.A., and O'Leary, D.H.: White matter lucencies on computed tomography, subacute arteriosclerotic encephalopathy (Binswanger's disease), and blood pressure. Stroke, 18:900, 1987.

262. Awad, I.A., Johnson, P.C., Spetzler, R.F., et al.: Incidental subcortical lesions identified on magnetic resonance imaging in the elderly. II. Postmortem pathological correlations. Stroke, 17:1090, 1986.

263. Hachinski, V.C., Potter, P., and Merskey, H.: Leuko-araiosis. Arch. Neurol., 44:21, 1987.

264. Steingart, A., et al.: Cognitive and neurologic findings in subjects with diffuse white matter lucencies on computed tomographic scan (leuko-araiosis). Arch. Neurol., 44:32, 1987.

265. Steingart, A., et al.: Cognitive and neurologic findings in demented patients with diffuse white matter lucencies on computed tomographic scan (leuko-araiosis). Arch. Neurol., 44:36, 1987.

266. Inzitari, D., et al.: Vascular risk factors and leuko-araiosis. Arch. Neurol., 44:42, 1987.

267. Ishii, N., Nishihara, Y., and Imamura, T.: Why do frontal lobe symptoms predominate in vascular dementia with lacunes? Neurology, 36:340, 1986.

268. Ishii, N., and Nishihara, Y.: Vascular dementia: Correlation between the clinical manifestations and the localization of lesions. Progress Clin. Neurosciences, 1:105, 1987.

269. Liston, E.H., and La Rue, A.: Clinical differentiation of primary degenerative and multi-infarct dementia: A critical review of the evidence. Part I: Clinical studies. Biol. Psychiatry, 18:1451, 1983.

270. Liston, E.H., and La Rue, A.: Clinical differentiation of primary degenerative and multi-infarct dementia: A critical review of the evidence. Part II: Pathological studies. Biol. Psychiatry, 18:1467, 1983.

271. O'Brien, M.D.: Vascular dementia is underdiagnosed. Arch. Neurol., 45:797, 1988.

272. Brust, J.C.M.: Vascular dementia is overdiagnosed. Arch. Neurol., 45:799, 1988.

273. Grotta, J.C.: Current medical and surgical therapy for cerebrovascular disease. N. Engl. J. Med., 317:1505, 1987.

CHAPTER 3

Dementia

SERGE BRION
JACQUELINE MIKOL
JOEL PLAS
ANCA BEREANU

Vascular Dementia

JACQUELINE MIKOL

It has been known for nearly a century and a half that dementia can be caused by vascular pathology of the brain.[1] One of the causes of dementia, according to Klippel,[2] is atherosclerosis of cerebral blood vessels. Binswanger agreed with Klippel's view and described a form of dementia caused by cerebral arteriosclerotic degeneration.[3] In those early days the word dementia was a general term which included a multitude of diseases with loosely defined etiologies. With time the clinicopathologic characteristics of separate diseases such as Alzheimer's disease were clearly delineated from the large group of undifferentiated dementia.[4] The importance of lacunes (holes) in the brain caused by vascular pathologic disorders and their association with neurologic diseases was underlined at the turn of the century by Pierre Marie.[5,6] During the following decades the clinical diagnosis of vascular and arteriopathic dementia was frequently noted but few reports on the subject were published until the 60s.[7,8]

Tomlinson, Blessed, and Roth[9] reported that in a large series of elderly demented patients the most frequent neuropathologic lesion was that of multiple small or large cerebral infarcts. Such studies resulted in the definition of multi-infarct dementia (MID)[10] [Figs. 3–1 and 3–2]. Many MIDs are caused not by intracerebral but by extracranial vascular disease due to thrombosis, embolism, or heart disease.

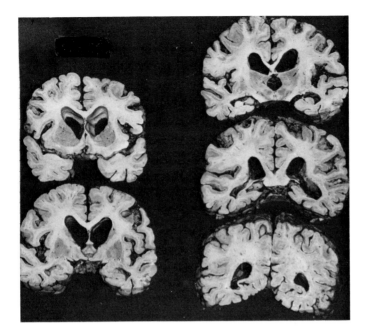

Fig. 3-1. Multiple infarct dementia. Coronal section of the cerebral hemispheres showing infarcts involving superficial gyri, basal ganglia and thalami; note the enlarged ventricles. Myelin, Wolcke stain.

Neuro-imaging has given new insight into the different aspects of MID. The concept that dementia can be caused by cerebral arteriosclerosis is still a matter of debate.[11,12] Different subgroups of MID have been established.[9,10]

In an extensive study of the literature,[16] a constant relationship between the prevalence of vascular disease and age has been found with an estimated prevalence rate doubling every 5.1 years up to the age of about 95. The rates tend to be higher among males. MID accounts for approximately 12 to 20% of dementia of advanced age, while associated forms with Alzheimer's disease (AD) represent 16 to 20% of the patients.[9,15,17]

We will briefly review the neuropathology of the various causes or associations of MIDs, such as the diffuse and focal lesions, the cardiovascular causes, and the associations of MID with other diseases.

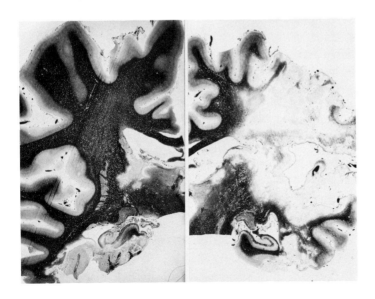

Fig. 3-2. Multiple infarcts. Myelin preparations showing infarcts in both cerebral hemispheres of the same brain. Celloidin. Wolcke stain. ×1.75.

PATHOLOGY

DIFFUSE FORMS OF VASCULAR PATHOLOGY

Multiple Infarcts as a Cause of Dementia. Large cerebral infarcts that destroy cortical connections are sometimes observed in MID.[18] A volume of more than 100 ml of cerebral softening, whatever its distribution, may be present in demented patients.[9] There is a positive correlation between reduced cerebral blood flow and the degree of dementia.[19] The lesions are situated bilaterally in the cortex, the white matter, the basal ganglia, the brainstem, and rarely, a laminar cortical distribution[8] [case 3 V] [Fig. 3–3]. Delay and Brion [8] have described two groups of changes; in older patients the infarcts were diffuse, predominant in the periventricular white matter; clinically, the psychiatric features were similar to those observed in senile dementia, but a history of strokes with higher function disturbances was noted; in the younger patients (presenile dementia) ischemic lesions were multiple but not diffuse, usually present at the base of the brain.

Granular Atrophy of the Cerebral Cortex. Cortical granular atrophy is a rare form of MID present in middle-aged or younger persons with a recurrent clinical course of long duration characterized by intellectual impairment and episodes of weakness or numbness of arms or arms and legs; the face is spared.[20,21] On gross examination, some gyri appear shrunken and punctuated with many small depressions [Fig. 3–4A]. The lesions are bilaterally symmetrical and located mainly along "the border zone" (watershed infarct) between the cortical areas of supply of the large cerebral arteries [Fig. 3–4B]. The cortical gyri affected include the middle frontal, the middle part of the ascending frontal and parietal, the posterior part of the superior parietal, the middle temporal, the middle and inferior occipital gyri; the cerebellar cortex is rarely involved. Microscopically, the lesions correspond to small punctate areas of necrosis of the cortex that accompany occlusion of small overlying leptomeningeal arteries[20-22] [Fig. 3–5]. Lower motor neuron lesions and neurogenic muscle atrophy have also been observed.[25] Lacunes may be present. The original reports of dementia associated with granular cortical atrophy designated thromboangiitis obliterans as the basic vascular pathology [see below]. Subsequently, it was shown that stagnation or reduction in cerebral blood flow in relation

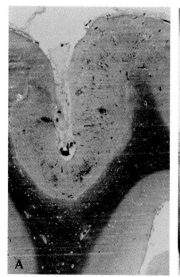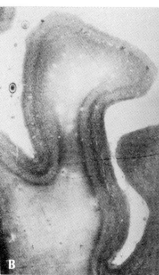

Fig. 3–3.   Multiple infarcts. A. Myelin preparation showing cortical hemorrhagic infarct. Celloidin. Wolcke. × 8.4. B. Infarcted white and gray matter: the spared IV lamina appears as a black line. Celloidin. Hematein-Phloxine-Luxol fast blue (H.P.L.) . ×5.6. C. Microscopic appearance of pale-staining area of cortical infarction. Celloidin. Nissl . ×82.5.

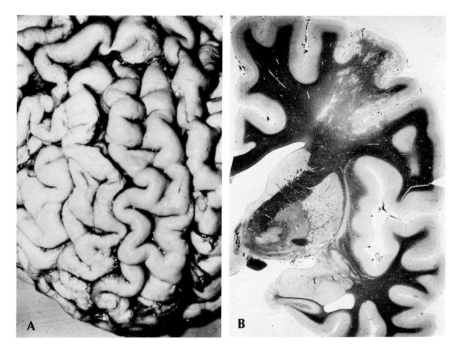

Fig. 3-4. Granular atrophy of the cortex. A. Note the depressions of the surface after removal of the meninges. B. Myelin preparation showing numerous small infarcts in the boundary zone between the cortical territories of the anterior and middle cerebral arteries. Celloidin. Wolcke.

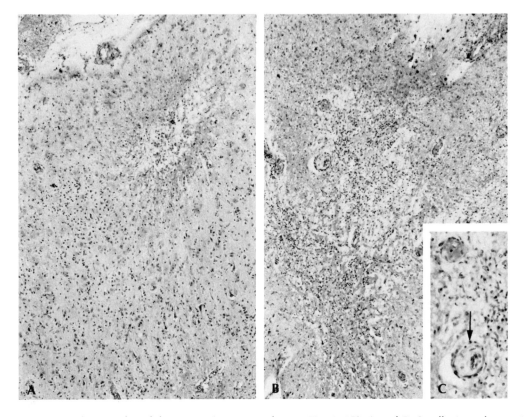

Fig. 3-5. Granular atrophy of the cortex (corresponding to Fig. 3-4B). A and B. Small triangular cortical infarcts under the surface. ×175. C. Note the endarteritis in the vessels observed on figure B. Celloidin. Hematoxylin-eosin (H&E). A, B. ×87.5.

with cardiac disturbances or atherosclerosis would also result in occlusion of the microvasculature.[26-28] Such lesions have been noted in 3 cases of generalized small vessel thrombosis (arteries and veins) in patients under 60 years of age;[29] the main ischemic lesions were found in the brain and the main symptom was a progressive dementia. Sourander and Walinder[20] described a similar vasculopathy in young adults of the same family characterized by autosomal dominant transmission; small arterial vessels in the pia-arachnoid and in the deep cerebral regions were affected and contained PAS+ deposits in the thickened intima and the media. Another family of 16 patients was studied by Sonninen et al.:[31] in the one postmortem study, the lesions involved the basal ganglia, the thalamus, the periventricular matter and were limited to a small occipital cyst in the cortex. The recent review of the 25 reported cases[25] has emphasized the frequency of valvular or ischemic heart disease. Furthermore, it appears to be difficult to integrate the observations of arterial hyalinosis distributed in the border zone associated with or different from arteriosclerosis and dyshoric angiopathy.[32]

Lacunes. The frequency of lacunes as a cause of dementia has been inconsistently confirmed. Some degree of dementia was recognized in the description of "l'etat lacunaire" of Pierre Marie.[5] Lacunes correspond to small infarcts that lie in the deeper part of the cerebrum and brainstem. The reports of Fisher[33] have demonstrated their characteristics: they range in size from large (1.5 to 2 cm) to small (3 to 4 mm); they are often multiple. The most common sites are the putamen, caudate, thalamus, pons, internal capsule, and the white matter [Fig. 3–6]. In large lacunes, the cause of the vascular occlusion is more often an occlusion of a penetrating branch or an atheromatous plaque. In small lacunes, the occlusion may be due to an embolus, a segmental arterial disorganization with or without enlargement, lipohyalinosis or thrombosis of a fusiform microaneurysm.[33,34] A new classification of the lacunes has been proposed.[25] Fisher has described three types of lacunes:[33,34] lacunes type I, containing non-occluded small vessels passing through; lacunes type II, which are the result of small hemorrhages, are unique and situated in basal ganglia or cerebral white matter; and lacunes type III, which are dilatations of the perivascular spaces, ranging in size from a few microns to large space occupying lesions.[36,37] In the patients, dementia cannot always be correlated with the number and situation of the lacunes. In 90% of the cases, lacunar infarcts are associated with systemic arterial hypertension.[34] Other vasculopathies such as Sneddon syndrome or thromboangiitis obliterans cerebri and sickle cell disease have been shown associated with dementia due to lacunar infarcts.[38]

Binswanger Disease (BD). BD is a progressive disease characterized by an early onset at age 25 to 30, dementia and pyramidal signs, inconstant hypertension, diffuse alopecia since youth and spondylitis deformans. Before the introduction of modern neuroimaging techniques, arteriosclerotic encephalopathy was diagnosed only at necropsy. The main clinical symptoms are acute strokes, seizures, subacute accumulation of focal deficits including pseudobulbar palsy, and pyramidal signs that develop into dementia. Pre-existing hypertension and other factors known to predispose to vascular disease are noted. A lengthy clinical course with clinical plateaus or improvement is usually observed.[39,42]

On gross examination there may be evidence of atheroma in the cervical extracranial vessels, the circle of Willis and its distal branches with a variable reduction of the lumen. A 75% reduction of the lumina of carotid vessels as well as a fresh thrombus of the vertebral arteries have been observed.[43] Examination of gross sections of the brain shows bilateral large patchy soft regions of the white matter which appear whitish or yellow [Fig. 3–7]. The lesions are situated primarily in the occipital or frontal lobe, exceptionally unilateral.[44] The ventricles are enlarged.

Histologic studies show variable pathologic changes of the white matter displaying chronic progressive ischemia from small areas of necrosis to large areas of pallor of myelin and gliosis; the arcuate U fibers are usually spared as well as the cortex[41,45-47] [Figs. 3–8A and B]. The terminal deep white matter arteries appear thickened, hyalinized with hypertrophy of the media and are often obliterated[48] [Fig. 3–8C]. Roman[49] considers that BD and lacunes are the

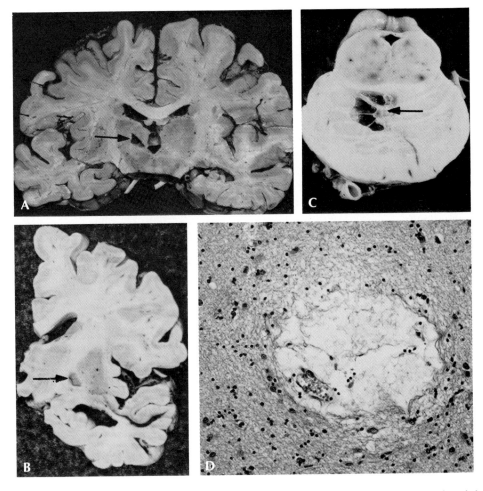

Fig. 3–6. Lacunes. Coronal slices of the brain showing large lacunes in the thalamus (A), the globus pallidus (B), and the pons (C). D. Lacune (etat crible) in the putamen. Paraffin. H&E . × 175.

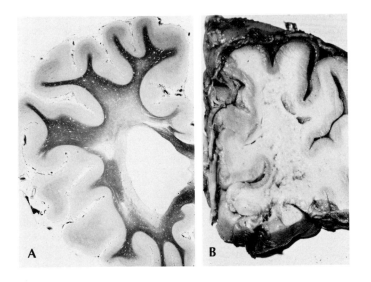

Fig. 3–7. Binswanger's disease. A. Myelin preparation showing patchy demyelination of white matter in the frontal lobe. Celloidin. Wolcke. B. Cavitations and softenings of the white matter (occipital lobe).

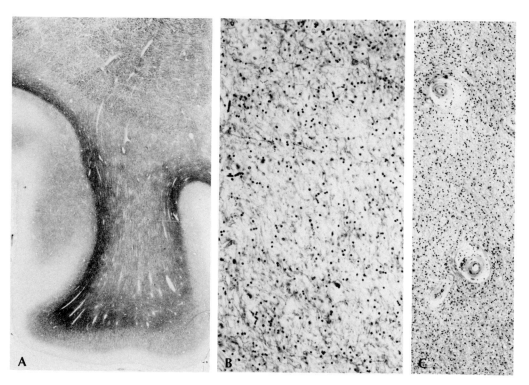

Fig. 3–8. Binswanger's disease. A. Myelin preparation showing pallor of the white matter with sparing of the arcuate U fibers. Celloidin. Wolcke . × 4. B. Demyelination of the white matter. Celloidin. Wolcke . × 100. C. Arteriosclerotic vessels in the white matter. Celloidin. H&E . × 100.

same disease, i.e., a lacunar dementia or a small-vessel dementia. Lacunes are specially frequent in the basal ganglia and thalamus [Fig. 3–9].

Different hypotheses have been considered concerning BD.[42,50] The disorder is a special vascular disease with tissue changes which are identical to those described in hypertensive arteriopathy with a more important alteration of the vessels. The hypertensive encephalopathy would be a factor in the genesis of the edema leading to fluid transudation and demyelinization. Recently, the role of poor perfusion of the white matter caused by a drop of blood pressure, cardiac failure or stenosis of large vessels, in the presence of a wide zone of ischemia has been emphasized.[42] Repeated episodes of chronic or acute hypo-and hyperfusion, alteration of the blood-brain barrier common to cerebral arteriopathic, and amyloid angiopathies have been suggested as the cause of BD.[51] Loss of myelin around the ventricles in the border zones and in the centrum semiovale appears to be due to transient episodes of cardiac failure

and chronic hypoxemia.[52,53] The cause of BD is unknown, but it has been suggested that BD is the result of a defective regulation of blood flow and microcirculation.[50,54–56]

Neuro-imaging studies (translucencies on CT scan, lesions of high signal intensity on MRI) have shown that patchy white matter changes are seen in BD and in normal aging.[57–61] Subcortical MRI lesions are present in arteriosclerosis, dilated perivascular spaces, and vascular ectasia.[59] These changes have been observed in BD and also in the lacunar state, systemic hypoperfusion, and multiple strokes.[62–67] The descriptive term of leukoaraiosis was proposed,[68] meaning a diminution of the density of representation of the white matter; in physical terms, it represents an accumulation of extra- and intracellular water and of small protein molecules in the brain lattice.[69] Its morphologic counterpart consists of paraventricular loss of white matter, axonal degeneration, secondary demyelination, multiple microinfarcts, and perifocal gliosis.[70–73] These data support "the uniform hypothesis

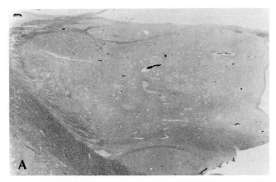

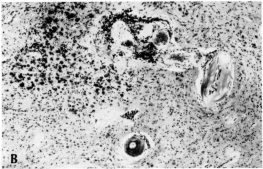

Fig. 3–9. A. Note several small infarcts or hemorrhage in the thalamus. B. Higher power view of a small hemorrhagic focus with hyaline thickening of the vessels. Celloidin. H&E. A . ×6.3; B . ×87.5.

that MRI provides a non-specific index of brain parenchymal alterations caused by aging and chronic vascular disease."[59] Hachinski[68] has shown that white matter changes are associated with intellectual impairment. Aharon-Peretz et al.[74] using quantitative studies have correlated this impairment with the enlargement of the third and lateral ventricles. A possible autosomal recessive transmission has been proposed.[75,76]

FOCAL FORMS OF VASCULAR PATHOLOGY

Dementia is not necessarily correlated with the destruction of a large amount of tissue and it can be caused by focal lesions in relevant cerebral territories. The existence of asymmetrical or unilateral forms is not as well documented as the bilateral lesions in the brain.

Bilateral Lesions of the Brain. Most of the bilateral lesions of the localized forms are situated in the territory of the posterior cerebral artery. However, as the exact topography

of the territory supplied by the intrinsic thalamic arteries is not individualized precisely, the occipital, temporal, and thalamic dementias will be described separately.

Occipital Vascular Lesions as a Cause of Dementia. Few observations have been reported. The patient described by Dide and Botcazo[77] had a Korsakoff syndrome with spatial disorientation, alexia, astereognosia, and hemianopsia; a bilateral infarct of the lingual lobe was present with an extension to the left postero-lateral thalamus. The patient described by Boudin et al.[78] had a cortical blindness in addition to Korsakoff syndrome; anatomically bilateral inferomesial occipital infarcts were associated with lesions of the splenium of the corpus callosum and of the fornices.

Temporal Vascular Lesions as a Cause of Dementia. There are reports of demented patients with partial or complete lesions of the hippocampi extending into neighboring temporal tissue sometimes associated with other degenerative disorders.[79–81] The distinction between dementia and amnesia in such cases is said to be difficult to establish clearly.[8,82–87]

Thalamic Vascular Lesions as a Cause of Dementia [Fig. 3–10]. There are several classical studies in which damage of the mediodorsal nucleus of the thalamus is regarded to be primarily responsible for amnesic or affective disorders;[88–90] the role of the mammillo-thalamic bundle of Vicq-d'Azyr has also been discussed.[8] Clinical features of thalamic dementia have been identified on the basis of anatomic or neuro-imaging correlations of published cases.[91–96] The behavioral disturbances are characterized by apathy, motor and verbal lack of spontaneity and responsiveness, affective indifference, and amnesia. Impaired attention may be present. Confabulation may be more prominent than dysphasia.[97] The patient reported by Bogaert et al.[98] had delusions without loss of memory and a bilateral degenerative lesion of the mediodorsal nucleus. Such findings accompany selective vascular or degenerative lesions of the thalamus involving the paramedian territories.[8,36,99] Castaigne et al.[91,100] have summarized the findings of the published pathologic cases and 6 personal cases.[36] In 75% of the cases paramedian infarcts affect the intraluminar and parafascicu-

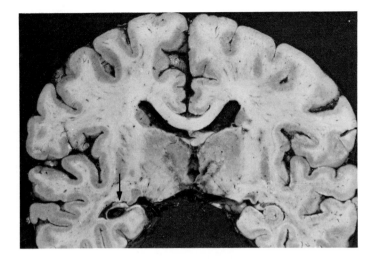

Fig. 3–10. Focal form of vascular dementia. Coronal section of cerebral hemispheres showing bilateral paramedian infarcts in the thalami and hemorrhagic lesion of the Ammon's horn (arrow).

lar nuclei, the inferior internal region of the mediodorsal nucleus, the inferior internal region of the central nucleus as well as the superior internal pole of the red nucleus[100] [Fig. 3–10].

Fronto-Cingulate Vascular Lesions as a Cause of Dementia. Dementia is frequently the clinical manifestation of primary cerebral degenerations or cerebral infections involving the fronto-cingulate gyrus, whereas it is rare in vascular lesions affecting this gyrus. The clinical manifestations are the result of infarcts in territories supplied by the anterior cerebral arteries. Clinically, in addition to paresis of lower limbs, there is some degree of mental disturbance, complex behavioral changes associated with the Korsakoff syndrome,[101] mutism, akinesia,[102] loss of empathy, and lack of attention.[103] Clinicopathologic correlations of the published cases reviewed by Escourolle and Gray[104] have emphasized the role of the complete disconnection between frontal lobes and the components of the limbic system. The relevance of the circuitry of the frontal association cortex to dementia has been analyzed recently.[105] The memory disturbances may be explained by the damage of the fornices. The lesions are due to arteriosclerosis of the anterior cerebral artery,[101–106] complications of aneurysms of the anterior communicating artery,[102,107–109] and surgery of tumors or arteriovenous malformations situated at the anterior part of the skull related to the vessels of the frontal lobe.[102,104,110]

Asymmetrical Vascular Lesions as a Cause of Dementia. The asymmetrical forms are rare and the analysis of the topography of the lesions has supported the notion of circuitry of the limbic system. The first case of Dide and Pezet[111] included a left occipital infarct and a right thalamic lesion. The case of Victor[80] was bitemporal, mostly confined to the left side with a bilateral destruction of hippocampo-mammillary connections. The case of Delay et al.[112] had a left temporo-occipital infarct with secondary degeneration of the left mammillary body and a lesion of the right mammillo-thalamic bundle. An asymmetry of lesions was also found in the case of Schenk who described a destruction of the posterior right hippocampus and the left frontal lobe from the pre-central areas to the cingulate gyrus. Boudin et al.[113] reported a case of dementia with involvement of the posterior left pillar of the fornix and the right cingulate gyrus.

Unilateral Forms of Cerebral Vascular Pathology As a Cause of Dementia. These are exceptional. The memory disturbances of the patient of Geschwind and Fusillo[114] disappeared after 2 months even though he had a right hippocampal lesion. A minute contralateral lesion of the laterodorsal nucleus of the thalamus was noted in a number of cases.[115–118]

Unilateral lesions more often give rise to psychic disturbances than to real dementia states. Such is the case, for instance, in the unilateral vascular lesions of the posterior part of the non-dominant hemisphere which produce a pseudo-dementia of depressive type.[119]

PATHOGENESIS OF VASCULAR DEMENTIA

A review of this subject is found in Chapter 2, hence, only a brief description is given here focused on points highlighted by Feigin and Budzilovich.[120] The vascular diseases which cause dysfunction of the CNS may simply be a manifestation of a systemic disease. Atherosclerosis is a disease process which most commonly affects the larger arteries of the CNS. Recent concepts emphasize some of the similarities between its pathogenesis and that of inflammation.[121]

Different categories of risk factors have been postulated: age, inheritance, sex, arterial hypertension, abnormalities of plasma lipids, diabetes, life style; thus the treatment of early factors may prevent the development of the disease, and the treatment of later factors responsible for the complications, may decrease the extent and severity of vascular dementia.[122]

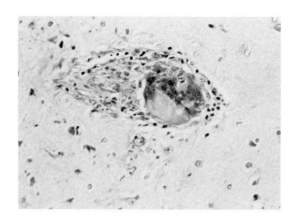

Fig. 3–11. Granulomatous angiitis. Cortical artery showing cellular infiltration including multinucleated giant cell. Paraffin. H&E . × 330.

Thus, hypertensive fibrinoid arteritis is less frequently a cause of vascular dementia because of the important progress of therapy. Fisher[34] has attributed the decreasing frequency of lacunes observed at postmortem examination to the effective treatment of hypertension.

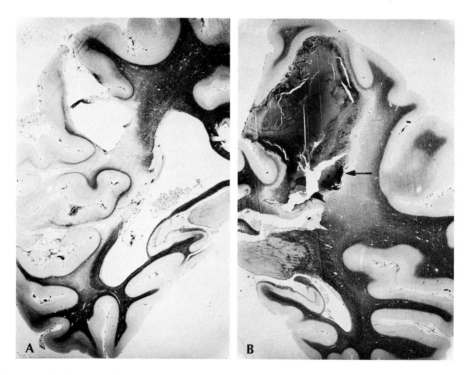

Fig. 3–12. Amyloid angiopathy. Myelin preparations showing bilateral associated lesions in a demented patient: middle artery cerebral infarct on the left (A) and fronto-parietal hematoma on the right (B). Celloidin. Wolcke . × 1.7.

The association of dementia and angiitis has recently been reviewed extensively.[123,124] Angiitis is an inflammatory pathologic condition of small arteries and arterioles (200 to 500 μm in diameter). [Fig. 3–11]. Parenchymal biopsy is sometimes necessary to confirm isolated cerebral angiitis before successful treatment.[125] Among the systemic necrotizing vasculitides, the most frequently observed is polyarteritis nodosa. Dementia related to giant cell arteritis was observed only in 1 out of 51 patients in a recent study.[126] Dementia was also seen in patients with rheumatoid arthritis[127] or systemic lupus erythematosis (SLE).[128,129] In a few cases it has been shown that MID in SLE was associated with antiphospholipid antibodies.[130] This association has also been recognized recently without evidence of systemic vasculitis or inflammatory condition.[131] Nearly half of a group of 61 patients with Cogan's syndrome had a psychiatric disorder.[123]

The role of cerebral amyloid angiopathy in dementia has been the subject of great interest to neuropathologists, geneticists, and molecular biologists [see Chaps. 2 and 13]. Recent studies on AD have permitted important progress in the knowledge of the structure of amyloid, the analysis of the A4 amyloid gene, and its relationship with abnormal protease inhibition.[132] Familial forms of hereditary cerebral hemorrhage with amyloidosis and dementia with dominant autosomic transmission have also been individualized. The frequency and importance of leukoencephalopathy in diffuse hemorrhagic cerebral amyloid angiopathy have been underlined[133,134] [Figs. 3–12 and 3–13].

Dementia is rarely observed in fibromuscular dysplasia.[135,136] It is present in Moya-Moya disease which affects mostly young people. Recently, several reports have discussed the common pathologic features present in throm-

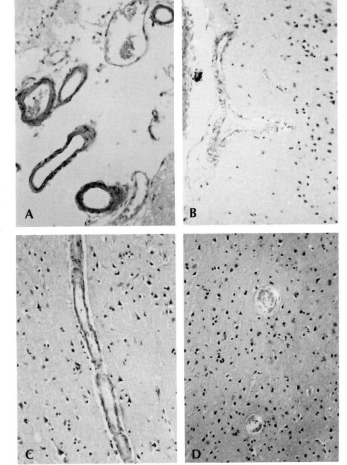

Fig. 3–13. Amyloid angiopathy. Leptomeningeal (A and B) and cortical arterioles (C and D) stained with Congo red, taken without (A and C) and with polarized light (B and D). Paraffin. Congo red. A . ×175; B. ×87.5; C . ×350; D .× 330.

boangiitis obliterans cerebri, Sneddon syndrome and cortico-meningeal angiomatosis of Divry and Van Bogaert.[38, 137-140] Neoplastic angioendotheliomatosis, a cause of subacute dementia, is now recognized as a true lymphoma.[141-145] Mitochondrial encephalomyopathy could be explained by a sporadic or familial mitochondrial angiopathy of the pial arterioles and small arteries.[143-145] Dementia due to a thrombophlebitis of the superior sagittal sinus has also been observed.[146]

The cardiac diseases which can result in dementia include myxoma, infections, and marantic endocarditis.[147,148] Vascular dementia of the hemodynamic type due to cardiac arrhythmias and systemic hypotension has been described.[149]

The association of Alzheimer-type senile dementia (SDAT) and vascular dementia has been reported. However, the loss of noradrenaline containing neurones may occur in Alzheimer disease but not in vascular dementia.[150] The nucleus basalis of Meynert is intact in MID but not in Alzheimer disease (AD).[151] It should also be noted that vascular lesions, except amyloid angiopathy, are rare in AD, and that senile plaques and neurofibrillary degeneration are present in old patients.

Degenerative Dementias

SERGE BRION,
JOEL PLAS, and
ANCA BEREANU

PICK'S DISEASE

Pick's disease is characterized clinically by a dementia usually without aphasia, agnosia, or apraxia and atrophy of the frontal and temporal lobes [Fig. 3–14]. There are variants of Pick's disease. Arnold Pick was interested in the symptomatology of all atrophies, whatever the anatomic substrata. Between 1892 and 1906 he described a total of 6 cases of focal atrophy. Two of these 6 cases were Alzheimer's disease, one was a vascular lesion resulting in a hemiplegia, another case was a Lissauer general paralysis, while only 2 cases corresponded to what would later be called Pick's disease.[152-156] Pick's disease was individualized and named in 1926 by Onari and Spatz.[157]

CLINICAL PRESENTATION[158-162]

The age of onset is mainly between 45 and 65 years, with exceptions at each end. There are reports of familial distribution.

THE FRONTAL AND TEMPORAL FORMS

The clinical signs at the onset are subtle but specific consisting of frontal deficits—apathy, indifference, and apragmatism. The absence of the aphasia, apraxia and agnosia, disturbed orientation and psychotic manifestations, features characteristic of Alzheimer's disease, differentiate the two entities. The specific features consist of gluttony, inappropriate jocularity and loss of the usual social restraints.

The onset is marked by stereotypes of language and behavior such as echolalia. There is also an abnormal behavior regarding food with gluttony-bulimia and ingestion of unusual matter. As the disease progresses, the patient may do stereotypical and absurd acts (i.e. the repeated purchase of orchestra tickets for the same show, attendance at all the encountered funerals in town, etc.).

The florid stage is characterized by an important global deficit. There is no significant disturbance of the symbolic functions except

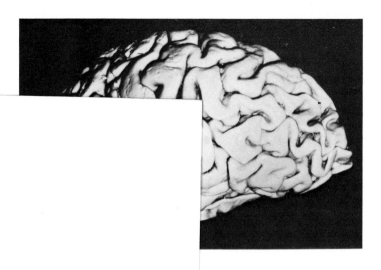

Fig. 3–14. P
view of the
and temporal

for occasional   sm and an apathy difficult to
nal aphasia" n   l et al.[163] described a syndrome
objects withou   ll the general aspects of these
defined by their   e acronym, PEMA, for palila-
or by another ot   utism, and amimia. The pa-
gory of a more g   cerebrate and comatose in the
called "the hand"), or by a universal word for   terminal stages and death is due to cachexia.
anything defined as "thing." The language def-   Rigidity occurs rarely and late in the course of
icit is also manifested by encephalopathy and   this disease, as opposed to Alzheimer's dis-
echolalic repetition of the last fragments of a   ease, despite the early involvement of the cau-
phrase spoken by the subject or others.   date nucleus. The evolution lasts 5 to 15 years
   There is no constructional apraxia and no vi-   and sometimes more. Diagnostic imaging stud-
sual agnosia. Ideomotor apraxia is encountered   ies are helpful: the CT scan shows a specific
only late in the disease, so that the patients   image of the frontal horn which has a globular
preserve praxia for a long time. They also   shape due to the cortical-subcortical atrophy
maintain correctly spatial dimensions and   and loss of relief of the atrophied caudate nu-
space construction, while these capabilities are   cleus. The enlarged frontal ventricles are as-
lost early in Alzheimer's disease. Memory is   sociated with a dilation of the corresponding
practically spared for a long time and the pa-   superficial sulci and the second typical element
tients maintain a certain amnesic knowledge   on the CT scan is the enlargement of the an-
and a temporospatial orientation quite surpris-   terior part of the temporal ventricle in contrast
ing for their advanced degree of global intel-   with a normal posterior. There is marked at-
lectual deficits. There are a considerable num-   rophy of the frontal-temporal poles and of the
ber of negative signs worth mentioning. The   lateral temporal gyri. The occipital horn and
usual forms have no long tract involvement,   the posterior aspects of the cortex are normal.
which means no pyramidal or visual field def-   MRI shows the same changes as the CT scan,
icits. Also, there are no psychotic changes, de-   but in more detail.[161] Psychomotor testing re-
lirious ideas of prejudice, or visual hallucina-   veals a pure frontal lobe syndrome with pres-
tions that are so typical for Alzheimer's   ervation of most of the language and memory
disease. Finally, there are no epileptic seizures functions. EEG is normal throughout the dis-
and the EEG maintains a normal tracing   ease and represents one of the strong negative
throughout the course of the disease. The   signs for Pick's disease, even in the terminal
course is relentlessly progressive and culmi-   stages.

PARIETAL FORMS

Pure parietal forms of Pick's disease have been described but their anatomic substratum remains debatable.[164] Recently, Cambier et al.[165] have reported such a pure form without dementia in a 57-year-old female with specific Pick's disease histologic findings predominant in the parietal lobe, whereas the classical forms show only late and secondary parietal lesions. There were no occipital lesions.

PICK'S DISEASE AND AMYOTROPHIC LATERAL SCLEROSIS (ALS)[166–168]

Twelve cases have been reported so far in the literature. This is a rare association that comprises specific Pick's disease and ALS lesions consisting of anterior horn and pyramidal tract involvement and in the cerebral cortex there is subcortical gliosis, neuronal loss without ballooning, without spongiform changes of the second cortical layer. It is difficult to decide whether this is an extension of Pick's disease over the ascending frontal area or just the fortuitous association of Pick's disease and ALS.

FAMILIAL CASES OF PICK'S DISEASE

Many familial cases were reported particularly in the German literature, and the topic was reviewed by Wilson and Bruce[160] and by Jervis.[169] Schmitz and Meyer[170] reported 3 sisters (the whole sibship) presenting the clinical signs of Pick's disease, confirmed at postmortem in one of the sisters. Malamud and Waggoner[169] described 15 affected members in 4 generations of the same family. Sjogren et al.[170] suggested that the cause of Pick's disease was genetic on the basis of a detailed genetic investigation of 18 cases of histologically verified Pick's disease.

JUVENILE CASES OF PICK'S DISEASE

Sjogren and his associates[170] diagnosed Pick's disease in adolescents in the families described above. We observed a 26-year-old woman, with typical clinical, radiologic, and histologic findings of Pick's disease.

THE ASSOCIATION OF PICK'S AND ALZHEIMER'S DISEASE IN THE SAME PATIENT

Cases having the clinical manifestations and the typical histologic findings of both Pick's and Alzheimer's disease have been reported.[173–175]

Pathology.[160,170,179] The atrophy is bilateral and involves the frontal lobe from the pole to the central sulcus [Fig. 3–14] particularly the middle frontal gyrus. The pathologic condition also involves all of the temporal lobes particularly at the poles, while the posterior two-thirds of superior temporal gyrus is spared. The parietal lobes have a late and more discrete involvement with diffuse lesions of the inferior parietal gyrus. The ascending parietal gyrus is always intact. The occipital lobe is always intact. The motor, sensory, visual, and auditory projections are spared except in those

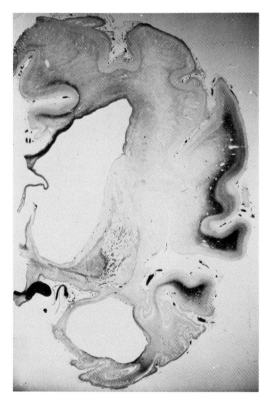

Fig. 3–15. Pick's disease. Myelin preparation showing gross fronto-temporal atrophy with marked enlargement of the ventricles and atrophy of the caudatus nucleus. The sparing of the posterior part of the superior temporal gyrus and of FA is noteworthy. Celloidin. Wolcke.

cases associating Pick's disease and ALS. There is a marked early atrophy of the caudate nucleus [Fig. 3–15].

Histologic studies underline the pathologic condition in the cerebral cortex, white matter, Ammon's horn, and basal ganglia. In the cortex there is a marked neuronal loss with gliosis and spongiosis severe in the advanced forms but limited to the second and third laminae in the milder forms[177] [Fig. 3–16]. The cellular changes consist of ballooning with cytoplasmic pallor and displacement of the nucleus in the large pyramidal neurons of the third and fifth laminae [Fig. 3–16]. Small argentophilic bodies are present in the cytoplasm in the later stages of the disease [Fig. 3–17]. The small neurons of the superficial cortex have less obvious globular changes, and also contain a small argentophilic cytoplasmic body named Pick's body, a homogeneous fine fibrillary structure. Pick's bodies are demonstrated also with H&E stain as pale homogeneous bodies. Pick's bodies are present in the pyramidal cells of Am-

mon's horn, the dentate gyrus, amygdala and the small pyramidal cells of the fronto-temporal cortex[177] [Fig. 3–17].

Hirano bodies are frequently seen in the hippocampus. These are club-shaped bodies, bright red colored with H&E and brown with silver stain situated among the matrix cells [Fig. 3–18]. The white matter involvement in the early stages consists of a diffuse gliosis and demyelination, particularly evident in the subcortical area. The early gliotic changes have suggested that the origin of the disease is in the white matter.[178] Certain white matter tracts are more involved by this process notably the frontopontine and temporopontine tracts. The involvement of fronto temporopontine fascicles does not involve the nuclei pontis[179] [Fig. 3–19A]. As opposed to Alzheimer's disease, there are no senile plaques or neurofibrillary tangles present in Pick's disease.

In rare cases there is a massive, total neuronal loss in Ammon's horn with spongiogliosis similar to the cortex[180] [Fig. 3–19B]. The patho-

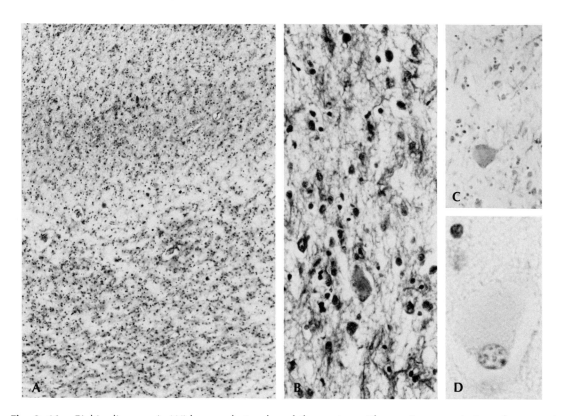

Fig. 3–16. Pick's disease. A. Widespread atrophy of the cortex with massive spongiosis and neuronal rarefaction. Celloidin. Nissl . × 87.5. B.—D. Different ballooned cells. B. Paraffin. Bodian silver stain . × 350. C. Celloidin. Nissl . × 350. D. Paraffin. Nissl . × 1230.

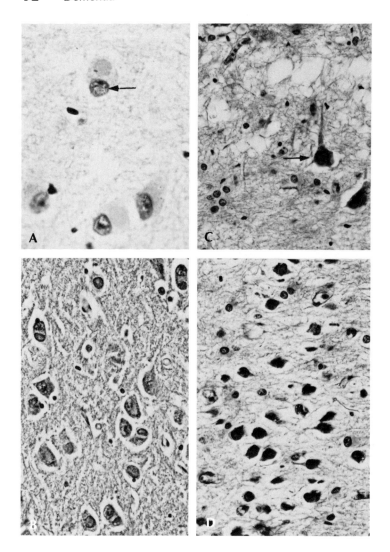

Fig. 3–17. Pick's disease. A. Pick's bodies in pyramidal cells. Note the presence of granulovacuolar degeneration appearing as small "beads" (arrow). B., C. Pick's bodies of different shapes and sizes in pyramidal cells. D. Round Pick's bodies in the cells of the gyrus dentatus. A. H&E . ×1200. B–D. Bodian. ×350.

logic condition in basal nuclei is particularly evident in the amygdala where many cells are ballooned and contain Pick's bodies, along with neuronal loss and diffuse gliosis, and in the caudate nuclei which shows a diffuse atrophic process and neuronal loss but less ballooning. Other regions, such as the thalamus, show little involvement except for occasional neuronal loss and gliosis.[181]

It has been shown by light microscopy immunocytochemistry that filaments inconstantly present in ballooned cells are antigenically normal neurofilaments,[182] with phosphorylated epitopes;[183] in our material no immunostaining of filaments was observed.[184] Studies with light microscopy immunocytochemistry have demonstrated that the Pick's

bodies share epitopes with neurofilaments,[182, 185–187] microtubules,[185] paired helical filaments[182,188,184,189] and tau proteins[190–192] [Fig. 3–20]. The same antigenic determinants have been demonstrated at ultrastructural level.[193] However, several polyclonal and monoclonal antibodies developed against neurofilaments do not recognize the Pick's bodies indicating that some neurofilament epitopes are either absent or inaccessible in these inclusions.[182,184,193] Recently ubiquitin, a protein involved in the degradation of short-lived and abnormal proteins has also been shown with light and electron microscopy immunocytochemistry in Pick's body.[294] Furthermore, Pick's filaments were resistant to the ionic detergent, sodium dodecyl sulfate, a solvent of

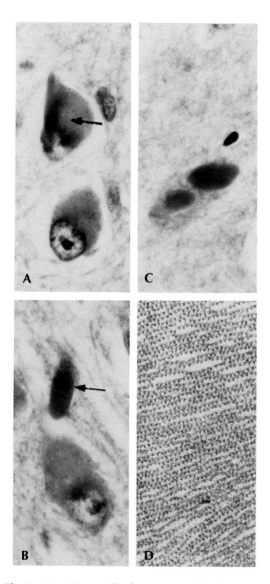

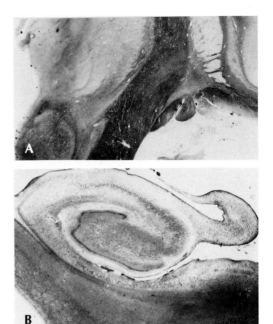

Fig. 3–19. Pick's disease. A. Myelin preparation. Note degeneration of the temporo-pontine tract close to the inferior part of the globus pallidus. Celloidin. Wolcke . ×12.5. B. Rarefaction of the neurons of CA1 (N-LFB) . ×6.2.

Fig. 3–18. Hirano's body. A. Hirano body stuck in the cytoplasm of a pyramidal neuron (arrow). B. Two bodies of different size in the same perikaryon. C. Hirano body free in the neuropile. D. Electron micrograph of a Hirano body showing a regular lattice punctated by regularly spaced dark dots. A.B.D. paraffin. H × E × 825. D. Uranyl acetate. Lead citrate × 70 000.

the normal neuronal cytoskeleton.[193] These insolubility characteristics and the results of immunostainings are similar to those of the paired helical filaments of Alzheimer's disease. Both involve altered components of the normal neuronal cytoskeleton. The chemical composition of Hirano bodies is not known. Epitopes of actin have been demonstrated in these structures[195] as well as actinin, vinculin, tropomyosin,[196] and tau protein.[197] These findings suggest that Hirano bodies are derived from neuronal microfilaments.

The electron microscopy studies[198–201] of biopsied specimens from the brain of patients with Pick's disease show that the large abnormally ballooned neurons show a loss of the usual organelles such as endoplasmic reticulum and mitochondria. These ballooned neurons contain variable amounts of abnormal neurofilaments.[182,202] The characteristic Pick's bodies present in small neurons consist of filaments measuring 10 to 12 nm in the cytoplasm and often surrounded by lipofuscin [Fig. 3–21].

PROGRESSIVE SUBCORTICAL GLIOSIS (PSG)

Progressive subcortical gliosis is an organic disease of the presenile dementia group manifested clinically by depressive psychosis with a frontal lobe syndrome.[174,203–205] Anatomically, there is a subcortical gliosis of the frontal, tem-

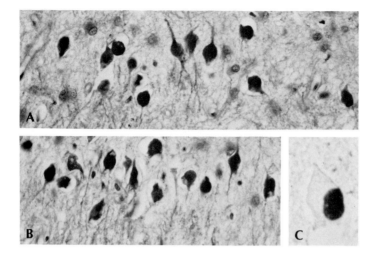

Fig. 3-20. Pick's disease. A.—B. Immunostaining of Pick's bodies of the gyrus dentatus (same case as 17 D) using the 85 to 45 antisera (kindly given by C. Masters), developed against amyloid core of senile plaques and amyloid congophilic angiopathy. C. Immunostaining of Pick's body by anti-tau. Paraffin. Avidin-Biotin-Complex-HRP or AEC. A.-B. ×350; C . ×670.

poral, and occasionally, of the parietal areas. The disease was described in 1949 by Neumann.[174] Pick's disease and PSG have a common anatomical involvement but important clinical differences. The disease was described by Oksala[212] in 1920 under the name of pre-senile pernicious psychosis or Kraepelin's disease. Oksala noted the organic depressive picture and the neuronal pyknosis in the cerebral cortex but not the subcortical gliosis. It is difficult to determine whether this disease is a separate disease; familial and sporadic forms

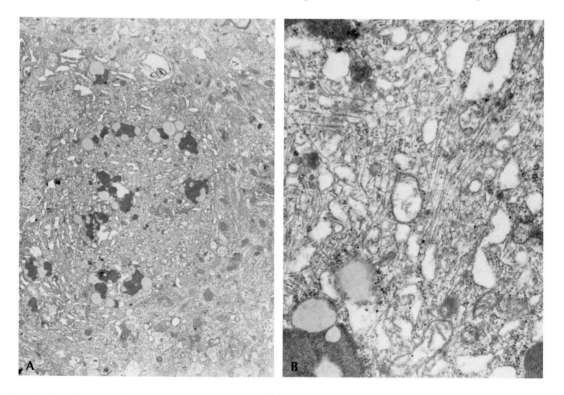

Fig. 3-21. Electron microscopy photographs of Pick's body (cortical biopsy in the right superior frontal gyrus). A. Cluster of filaments surrounded by lipofuscin deposits, without limiting membrane, in the perikaryon of a small neuron. B. Higher power view showing the straight filaments, 12 nm wide, mixed with vacuoles, lipofuscin and core dense vesicles. Uranyl acetate—lead citrate. A . ×4500. B . ×31.700.

have been described.[207,208] The incidence may be higher than thought previously according to Brun and Englund[215] who reported 10 cases in 1987 indicating that there may be many psychiatric patients with the disease that have not been diagnosed.

CLINICAL PRESENTATION

The clinical manifestations include depression accompanied by a frontal lobe syndrome often associated with disorientation, a feature absent from the pure frontal lobe syndrome. Psychosis may also be encountered. The symptomatology is thus a mixture of Pick's and Alzheimer's disease features. The CT is usually normal and is without the ventricular enlargement or atrophy seen in the other presenile dementias. The EEG frequently shows abnormal waves and spikes in contrast to Pick's disease where the EEG is normal. Besides the classical forms with frontal predominance, there are pure temporal forms with progressive aphasia. These are often erroneously considered typical Pick's disease since the underlying process is a subcortical gliosis.

PATHOLOGY

The main lesion is a superficial subcortical gliosis in the frontal, temporal and sometimes parietal lobes and a patchy loss of cortical neurons[206] [Fig. 3–22]. Later a cortical laminar spongiosis appears between the first and the second cortical layers with small aligned vacuoles representing degenerated dendritic processes [Fig. 3–23].[209] Verity[210] reported gliosis in the thalamus and olivary complex of the medulla. Electron microscopic changes are nonspecific. A familial form [208,211] of progressive subcortical gliosis has been described as well as sporadic and partial forms.[209,210] Congophilic vasculopathy has been described in one sporadic case of this disease.[212]

AMYOTROPHIC LATERAL SCLEROSIS (ALS) AND DEMENTIA

There are different clinical presentations of the association of ALS and dementia: (1) Pick's or Alzheimer's presenile dementia preceding ALS, (2) Creutzfeldt-Jakob's disease with amy-

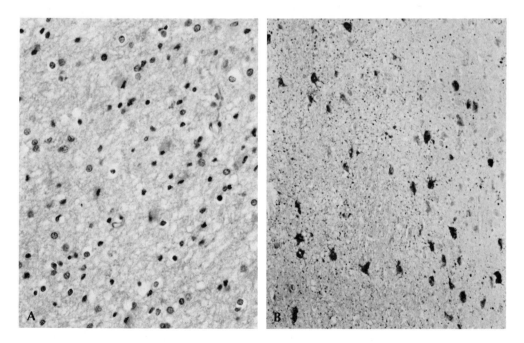

Fig. 3–22. Progressive subcortical gliosis. A. Astrocytosis with mild spongiosis of the white matter. B. Immunostaining of astrocytes of the white matter using antibodies developed against the glial fibrillary acidic protein. Paraffin. HPL. A . × 330—B . × 165.

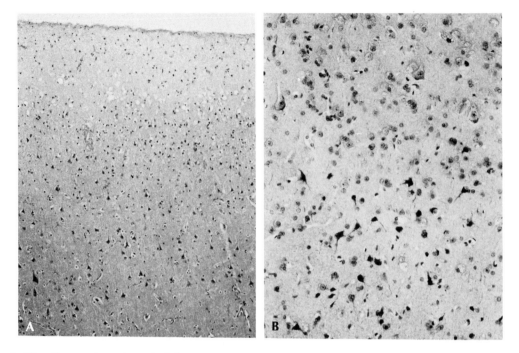

Fig. 3–23.   Progressive subcortical gliosis. Postmortem examination. A. Laminar spongiosis of cortico-frontal layer II. B. Pyknotic cortical neurons. Paraffin. HPL. A . × 82.5—B . × 165.

otrophy, (3) ALS preceding dementia, and (4) the ALS-Parkinson-dementia of Guam.[213]

PICK'S, ALZHEIMER'S DISEASE AND ALS

Three reports concern an association of Alzheimer's disease and ALS.[221-223] The dementia began in the fourth decade of life. At postmortem there were numerous neurofibrillary tangles and senile plaques throughout the cortex. Lowenberg and Waggoner[214] noted the presence of senile plaques in the gray substance of the spinal cord. Barret[215] noted lesions of the cortical spinal tracts.

The association of Pick's disease with ALS is more frequent.[167] In such cases the dementia begins in the fourth and fifth decades and eventually the clinical manifestations of ALS are present. The histologic lesions are typical of Pick's disease, as described above and tend to be present in the hippocampal uncus or in the frontal and temporal lobe. The lesions in the cortex and in the spinal cord are evident though dispersed. Recently, the following case was reported. A 46-year-old woman began with paranoia and eventually the clinical man-

ifestations of ALS. On postmortem there was noted an important lesion of the dorsal medium nucleus of the thalamus and a loss of neurons and gliosis[216] [Fig. 3–24].

CREUTZFELDT-JAKOB DISEASE AND AMYOTROPHY

This is a rare and debated clinicopathologic association noted for the length of its evolution associated with discrete gliosis and spongiosis limited to the superficial lamina of the cerebral cortex.[217,218] Masses of glial nodules have been noted in the spinal cord in one case.

AMYOTROPHIC LATERAL SCLEROSIS PRECEDING DEMENTIA

There are a number of cases where the patient first has a dementia, later with evidence of the amyotrophic lateral sclerosis disease. The cerebral lesions are in the frontal temporal lobes. Histologic examination shows spongiosis, gliosis, and loss of neurons in the second and third laminae [Fig. 3–25]. This is associated with lesions in the medulla oblongata and in the spinal cord, such as loss of interior horn

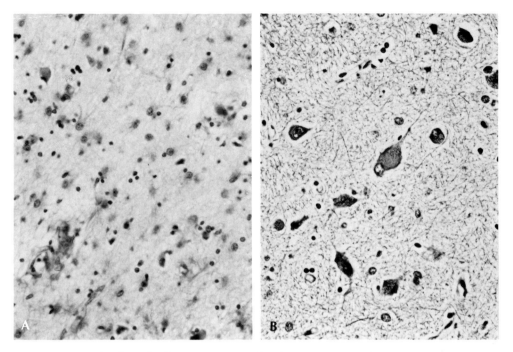

Fig. 3–24. Amyotrophic lateral sclerosis (ALS)—Pick's disease. A. Note the swollen neurons and gliosis. B. Pick's bodies in neurons in the temporal cortex. A. Celloidin. HPL . × 175. B. paraffin. Bodian . × 330.

Fig. 3–25. ALS—Dementia. A. Frontal cortical spongiosis. B. Higher power view of the spongiosis of layer II overlined by gliosis of the subpial layer. Celloidin. HPL. A . ×35—B . ×202.

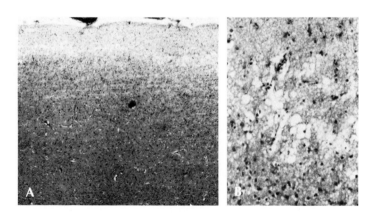

cells and in the motor neurons of the medulla oblongata and involvement of the cortical spinal tracts. On the basis of the clinical evolution it would appear that the cerebral lesions appear first followed by those in the brainstem and the spinal cord unless these were examples of an association of two separate diseases.[217,219]

PARKINSON DEMENTIA COMPLEX OF GUAM

This disease afflicts the Chamorro population of Guam and consists of parkinsonism as-

sociated with dementia and/or a variant of amyotrophic lateral sclerosis. The disease afflicts mostly males between the ages of 50 to 60. The presentation is usually that of Alzheimer type dementia and loss of cortico-spinal function. Death occurs within 4 years. Gross examination of the brain reveals frontal temporal cortical atrophy and depigmentation of the substantia nigra. On histologic examination one sees the widespread presence of neurofibrillary tangles and neuronal loss throughout the CNS. Interestingly enough, there are neither senile plaques nor Lewy bodies present in the tissues. Neuronal cytoplasmic inclusions, sometimes referred to as Hirano bodies are present in neurons, particularly in the hippocampus.[220,221]

CREUTZFELDT-JAKOB DISEASE (CJD)

INTRODUCTION

In 1920 and 1921 H.G. Creutzfeldt and Alfons Jakob separately described 4 demented patients with a subacute or chronic diffuse encephalomyelopathy of unknown origin with an affinity for the cerebral cortex, pyramidal tracts and extrapyramidal system, and a lethal course of 3 months to 3 years.[222,223] The clinical symptoms of the original cases so reminded Jakob of Wilson's disease, Westphal-Strumpell disease, and amyotrophic lateral sclerosis that he named the disease spastic pseudosclerosis; eventually this name was changed to Creutzfeldt-Jakob or Jakob-Creutzfeldt disease. Following these early descriptions, there appeared numerous descriptions of this disease many of which differed from the original and were described as variants.[224] Yet there is a clinical presentation of CJD whose clinical manifestations are evident to the experienced physician according to Denny-Brown.[225]

CLINICAL PRESENTATION

The majority of cases of CJD are sporadic but familial forms have been described.[224] The onset of the disease is in middle life notably during the fifth and sixth decades with extensions to 70 and 80 years of age.[226] The course of the disease is subacute and death comes within a few months to 3 years; longer survivals have been described particularly in association with the amyotrophic form of CJD.[227] The first clinical evidence of the disease is anxiety, irritability, and apathy quickly followed by a rapid progressive mental deterioration with memory losses, delirium, and confusion. This dementia is associated with neurologic signs which indicate the anatomic location of the lesions, most frequently rigidity, tremors, choreiform movements, stiffness of limbs, dysarthria, myoclonic jerks and myoclonic epilepsy, cerebellar signs, muscular wasting and blindness in the Heidenhaim variant of CJD.[228] The EEG frequently shows paroxysmal discharges of high-voltage bilateral, synchronous, and rhythmic and spike complexes.

PATHOLOGY

The gross examination of the brain usually is normal in appearance weighing between 1000 and 1450 g. Sometimes cortical atrophy is evident. Lateral ventricles are enlarged. Cortical involvement is more prominent on the inferior aspect of the hemispheres in the frontal temporal and temporal parietal insular zones bilaterally and symmetrically. The cerebellum, the putamen, the caudate, and the hippocampus may be involved. In some cases, the cortical areas most affected are in the occipital and parietal area (Heidenhaim form).

The distribution of the pathologic condition in the gray matter is often diffuse with patchy cell loss [Fig. 3–26]. The histologic picture varies but usually it consists of a loss of neurons, spongiosis, and gliosis primarily in the deeper layers of the cortex. The affected neurons may be retracted, dense with a darkly stained nucleus or bizarre shaped, swollen, pale, without Nissl substance, chromatolyzed. There is frequent satellitosis and neurophagia. The gliosis is more diffuse than the neuronal loss and particularly evident with the stain for glial fibrillary acid proteins (GFAP). The spongiosis consists of tiny vacuoles, individualized or grouped, evident with light microscopy. Senile lesions, that is neurofibrillary tangles, plaques, and cellular lipofuscin deposits, are considered to be coincidental.

The electron microscopy studies of biopsies of cerebral cortex have resulted in a more specific morphologic description of the vacuoles which are of regular shape, round or oval, 10 to 20 μ in diameter [Fig. 3–27B]. The smaller vacuoles are situated in the cytoplasm or processes of neurons and glial cells. There have been descriptions of modifications of postsynaptic dendrites and accumulations of filaments within astrocytes, while others have insisted on the membrane proliferation with multilaminar appearance in association with the spongiosis.[229,230]

The thalamic form of CJD is rare.[231,232] Histologically the same cellular lesions are present with severe neuronal loss and bilateral symmetrical involvement of the thalamus. The rest

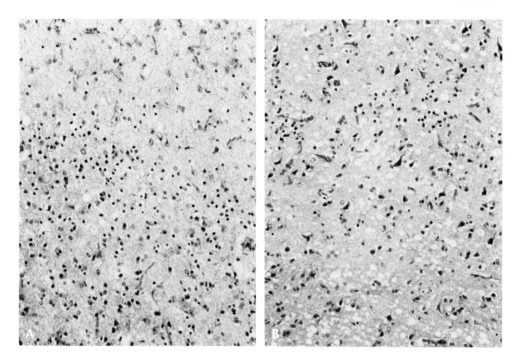

Fig. 3-26. Creutzfeldt-Jakob disease. A. Note the loss of neurons associated with gliosis in the superficial cortex. B. Gliosis and microspongiosis of the underlying cortex. Celloidin. H&E. A.—B . × 165.

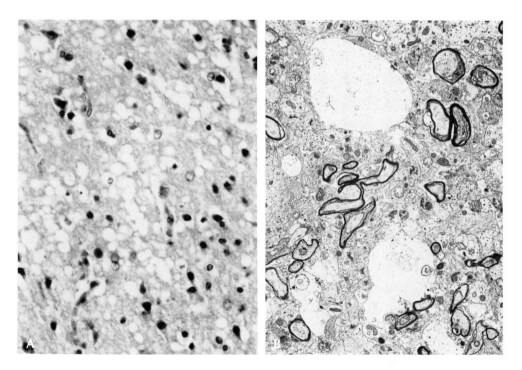

Fig. 3-27. Creutzfeldt-Jakob disease. A. Numerous vacuoles (spongiosis) in the deep layers of the cortex. Celloidin. H&E . × 330. B. Frontal cortical biopsy. Electron micrograph. Vacuolization of post-synaptic processes. Uranyl acetate—lead citrate . × 4500.

of the brain has few and minimal lesions. The cerebellar form associated with ataxia is more common. Brownell[233] reported 4 cases together with 6 other cases previously described in the literature. The cerebellar involvement was massive with a gross microscopic atrophy of the vermis. There was an atrophy of the folia, dense gliosis, and spongiosis of the molecular layer. The rest of the brain contained minimal lesions. The "authenticity" of the amyotrophic form has been questioned by many authors usually because of the different anatomo-clinical presentations of the cases.[224] Clinically, the course of the disease exceeds 1 year; the abnormal movements are not always present. There may be a typical atrophy of the Aran-Duchenne type and pyramidal signs. Associated senile lesions such as neurofibrillary tangles and senile plaques have been described.[234] Gliotic nodules in areas of spongiosis have been described in the spinal cord.[227]

Recently a panencephalitic form of CJD has been described in which the white matter is particularly involved.[235] Any part of the myelinated areas of the CNS may be involved particularly the cortical spinal tracts. The ultrastructural studies of the white matter reveal a spongiosis similar to that seen in the cortex in the more classical forms of CJD.[236]

PATHOGENESIS

Numerous variants, subdivisions, and causes have been proposed for CJD. Originally, Jakob proposed hereditary predispositions, endogenous and exogenous factors. A metabolic cause such as pellagra was considered.[237] Nevin and his colleagues then suggested CJD was due to a vascular dysfunction.[238,239] More recently it has been proposed that CJD is caused by an infectious organism. A slow virus was first implicated, shown to be transmissible but never seen. Currently, it has been proposed that prions are the agents which cause not only CJD but Alzheimer, Kuru, Gerstmann-Straussler-Scheinker disease.[240] Prions are said to be infectious organisms derived from a normal glycoprotein present in human tissues. The theory that an infectious organism causes CJD, such as a slow

virus, scrapie fibril or prion, is primarily based on the work of Gibbs and his colleagues who have reported that brain extracts of human cases of CJD cause a similar pathologic condition when injected into the brains of monkeys.[241-242]

GERSTMANN-STRAUSSLER-SCHEINKER DISEASE (GSS)

This rare familial disease was identified in 1936[243] by Gerstmann, Straussler, and Scheinker. Recently Seitelberger[244] has related it to Kuru disease and the spongiform encephalopathies.

CLINICAL PRESENTATION

The onset is during the fifth and sixth decades, marked by cerebellar ataxia, slurred speech, and muscle atrophy. The evolution is progressive or in stages with severe mental deterioration: Death occurs 2 to 7 years after onset due to a slowly progressive cachexia.

PATHOLOGY

On gross examination the brain usually appears to be normal. There may be a diffuse atrophy of the cerebral cortex and of the cerebellar vermis. The histologic features include a varied morphologic spectrum of plaques extending from a single or multiple amyloid deposit [Fig. 3–28], a typical senile plaque, Kuru "stellate" plaque consisting of a dense amyloid center from which radiates interwoven fibrils. The plaques may vary in size from 10 to 60 μ. There are abnormal astrocytes and diffuse gliosis in areas with the plaques. The nerve cells are relatively intact and the spongioform changes are discrete, if present, located in the superficial layers of the cerebral cortex or around plaques. There is a diffused loss of myelin which affects one or other regions of the CNS, in particular, the centrum ovale, the cortical spinal tracts, the cerebellum, the brainstem, and sometimes the spinal cord.[245]

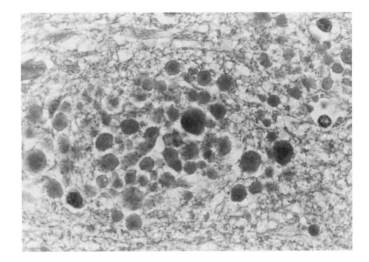

Fig. 3–28. Gerstmann-Straussler-Scheinker disease. Multicentric amyloid plaques in the cerebellar cortex. Masson's trichrome. ×500 (Courtesy of Dr. C. Fallet-Blanco).

THE ASSOCIATION OF CORPUS CALLOSUM NECROSIS (MARCHIAFAVA-BIGNAMI DISEASE) AND LAMINAR SCLEROSIS OF MOREL

Marchiafava-Bignami disease is a rare disease caused by alcoholism which results in a central necrosis of the corpus callosum,[246] often associated with laminar sclerosis in the cerebral cortex.[247,248]

CLINICAL PRESENTATION

The clinical picture is that of a sudden onset of loss of consciousness followed by seizures after an episode of excessive alcohol intake in a known drinker. Upon awakening the subject has demential behavior and specific rigidity with upper and lower extremities in flexion. The evolution is variable. Sometimes death intervenes in several weeks to months; in other cases, the evolution may take the aspect of recovery with recurrent attacks followed by rigidity. When the subject has a mild dementia and is able to speak, he usually has frontal dysarthria, characterized by hesitations in the middle of the words.[249–251]

Mild forms are manifested by disturbance of gait, rigidity, and frontal dysarthria. In more severe forms with acute episodes followed by remission and recurrence, the evolution is usually fatal after several episodes. There are some forms with signs of callosal disconnection. Lechevalier and Anderson[252] described such a case in a heavy alcoholic with necrosis of the corpus callosum, who manifested a peculiar ideomotor apraxia of both hands.

PATHOLOGY

The necrosis of the corpus callosum is seen macroscopically and involves the central portion of the structure along its entire length [Fig. 3–29A and B]. Laterally, it extends to the origin of the centrum ovale. Microscopically, the necrotic area consists of numerous macrophages with a moderate gliosis [Fig. 3–29C]. Vascular proliferation remains moderate. Cortical laminar sclerosis accompanies the necrosis of the callosum. It is characterized with myelin stains by pallor of the third cortical layer which appears as a light band between the second and fourth layers. Histologically, the pathologic area is characterized by a more or less complete neuronal loss in the third layer associated to a diffused fibrillary gliosis [Fig. 3–30]. The association between the laminar sclerosis and the necrosis of the callosum is frequent.[248–249] The pathologic condition of the laminar sclerosis does not appear to be of vascular origin (anoxia) as suggested by certain authors.[253] The location of the laminar sclerosis is possibly explained by the anatomy of the callosum fibers, since these originate in the third cortical layers of the opposite cortex.

PATHOGENESIS

The pathophysiology of corpus callosum necrosis is unknown. The hypothesis of a

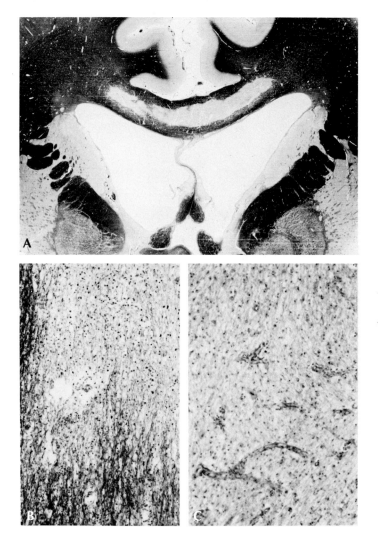

Fig. 3–29. Marchiafava Bignami disease. A. Myelin preparation showing the degeneration of the central fibers of the corpus callosum. Celloidin. Wolcke. ×2.5. B. Higher power view of A showing the margins of the lesion. Wolcke. ×87.5. C. Macrophages occupying the necrotic area. Celloidin. H&E. ×87.5.

cyanide intoxication due to the presence of cyanide in the ingested wines has been corroborated by some authors by comparison to experimental lesions induced in rats. There appeared to be disturbed metabolism of the vitamin B_{12} which contains cyanocobalamin.[254]

DIAGNOSIS

The diagnosis is usually evident. The differential diagnosis is limited to the alcoholic pseudo-pellagra caused by nicotinic acid deficiency, which is rare and presents with rigidity absolutely identical to the rigidity of corpus callosum necrosis. However, there is no dementia. The patients appear mean and hostile.

The differential is important because the hypovitaminosis is easily corrected with vitamin supplementation.[254]

NORMAL PRESSURE HYDROCEPHALUS (NPH)

Normal pressure hydrocephalus is a clinical syndrome that usually defies pathologic explanation. It can be considered one of the curable dementias, so much so as to raise the question whether it is true dementia. It is characterized by a progressive, slow, ventricular enlargement, sometimes following a post-traumatic or post-meningitic event, that leads to a loss of CSF re-absorption expressed anatomically by a

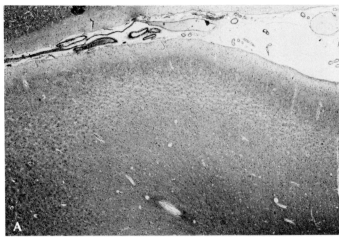

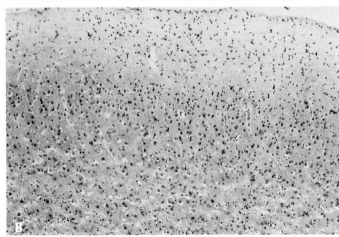

Fig. 3–30. Laminar sclerosis of Morel. A. Cortical laminar necrosis affecting the third layer. Celloidin. HPL. ×21. B. Higher power view showing the loss of neurons and the gliosis of the third layer. ×82.5.

communicating hydrocephalus without significant increase in intracranial pressure (ICP). The disease was first described in 1965 by Adams et al.[255] and Hakim and Adams[256] and its discovery was more or less accidental, the second case being one of supposed carcinomatous meningitis who did not die as predicted. Other psychiatric patients who underwent lumbar punctures or encephalograms showed an unexplained clinical improvement. It was then realized that the extraction of CSF sometimes led to clinical improvement in patients who had no signs of increased intracranial pressure.[255]

"Normal pressure hydrocephalus" is an interesting and challenging diagnosis, interesting because its treatment frequently produces an improvement in the degree of dementia, challenging because even after 25 years of study it is impossible to predict which patients will show such an improvement. "Normal pressure hydrocephalus" must be differentiated from the much more common "hydrocephalus ex vacuo" but both are heterogeneous groups of diseases with varying degrees of dementia and/or other signs. The attempt to define "normal pressure hydrocephalus" as dementia with dilated ventricles accompanied by various incidences and degrees of gait disturbances and incontinence has not been completely successful since no really accurate predictive or diagnostic features exist. Significant improvement in the dementia following shunting of the dilated ventricles may occur no matter what the underlying disease(s) may be: Alzheimer's, Pick's, chronic (fibrotic) meningitis, cerebrovascular disease, etc., including none of the above (i.e., "idiopathic"). In Salman's study of 80 consecutive patients[257] about 20% showed moderate to marked improvement regardless of the underlying disease; only those with a history of head injury responded to the shunting of CSF less frequently.

To begin near the beginning, one must recognize that the diagnosis "normal pressure" is wrong; if prolonged measurements are made over 24 hours or more, the pressure will be found to be intermittently elevated, leading to the proposal that it be called "variotensive" hydrocephalus.[258] The classic requirements for the diagnosis and treatment are dementia, gait ataxia, urinary incontinence and CT evidence of ventricular dilatation out of proportion to sulcal widening.[259] However, only a therapeutic trial seems to be able to differentiate "normal pressure hydrocephalus" from "hydrocephalus ex vacuo," but few physicians seem to want to expose the large number of Alzheimer suspects to such a surgical procedure!

CLINICAL PRESENTATION

The major manifestations are pyramidal signs and urinary disturbances. All these manifestations are curable by treatment.

PATHOLOGY

The ventricular system is dilated involving the lateral ventricles, the third and fourth ventricles, and the Sylvian aqueduct [Fig. 3–31]. In some cases the fluid is entrapped in thickened meninges that obstruct drainage, in others no obvious obstruction can be seen. The histologic examination sometimes confirms the meningeal thickening, and in most cases that respond to treatment by ventricular shunting there are no parenchymal lesions, specifically no Alzheimer-type senile lesions. However, about 20% of cases of Alzheimer's or Pick's diseases respond temporarily to shunts, only to progress again to disclose their underlying disease.[257] There may also be abnormalities of the lining of the ventricular cavity. The ependymal wall may be interrupted by fractures or thickened in granulations consisting of a mixture of ependymal cells and glia, especially in the ventricular floor. There may also be diffuse increase of the subependymal glia. All of these changes are difficult to define quantitatively and may be seen in many adults without ven-

tricular enlargement. In the advanced forms the white matter is altered by diffuse axonal destruction with moderate gliosis of the frontal and temporal regions, centrum semiovale, and corpus callosum but with relative sparing of the subcortical arcuate fibers.[260] Electron microscopic studies of biopsy specimens show the normal cortical architecture, as well as empty synaptic terminations that may not be differentiated from artifact. In 40% of cases no etiologic factor, such as hemorrhage or meningitis, could be found.

DIFFERENTIAL DIAGNOSIS

There is a rare cerebellovestibular form that corresponds anatomically to a marked enlargement of the fourth ventricle and is demonstrated clinically by cerebellar signs, usually bilateral, associated with central vestibular symptoms.

The differential diagnosis of the usual case includes the other major dementias:

- Alzheimer's disease has a different clinical picture with absence of pyramidal signs and the late development of urinary incontinence. The CT scan shows an enlargement of "sillons" which are always occluded in NPH.
- Pick's disease has a similar frontal lobe syndrome in the clinical presentation without the pyramidal and extrapyramidal signs, again with late urinary incontinence.
- Other dementias: There are some reports in the literature of Alzheimer's disease cured or improved temporarily by diversion of CSF. Those probably represent cases of NPH combined with the early stage of the primary dementia. Adams[256] estimated that ventricular enlargement, even due to atrophy as in Alzheimer's disease, increases due to the phenomenon of mariot (PV = K), where a minimum pressure over a large ventricular area results in a marked increase in dilatation. If this hypothesis is correct, all severe ventricular enlargements would have a secondary component in addition to the primary atrophy.

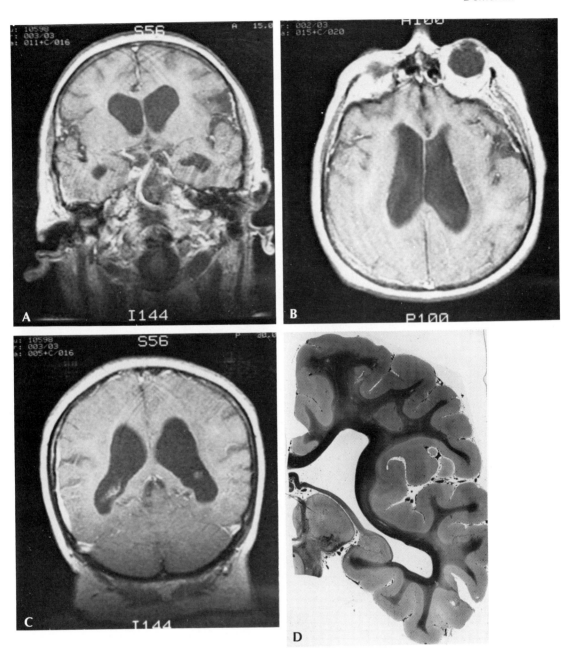

Fig. 3–31. A, B, and C are photographs of MRIs of the brain of a case of normal pressure hydrocephalus. A is an anterior coronal section in the fronto-tempero region. B is a longitudinal section extending from the frontal to the occipital poles. C is a posterior coronal section through the occipital parietal regions and cerebellum. D is a myelin (Loyez) stained section of the posterior portion of a cerebral hemisphere, at the level of the pulvinar, of a case of normal pressure hydrocephalus.

PROGNOSIS AND TREATMENT

Cases of true NPH are correctable (by definition) and have a good prognosis when the proper therapy (CSF diversion) is instituted. Other disorders may show a transient improvement.

Ventriculo-atrial or ventriculo-peritoneal shunting usually produces excellent results with fast resolution of the symptoms. It is always important to biopsy the cerebral cortex when placing a shunt in order to determine the presence of an underlying cortical atrophy which may predict a clinical relapse.

REFERENCES

1. Durand-Farde, M.: *Traite clinique et pratique des malades des vieillards.* Paris, J.B. Bailliere, 1854.
2. Klippel, M.: Caracteres histologiques differentiels de la PG. Classification histologique des paralysies generales. Arch. Med. Exp., 3:660, 1891.
3. Binswanger, D.: Die abgrenzung der aligemeinen progressiven paralysie. Berl. Klin. Wochenschr., 31:1103;1137;1180, 1894.
4. Alzheimer, A.: Neuere arbeiten uber die dementia senilis und die auf atheromatosen gefasserkrankung banerenden gehirn krankheiten. Moshr. Psychiat. Neurol. 3:101, 1898.
5. Marie, P.: Des foyers lacunaires de desintegration et de differents autres etats cavitaires du cerveau. Rev. Med., 21:281, 1901.
6. Ferrand, J.: *Essai sur l'hemiplegie des vieillards: les lacunes de desintegration cerebrale.* Paris, These, 1902.
7. Fisher, C.M.: Lacunes: small deep cerebral infarcts. Neurology (Minn.), 15:774, 1965.
8. Delay, J., and Brion, S.: *Les demences tardives.* Paris, Masson, 1962.
9. Tomlinson, B.E., Blessed, G., and Roth, M.: Observations on the brains of demented old people. J. Neurol. Sci., 11:205, 1970.
10. Hachinski, V.C., Lassen, N.A., and Marshall, J.: Multi-infarct dementia. A cause of mental deterioration in the elderly. Lancet, 2:207, 1974.
11. Brust, J.C.M.: Vascular dementia is overdiagnosed. Arch. Neurol. (Chic.), 45:799, 1988.
12. O'Brien, M.D.: Vascular dementia is underdiagnosed. Arch. Neurol. (Chic.), 45:797, 1988.
13. Jellinger, K.: Neuropathological aspects of dementias resulting from abnormal blood and cerebral fluid dynamics. Acta. Neurol. (Belg.), 76:83, 1976.
14. Erkinjuntti, T.: Types of multi-infarct dementia. Acta. Neurol. Scand., 75:391, 1987.
15. Jorm, A.F., Korten, A.E., and Henderson, A.S.: The prevalance of dementia: a quantitative integration of the literature. Acta. Psychiat. Scand., 76:465, 1987.
16. Alafuzoof, I., et al.: Histopathological criteria for progressive dementia disorders: clinical-pathological correlation and classification by multivariate data analysis. Acta. Neuropathol. (Berl.) 74:209, 1987.
17. Rosen, W.G., et al.: Pathological verification of ischemic score in differentiation of dementias. Ann. Neurol., 7:486, 1980.
18. Mc Menemy, W.H.: The dementias and progressive diseases of the basal ganglia. In: *Neuropathology,* 3rd Ed., Edited by J.G. Greenfield, et al. London, E. Arnold, 1961.
19. Hachinski, V.C., et al.: Cerebral blood flow in dementia. Arch. Neurol., 32:632, 1975.
20. Lindenberg, R., and Spatz, H.: Uber die thromboendarteriitis obliterans der Hirngefasse (cerebrale form der V. Winiwarter-Buergerschen Krankheit), Virch. Arch. Patho. Anat., 305:531, 1939.
21. Jellinger, K.: Die sogennante cerebrale form der Endangitis obliterans. Nervenarzt., 42:397, 1971.
22. Pentschew, A.: Die granulare atrophie der groshirnrinde. Arch. Psychiat. Nervenkr., 101:80, 1933.
23. Morel, F., and Meyra, G.: L'atrophie granulaire de l'ecorce cerebrale. Contribution a l'etude de la forme systematisee de cette affection. Schweitz. Arch. Neurol. Psychiatr., 53:315, 1944.
24. Wildi, E.: Etat granulaire systematise cardiopathique de l'ecorce cerebrale (atrophie granulaire). Etude anatomo-clinique. Bull. Acad. Suisse Sci. Med. 15:18, 1959.
25. Kaplan, J.G., et al.: Progressive dementia, visual deficits, amyotrophy, and microinfarcts. Neurology (Minn.) 35:789, 1985.
26. Romanul, F.C.A, and Abramowicz, A.: Changes in brain and pial vessels in arterial border zones. A study of 13 cases. Arch. Neurol. (Chic.), 11:40, 1961.
27. Fischer, C.M.: Cerebral thromboangiitis obliterans. Medicine (Balt.), 35:169, 1957.
28. Adams, J.H., Brierley, J.B., Connor R.C., et al.: The effects of systemic hypotension upon the human brain. Clinical and neuropathological observation in 11 cases. Brain, 89:235, 1966.
29. Torvik, A., Endresen, G.K.M., Abrahamsen, A.F., et al.: Progressive dementia caused by an unusual type of generalized small vessel thrombosis. Acta. Neurol. Scand., 47:137, 1971.
30. Sourander, P., and Walinder, J.: Hereditary multi-infarct dementia. Morphological and clinical studies of a new disease. Acta. Neuropath. (Berl.), 39:247, 1977.
31. Sonninen, V., and Savontaus, M.L.: Hereditary multi-infarct dementia. Europ. Neurol., 27:209, 1987.
32. Arab, A.: Arteriosclerose cerebrale scalariforme hypertensive. Etude anatomo-clinique. Psychiat. Neurol., 134:175, 1957.
33. Fisher, C.M.: The arterial lesions underlying lacunes. Acta Neuropath. (Berl.), 12:1, 1969.
34. Fisher, C.M.: Lacunar strokes and infarcts: a review. Neurology (Minn), 32:871, 1982.
35. Poirier, J., Gray, F., Gherardi, R., et al.: Cerebral lacunae. A new neuropathological classification. J. Neuropath. Exp. Neurol., 44:312, 1985.
36. Poirier, J., Barbizet, J., Gaston, A., et al.: Demence thalamique. Lacunes expansives du territoire thalamo-mesencephalique paramedian. Hydrocephalie par stenose de l'acqueduc de Sylvius. Rev. Neurol. (Paris), 139:349, 1983.
37. Benhaiem-Sigaux, N., et al.: Expanding cerebellar lacunes due to dilatation of the perivascular space associated with Binswanger's subcortical arteriosclerotic encephalopathy. Stroke, 18:1087, 1987.
38. Molaie, M., and Collins, G.H.: Systemic non-inflammatory vasculopathy with prominent CNS involvement. A case report. Angiology, 38:686, 1987.
39. Olszewski, J.: Subcortical arteriosclerotic encephalopathy. World Neurol., 3:359, 1962.

40. Garcin, R., Lapresle, J., and Lyon, G.: Encephalopathie sous-corticale chroniquede Binswanger. Etude anatomo-clinique de trois observations. Rev. Neurol., 102:423, 1960.

41. Mikol, J.: Maladie de Binswanger et formes apparentees. Rev. Neurol., 118:111, 1968.

42. Caplan, L.R., and Schoene, W.C.: Clinical features of arteriosclerotic encephalopathy (Binswanger's disease). Neurology (Minn.), 28:1206, 1978.

43. Rosenberg, G.A., Kornfeld M., Stovring, J., et al.: Subcortical arteriosclerotic encephalopathy (Binswanger): computerized tomography. Neurology (Minn.), 29:1106, 1979.

44. Ali Cherif, A., et al.: Encephalopathie sous-corticale de Binswanger. Rev. Neurol., 135:665, 1979.

45. Davison, C.: Progressive subcortical encephalopathy (Binswanger's disease). J. Neuropath. Exp. Neurol., 1:42, 1942.

46. Neumann, M.A.: Chronic progressive subcortical encephalopathy: Report of a case, J. Gerontol., 2:57, 1947.

47. Dupuis, M., Brucher, J.M., and Gonsette, R.E.: Observation anatomo-clinique d'une encephalopathie sous-corticale arterisclereuse ("maladie de Binswanger") avec hypodensite de la substance blanche au scanner cerebral. Acta Neurol. (Belg.), 84:131, 1984.

48. Okeda, R.: Correlative morphometric studies of cerebral arteries in Binswanger's encephalopathy and hypertensive encephalopathy. Acta Neuropath. (Berl.), 26:23, 1973.

49. Roman, G.C.: Lacunar dementia. In: Senile Dementia of the Alzheimer's Type. Edited by J.T. Hutton and A.D. Kenny. New York, Alan R. Liss, 1985.c

50. Bogousslavsky, J.: Leucoencephalopathie, leucoaraiose et infarctus cerebral. Rev. Neurol., 144:11, 1988.

51. Dubas, F., Gray, F., Roullet, E., et al.: Leucoencephalopathies arteriopathiques (17 cas anatomo-cliniques). Rev. Neurol., 141:93, 1985.

52. De Reuck, J., and Vander Eecken, H.M.: Periventricular leukomalacia in adults. Clinico-pathological study of four cases. Arch. Neurol. (Chic). 35:517, 1978.

53. De Reuck, J., et al.: Pathogenesis of Binswanger chronic progressive subcortical encephalopathy. Neurology (Minn.). 30:920, 1980.

54. Garcia-Albea, E., Cabello, A., and Franch, O.: Subcortical arteriosclerotic encephalopathy (Binswanger's disease): a report of five patients. Acta Neurol. Scand., 75:295, 1987.

55. Artigas, J., et al.: Light microscopical and ultrastructural findings in diffuse subcortical angiopathy. In: Stroke and Microcirculation. Edited by J. Cervos-Navarro and R. Ferszt. New York, Raven Press, 1987.

56. Nichols, III, F.T., Mohr, J.P.: Binswanger's subacute arteriosclerotic encephalopathy. In: Stroke, Pathophysiology. Diagnosis and Management (vol. 2). Edited by H.J.M. Barnett, B.M. Stein, J.P. Mohr, and F.M. Yatsu. New York, Churchill Livingstone, 1987.

57. Rezak, D.L., Morris, J.C., Fulling, K.H. et al.: Periventricular white matter lucencies in senile dementia of the Alzheimer type and in normal aging. Neurology (Minn.), 37:1365, 1987.

58. Awad, I.A., et al.: Incidental subcortical lesions identified on magnetic resonance imaging in the elderly. I. Correlation with age and cerebrovascular risk factors. Stroke, 17:1090, 1986.

59. Awad, I.A., Johnson, P.C., Spetzler, R.F., et al.: II Post-mortem pathological correlations. Stroke, 17:1090, 1986.

60. Tomonaga, M., Yamanouchi, H., Toghi, H., et al.: Clinico-pathological study of progressive vascular encephalopathy (Binswanger type) in the elderly. J. Am. Geriatr. Soc., 30:524, 1982.

61. Malone, M.J., and Szoke, M.C.: Neurochemical changes in white matter aged human brain and Alzheimer's disease. Arch. Neurol. (Chic), 42:1063, 1985.

62. Loizou, L.A., Kendall, B.E., and Marshall, J.: Subcortical arteriosclerotic encephalopathy: a clinical and radiological investigation. J. Neurol. Neurosurg. Psychiat., 44:294, 1981.

63. Inzitari, D., et al.: Vascular risk factors and leukoaraiosis. Arch. Neurol., 44:42, 1987.

64. Erkinguntti, T., et al.: Do white matter changes on MRI and CT differentiate vascular dementia from Alzheimer's disease. J. Neurol. Neurosurg. Psychiat., 50:37, 1987.

65. Steingart, A., et al.: Cognitive and neurologic findings in demented patients with diffuse white matter lucencies on computed tomographic scan (leuko-araiosis). Arch. Neurol. (Chic.), 44:36, 1987.

66. Zeumer, H., Schonsky, B., and Sturm, K.W.: Predominant white matter involvement in subcortical arteriosclerotic encephalopathy (Binswanger disease). J. Comput. Assist. Tomograph., 4:14, 1980.

67. McQuinn, B.A., and O'Leary, D.H.: White matter lucencies on computed tomography, subacute arteriosclerotic encephalopathy (Binswanger's disease), and blood pressure. Stroke, 18:900, 1987.

68. Hachinski, V.C., Potter, P., and Merskey, H.: Leukoaraiosis. Arch. Neurol. (Chic.), 44:21, 1987.

69. Kowalski, H., et al.: Regional cerebral MRI T2 values. Effects of normal aging. Neurology (Minn.), 38(1):371, 1988.

70. Ferszt, R., Bradac, G.B., and Nassel, F.: Stroke and microcirculation. In: Value of MRI in Diagnosing Alzheimer Versus Vascular Dementia. Edited by J. Cervos-Navarro and R. Ferszt. New York, Raven Press, 1987.

71. Gupta, S.R., et al.: Periventricular white matter changes and dementia. Clinical, neuropsychological, radiological, and pathological correlation. Arch. Neurol. (Chic.), 45:637, 1988.

72. Morgello, S., Farrar, J.T., and Heier, L.A.: Periventricular hyperintense lesions on magnetic resonance scans. Neurology (Minn.), 38:suppl 1, 1988.

73. Ball, M.J.: Ischemic axonopathy: further evidence that neocortical pathology accompanying cerebral hypoperfusion during systemic hypotension causes white matter rarefaction in the elderly and some people with Alzheimer dementia. J. Neuropath. Exp. Neurol., 47:338, 1988.

74. Aharon-Peretz, J., Cummings, J.L., and Hill, M.A.: Vascular dementia and dementia of the Alzheimer type. Cognition, ventricular size and leuko-araiosis. Arch. Neurol. (Chic.), 45:719, 1988.

75. Yamamura, T., Nishimura, M., Shirabe, T., et al.: Subcortical vascular encephalopathy in a normotensive, young adult with premature baldness and spondylitis deformans. A clinopathological study and review of the literature. J. Neurol. Sci., 78:175, 1987.

76. Yokoi, S., and Nakoyama, H.: Chronic progressive leukoencephalopathy with systemic arteriosclerosis in young adults. Clin. Neuropath., 4:165, 1985.

77. Dide, H., and Botcazo, E.: Amnesie continue, cecite verbale pure, perte du sens topographique, ramollissement double lobe lingual. Rev. Neurol., *10*:676, 1902.

78. Boudin, G., Barbizet, J., Derouesne, C., et al.: Cecite corticale et probleme des "amnesies occipitales." Rev. Neurol., *116*:89, 1967.

79. Glees, P., and Griffith, H.G.: Bilateral destruction of hippocampus (Cornu Ammonis) in a case of dementia. Mschr. Psychiat. Neurol., *123*:193, 1952.

80. Victor, M., Angevine, J.B., Mancall, E.J., et al.: Memory loss with lesions of hippocampal formation. Report of a case with some remarks on the anatomical basis of memory. Arch. Neurol., *5*:244, 1965.

81. Nomura, H., and Ishikawa, T.: Bilateral temporal softening found at autopsy in a patient with peculiar mental symptoms. Amsterdam Excerpta Medica Section VIII, nᵒ 4421:970, 1951.

82. Grunthal, E.: Lieber das Klinische bild nach unschriebenem beiderseitigem Ausfall der Ammonshornrinde ein beitrag sur Kentniss der funktion des ammonshorns. Mschr. Psychiat. Neurol., *113*:1, 1947.

83. Delay, J., and Brion, S.: *Le syndrome de Korsakoff.* Paris, Masson, 1969.

84. Van Buren, J.M., and Borke, R.C.: The medial temporal substratum of memory. Brain, *95*:599, 1972.

85. Horel, J.A.: The neuroanatomy of amnesia. A critique of the hippocampal memory hypothesis. Brain, *101*:403, 1978.

86. Squire, L.R.: The anatomy of amnesia. TINS, *3*:52, 1980.

87. Brion, S., Mikol, J., and Plas, J.: Neuropathologie des syndromes amnesiques chez l'homme. Rev. Neurol., *141*:627, 1985.

88. Schuster, P.: Beitrage zur pathologie des thalamus opticus. Arch. Psychiat. Nervenkr., *105*:550, 1936.

89. Grunthal, E.: Ueber thalamische demenz. Mschr. Psych. Neurol., *106*:114, 1942.

90. Van Bogaert, L.: Approche d'une pathologie de la couche optique. IVe Congres Neurologique International, Paris, *1*:61, 1949.

91. Castaigne, P., et al: Paramedian thalamic and midbrain infarcts: clinical and neuropathological study. Ann. Neurol., *10*:127, 1981.

92. Markowitsch, H.J.: Thalamic mediodorsal nucleus and memory: a critical evaluation of studies in animals and man. Neurosci. Biobehav. Rev., *6*:351, 1982.

93. Guberman, A., and Stuss, D.: The syndrome of bilateral paramedian thalamic infarction. Neurology (Minn.), *33*:540, 1983.

94. Von Cramon, D.Y., Hebel, N., and Schuri, U.: A contribution to the anatomical basis of thalamic amnesia. Brain, *108*:993, 1985.

95. Gentilini, M., De Renzi, E., and Crisi, G.: Bilateral paramedian thalamic artery infarcts: report of eight cases. J. Neurol. Neurosurg. Psychiat., *50*:900, 1987.

96. Katz, D.I., Alexander, M.P., and Mandell, A.M.: Dementia following strokes in the mesencephalon and diencephalon. Arch. Neurol. (Chic.), *44*:1127, 1987.

97. Bogousslavsky, J., Regli, F., and Uske, A.: Thalamic infarcts; clinical syndromes, etiology, and prognosis. Neurology (Minn.), *38*:837, 1988.

98. Van Bogaert, L., Martin, L., and Martin, J.J.: Sclerose laterale amyotrophique avec degenerescence spinocerebelleuse et delire epileptique. Contribution a l'etude des formes de passage des atrophies thalamiques medianes. Acta. Neurol. Belg., *65*:845, 1965.

99. Warrington, E.K., and Weiskrantz, L.: Amnesia: a disconnection syndrome? Neuropsychologia, *20*:233, 1982.

100. Castaigne, P.: Demence thalamique d'origine vasculaire par ramollissement bilateral limite au territoire du pedicule retro-mamillaire. A propos de deux observations anatomo-cliniques. Rev. Neurol., *114*:89, 1966.

101. Mabille, H., and Pitres A.: Amnesie de fixation postapoplectique. Rev. Med., *33*:257, 1913.

102. Buge, A., Escourolle, R., Rancurel, G., et al.: "Mutisme akcinetique" et ramollissement bicingulaire. Trois observations anatomo-cliniques. Rev. Neurol., *131*:121, 1975.

103. Laplane, D., Degos, J.D., Baulac, M., et al.: Bilateral infarction of the anterior cingulate gyri and the fornices. Report of a case. J. Neurol. Sci., *51*:289, 1981.

104. Escourolle, R., and Gray, F.: Les accidents vasculaires du systeme limbique. In: *Proceedings of the VIIth International Congress of Neuropathology.* Vol. II. Edited by St. Kornyey, St. Tariska, G. Gosztonyi. Amsterdam, Excerpta Medica, 1975.

105. Goldman-Rakic, P.S.: Circuitry of the frontal association cortex and its relevance to dementia. Arch. Gerontol. Geriatr., *6*:299, 1987.

106. Brion, S., Pragier, G., Guerin, R., et al.: Syndrome de Korsakoff par ramollissment bilateral du fornix. Le probleme des syndrome amnesiques par lesion vasculaire unilaterale. Rev. Neurol., *120*:255, 1969.

107. Lindqiost, G., and Norlen, G.: Korsakoff's syndrome after operation on ruptured aneurysm of the anterior communications artery. Acta Psychiat. Scand., *42*:24, 1966.

108. Brion, S., Derome, P., Guiot, G., et al.: Syndrome de Korsakoff par anevryzme de l'artere communicante anterieure; le probleme des syndromes de Korsakoff meninges. Rev. Neurol., *118*:293, 1968.

109. Faris, A.A.: Limbic system infarction. A report of two cases. Neurology (Minn.), *19*:91, 1969.

110. Damasio, A. R., et al.: Amnesia following basal forebrain lesions. Arch. Neurol. (Chic.), *42*:263, 1985.

111. Dide, M., and Pezet, Ch.: Syndrome occipital avec dyspraxie complete surajoutee. Bull. Soc. Clin. Med. Ment., *6*:279, 1913.

112. Delay, J., Brion, S., Escourolle, R., et al.: Demences arteriopathiques. Lesions du systeme hippocampo-mamillo-thalamique dans le determinisme des troubles mnesiques. Rev. Neurol., *105*:22, 1961.

113. Boudin, G., Brion, S., Pepin, B., et al.: Syndrome de Korsakoff d'etiologie arteriopathique par lesion bilaterale asymetrique du systeme limbique. Rev. Neurol., *119*:341, 1968.

114. Geschwind, N., and Fusillo, M.: Color-naming defects in association with alexia. Arch. Neurol. (Chic.), *15*:137, 1966.

115. Mohr, J.P., Leicester, J., Stoddard, L.J., et al.: Right hemianopsia with memory and color deficit, in circumscribed left posterior cerebral artery territory infarction. Neurology (Minn.), *21*:1104, 1971.

116. Mikol, J., Brion, S.: Connexions du noyau latero-dorsal du thalamus et du circuit limbique chez l'homme. Etude de douze documents anatomo-cliniques d'etiologie vasculaire. Rev. Neurol., *131*:475, 1975.

117. Mikol, J., et al.: Connections of the latero-dorsal nucleus of the thalamus. II Experimental studies in Papio-Papio. Brain Res., *138*:1, 1977.

118. Mikol, J., Menini, M., Brion, S., et al.: Connexions du noyau latero-dorsal du thalamus chez le singe. III Etude de ses efferences. Rev. Neurol., *140*:615, 1984.

119. Brion, S., Chevalier, J.F., and Gueriot-Colasse, C.: Syndromes pseudo-dementiels par lesions de la partie posterieure de l'hemisphere mineur. In: *L'actualite en Gerontologie*. IVe Congres de Neuro-Geriatrie et Geronto-Psychiatrie. Edited by J. Bille. Paris. Sandoz, 1980.

120. Feigin, I., and Budzilovich, G.N.: The general pathology of cerebrovascular disease. In: *Handbook of Clinical Neurology* (vol 2). Vascular diseases of the nervous system. Edited by P.J. Vinken and G.W. Bruyn. Amsterdam, North Holland Publ. Co., 1972.

121. Munro, J.M., and Cotran, R.S.: The pathogenesis of atherosclerosis: atherogenesis and inflammation. Lab. Invest, 58:249, 1988.

122. Capron, L.: Atherosclerose. I Description. II Mecanismes. Rev. Neurol., 139:167, 239, 1983.

123. Sigal, L.H.: The neurologic presentation of vasculitic and rheumatologic syndromes. A review. Medicine, 67:20, 1987.

124. Calabresse, L.H., and Mallek, J.A.: Primary angiitis of the central nervous system. Report of 8 new cases, review of the literature, and proposal for diagnostic criteria. Medicine, 67:20, 1987.

125. Vanderzant, C., Bromberg, M., MacGuire, A., et al.: Isolated small vessel angiitis of the central nervous system. Arch. Neurol. (Chic.), 45:683, 1988.

126. Caselli, R.J., Hinder, G.G., and Whisnant, J.P.: Neurologic disease in biopsy-proven giant cell (temporal) arteritis. Neurology (Minn.), 38:352, 1988.

127. Ramos, M., and Mandybur, T.I.: Cerebral vasculitis in rheumatoid arthritis. Arch. Neurol. (Chic.), 32:271, 1975.

128. Ellis, S.G., and Verity, M.A.: Central nervous system involvement in systemic lupus erythematosus. Semin. Arthritis Rheum., 8:212, 1979.

129. Devinsky, O., Petito, C.K., and Alonso D.R.: Clinical and neuropathological findings in systemic lupus erythematosus: the role of vasculitis, heart emboli and thrombotic thrombocytopenic purpura. Ann. Neurol., 23:380, 1988.

130. Asherson, R.A., et al.: Recurrent stroke and multi-infarct dementia in systemic lupus erythematosus: association with antiphospholipid antibodies. Ann. Rheum. Dis., 46:605, 1987.

131. Coull, B.M., et al.: Multiple cerebral infarctions and dementia associated with anticardiolipin antibodies. Stroke, 18:1107, 1987.

132. Hardy, J.: Molecular biology and Alzheimer's disease: more questions than answers. TINS, 11:293, 1988.

133. Gray, F., Dubas, F., Roullet, E., et al.: Leukoencephalopathy in diffuse hemorrhagic cerebral amyloid angiopathy. Ann. Neurol., 18:54, 1985.

134. Roullet, E., et al.: Leukoencephalopathy in cerebral amyloid angiopathy: clinical, radiologic and pathologic study of six cases. Neurology (Minn.), 38(1):325, 1988.

135. Mettinger, K.L., and Ericson, K.: Fibromuscular dysplasia and the brain. Observations on angiographic, clinical and genetic characteristics. Stroke, 13:46, 1982.

136. Mettinger, K.L.: Fibromuscular dysplasia and the brain. II Current concept of the disease. Stroke, 13:53, 1982.

137. Rebollo, M., et al.: Livedo reticularis and cerebrovascular lesions (Sneddon's syndrome). Clinical, radiological and pathological features in eight cases. Brain, 106:965, 1983.

138. Bruyn, R.L.M., et al.: Sneddon's syndrome. Case report and literature review. J. Neurol. Sci., 79:243, 1987.

139. Ellie, E., et al.: Angiomatose cortico-meningee de Divry et Van Bogaert et syndrome de Sneddon. A propos de 4 cas. Rev. Neurol., 143:798, 1987.

140. Blackwood, W.: Vascular diseases of the central nervous system. In: *Neuropathology*, 3rd ed., Edited by J.G. Greenfield, et al.: London, E. Arnold, 1961.

141. Daniel, S.E., Rudge, P., and Scaravilli, F.: Malignant angioendotheliosis involving the nervous system: support for a lymphoid origin of the neoplastic cells. J. Neurol. Neurosurg. Psychiat., 50:1173, 1987.

142. Knight, R.S.G., Anslow, P., and Theaker, J.M.: Neoplastic angioendotheliosis: a case of subacute dementia with unusual cerebral CT appearances and a review of the literature. J. Neurol. Neurosurg., Psychiat., 50:1022, 1987.

143. Lach, B., et al.: Maternally inherited mitochondrial encephalomyopathy. A vasculopathy. Muscle and Nerve, 9:55, 180, 1986.

144. Ohama, E., et al.: Mitochondrial angiopathy in cerebral blood vessels of mitochondrial encephalomyopathy. Acta Neuropathol. (Berl.), 74:226, 1987.

145. Vilming, S.T., et al.: Late-onset hereditary myopathy with abnormal mitochondria and progressive dementia. Acta Neurol. Scand., 73:502, 1986.

146. Arne, L., Guerin, A., Julien, J., et al.: Sur un cas de leucoencephalopathie subaigue chez une malade ayant presente une thrombophlebite des membres inferieurs. Rev. Neurol., 112:560, 1965.

147. Damasio, H., et al.: Multiple cerebral aneurysms and cardiac myxoma. Arch. Neurol. (Chic.), 32:269, 1975.

148. Reagan, T.J., and Okazaki, H.: The thrombotic syndrome associated with carcinoma. A clinical and neuropathologic study. Arch. Neurol. (Chic.), 31:390, 1974.

149. Sulkava, R., and Erkinjuntti, T.: Vascular dementia due to cardiac arrhythmias and systemic hypotension. Acta. Neurol. Scand., 76:123, 1987.

150. Mann, D.M.A., Yates, P.O., and Hawkes, J.: The noradrenergic system in Alzheimer and multi-infarct dementias. J. Neurol., Neurosurg., Psychiat., 45:113, 1982.

151. Mann, D.M.A., Yates, P.O., and Marcyniuk, B.: The nucleus basalis of Meynert in multi-infarct (vascular) dementia. Acta. Neuropathol. (Berl.), 71:332, 1986.

152. Pick, A.: Weber die Beziehungen der senilen Hirnatrophie zur Aphasie, Prag. Med. Wschr., 17:165, 1892.

153. Pick, A.: Senile Hirnatrophie als Grundlage von Hederscheinungen, Wien, Klin. Wschr., 14:403, 1901.

154. Pick, A.: Ueber Symptomenkomplexe bedingt durch die Kombination sub-corticaler Herdaffektionen mit seniler Hirnatrophie, Wein, Klin. Wschr., 46:1121, 1901.

155. Pick, A.: Zur Symptomatologie der linksseitigen Schlafenlappenatrophie. Mschr. Psychiat. Neurol., 16(4):378, 1904.

156. Pick, A.: Ueber einenweiteren symptomenkomplex in Rahmen der Dementia senilis, bedingt durch umschriebene starkere Hirnatophie (gemischte Apraxie). Mschr. Psychiat. Neurol., 19(97):1906.

157. Onari, K., and Spatz, H.: Anatomische Beitrage zur lehre von den Pickschen umschriebenen Grosshirnrindenatrophie (Pickshe Krankheit). Z. ges. Neurol. Psychiat., 101:470, 1926.

158. Horn, L., and Stengel, E.: Zur Klinik und Pathologie der Pickschen Atrophie, Ueber die nosologisch Stel-

lung der Pickschen Krankheit. Z. ges. Neurol. Psychiat., *128*:673, 1930.

159. Van Mansvelt, J.: Pick's disease. A syndrome of lobar cerebral atrophy, its clinico-anatomical and histopathological types. Theses, Van der Loeff, 1954.

160. Wilson, A.K.: *Neurology* (vol. 2), Edited by A.N. Bruce. Baltimore, Williams & Wilkins, 1955.

161. Knopman, D.S., et al.: The spectrum of imaging and neuropsychological findings in Pick's disease. Neurology, *39*(3):362, 1989.

162. Adams, R.D., and Victor, M.: Degenerative Diseases of the Nervous System. In: *Principles of Neurology.* New York, Mc Graw-Hill, 1981.

163. Guiraud, P.: *Demences degeneratives (maladie de Pick—maladie d'Alzheimer).* In Psychiatrie clinique. Paris, Le Francois, 1956.

164. Lhermitte, J., and Trelles, J.O.: Sur l'apraxie pure constructive. Les troubles de la pensee spatiale et de la somatognosie dans l'apraxie. Encephale, *28*(6):413, 1933.

165. Cambier, J., Masson, M., Dairou, R., et al.: Etude anatomo-clinique d'une forme parietale de maladie de Pick. Rev. Neurol. (Paris), *137*(1):33, 1981.

166. de Morsier, G.: Un cas de maladie de Pick avec sclerose laterale amyotrophique terminale. Contribution a la semiologie temporale. Rev. Neurol. (Paris), *116*(5):373, 1967.

167. Brion, S., et al.: L'association maladie de Pick et sclerose laterale amyotrophique. L'Encephale, *VI*:259, 1980.

168. Constantinidis, J.: A familial syndrome: a combination of Pick's disease and amyotrophic lateral sclerosis. Encephale, *13*(5):285, 1987.

169. Jarvis, G.A.: Pick's Disease. In: *Pathology of the Nervous System* (vol. 2). Edited by J. Minckler. New York, Mc Graw-Hill, 1971.

170. Schmitz, H.A., and Meyer, A.: Uber die Picksche Krankheit, mit besonderer rerucesicutigung der Eeblichkeit. Arch. Psychiat., *99*:744, 1933.

171. Malamud, M., and Waggoner, R.W.: Genealogic and clinicopathologic study of Pick's disease. Arch. Neurol. Psychiat., *50*:228, 1943.

172. Sjogren, T., Sjogren, H., and Lindgren, A.G.H.: Morbus Alzheimer and Morbus Pick (A genetic, clinical and patho-anatomical study). Acta Psychiat. Scand., *82*:152, 1952.

173. Berlin, L.: Presenile sclerosis (Alzheimer's disease) with features resembling Pick's disease. Arch. Neurol. Psychiat. (Chic.), *61*(4):369, 1949.

174. Neumann, M.A.: Pick's disease. J. Neuropath. Exp. Neurol., *8*:255, 1949.

175. Oyanagi, S., Maeda, T., Ikuta., F., et al.: An autopsy case of presenile dementia with morphological features of Alzheimer's disease and Pick's disease. Psychiat. Neurol. Jpn., *75*:18, 1975.

176. Yoshimura, N.: Topography of Pick body distribution in Pick's disease: a contribution to understanding the relationship between Pick's and Alzheimer's diseases. Clin. Neuropath., *8*(1):1, 1989.

177. Arima, K., Oyanagi, S., Kosaka, K., et al.: Distribution of Pick bodies in the central nervous system of the Pick's disease with a special reference to their association with neuronal loss. Psychiat. Neurol. Jpn., *89*:43, 1987.

178. Williams H.: The peculiar cells of Pick's disease. Arch. Neurol. Psychiat. (Chicago), *34*(3):508, 1935.

179. Van Bogaert, L.: Syndrome extrapyramidal au cours d'une maladie de Pick. J. Belge Neurol. Psychiat., *34*:315, 1934.

180. Brion, S., Mikol, J., and Plas, J.: Neuropathologie des syndromes amnesiques chez l'homme. Rev. Neurol. (Paris), *141*(10):627, 1985.

181. Brion, S., Mikol, J., and Psimaras, A.: Recent findings in Pick's disease. In: *Progress in Neuropathology,* Edited by H.M. Zimmermann. New York, Grune & Stratton, 1973.

182. Probst, A., et al.: Pick's disease: an immunocytochemical study of neuronal changes. Monoclonal antibodies show that Pick bodies share antigenic determinants with neurofibrillary tangles and neurofilaments. Acta Neuropath. (Berl.), *60*:175, 1983.

183. Dickson, D.W., et al.: Ballooned neurons in select neurodegenerative diseases contain phosphorylated neurofilament epitopes. Acta Neuropath. (Berl.), *71*:216, 1986.

184. Mikol, J., Masters, C.L., Brion, S., et al.: Immunocytochemical studies of Pick's bodies. International Congress Neuropathology. Stockholm, 1986.

185. Munoz-Garcia, D., and Ludwin, S.K.: Classic and generalized variants of Pick's disease : a clinicopathological ultrastructural and immunocytochemical comparative study. Ann. Neurol., *16*:467, 1984.

186. Gambetti, P., et al.: Neurofibrillary changes in human brain: an immunocytochemical study with a neurofilament antiserum. J. Neuropath. Exp. Neurol., *42*:69, 1983.

187. Anderton, B.H., Calvert, R., Probst, A., et al.: Antibody studies of neurofilaments and neurofibrillary tangles. J. Submicrox. Cytol., *16*:63, 1984.

188. Rasool, C.G., and Selkol, D.J.: Sharing of specific antigens by degenerating neurons in Pick's disease and Alzheimer's disease. New Engl. J. Med., *312*:700, 1985.

189. Ulrich, J., et al.: Alzheimer dementia and Pick's disease: neurofibrillary tangles and Pick bodies are associated with identical phosphorylated neurofilament epitopes. Acta Neuropath. (Berl.), *73*:240, 1987.

190. Murayama, S., et al.: An autopsy case of a generalized variant of Pick's disease. Clin. Neurol., *26*:1051, 1986.

191. Pollock, N.J., et al.: Filamentous aggregates in Pick's disease, progressive supranuclear palsy and Alzheimer's disease share antigenic determinants with microtubule-associated protein tau. Lancet, 2:1211, 1986.

192. Joachim, C.L., Morris, J.H., Kosik, K.S., et al.: Tau antisera recognize neurofibrillary tangles in a range of neurodegenerative disorders. Ann. Neurol., *22*:514, 1987.

193. Perry, G., et al.: Filaments of Pick's bodies contain altered cytoskeletal elements. Ann. J. Pathol., *127*:559, 1987.

194. Manetto, V., et al.: Ubiquitin is associated with abnormal cytoplasmic filaments characteristic of neurodegenerative diseases. Proc. Natl. Acad. Sci. (USA), *85*:4501, 1988.

195. Goldman, J.E.: The association of actin with Hirano bodies. J. Neuropath. Exp. Neurol., *42*:146, 1983.

196. Galloway, P.G., Perry, G., and Gambetti, P.: Hirano body filaments contain actin and actin-associated proteins. J. Neuropath. Exp. Neurol., *46*:185, 1987.

197. Galloway, P.G., Perry, G., Kosik, K.S., et al.: Hirano bodies contain tau protein. Brain Res., *403*:337, 1987.

198. Brion, S., and Mikol, J.: Etude ultrastructurale de la maladie de Pick. A propos de trois cas. Rev. Neurol. (Paris), *125*:273, 1971.

199. Brion, S., Mikol, J., and Plas, J.: Renseignements

fournis par les biopsies cerebrales des demences chez l'adulte. In: *Investigations cliniques et para-cliniques dans le vieillissement cerebral*. Collection de l'Institut de Recherches Internationales Servier, Doin. Paris, 1987.

200. Brion, S., Mikol, J., and Psimaras, A.: Problemes concernant la maladie de Pick. In: *Excerpta Medica International Congress*, Series N° 274, Psychiatry (Part 2), 1971.

201. Kato, S., Nakamura, H., and Otomo, E.: Reappraisal of neurofibrillary tangles. Immunohistochemical, ultrastructural, and immunoelectron microscopical studies. Acta Neuropath., 77(3):258, 1989.

202. Arima, K., and Miyasaka, Y.: An autopsy case of Pick's disease, with special reference to light and electron microscopical findings of Pick bodies and ballooned neurons. Neuropath., 6:325, 1985.

203. Neumann, M.A., and Cohn, R.: A rare form of slowly progressive "presenile" dementia. J. Neuropath. Exp. Neurol., 25:122, 1966.

204. Neumann, M.A., and Cohn R.: Progressive subcortical gliosis. A rare form of presenile dementia. Brain, 90:405, 1967.

205. Morita, K., Kaiya, H., Ikeda, T., et al.: Presenile dementia combined with amyotrophy: a review of 34 Japanese cases. Arch. Gerontol. Geriat., 6(3):263, 1987.

206. Oksala, D.: Ein Beitrag zur Kenntnis der praesenilen Psychosen. Z. ges. Neurol. Psychiat., 81:1, 1923.

207. Schaumburg, H.H., and Suzuki, K.: Non-specific familial presenile dementia. J. Neurol. Neurosurg. Psychiat., 31:479, 1968.

208. Kim, R.C., et al.: Familial dementia of adult onset with pathological findings of a "non specific" nature. Brain, 104:61, 1981.

209. Masse, G., Mikol, J., and Brion, S.: Atypical Presenile Dementia. Report of an Anatomo-clinical Case and Review of the Literature. J. Neurol. Sci., 52:245, 1981.

210. Verity, A.: Progressive subcortical sclerosis : Nosology, Neuropathology and review. Eric K. Fernstrom Symposium. Frontal non-Alzheimer Dementia. Lund, Sweden, 1986.

211. Khoubesserian, P., et al.: Demence familiale de type Neumann (gliose sous corticale). Rev. Neurol. (Paris), 141:706, 1985.

212. Nadeau, S.E., Bebin, J., and Smith, E.: Non-specific dementia, cortical blindness and congophilic angiopathy. A clinicopathological report. J. Neurol., 234:14, 1987.

213. Spencer, P., et al.: Motorneurone disease on Guam: possible role of a food neurotoxin. Lancet, i:965, 1986.

214. Lowenberg, K., and Waggoner, R.W.: Familial organic psychosis (Alzheimer's type). Arch. Neurol. Psychiatr. (Chic.), 31:737, 1934.

215. Barret, A.: A case of Alzheimer's disease with unusual neurological disturbance. J. Nerv. Ment. Dis., 40(6):361, 1913.

216. Deymeer, F., Smith, T.W., De Girolami, U., et al.: Thalamic dementia and motor neuron disease. Neurology, 39:58, 1989.

217. Plas, J.: Les lesions corticales dans la sclerose laterale amyotrophique: (consequences sur l'interpretation des formes dementielles de la maladie). These Medecine, Paris, 1979.

218. Brion, S.: Amyotrophic forms of Creutzfeldt-Jakob disease. Afri. J. Neurol. Sci., 2:20, 1983.

219. Brion, S., and Plas, J.: Les lesions du cortex moteur dans la sclerose laterale amyotrophique. L'Encephale, 12:81, 1986.

220. Hirano, A., Malamud, N., Elizan, T., et al.: Parkinsonism-dementia complex, an endemic disease of the island of Guam. II. Pathological features. Brain, 84:662, 1961.

221. Hirano, A., Malamud, N., and Kurland, L.T.: Amyotrophic lateral sclerosis and Parkinsonism Dementia complex of Guam. Arch. Neurol., 15:35, 1966.

222. Creutzfeldt, H.G.: Uber eine eigenartige herdformige Erkrankung des Zentralnervensystems. Preliminary communication. Z. ges. Neurol. Psychiat., 57:1, 1920.

223. Jacob, A.: Uber eigenartige Erkrankungen des Zentralnervensystems mit bemerkenswertem anatomischen Befunde (spastische Pseudosclerose-encephalomyelopathie mit disseminierten Degenerationsherden). Z. ges. Neurol. Psychiat., 64:147, 1921.

224. Kirschbaum, W.R.: Jakob-Creutzfeldt Disease. New York, London, Amsterdam, Elsevier, 1968.

225. Denny-Brown, D.: *The Basal Ganglia*. Oxford, Oxford University Press, 1962.

226. Harris-Jones, R., et al.: Creutzfeldt-Jakob disease in England and Wales, 1980–1984: a case control study of potential risk factors. J. Neurol., Neurosurg., Psychiat., 51(9):1113, 1988.

227. Chateau, R., et al.: Amyotrophie distale lente des quatre membres avec evolution dementielle (forme amyotrophique du syndrome de Creutzfeldt-Jakob?). Etude anatomo-clinique. Rev. Neurol. (Paris), 115:955, 1966.

228. Meyer, A., Leigh, D., and Bagg, C.E.: A rare presenile dementia associated with cortical blindness (Heidenhain's syndrome). J. Neurol. Neurosurg. Psychiat., 17:129, 1954.

229. Marin, O., and Vial, J.D.: Neuropathological and ultrastructural findings in two cases of subacute spongiform encephalopathy. Acta Neuropathol., 4:218, 1964.

230. Gonatas, N.K., Terry, R.D., and Weiss, M.: Electron Microscopic Study in Two Cases of Jakob-Creutzfeldt Disease. Trans. Am. Neurol. Assoc., 89:13, 1964.

231. Stern, K.: Severe dementia associated with bilateral symmetrical degeneration of the thalamus. Brain, 62:157, 1939.

232. Macchi, G., Abbamondi, A.L., and Arnetoli, G., Toscani, L.: On the diffuse degeneration of the thalamus and the striatum. Clinico-pathological study of a case. Xth International Congress of Neuropathology, Stockholm, 1986.

233. Brownell, B., and Oppenheimer, D.R.: An ataxic form of subacute presenile polioencephalopathy (Jakob-Creutzfeldt disease). J. Neurol. Neurosurg. Psychiat., 28:350, 1965.

234. de Ajuriaguerra, J., Hacaen, H., Layani, F., et al.: Degeneration cortico-strio-spinale, etude anatomo-clinique a propos de la maladie de Creutzfeldt-Jakob. Rev. Neurol., 89:81, 1953.

235. Mizutani, T., Okumara, A., Oda, M., et al.: Panencephalopathic type of CJD. Primary involvement of the cerebral white matter. J. Neurol. Neurosurg. Psychiat., 44:103, 1981.

236. Cruz-Sanchez, F., Lafriente, J., Gertz, H.J., et al.: Spongiform encephalopathy with extensive involvement of white matter. J. Neurol. Sci., 82:1, 81:7, 1987.

237. Josephy, H.: Jakob-Creutzfeldt Krankheit, "spastische Pseudosklerose Jakob". In Handbuch der Neu-

rologie. Edited by O. Bunke, O. Foerster. Berlin, Springer, 1936.

238. Jones, D.P., and Nevin, S.: Rapidly progressive cerebral degeneration (subacute vascular encephalopathy) with mental disorder, focal disturbances and myoclonic epilepsy. J. Neurol., Neurosurg., Psychiat., 17:148, 1954.

239. Nevin, S., McMenemey, W.H., Gehrman, S., et al.: Subacute spongiform encephalopathy. A subacute form of encephalopathy attributable to vascular dysfunction (spongiform cerebral atrophy). Brain, 83:519, 1960.

240. Prusiner, S.B.: Creutzfeldt-Jakob disease and scrapie prions (review). Alzheimer Disease and Associated Disorders, 31(1–2):52, 1989.

241. Gibbs, C.J., et al.: Creutzfeldt-Jakob disease (spongioform encephalopathy). Transmission to chimpanzee. Science, 161:388, 1968.

242. Masters, C.L., Gajdusek, D.C., and Gibbs, Jr., C.: CJD virus isolations from the Gerstmann Straussler syndrome. Brain, 104:559, 1981.

243. Gerstmann, J., Straussler, E., and Scheinker, I.: Uber eine eigenartige hereditar-familiare Erkrankung des Zentralnervensystems. Zugleich ein Beitrag zur Frage des vorzeitigen lokalen Alterns. Z. Neurol., 154:736, 1936.

244. Seitelberger, F.: Eigenartige familiare-hereditare Krankheit des Zentralnervensystems in einer niederosterrichischen Sippe (Zugleich ein Beitrag zur vergleichenden Neuropathologie des Kuru). Weiner Klinische Wochenschrift, 74:681, 1962.

245. Schlot, W., Boellaard, W., Schumm, F., et al.: Gerstmann-Straussler-Scheinker's Disease. Acta Neuropathol. (Berl.), 12:208, 1980.

246. Marchiafava, E., and Bignami, A.: Sopra un alterzione del corpo calloso osservata in soggetti alcoolistti. Riv. Pat. Nerv. Ment., 8:544, 1903.

247. Morel, F.: Une forme anatomo-clinique particuliere de l'alcoolisme chronique rappelant cliniquement la pseudo-paralysie des anciens auteurs, anatomiquement presentant une sclerose laminaire corticale. Schweiz. Arch. Neurol. Psychiat., 44(2):305, 1939.

248. Jequier, M., and Wildi, E.: Deux cas de syndrome de Marchiafava-Bignami et de sclerose laminaire de Morel associes. Schweiz. Arch Neurol. Psychiat. 75(1/2):77, 1955.

249. Brion, S.: Marchiafava-Bignami Syndrome. In: Handbook of Clinical Neurology. New York, Vinken, W. Bruyn, 1976.

250. Delay, J., Brion, S., Escourolle, R., et al.: Rapports entre la degenerescence du corps calleux de Marchiafava-Bignami et la sclerose laminaire corticale de Morel. Encephale, 48:281, 1959.

251. Delay, J. Brion, S., Escourolle, R., et al.: Demences alcooliques. Pseudoparalysie generale alcoolique et lesions-cortico calleuses. Presse med. 68(19):715, 1960.

252. Lechevalier, B., and Anderson, J.C.: Cited by S. Brion et C.S. Jedynak. Les troubles du transfert interhemispheriques.

253. Mc Lardy, T.: Primary degeneration of the corpus callosum. Proc. Roy. Soc. Med., 44:685, 1951.

254. Smith, A.D., Duckett, S., and Waters, A.H.: Neuropathological changes in chronic cyanide intoxication. Nature (Lond.), 200:179, 1963.

255. Adams, R.D., et al.: Symptomatic occult hydrocephalus with "normal" cerebrospinal fluid pressure. N. Engl. J. Med., 273:117, 1965.

256. Hakim, S., and Adams, R.D.: The special clinical problems of symptomatic hydrocephalus with normal cerebrospinal fluid pressure. J. Neurol. Sci., 2:307, 1965.

257. Salmon, J.H.: Adult hydrocephalus. Evaluation of shunt therapy in 80 patients. J. Neurosurg., 37:423, 1972.

258. Friedland, R.P.: Normal-pressure Hydrocephalus and the Saga of the Treatable Dementias. JAMA, 262(18), 2577.

259. Clarfield, A.M.: Normal-pressure Hydrocephalus: Saga or Swamp? JAMA, 262(18), 2592.

260. Probst, A., Fordglou G., Zander, E.: Lesions neuropathologiques lors de l'hydrocephalie interne posttraumatique. Schw. Arch. Neurol. Neurochir. Psychiatr., 116:135, 1975.

ACKNOWLEDGMENT

We wish to thank J. Dellanave (Hôpital Lariboisière), the technicians of Sainte Anne Hospital (Faculty of Medicine) for excellent technical work, I. Coquart and V. Deprat for typing the manuscript.

4

Alzheimer's Disease

JEAN-JACQUES HAUW
CHARLES DUYCKAERTS and
PIA DELAERE

Alzheimer disease (AD)[1] is the most common form of dementia in adults in the industrialized world; it accounts for around 50% of all cases of dementia. In elderly women, AD predominates even more markedly over the other causes of dementia. Dementia increases dramatically with age, reaching 10 to 20% and more in the ninth decade, consequently, the number of cases of AD has increased steadily in countries, where more people survive into old age[2] [See Chap. 1]. AD begins usually with disturbance in recent memory, and a loss of initiative in an otherwise alert patient. Affective problems, such as depression, and disorientation in time and place may appear early in the course. Since similar symptoms can be produced by other types of pathologic situations, an early and important diagnostic consideration should be a search for various treatable disorders.[3,4] The loss of intellectual abilities in AD progresses steadily (although occasional

plateaus and even momentary improvements are possible) to the point that it interferes with social and occupational functions. Focal neurologic signs and symptoms are rare early in the course of the disease, but aphasia, apraxia, and agnosia may predominate in some cases. Seizures and myoclonus may be present in the later stages of the disease. The course of the disease is usually long (6 to 10 years on average) and death is usually caused by an intercurrent infection such as bronchopneumonia.

Clinical diagnosis of AD has improved in recent years with the wider use of diagnostic criteria, especially the DSM-III[5,6,7] Autopsy studies had shown inaccuracy in the antemortem diagnosis ranging from 18 to 45%.[8] There is now a 90% clinical accuracy in cases diagnosed by DSM-III criteria of Primary Degenerative Dementia.[4] In a recent neuropathologic study, 87% of 150 brains of patients diagnosed as AD presented morphologic evidence of the disease.[9] Seventeen of 26 cases diagnosed after postmortem as AD had been diagnosed clinically during life as only mildly retarded.[10]

Some authors distinguish AD from senile dementia of the Alzheimer type (SDAT) on the basis of age of onset, before age 65,[11,12] before age 70,[13] before and after 80,[14] and/or clinical patterns.[11,15,16] These distinctions are still regularly maintained in Europe,[17] while neurologists in the U.S. tend to lump both diseases.[4,12,16] Up to now, epidemiologic studies, clinical or pathologic have failed to disclose different peaks of incidence for AD and SDAT, based on age. Therefore unless specified in this text, we shall use the term AD for both AD and SDAT.

Pathologic changes observed in AD are qualitatively similar to some of those seen in so-called normal aging but then normality of an aged brain is often hard to define. It is often difficult to determine if the changes commonly seen in the brain of the elderly are the pathologic manifestations of an actual disease. Part of the problem is semantic and depends on the definition of normality.[19] The "probable" diagnosis can be made on the basis of clinical or pathologic evidence.[20] We consider that the diagnosis of "definite" AD is best assured by a clinicopathologic correlation.[6] Finally, the diagnosis of dementia according to DSM-III[5] or of AD[6] has been restrictive. This procedure leaves some clinical situation unlabeled: e.g. memory trouble without cognitive changes and with numerous Alzheimer lesions in the hippocampus. Isolated memory problems are not evidence of dementia or of AD.

CASE SELECTION IN NEUROPATHOLOGIC STUDIES

Most of the neuropathologic studies reported in the literature have been cross-sectional and retrospective. Their conclusions were probably valid for the deeply demented patients, but questions arise concerning the diagnosis in the control groups. The frequency of SDAT is high in the general population, especially in institutions where anatomic cases are generally recruited, and where it may be over 50%.[21] The first symptoms and signs can be moderate and not easily recognized unless specifically looked for in a prospective way. Classical and recent studies planned in a prospective manner have taught us much about the neuropathology of the disease.[22-27]

GROSS EXAMINATION OF THE BRAIN

Often the brain appears normal on examination. In some cases, there is cerebral atrophy as shown by the small widened sulci and dilated lateral ventricles, contrasting with the normal configuration of the cerebellum. The atrophy usually involves the frontal, temporal and/or parietal lobes, and it may be symmetric, asymmetric or even focal.[11,12,20]

CEREBRAL ATROPHY

Loss of Brain Weight and Volume. The age-related decrease in normal adult brain weight was incorrectly estimated in many earlier studies.[29] It has recently been shown that if the proportion of body size and brain weight are taken into account, the volume of the cerebral hemispheres does not change significantly until age 50; after which it decreases 2% per decade.[30,31] Thus, decline occurred most frequently after 55 in one series of 51 normal carefully selected brains.[27] Atrophy may be assessed by comparing the volume of a brain to its own cranial capacity.[32] The brain fills about 92% of the cavity in the sixth decade, 83% in the ninth and 81% in the tenth. The loss of brain weight is particularly severe in AD of early onset: 200 to 300 g, i.e. 15 to 25% for most authors. It is usually less severe in SDAT (less than 10%), with a wide range and frequent overlaps with age-matched controls. However, large series have shown clear differences between the mean weight of brains with microscopic changes and those without.

Gyral Atrophy. Tomlinson et al.[22] found no case with marked or generalized cortical atrophy in elderly normal individuals; a slight atrophy of the parasagittal gyri of the frontal and parietal lobes, generalized or isolated frontal atrophy was sometimes observed. With CT scan, gyral atrophy is first seen at about age 40 and increases thereafter.[34,35] However, brains at autopsy sometimes fail to exhibit the atrophy which had been noted with CT. The volume of the brain in vivo is indeed highly dependent on the hydration status and can thus fluctuate.

Gyral atrophy [Fig. 4–1] is usually less marked in SDAT than in early onset AD. Recognizable atrophy is lacking in some patients with SDAT or AD (40% in some series). When present, gyral atrophy is prominent in the par-

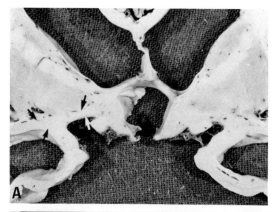

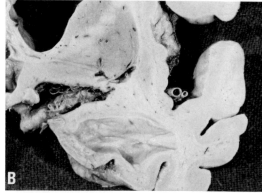

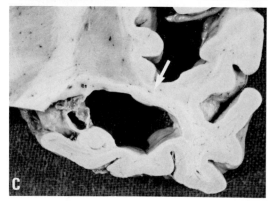

Fig. 4–2. Gross appearance of coronal sections of the brain in a case of severe Alzheimer's disease demonstrating: A. The topography of the sublenticular area where the nucleus basalis of Meynert is located (arrows) B. The atrophy of the amygdaloid body and of the hippocampal uncus and C. The atrophy of the hippocampus and the thinning of the temporal stem (arrow).

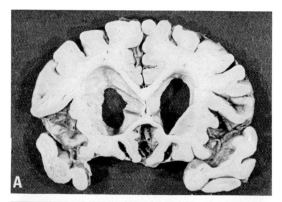

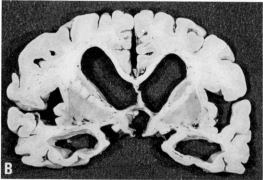

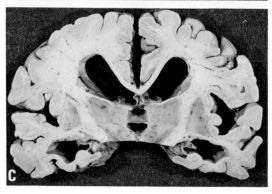

Fig. 4–1. Gross appearance of coronal sections of the brain involving: A. Prefrontal cortex B. Anterior part of the basal ganglia C. Their posterior part in a case of severe Alzheimer's disease. Gyral atrophy, enlargement of the sylvian fissure and ventricular dilation are seen.

asagittal areas and especially in the temporal lobes [Fig. 4–2]. Involvement of the associative cortices has been said to be particularly severe. This remains controversial.[28,33]

The thickness of the neocortex is only

slightly affected by normal aging.[33] Terry et al.[27] showed a moderate but significant decrease of the cortical thickness in the midfrontal and superior temporal areas but not in the inferior parietal areas associated with age. Decrease of 28% in the thickness of the subiculum was observed in 65+ individuals (1933). In AD, the neocortical area of all the cerebral lobes was significantly decreased in early onset forms, whereas only the temporal lobe was atrophic in cases of SDAT over the age of 80.[36] Decrease in the thickness of the neocortex is moderate in AD and SDAT[28,33,37] and not directly proportional to the atrophy. It has been proposed that the decrease of the cortical area on sections of the brain (i.e. atrophy) could be mainly due to a decrease in the length of the cortical ribbon when measured in coronal sections, whereas its thickness did not vary significantly at least in the early stages of the disease. A correlation was reported between the length—and not thickness—of the cortical ribbon and the premortem mental score in a series including patients with SDAT of varying degrees of severity and normal or little affected persons of the same age range in the same institution.[38] These data suggest a loss of columns of neurons or of fibers, arranged perpendicularly to the surface of the cortex [Fig. 4–3]. These columns could correspond to the developmental columns described by Rakic.[39] The loss of selective layers of the neocortex (laminar loss) would rather alter the thickness of the cortical ribbon [Fig. 4–3]. The latter is detectable only in the most affected cases, when it can be seen at gross examination, especially in the temporal cortex.

Ventricular Dilation. Ventricular size increases after age 45.[40] Ventricular size is larger on average in SDAT, compared to an age matched normal control group. Only 13 (57%) of the 23 dements showing the microscopical changes of SDAT had a ventricular volume above the upper limit of normal in the series of Hubbard and Anderson.[36] CT scan measurements of ventricular size as a function of age and of mental impairment have provided conflicting results, even with volumetric measurements. However, quantitative methods confirmed that brain atrophy and ventricular dilation were related to the severity of dementia in patients, provided that strict age- and sex-matched controls were used.[35]

NEURONAL LOSS AND PERIKARYAL ATROPHY[33,41–44]

Some brain stem nuclei: ventral cochlear,[45] trochlear,[46] abducens,[47] inferior olive,[48] show no cell loss with age. For the facial nerve nu-

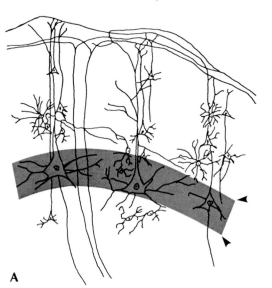

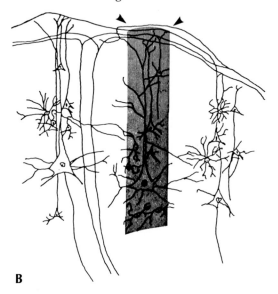

Fig. 4–3. Models of cortical atrophy in aging and Alzheimer's disease. A. Laminar distribution of changes causing a decrease in the thickness of the cortical ribbon. B. Columnar distribution of changes causing a decrease in the length of the cortical ribbon without thinning. The latter seems to predominate at least in the early stages of Alzheimer's disease.

cleus, data are conflicting: some authors consider it is stable with age,[42] whereas according to Hanley's[49] recalculation of Maleci's data[50] a significant 15% loss takes place between the third and the ninth decade (quoted[33]). The number of neurons decreases in the locus ceruleus,[46,51,52,53] substantia nigra[54,55] and Purkinje cell layer.[56] Neuronal loss has also been documented in the thalamus,[57] putamen,[58,59] and the phylogenetically older regions of the amygdala,[60] the basal magnocellular complex (nucleus basalis of Meynert, nucleus of the diagonal band, septal nucleus) and the medial mamillary nucleus.[33] Both Ball[61] and Dam[62] noted a neuronal loss of around 25% in the hippocampus.

The classic literature concerning the loss of neocortical neurons with aging has been evaluated by Brody.[41] Burns,[63] combined the data of Brody (showing a decrease in neuronal density) and that of Leboucq[64] and concluded that there was a 10% decrease in the surface area of the brain between the third and ninth decades.[42] The proposition that there is neuronal loss in the aging brain "is certainly not scientifically accurate" according to Brody and should not be uncritically accepted.[42] Methodologic difficulties are indeed numerous: neuronal counts are expressed by the ratio: number of neurons/unit volume. The counts are performed in a given test volume which is considered a constant fraction of the total volume of the brain. This assumption ignores atrophy, changes in the neuropil volume in connection with hydration, regional differences, etc. Counts of cells in a given area of observation yield a density expressed per unit area. The significant value is the number of cells per unit volume. Calculation of the density per volume given the density per area has to take into account the size and shape of the neurons, and the thickness of the section: the area density of large cells is higher than the area density of small ones when density of their volume is equal. The overestimation of large cell density decreases in proportion to the thickness of the microscopical section. Atrophy of the neurons decreases their density per unit area (i.e. evaluated on the microscopic section), whereas their density per unit volume remains constant. All these difficulties hinder the conclusions which can be drawn from a single value

of neuronal density per unit area.[65] The areal density of neurons of various sizes can be depicted by a histogram. Atrophy of a neuron leads to an increase of some of the smaller size classes at the expense of one class of larger neurons. Decrease of some classes without parallel increase in smaller ones is the consequence of neuronal loss. The shape of the histogram remains unchanged if an equal number of neurons disappears in each size class. This would occur if a loss of cortical columns would have taken place. The interpretation of the histogram becomes complicated as soon as atrophy and loss are combined.

Data concerning quantitative assessments of the cellular population in the brain in normal aging are controversial: some authors emphasize the relative stability of neuronal density: Haug et al.[66] did not find any decrease in the neuronal density of areas 11 (prefrontal) where neurons atrophy, and 17 (occipital) in patients up to 111 years of age when the differences in shrinkage of the microscopic specimen and variability of age are taken into account. Meyer-Ruge et al.[67] showed that the size and shape of neuronal perikarya did not change significantly up to age 75. Later on, decrease in perikaryal area was observed in the pyramidal layers, particularly in layers II and III. Terry et al.[27] found a decrease in the proportion of large neurons balanced by an increase of the small ones in midfrontal and superior temporal gyri. This was interpreted as atrophy without cellular loss. Brody[41,42] found a significant loss in the superior frontal, superior temporal and precentral gyri as well as in the visual cortex. The decrease in neuronal density was not significant in the postcentral and inferior temporal gyri. On the contrary, Henderson et al.[68] using an automatic image analyzer showed a decrease of all size classes in the precentral, postcentral and superior temporal gyri. A 27% loss of neurons in the hippocampus has been noted by Ball.[61] Neocortical neuronal loss in aging preferentially involves granule cells of layers II and IV.[42] Large neurons are less affected than small ones and glial cells according to Henderson et al.[68] Braak and Braak[69] have found a severe and preferential loss of non-pyramidal neurons.

The assertion that neuronal loss in the normal aging cortex is still debated and far from being generally accepted. The "normal" neuronal loss does not seem to generally involve the neurons destroyed in AD and SDAT (small, granular neurons in normal aging, versus middle-sized pyramidal neurons in AD; cf infra). This argues against AD and SDAT being a non specific premature aging and for a distinct, abnormal process occurring in these diseases.[37,70]

Neuronal loss in the cerebral cortex is more evident in AD and SDAT. In the latter, Terry et al.[71] found a 36 to 46% decrease in the density of neurons larger than 90 μm^2 in three neocortical regions. This was subsequently confirmed: morphometric data on a larger number of cases[73] of AD of various ages revealed a spectrum of graded pathologic severity inversely proportional to age, including the decrease of neuronal density in the midfrontal and superior temporal (but not in the inferior temporal) neocortices.[37] Mountjoy et al.[72] have also noted that the neuronal density was smaller in the inferior frontal and superior temporal gyri in the whole demented group of patients and in the under 80s. The decrease in the absolute number of neurons in four columns extending from the pial surface to the white matter was more severe than the changes in neuronal density. This could have been the consequence of a reduction of the thickness of the cortex in the demented group. In the hippocampus, the neuronal fall-out reached 57%.[61] Mann et al.[73] found an overall 40% reduction in number of pyramidal neurons in area H1. Significant neuronal loss was observed in Rose's H1 field and the subiculum but not in the end-plate or Rose's H2 field. However, quantitative cytochemical techniques showed that pyramidal neuronal RNA was depressed in all areas of the hippocampus examined.[74] This loss has been found to be correlated with the number of tangle-bearing cells.[61,74] A marked cell loss is also seen in the entorhinal cortex[75] and in the amygdala.[60,76]

Cellular loss in the cerebral cortex in AD/SDAT has also been shown in the cholinergic basal magno-cellular complex: nucleus basalis of Meynert and septal nucleus.[78,79] The results of the numerous studies of cholinergic neurons in the nucleus basalis of Meynert suggest that cell loss is mild, and undetectable in some cases.[79] This could be due to technical factors

since numeration of the whole nucleus is difficult and since only the anterior parts are affected in mildly affected patients.[80] In addition, neuronal loss in this nucleus seems to be a late phenomenon in the course of the disease.[81] Cell loss is better documented in the noradrenergic locus coeruleus, where it affects mainly the dorsal and oral parts,[82] and to a lesser extent the serotoninergic raphe nuclei.[83] The loss of aminergic neurons could be correlated with the depression which sometimes occurs in the course of AD.[84] As a rule, the substantia nigra is preserved, although it has been reported to be affected in some younger patients.[76] Neuronal loss has also been documented in the anterior olfactory nucleus,[85] the paraventricular nucleus of the hypothalamus, particularly in the younger patients,[86] and in the suprachiasmatic nucleus.[87] A significant loss of the ganglion cells in the retina has been described in AD.[88] The lesion may differentially affect the large ganglion cells and may have a greater effect on centrally placed ganglion cells of the macula.[89] This loss would suggest that neurons can disappear in regions known to be devoid of NFT. Other areas although affected by age-related neuronal loss e.g. basal ganglia and cerebellar cortex, are not greatly altered in AD and SDAT. It is generally thought that the neuronal loss as well as much of the biochemical and pathologic changes is much more significant and widespread during AD than during SDAT.[86,90,91]

DENDRITIC CHANGES

The Golgi method has been used to study dendritic morphology in aging, AD and SDAT. Postmortem delay was shown to cause artifactual changes.[92,93] Some aspects once thought to be typical of aging are now considered mere artifacts. However, disorganization of the fibers of the cerebral cortex is seen by silver impregnations and immunocytochemistry. This is possibly due to regressive changes of the processes of degenerating neurons and cells. The diffuse meshwork of dystrophic nerve fibers in the neuropil is labeled by a monoclonal antibody directed against a group of proteins named tau (tubulin associated proteins)[94] which labels also neurofibrillary tangles located inside the neuronal soma.[95] Braak et al.[96]

observed some abnormal fibers impregnated with Gallyas silver method at a distance from the neuronal body which he named neuropil threads. The same team showed that some of these neuropil threads were located in dendritic processes of neurons bearing neurofibrillary tangles.[97] Morphometric studies of the alterations in the length and in the orientation of neocortical fibers confirmed that they were correlated with the density of senile plaques and of neurofibrillary tangles.[98] The reduction in synaptic density reported in the neocortex in AD[99] can be related to these regressive changes and to neuronal loss. In addition, carefully controlled studies suggested that dendritic spatial extension increases with age in pyramidal cells of the parahippocampal gyrus, granule cells of the dentate gyrus and reticular neurons of the basal magnocellular complex. Small excrescences from the neuronal body ("perisomatic filopodia") testify to a persistent neural plasticity in aging.[100]

Cellular regeneration in AD/SDAT is seldom observed except in certain types of cells such as the reticular neurons of the basal nucleus.[100,101] The distribution of receptors for kainic acid and of acetylcholinesterase in early cases of AD indicated the persistence of some plasticity of the hippocampus.[102] This was not the case in late onset cases.[103,104]

SENILE CHANGES

These pathologic structures are seen in the so-called normal elderly brain, AD, middle-age Down syndrome, and some cases of Parkinson's disease. These changes are neurofibrillary tangles (NFT), senile plaques (SP) [Fig. 4-4] and granulovacuolar degenerations (GVD). NFT are present and SP are absent in Guam ALS-Parkinson dementia complex and in dementia pugilistica.

NEUROFIBRILLARY TANGLES AND PAIRED HELICAL FILAMENTS

Neurofibrillary tangles (NFT) are torchlike or globose inclusions located in the neuronal perisoma containing paired helical filaments (PHF). Sometimes these are found free in the neuropil, especially in the hippocampus[12] [Fig. 4-5]. NFT are impregnated by silver methods

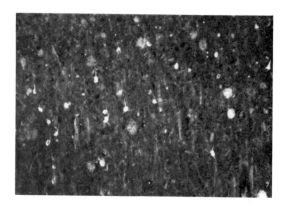

Fig. 4-4. Numerous senile changes (senile plaques and neurofibrillary tangles) in the supramarginal gyrus (objective ×10; thioflavin S).

(such as Bodian's, Bielschowsky's, Holmes', Gallyas', Palmgren's), thioflavin S and less regularly Congo red results in a birefringence with polarized light. Congophilia and stainability by thioflavin are the tinctorial characteristics of amyloid substance. X ray diffraction has shown these characteristics to be usually linked with a special type of protein spatial configuration, i.e. B-pleated sheet which seems indeed the structure exhibited by PHF with x ray diffraction procedure.[105] In electron microscopy, NFT are constituted of fibrils with constrictions located at 79 nm intervals on average range: 50 to 105 nm.[106] At the constrictions, the fibrils are 10 nm wide and 20 to 25 nm wide midway between constrictions.[107] There are various interpretations of this morphology: Kidd[108] suggested that they were made up of two filaments 10 nm wide, twisted in a helical structure (paired helical filaments, PHF), which was confirmed later. Wisniewski et al.,[109] using tilt analysis, thought that they were made of four protofilaments 3 to 5 nm wide [Fig. 4-6]. Image reconstruction[110] suggested that a set of six spherical subunits (axial dimension 4 nm) overlapped to form a ribbon twisted in a left-handed helix. The PHF can exist in both right-handed and left-handed configurations.[111] In addition to these elements, straight tubules, 15 nm in diameter can be seen, either constituting the entire tangle or coexisting with the PHF.[107] A mixture of normal neurofilaments has also been observed.[12]

The biochemical nature of NFT remains unknown. Their insolubility in most solvents is

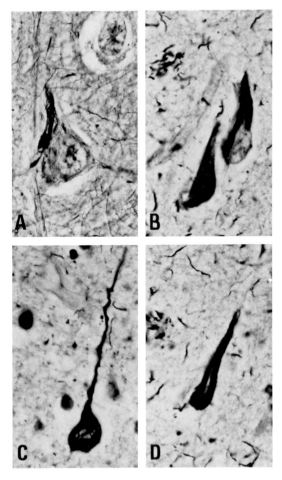

Fig. 4-5. Neurofibrillary tangles. A. Palmgren method (mod Cross): discrete argyrophilic tangles in a pyramidal neuron. B. Torchlike, C. Plump, D. Extracellular neurofibrillary tangle. (Bodian stain and Luxol fast blue; ×100)

used to isolate them[112] but precludes protein sequencing. NFT are also resistant to most proteolytic digestion.[113] Recently, a new technique was proposed to solubilize NFT thus the sequencing of NFT may be soon available.[114,155] There is no doubt that this would clarify the controversies about the nature and origin of this structure. The chemical nature of PHF based on immunochemical studies is incomplete but promising at this time.

Antibodies to neurofilament constituents have been repeatedly shown to label NFT.[116,117] Antibodies against phosphorylated neurofilaments were demonstrated by Sternberger to abnormally label the soma of the neurons with

NFT.[118] The most regular results were obtained with antibodies directed against tau.[95] Tau seems abnormally phosphorylated.[119,120] Anti-tau antibody labels NFT but also an abnormal meshwork of neurites. Before the finding of tau epitopes within the PHF, it had been noticed that the density of neurotubules was ab-

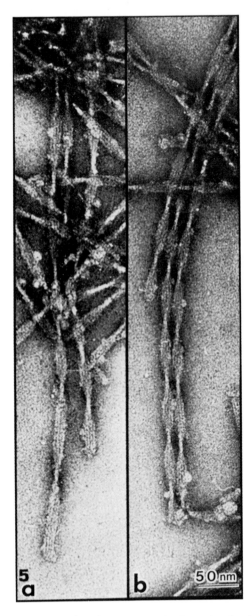

Fig. 4-6. Isolated PHF negatively stained with phosphotungstic acid, (a) and (b). These micrographs illustrate four protofilaments of a PHF along its length. (×215,000). From Wisniewski et al., J. Neuropathol. Exp. Neurol. *43*:643, 1984. (with permission)

normally low in neurons containing PHF[121,122] and a possible relation had been suggested at that time between tubules and PHF.[12] Antibodies raised against ubiquitin linked to subcellular components destined for proteolysis, label NFT.[124,125] It is not known if ubiquitin epitopes are integrated in the NFT or if they are secondarily linked to this structure in order to initiate proteolysis. Some antibodies, generally polyclonal, have been raised against enriched fraction of NFT.[95,126–128] These antibodies generally exhibit a high anti-tau activity, which, however, is probably not exclusive. Gambetti et al.[129] found that tau proteins and high-molecular-weight microtubule associated proteins were not stained with Bodian silver. On the other hand, Bodian's technique and anti-NFT antiserum were not labeling the same number of alterations on alternative slides of 15 cases with graded intellectual deficit:[130] it is thus probable that anti-NFT and Bodian's technique label different epitopes. Finally an antibody (Alz50) was claimed to label a protein (A 68) located in the NFT but also in the vulnerable neurons before NFT become visible.[131,132] Relationships of this protein and of tau remain controversial.[133] A monoclonal antibody directed towards GQ1b and minor gangliosides (A2B5) were also shown to label NFT. The A2B5 reactive epitope is noncovalently bound to the NFT.[134] Cholinesterase activity within NFT related to age and Alzheimer disease has also been mentioned.[135]

A few NFT are seen during normal aging in the hippocampus (CA1 and the subiculum), the entorhinal cortex, parahippocampal gyrus, and in the amygdala. Rare NFT can be found in other neocortical areas, in the olfactory bulb,[136] in some basal ganglia such as the basal magnocellular complex and in the brainstem, especially in the locus ceruleus and in the substantia nigra, where they affect the most medial extremity.[28] NFT are sometimes seen in apparently normal persons less than 40. They were present in about 5% of individuals age 50 to 60% in 70 years old population in autopsies of a non selected population.[137–139] NFT were constant in a non-selected series of institutionalized centenarians.[140] However, the percentage of brains with a high density of NFT has been reported to decrease from the ninth to the tenth decade.[33] Three out of 9 brains of non-demented individuals of the eleventh decade had few NFT among the 11 samples examined. NFT were constantly present in the hippocampus, the temporal cortex (parahippocampal gyrus and adjacent neocortex), less frequent in the cingulate cortex (4/9) and the prefrontal cortex (1/9) and were absent in the occipital cortex. They were seen in 8 cases in the nucleus basalis of Meynert, in 3 in the septal nuclei, in 4 in the other basal ganglia and in the brainstem.[140] Various opinions are held about the significance of these changes, seen in apparently normal persons: for some authors, they are the consequence of a disease stopped at various stages of its course. Others believe that NFT are the mere consequence of physiologic aging, dramatically accelerated in AD and SDAT. Part of the question is semantic but it is clear at the present time that NFT seen in normal aging can not be morphologically distinguished from those seen in AD or in SDAT, except for their density and distribution. NFT have been noted in neurons of the upper cervical ganglia, i.e. in the peripheral nervous system.[141] Although structures bearing some similarities with PHF have been described in various animal species.[142] There are various presentations of NFT. NFT seen in supranuclear palsy (and probably in postencephalitic Parkinson's disease) are mainly composed of straight 15 nm tubule-like structures; phosphorylated tau polypeptides are also a major antigenic determinant of NFT in supranuclear palsy. One epitope in AD tangle seems absent on, or at least inaccessible in, the 15 nm straight fibrils of supranuclear palsy.[143] Comparison of the antigenic properties of NFT in AD and in supranuclear palsy has recently shown that some antigenic determinants depended upon the location of the tangle-bearing neuron and not of the disease or of the main ultrastructural appearance of the filaments. It is tempting to speculate that the epitopes examined (a phosphorylated epitope of the 200 kDa protein of neurofilament, and various epitopes of ubiquitin) belong to cell constituents that become associated with a core element.[144] NFT seen in experimental aluminum intoxication are made of bundles of intermediate filaments, 10 nm wide. NFT are present in AD, Guam ALS-Parkinson dementia complex, dementia pugilistica, aged Down syndrome, and some forms of Parkinson's disease, subacute sclerosing panencephalitis, adult lipofuscinosis, sudanophilic leukodystrophy, tuberous sclerosis, juvenile dystonic lipidosis, advanced hydrocephalus, lead encephalopathy.[145-148] It has been recently confirmed that NFT may be present in the nucleus basalis of Meynert as early as 5 years after a massive cerebral infarct. This suggests that NFT could occur as a retrograde reaction in some neurons.[146] Some cases of AD and SDAT do not have NFT when SP are numerous.[149] Some authors[150] tend to consider SP more specific a change than NFT which are, in their view, more contingent and common. Wilcock and Esiri,[151] using silver impregnation, found NFT to be better correlated with the intellectual status than SP. Differences in the techniques which are used to reveal SP and NFT could possibly explain part of these discrepancies.[130,152]

In AD and SDAT, NFT are not as widespread in the cortex as senile plaques [See below]. Only some categories of middle-sized neurons are affected: pyramidal in the cortex, multipolar in the basal magnocellular complex and in the brainstem. Granule cells (layer IV of the neocortex; fascia dentata) and giant pyramidal cells (Betz cells) are most generally spared. The distribution of NFT in the hippocampus and amygdala has been thoroughly studied.[33,153] NFT are numerous in the pyramidal neurons of the hippocampus. The ranking order of predilection is: entorhinal cortex > subiculum > H1 > end-plate > presubiculum > H2.[154] The parahippocampal gyrus, amygdala,[60] olfactory bulb[155] and most of neocortical areas (the primary motor and sensory cortices being relatively spared) are also affected. Their laminar distribution was shown to be nonrandom. They are more numerous in the pyramidal neurons of layers III and V.[156] Some neurons having expressed an epitope of a non-phosphorylated neurofilament seem more often affected.[157] The density of neocortical NFT is correlated with the degree of mental impairment.[151] They are also seen in some deep nuclei, most of them projecting to the cerebral cortex: the basal magnocellular complex, the hypothalamus (especially the medial part of the posterior lateral hypothalamic area), the midline area of the thalamus, the an-

terior olfactory nucleus, the peripeduncular nucleus, the pedunculopontine and dorsal tegmental nuclei, the pontine tegmentum and especially the medial parabrachial nucleus, the dorsal and median raphe nuclei, the ventral tegmental area, the locus ceruleus, substantia nigra, the other areas of the reticular formation, and seldom in medulla and cerebellum.[33,76,153]

SENILE PLAQUES

These are spherical lesions constituted of a crown of argyrophilic debris and an amyloid core [Fig. 4–7]. Such plaques have been named neuritic by Wisniewski and Terry.[158] The mean diameter of the SP has been variously estimated as 36 to 200 μm.[12,152,159] The amyloid core is visible after staining with hemateineosin, PAS, Alcyan blue, Masson's trichromic method, thioflavin S, and anti-A4 antibodies. The abnormal crown which surrounds SP is impregnated by various silver techniques such as von Braunmuhl's method. The crown of the SP is labeled with anti-NFT and anti-tau markers. Most of the debris in the crown consists of axonal processes identified by the presence of presynaptic vesicles;[158] some are dendritic as seen with Golgi impregnation,[160] astroglial[126,161-163] and of microglial origin.[164] Axonal processes at the periphery of the SP are massively enlarged and contain PHF identical to those found in NFT, granular degenerating mitochondria and many lysosomes.[12]

Acetyl cholinesterase activity was shown by histochemistry to be present in some of the fibers of the crown of the SP[165] and accepted as evidence for the presence of cholinergic fibers, originating in the nucleus basalis of Meynert. This innervation was considered supportive of the "cholinergic hypothesis", according to which the main disturbances were located in the nucleus basalis of Meynert and in its cholinergic fibers.[166,167] Numerous other neurotransmitters have since been demonstrated in the SP: neuropeptide Y, substance P, neurotensin, cholecystokinin, catecholamine, and somatostatin.[168] The neuromediator content depends on the location of the SP: an antibody against tyrosine hydroxylase labeled most of the SP seen in the amygdala but almost none of the SP located in the nearby neocortex.[169]

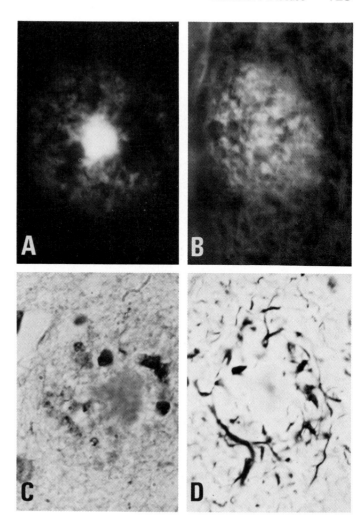

Fig. 4–7. Senile plaques: A- Dense core of amyloid (thioflavin S), B. Amyloid wisp without dense core (thioflavin S). C. Anti-PHF labeled processes surrounding a core of amyloid substance. D. Neurites impregnated by silver. Bodian stain and luxol fast blue. ×100.

The amyloid core consists of 5 to 10 nm filaments. It contains a 4.2 kD hydrophobic protein which has been completely sequenced[170] and called A4 B protein (because of its B-pleated structure), the gene of which is located on the long arm of chromosome 21 [see later]. The cloning of A4 amyloid gene enabled the clone sequencing of the precursor of A4.[171] This 695 amino-acid glycoprotein has a single predicted transmembrane domain, most of which is present in the 42 amino-acid peptide deposited in SP vessels. It is believed to be a membrane protein with a carboxyterminal intracellular portion and a large amino-terminal extracellular portion. It has therefore been suggested that amyloid formation may arise as a consequence of membrane damage.[172] There are at least two alternatively spliced products of the A4 precursor gene. The two longer forms carry an additional domain with probably a protease inhibitor function.[173–175] These could act either as inhibitor of the proteolytic processing of the amyloid precursor or as a membrane-bound inhibitor involved in cell growth and differentiation.[173] The isolation, partial amino acid sequencing and immunocytochemical characterization of amyloid P component (a serum protein found in association with almost all types of amyloid deposit) in SP has also been reported.[176]

Some SP contain only argyrophilic fibers and have been identified as "immature" plaques,[158] some have both an amyloid center and a neuritic crown and are named "classical" or "mature" plaques, and some appear to contain only amyloid, and are referred to as "burn out" or "hypermature" plaques. This terminology suggests a sequence of morpho-

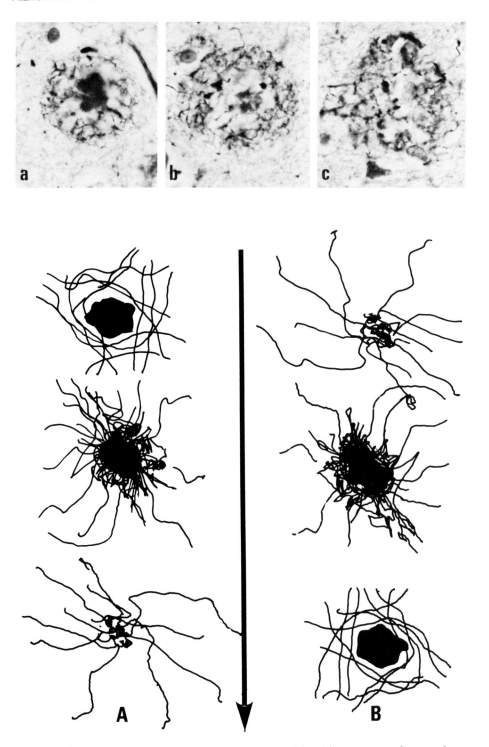

Fig. 4–8.   The 3 types of senile plaque. Bodian stain and luxol fast blue. a, Burned-out or hypermature, b, Classical or mature, c, Neuritic. These 3 types could represent various stages: amyloid, amyloid and neurites, resorption of amyloid leaving abnormal neurites (model A); neurites, amyloid and neurites, resorption of neurites leaving amyloid (model B). See text for explanation. ×100.

logical changes [Fig. 4–8]. The relationship between neurites and the amyloid substance remains open to question: the amyloid may appear first and then be surrounded by neurites or it may occur secondary to degenerating neurites, as initially proposed by Wisniewski and Terry.[158]

The hypothesis of a disturbed metabolism of amyloidogenic or amyloid substance was suggested as the initial step of the formation of the SP.[177,178] This hypothesis has recently received some support: in the least affected patients of a series of 15 cases with graded intellectual deficit from the Charles Foix longitudinal study, SP revealed by thioflavin S were not immunolabeled by a polyclonal antibody against PHF. This could not be explained only by differences in sensitivity of the stains and was compatible with the hypothesis that amyloid was surrounded by anti-PHF positive neurites only in the latest stages of the SP.[152] In addition to the classic senile plaques, A4 immunocytochemistry permits identification of diffuse afibrillar deposits of A4 protein that are not observed by conventional methods. The discovery of protease inhibitor-like domains (which could be growth factors) in the proposed extracellular portion of the amyloid precursor protein would explain that amyloid could attract neighboring neurites to constitute an SP.[173] Similarities with a glycosylated cell surface receptor have been emphasized.[171] The m-RNA for B protein is found in many nonneural tissues in addition to brain.[179,180] The origin, cerebral or extracerebral, of this protein is unknown. Some authors have noted that a capillary was always present in the SP and suggested that the amyloidogenic substance could indeed originate from the vessels and precipitate around them.[181,182] Amyloid may be the product of proteolysis of a precursor by macrophages in systemic amyloidoses. The identification of ubiquitin in SP, a protein which acts as a signal for the degradation of abnormal proteins, and that of proteases inhibitors (-antichymotrypsin and, possible protease inhibitors) argues for a similar mechanism in the brain.[174] Some SP contain a microglial cell stained by a lectin and possibly this cell plays a crucial role in amyloidogenesis.[164] If amyloid precedes the neuritic changes, its absence from some senile plaques suggests

that it can be resorbed unlike systemic amyloid. Microglial or astrocytes could be candidates for this resorption which would be another example of regulation of amyloid deposit.[183]

Distribution of the SP is extremely diffuse in the cortex but concentrated in laminae II and III.[156,184–186] In the neocortex, SP are located between dendritic clusters, with pyramidal cell apical dendritic shafts extruding from the plaques.[187] SP are seen in regions usually devoid of NFT such as the occipital lobe. SP are numerous in the hippocampus, amygdala, hypothalamus,[153] basal ganglia,[188] the thalamus,[153] and in the substantia innominata.[189] SP are rare in the brainstem. In normal aging, SP occur in small numbers with increasing frequency from the fifth decade on, in the amygdala, the hippocampus and the neocortex,[136] with a predilection for the parahippocampal and occipitotemporal (fusiform) gyri and for the prefrontal cortex. The frequency of their distribution increases "monotically" after age 71 year in a general autopsy population.[138,139] In centenarians, SP were found in 8 of 9 nondemented individuals, mainly in the hippocampus (8/9), occipital cortex (6/9), parahippocampal gyrus and prefrontal cortices (5/9), the cingular cortex being less affected (2/9).[140] Blessed et al.[190] using a silver impregnation method to reveal the SP showed that there was a linear relationship between the intellectual status, as measured by a simple clinical scale and the number of SP. This has been confirmed by other studies.[151,185] Recently, a number of elderly people who were living in a nursing home and were considered intellectually normal were shown to exhibit a high density of SP at postmortem examination.[191] It was suggested that the density of SP was not a predictable variable for the intellectual status. The presence of neurites around the SP could play an important role in their contribution to the mental impairment.[152] It has been hypothesized that a threshold in the density of SP had to be reached before clinical consequences could occur (i.e. low threshold). On the other hand, the density of SP may well increase in certain advanced cases without causing any detectable worsening in patients with the most severe clinical score possible (high threshold effect).[190] SP identical to those of AD and aging are present in adults with Down syndrome and in some cases of Parkinson's disease. SP seen in slow virus diseases due to unconventional agents (Kuru, the Gerstmann-Straussler-Scheinker syndrome, and some cases of Creutzfeldt-Jakob disease) frequently occur in the cerebellum and are often purely amyloid without a crown of debris; such SP contain scrapie associated fibers and PrP amyloid.

AMYLOID ANGIOPATHY

In most cases of AD, amyloid substance infiltrates the wall of pial and penetrating small arteries or of parenchymatous small arterioles, capillaries and venules sometimes extending into surrounding cerebral tissues; this is referred to as dyshoric angiopathy [Fig. 4–9]. Dyshoric angiopathy is seen most frequently in lamina III of the calcarine gyrus and adja-

cent occipital cortex, occasionally in Ammon's horn and in the cerebellum. The amyloid substance in the vessel walls and in the core of the SP are morphologically alike biochemically similar (B protein and P component).[176] It is thus different from the amyloid substance seen in the senile type of cardiac or pancreatic amyloidosis, in chronic inflammatory disease, in plasma cells dyscrasia or in the disorders related to unconventional agents (Creutzfeldt-Jakob disease, Kuru and the Gerstmann-Straussler-Schinker syndrome). For most authors, NFT are biochemically different although some of them have amyloid tinctorial affinities.

Amyloid angiopathy is observed in three clinical settings: it can be found incidentally in apparently normal old individuals; it can be the cause of vascular lesions such as multiple hematomas, small infarcts[192] and transient

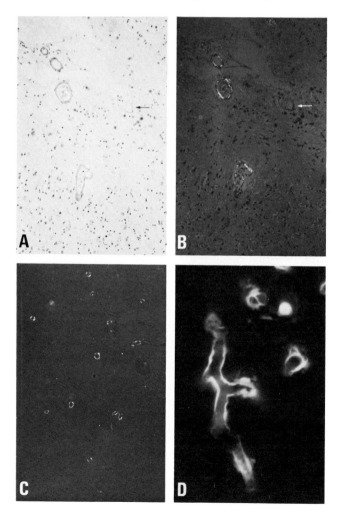

Fig. 4–9. Amyloid angiopathy: A and B: Congo red before (A) and after (B) polarization. Note the absence of amyloid angiopathy in one vessel shown by the arrow. ×10. C and D: Thioflavin S (C: ×10; D: ×63): amyloid deposit in the vessel walls. When the amyloid deposit is present in large vessels, some European authors use preferentially the term of congophilic angiopathy (A and B). In D, the amyloid deposit in small vessels also involves the adjoining parenchyma: dyshoric angiopathy for the same authors.

ischemic attacks[193] and it is frequently found in SDAT, AD and a few other related disorders such as Down syndrome, Guam-Parkinson-Dementia complex. Amyloid angiopathy is usually associated with SP and NFT.[192] With the exception of the type of amyloid related to unconventional agents (PrP), and of the amyloid of Icelandic hereditary cerebral hemorrhage (due to cystatin C), all cerebral amyloids are B-protein related. In normal aging, amyloid angiopathy is seen from the seventh decade on, sometimes in association with the senile type of cardiac or pancreatic amyloidosis. It has been reported in 8 to 50% of brains in the seventh decade, in 23 to 63% in the eighth and in 37 to 87% in the ninth.[33] Nine out of 12 centenarians we examined had vascular amyloid.[140] For most authors, AD or SDAT is not invariably associated with vascular amyloid,[12,28,194–196] but Joachim et al.[9] have claimed that it was constant in 100 consecutive cases of AD and not in age-matched controls. However, with conventional techniques marked vascular amyloid was seen only in about 50% of cases with AD. This frequency depends on the sensitivity of the staining method used to reveal amyloid. Amyloid angiopathy is considered much more frequent than previously thought when antibodies raised against epitopes of protein A4 are used.[197] The relationship between amyloid of vessels and of plaques is presumed. The vascular origin of cerebral amyloid has been hypothesized.[133,194,195] Most authors believe that there is no constant topographic relationship between SP and vascular amyloid, which is seen mostly in the occipital cortex. Mountjoy et al.[182] did not find a significant correlation between vascular amyloid and the severity of dementia in 15 cases of SDAT but there was a significant association between the presence of vascular amyloid and SP. A negative correlation was even found between the density of vascular amyloid and that of congophilic plaques or tangles in hippocampus. These data were less compatible with the hypothesis that the amyloid precursor protein first enters the vessel wall to produce amyloid there and then moves into the brain to produce amyloid of SP than with the reverse hypothesis.[198] In addition, during SP formation amyloid seems to precede neuritic changes, as already mentioned.[152]

GRANULOVACUOLAR DEGENERATION

Granulovacuolar degeneration (GVD) of neurones consists of the presence of vacuoles containing granules in the cytoplasm of pyramidal cells of the hippocampus [Fig. 4–10]. These granules are eosinophilic, argentophilic and indistinct with Nissl stain.[140] Whether the granules may contain tau protein is debated.[119,199] GVD is often present in association with NFT.[140] In Guam ALS-Parkinsonism dementia complex, Pick's disease, Down syndrome and in AD, the number of cells with GVD is markedly increased throughout the hippocampus, particularly the subiculum. GVD is rarely seen in the neocortex, amygdala, hypothalamus and in paramedian nuclei of the midbrain, and nowhere else in the brain.[28,200,201]

OTHER CHANGES IN GRAY MATTER

Reduction of the size of the nucleus and nucleolus and of the content of cytoplasmic RNA in AD appears early in the disease.[76,159] Accumulation of lipofuscin pigment within nerve cells in aging is usual. In AD, it has never been demonstrated to be linked to the level of dementia.[28,33,76,140] NFT-bearing neurons appear to contain more lipofuscin pigment than do the other cells.[202] Hirano bodies are short eosinophilic rod-like structures lying free or in the cytoplasm of neurones located almost exclusively in the Sommer's sector of the hippo-

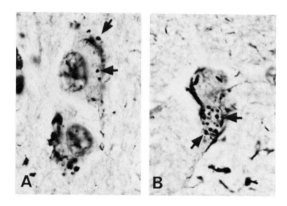

Fig. 4–10. A and B: Granulovacuolar degeneration: arrows (objective ×100; Bielschowsky's method).

campal pyramidal layer. These bodies are present in Guam-Parkinson-dementia complex, Pick's disease and AD.[107] Hirano bodies have a paracrystalline appearance in electron microscopy[12,107] and react with anti-actin sera[203] and with anti-tau.[204,205] Lewy bodies, considered for a long time to be pathognomonic of idiopathic Parkinson' disease,[12,91] are seen in some cases of AD, with or without parkinsonism. The significance of this association will be discussed later. A spongiform change in the upper neocortical layers can be seen especially in the more severe cases of AD.[121,206] Astrocytic hypertrophy and proliferation (gliosis) is diffuse in AD. A marked increase in the number of astrocytes in laminae II and VI without a change in the total number of glial cells has been noted in the cortex of frontal, temporal and parietal lobes.[162] An increase of the density of astrocytes has been found in the parietal, orbital, and occipital (visual) cortices.[66] Astrocytes participate in the constitution of SP as shown by electron microscopy[158] and immunocytochemistry[162] and in the processing of NFT after the neuronal death.[207] It has been suggested that astrocytes play a role in the regulation of amyloid deposit and resorption in SP.[183]

PROGRESSION OF THE PATHOLOGIC CHANGES IN THE GRAY MATTER

The progression of the lesions of AD as a function of time is difficult to assess. Recently, Mann et al.[159] compared the data of cerebral biopsies to the changes seen in the neighboring neocortical area at postmortem examination in the same patients affected with AD. In all 5 patients, the density and the nucleolar volume of pyramidal nerve cells fell significantly from biopsy to death, and SP density did not change. NFT density either did not change or decrease from the time of the biopsy to death.

CHANGES OF WHITE MATTER

The consequences of the loss of cortical neurons with long axons in AD on the morphologic characteristics of the centrum semi-ovale are not well known. The gray/white matter volume ratio was found to be 1:28 in individ-

uals born 20 years ago, 1:13 in those born 50 years ago and 1:55 in centenarians. This suggested a preferential loss of gray matter in quinquagenarians and of white matter later on if the fiber density of the white matter remained constant whatever the age.[30] Rarefaction of the white matter is observed on gross examination of the brain in the elderly.[208,209] Kemper considered that qualitatively the older normal brains of the Yakovlev collection showed a pallor of myelin staining of the forebrain that appeared to be confined to the corona radiata and stratum sagittale interna;[33] this observation suggested that fiber density decreased with age but awaits quantitative confirmation. A primary, age-related demyelination has been postulated for these changes that principally occur in late myelinated areas.[33] Loss of fibers secondary to neuronal degeneration is also plausible in the light of the present state of knowledge. In SDAT, rarefaction of the fibers and of oligodendroglia in the white matter was thought to be the consequence of vascular disturbances as suggested by hyalinosis of the vessel walls.[210] To our knowledge, the fiber loss in the white matter has not been quantified in the course of SDAT and compared to a control group and the hypothesis that it is a primary disease of the white matter awaits confirmation.[210] It is generally agreed that the disease process in AD (at least morphologically) is evident in the gray matter, much more so than in the white matter.

LEUKOARAIOSIS

CT scans sometimes show areas of hypodensity in the white matter. The word leukoaraiosis was coined to describe these changes.[211] It is a purely radiologic term and the pathology of this condition remains unknown. Vascular disorders such as lacunes or degeneration of myelinated fibers as seen in subcortical arteriosclerotic encephalopathy (Binswanger disease), and "etat cribe" of Durand-Fardel[208] can result in leukoaraiosis. Leukoaraiosis is present in the brains of normal old individuals but seems statistically correlated with intellectual impairment, mild neurologic signs and symptoms, and vascular risk factors.[212] The relationship between these radiologic aspects and Binswanger disease has been debated. Binswanger disease seems to be much more frequently diagnosed on radiologic grounds than at pathologic examination. It has been claimed that the decrease of the computerized tomography numbers in the gray and white matter was one of the best CT signs of AD and SDAT.[213–215] MRI hypersignals in T2-weighed sequences have been reported in the elderly on MRI and were associated at postmortem examination with enlarged perivascular spaces, characteristic of "etat crible"[216] [see Chap. 20].

TOPOGRAPHY OF THE CHANGES AND SELECTIVE VULNERABILITY

Does AD begin in one or different areas of the brain?

1. The selectivity of lesions in AD, affecting heavily some brain areas while sparing others a few microns distant, has given rise to many hypotheses.

The Olfactory Hypothesis. The strong involvement of the hippocampal-amygdaloid complex and the recent demonstration of lesions in olfactory bulbs and tracts suggested that the latter may be a portal of entry of the pathologic agent. This hypothesis is not supported by the morphologic studies which have shown that the lesions of entorhinal cortex and amygdala preceded those of the olfactory bulbs.[76]

The "Limbic" Hypothesis.[75] Changes in normal aging and in AD disrupt anatomical systems known from animal studies[217] and human pathology[218,219] to be involved in memory. Such structures, organized around the hippocampus, highly interconnected and linked with multimodal association cortices are said to be made of two parts:

• A "feed-forward" system stems from the primary sensory cortices and projects to association cortices and limbic structures through several synapses. It converges on lamina II of the entorhinal cortex (in the fifth temporal gyrus adjacent to the hippocampus) where the perforant path originates. This is the final common pathway for the neocortical inputs to the hippocampus.

• A "feedback" system starts in the subiculum, a pyramidal area of the hippocampal formation which it links to other parts of the limbic lobe and to subcortical targets such as the nucleus basalis of Meynert and the mamillary bodies. The limbic cortices finally project back to associative neocortical areas.

The amygdaloid body, located in the temporal pole, lies in the center of a similar network of connections. It has been suggested that the density of the changes conformed to a gradient parallel to this circuitry: the closer to the hippocampus and amygdala, the more severe the tissue alterations.[75,220,221]

The "Cortico-Cortical" Hypothesis. The topography of changes are interpreted in a slightly different way by Morrison et al.[222] The emphasis is not laid on the limbic system as such but on the long cortico-cortical connections. In these authors' view, neurons which are selectively involved in the disease are the pyramidal neurons that furnish the long cortico-cortical projections, which would explain the stereotypic distribution of SP and of NFT.[156,159,184,186] This way of explaining the topography of changes is obviously close to the "limbic" hypothesis since the limbic system is connected with the neocortex by long cortico-cortical fibers.

Cortico-Subcortical or Subcortico-Cortical Changes? The cholinergic hypothesis suggests that the cortical changes are secondary to the alterations of the substantia innominata (subcortico-cortical involvement). The primary involvement of the cortex with secondary involvement of the sub-cortex (cortico-subcortical involvement) is also a possible explanation.[153,167,223–227] The finding by Palmer et al.[227] of a group of patients without cholinergic deficit in the neocortex favors the cortico-subcortical series of event.

2. Selective vulnerability has been explained by various putative mechanisms:

A special metabolism or the specific vascularization of some areas or cell types in the brain have frequently been hypothesized as the cause of the selective vulnerability of AD. Some of the cell types actively involved in AD are also selectively injured in other pathologic processes such as cerebral anoxia. For example, the pyramidal cells in Ammon's horn, particularly in Sommer's sector (corresponding roughly to area CA1 of Lorente de No), or the pyramidal cells of laminae III and IV of the neocortex. Regional changes of the microvasculature in aging have indeed been described in the hippocampal areas selectively involved in AD.[226] However, this is not a general feature, and Purkinje cells of the cerebellum or the cells of the inferior olive, highly vulnerable to anoxia, are spared in AD.[91,229]

Neuromediator(s). The possibility that the topography of changes could be explained by the selective involvement of a specific neuromediator has been put forward several times: acetylcholine was once supposed to furnish such an unifying explanation (cfr supra). More recently, a high degree of correspondence between the anatomic localization of SP and NFT and the terminals of putative glutamatergic pathways has fostered the hypothesis of a possible role of glutamate in the pathology of AD, possibly through an excitotoxic mechanism.[230,231]

Amyloidogenesis. Regional variations of amyloidogenesis could explain selective involvement of some areas of the brain. Amyloid could originate from the blood or from the brain tissue itself. As A4 precursor protein is diffusely distributed in the body, it has been proposed that some local disturbances in the metabolism of this protein could explain the precipitation of the A4 protein; the microglia and/or astroglia could be the site of this altered metabolism.[183] In the nucleus basalis of Meynert, amyloid deposits conform to the topography of the changes.[189] The supporters of the "amyloid hypothesis" stress that selective vulnerability is also observed in systemic amyloidosis often without any clear explanation.

Vascular Permeability. The blood-brain barrier has been considered normal for a long time in AD. Some authors have recently emphasized alterations of CSF levels of albumin which could indicate a vascular defect. However, the specificity of these findings has not been confirmed by immunocytochemistry of postmortem specimens.[232] Regional variations of permeability (which could be due to loss of cholinergic or of monoaminergic influences on cerebral blood vessels) could explain the selective involvement of some vessels (and thus of some brain areas), but evidence is lacking. More research on the question of the anatomical and physiological integrity of the blood-brain barrier is needed to provide answers [For review see[76,233]].

Axonal Flow. Some authors[234] thought that neurons with long axons were more vulnerable because of the sensitivity of their axonal flow. This explanation can only be partial: Betz cells having probably the longest axons in the brain, remain untouched at least for a long time in the course of the disease.

Phylogeny. Rapoport[235] has suggested that the selective vulnerability of certain areas in the AD brain was bound to their more recent appearance during phylogeny.

Finally, the causes of selective vulnerability remain obscure and no definitive mechanism has been found in spite of the many hypotheses which have been put forward.

RELATIONSHIP BETWEEN AMYLOID ANGIOPATHY, PLAQUES, TANGLES, NERVE CELL ATROPHY AND LOSS, AND DEMENTIA

Although much has been written concerning the neuropathology and the pathogenesis of Alzheimer's disease, its cause is unknown.[12,28,70,90,153,166,175,177,236−240] As already mentioned, it has been hypothesized that SP may be derived from amyloid angiopathy on account of the morphologic and biochemical similarities of amyloid in the two lesions and of the constancy (or the high frequency) of the association of SP with capillaries. From a neuropathologic point of view, the lack of topographic relationship between both changes in some cases and in some areas does not favor this hypothesis (at least as the unique relationship between the two lesions). Conversely, amyloid angiopathy could be due to the sink effect of amyloid from the brain to the vessels. This does not seem likely since amyloid deposits are seen in small extraparenchymal meningeal arteries. At last, amyloid deposits of SP and of the cerebral vessels could be two distinct consequences of an overproduction or of a reduced degradation of the A4 precursor protein, SP seem to precede NFT, in AD, Down syndrome, and in old patients. NFT are less specific a change than SP, and can be seen alone in disorders other than AD. The presence of NFT is often linked with dementia.[151]

The simplest hypothesis is that neuronal atrophy and death are directly due to NFT formation. Most nerve cells do not contain NFT. These could be the mere side effect of a biochemical abnormality. The demonstration of cell loss in areas devoid of NFT (in the retina) favors this hypothesis, at least in some cell types. NFT could have other consequences for the cell, such as reduction of axonal transport. However, neuronal atrophy and loss (especially in the neocortex, where most detailed studies have been performed) are usually associated with dementia.

NEUROCHEMICAL DEFICITS

THE CHOLINERGIC HYPOTHESIS

The quest for a specific neurochemical deficit in AD/SDAT seemed to have reached its goal when a consistent decrease in the choline acetyl transferase (CAT) activity of the cortex was discovered in AD brain.[79,241-246] This disease in CAT activities was more marked in AD of early onset than in SDAT.[37] Other presynaptic cholinergic markers are affected: synaptosomal choline uptake is reduced;[247] acetylcholine synthesis and release from biopsy specimens are decreased;[248] synthesis and release of acetylcholine from nerve terminal is depressed.[249] These data demonstrate that the decrease in CAT activity is not purely an enzymatic deficit but is probably the direct consequence of the loss of cholinergic fibers. Most authors agree that postsynaptic cholinergic receptors (especially muscarinic binding sites and maybe low affinity nicotinic binding sites) are normal or increased.[79,244-246]

When the cholinergic deficit was discovered, the anatomy of the cholinergic pathways was poorly understood and relied mainly on the studies by Lewis and Shute[250] of the cholinergic pathways in the rat using acetylcholinesterase histochemistry. The finding of a cholinergic deficit in AD prompted a great number of studies concerning cholinergic pathways and functions in animals and man: the basal forebrain cholinergic neurons in the monkey form a continuum spreading at the ventral surface of the brain including the nucleus basalis of Meynert, the nucleus of the diagonal band and the medial septal nucleus. Neurons in a similar topography were known in the human brain under the name "basal magnocellular complex". It has been shown in man that 90% of the large neurons in the nucleus basalis of Meynert are cholinergic, 70% in the nucleus of the diagonal band, and 40% in the medial septal nucleus.[251] Tracing studies in animals have shown that the septal area and the nucleus basalis of Meynert are the major sources of cholinergic innervation of the hippocampus, whereas the neocortex is mainly innervated by the adjacent nucleus basalis of Meynert. The possibility has been suggested that cortical neurons are cholinergic.[252] The electrophysiologic effects of acetylcholine on sensitive neurons of the cortex and of the stimulation of basal forebrain neurons have been thoroughly studied in the rat[253] and seem mainly excitatory. The behavioral correlates of cholinergic blockade have been described in young volunteers and were said to mimic some clinical aspects of AD.[254]

Finally a massive neuronal loss was found in the basal forebrain of AD.[78,79] This set of data: neuronal loss in the basal forebrain, cortical cholinergic denervation, behavioral deficit was considered in the literature under the name of "cholinergic hypothesis". As some SP are innervated by cholinergic fibers and as there is a correlation between the number of SP in some cortical areas and the topographic arrangement of neurons in the nucleus basalis of Meynert,[255] it has also been suggested that the cholinergic fibers could initiate SP formation.[167] It is now generally accepted that the cholinergic hypothesis in its most radical version (i.e. AD results exclusively from a cholinergic defect) is not valid: a number of other neurotransmitters are affected; NFT are spread over much wider regions than the basal forebrain and microscopic changes in the cortex cannot be accounted for by cholinergic denervation; SP contain neurites belonging to several neurotransmitter systems; behavioral deficit is larger than the one obtained by cholinergic blockade. On the other hand the postulate of a connection between some of the cognitive impairments and a disturbance in cholinergic neurotransmission has been "reinforced and refined".[166] Through the cholinergic hypothesis, it was realized that AD and SDAT were not "neurotransmitter diseases" but diseases disturbing neurotransmission through cellular loss and dysfunction. In this respect, the observation by Perry et al.[256] that extensive loss of choline acetyltransferase activity was not reflected by neuronal loss in the nucleus basalis of Meynert in Alzheimer disease, although controversial, is of importance since it demonstrates that neuronal dysfunction could precede cellular loss for long. Now that the cholinergic deficit in the cerebral cortex is known to be only one of the neurochemical disturbances of AD and SDAT, it is also realized that it is not a necessary correlate of these diseases: Palmer et al.[227] isolated a group of old patients (with histologically assessed SDAT) who had no significant loss of CAT in the neocortex and in the hippocampus. In the 7 patients of this group CAT decrease was confined to the amygdala.

THE NORADRENERGIC SYSTEM

Animal studies have shown that the noradrenergic fibers stem mainly from the locus ceruleus, a pigmented nucleus located in the dorsal and upper pons: this is also the case in man but pathways are not known as precisely. The nucleus is made of a relatively small number of neurons, around 15,000.[51] It is thus possible to evaluate the total number of neurons of this small nucleus and this avoids some of the usual pitfalls of quantitative morphology. Significant reduced concentration of norepinephrine in the cerebral cortex of AD patients has been reported.[90] The activity of dopamine-B-hydroxylase, the enzyme which converts dopamine to noradrenaline, was found reduced in some but not all patients.[257] Berger et al.[258,259] using catecholamine fluorescence histochemistry of neurosurgical samples of the frontal cortex, noted that the number of fluorescent fibers was reduced and that the remaining fluorescent axons were paler and shorter than normally. Some were observed within SP. Postsynaptic adrenergic receptors were found spared in the study by Cross et al.[260]

The alterations in noradrenergic content of the cortex are thought to be the consequences of neuronal loss or dysfunction in the locus ceruleus. Neuronal loss has been found in a high percentage of cases in several studies.[53,261-263]

In some, generally older cases neuronal loss is lacking. The changes have a non-random distribution within the nucleus and seem to affect principally the dorsal level.[82] NFT have been noted in the locus ceruleus[264] and could be the cause of the neuronal loss.

THE SEROTONINERGIC SYSTEM

Animal tracing studies have shown that serotonin (5-HT) containing fibers originate from raphe nuclei: dorsalis and centralis superior.[265] NFT are frequently numerous in these nuclei.[266] The decrease in 5-HT and 5-HIAA concentrations in the cortex is generally agreed upon. Density of both S1 and S2 receptors is decreased. The location of these receptors is unknown. It was suggested that they could be located on vulnerable, cortical neurons [For review, see[76,251]].

THE DOPAMINERGIC SYSTEM

Changes in dopamine concentration, although observed by some authors and in various brain regions[267-270] are generally considered "minimal" or "secondary"[76] and correlated with the scarcity of NFT in the parent neurons of the substantia nigra.[264,271,272]

It should be noted, however, that in the primate, the cortical dopaminergic innervation does not arise from the substantia nigra but from the ventral tegmental area (VTA).[273] In man, NFT are frequently seen in this area.[226,272] The sparing of the substantia nigra projecting to the basal nuclei and the alterations of the VTA projecting to the cortex favors the hypothesis following which changes in the brainstem are secondary to the lesions of the cortex and affect the nuclei connected with it in a retrograde manner.[226] This pathogenetic mechanism has been discussed in another context by Mesulam[224] who supports it and Arendt and Bigl, who think it unlikely.[225,274]

NEUROPEPTIDES

Most studies (for review, see Rossor, et al.[245,275]) emphasize the relative sparing of most of the neuropeptides which have been studied: Met-enkephalin;[275] TRH;[276] LHRH;[276] neurotensin.[277-279] Cholecystokinin was found decreased in some cases by Perry et al.,[280] whereas no change was detected by Rossor et al.[281] and Ferrier et al.[278] Substance P was found decreased by Crystal and Davies[282] but other studies failed to duplicate these results.[276,278,280] Vasoactive intestinal polypeptide (VIP) concentration remains unchanged[280,283] but Swaab et al.[87] found a marked decrease in the total number of VIP neurons in suprachiasmatic nucleus of the hypothalamus.

Somatostatin has been found regularly[76] and sometimes in large amounts.[284] Somatostatin-like immunoreactivity (SRIF-IL) was found reduced in 7 papers quoted by Rossor et al.[275] on that topic. There is a marked decrease in severe examples of the disease.[285] SRIF-IL is located in middle-sized non-pyramidal neurons of layers II-III and IV.[286] Roberts et al.[287] localized NFT within SRIF-IL containing neurons. In some cortical neurons, neuropeptide Y (NPY) is co-localized with SRIF-IL.[288] Since SRIF-IL concentration was reduced in AD and SDAT, a parallel decrease of NPY was expected. However, Allen et al.,[289] Dawbarn et al.,[290] and Foster et al.[291] could not detect any decrease in NFY concentration, although alterations of NPY containing neurons were described using immunohistochemistry.[292–294] An explanation for this discrepancy is the observation by Gaspar et al.[286] that SRIF-IL containing neurons include two populations, one of which colocalized with NPY which is not sensitive to the disease process whereas the other is.

Corticotropin releasing factor (CRF)-like immunoreactivity is also reduced in cerebral cortex.[295,296] Receptors increase, suggesting a hypersensitivity due to denervation.[296]

AMINO ACIDS

Gamma-aminobutyric acid (GABA) and glutamic acid are thought to be cortical transmitters used by interneurons. GAD activity has been used as a marker of GABA neurons but is highly influenced at postmortem examination by the duration of terminal coma and postmortem delay before assay.[245,297] In AD, GABA concentration was decreased by about 30% in temporal cortex and in the younger patients in the study by Rossor et al.[298] The deficit seems mild and occurs in areas with severe pathologic changes. Lower et al.[285] measured the concentration of GABA in the cerebral cortex obtained at diagnostic craniotomy from patients with AD of 3 years' mean duration and compared these data with GABA content of five areas of the cerebral cortex and the cerebellar cortex from a large number of postmortem samples including specimens obtained within 3 hours of death with AD of 8 years' mean duration. This study confirmed that GABA concentrations were reduced in the superior parietal, frontal and temporal cortices in conventional autopsy specimen, but there was still a possibility that agonal state confounded the comparisons with controls. There was no deficit in GABA concentration in fresh cortical tissue from AD patients.[285] Presynaptic glutamate uptake sites are reduced in AD,[299] while postsynaptic NMDA receptor levels are unchanged.[300] The normal release of glutamate and aspartate from biopsy samples of cortex in AD[301] suggests a sparing of intrinsic cortical perikarya contrasting with loss of glutamergic nerve terminals. This could indicate a loss of cortico-cortical association fibers using GABA (intrinsic cells) or glutamate (projecting pyramidal neurons of layer III). In addition, there is indirect evidence of deficiency of the descending cortico-striatal pathways which are presumed to use glutamate and/or aspartate as transmitter.[76] The dementia score correlates with CAT activity in temporal cortex, but not with GABA levels.[245]

DOWN SYNDROME AND ALZHEIMER DISEASE

A large density of SP and NFT occur in the brain of most middle-aged patients with Down syndrome (trisomy 21).[302–305] In addition, some studies suggested a familial association between AD and Down syndrome. This has been recently challenged in a large case-control study.[306] Several studies have shown that such patients dying in their 30s and occasionally earlier develop SP and later on (10 to 20 years) NFT. These changes have been reported to be constant after 50. The selective reduction of cells in hippocampus and in cholinergic and noradrenergic forebrain neuronal systems is also found,[304,305] although this finding is disputed as far as the nucleus basalis is concerned.[307] The amino-acid sequences of the amyloid protein of AD (the gene of which is located on chromosome 21) and that of trisomy 21 are identical. The amyloid in SP in trisomy 21[308] may contain more sugar residues than observed in AD.[309] In some cases with Down syndrome, the clinical picture of AD appears. However, half or two thirds of elderly people with trisomy 21 are not demented; although they should be because of the high densities of SP and NFT in their brains.[305] Neuropathology could thus "antedate the appearance of clinical signs by a considerable margin of time", as emphasized by Sylvester[310] and Wisniewski et al.[305] This could be due to inadequate assessment of dementia in severely retarded person. On the other hand, it could indicate a dissociation between senile changes (especially SP) and mental impairment, as also hypothesized in AD.

DEMENTIA OF PARKINSON'S DISEASE

Although AD and Parkinson's disease are generally considered as separate conditions, an overlap between the two has been recently emphasized. The proportion of patients with Parkinson's disease who became demented is debated; between 20%[311] and 40%.[312] Clinical signs and symptoms usually include a milder degree of dementia than that which occurs in Alzheimer disease, without the aphasic, apraxic, and agnostic features common in that disorder. The term "subcortical dementia" coined for progressive supranuclear palsy was also used for this condition. However, severe dementia occurs in some cases. The examination of the substantia nigra in 40 cases of AD showed Lewy bodies in 14, most of them having had clinical signs of Parkinson's disease.[313] Conversely, neuropathologic evidence of changes of Alzheimer disease (SP and NFT in the cerebral cortex and some basal ganglia) coexistent to changes of Parkinson's disease (Lewy bodies in the brainstem) have been found in retrospective studies of demented cases of Parkinson's disease, and overall in severely demented patients.[314–317] In Parkinson's disease, the distribution of AD changes in the hippocampus and in the neocortex seems parallel though less severe than in AD milder. The dementia appears linked in some cases to the

AD changes of the neocortex. Mental changes could then be due to the loss of ascending fibers from some subcortical nuclei affected in Parkinson's disease, mainly the mesocortical and mesolimbic dopaminergic systems and the innominato-cortical cholinergic system. These lesions could also potentiate the affects of AD cortical changes.[318]

The relationship between AD and Parkinson's disease is debated. Some authors believe that there is no increased simultaneous occurrence of both diseases.[76,319] Some others think that the association between the two disorders may prove to be too frequent to be coincidental.[28,313] The difficulties come from the finding of changes characteristic of both disorders in so-called normal persons. Lewy bodies have been seen in old people, some of them clinically normal. Forno and Alvord found them in the substantia nigra in 7 to 10% of the general population over 60 (without evidence of either AD or Parkinson's disease) and in over 30% of cases over 80.[320] In a retrospective study of 314 continuous autopsy cases from a geriatric hospital, Lewy bodies have been found in the sympathetic ganglia (mostly in the stellate, upper cervical and celiac ganglia) in 41 cases:[321] they were never found under 60. From 60 to 69, they were found in 1 of 27 cases, in 17 of 110 cases (15%), from 80 to 89, in 20 of 141 cases (14%), over 90, in 3 of 25 cases (13%). These changes found in such population surveys may be the consequence of aging[76,322] or may indicate subclinical disease. Lewy bodies were not seen in a survey of the brain of 12 centenarians, favoring the second hypothesis.[140] If the Lewy body is a marker of Parkinson's disease then its absence suggests that it is possible that Parkinson's disease remains subclinical for some time. The prevalence of the disease (clinical and overall subclinical) could be evaluated from 10 to 30% in the elderly.

To explain the association of the two disorders, hypotheses have been made: AD and Parkinson's disease were said to be different consequences of the same basic defect affecting the cytoskeleton. Some authors proposed a continuum of dementing diseases: AD, SDAT, senile Parkinson's disease with dementia and AD changes, Parkinson's disease.[318] The common mechanism should be epigenetic since the study of a large twin cohort shows that Parkinson's disease is an acquired disease not caused by a hereditary process.[323] On the contrary, the high prevalence of both diseases (especially on neuropathologic grounds) in old patients and the similar age of their peak frequencies could well explain their coincidence: their prevalences in the elderly around 20% for AD,[324] around 15% for Parkinson's disease, preclinical or clinical, would indeed explain 20% of the autopsied Parkinsonian patients to suffer AD and 15% of AD cases to have Lewy bodies.

MIXED DEMENTIAS (COMBINED MULTI-INFARCT DEMENTIA AND AD)

The boundaries of AD and of multi-infarct (or vascular, or arteriosclerotic) dementia [See Chap. 4] are not clearly defined. Although most cases are easily classified into one of the two disorders, in some instances changes characteristic of both conditions are associated. These cases where the two processes are combined have been called mixed dementias.[11] Clinical diagnosis is difficult since patients with mixed dementia and those with pure multi-infarct dementia are similar.[4] Here again, even pathologic distinction can be difficult. The prevalence of mixed dementias has been variously estimated in autopsy series 17 of 31 (55%) in the series of Delay and Brion,[11] 32% for Constantinidis,[13] 10 to 25% as a function of the used criteria for Tomlinson et al.,[23] 13% for Jellinger et al.,[325] 10% for Buhl and Bojsen-Moller.[326] This could be due to sampling biases, different mean age of the cases and also to variations in the inclusion criteria. Two positions may be adopted and no consensus among neuropathologists has been reached: (1) to consider a mixed dementia only in those cases where both AD changes and cerebral infarction could be responsible for dementia. This would lead to the diagnosis in 10% of the cases of the series of Tomlinson et al.,[23] or (2) to extend this category to those cases where mild changes are associated: a few senile changes and some small infarcts, the effects of which could add up. This would increase the proportion of this diagnosis of 25% in the same series. Obviously, these difficulties

increase with the age of the patient, at the same rate as increases the proportion of mixed dementias: 0.6% before 70 to 12.2% after 70 in three pathologic series.[4]

DIAGNOSTIC CRITERIA

The neuropathologic diagnosis of AD is usually without full clinical information. The interpretation of the pathologic changes noted in a cerebral biopsy is usually easy in a presenile (before 65) demented patient. At that age, SP and NFT are diagnostic. NFT alone are seen in dementia pugilistica and Guam Parkinson-dementia complex. SP or amyloid angiopathy are found in cerebral amyloidosis, Gerstmann-Straussler-Scheinker disease and other related conditions. Plaques have a characteristic appearance. If SP or NFT are not present in the tissue examined, another cause of dementias must be considered (infective, metabolic, type). In our experience, cerebral biopsy has been diagnostic in 126 cases out of 168 in 6 series of demented patients.[4]

In autopsy situations, mild AD is sometimes difficult to distinguish from age-related changes, especially when the clinical picture has not been precisely assessed. Quantitative criteria have been formulated:

A work group of neuropathologists[327] has proposed that more than eight neocortical SP per mm^2 were needed in "any microscopic field encompassing 1 sq mm (microscopic magnification $\times$ 200 field) of tissue" between ages 50 and 65, more than 10 SP between 66 and 75, and more than 15 SP after 75 years of age. NFT were thought useful for the diagnosis but neither sufficient nor necessary to support it. Microscopic sections had to be 5 to 15 μm and stained by Bielschowsky silver method, thioflavin S or Congo red. Bodian stain was said to be "insensitive to the (senile) lesions". Some of these criteria, have been debated: (1) locations of the sample were not defined, (2) some neuropathologists prefer the Bodian stain rather than Congo red,[328] (3) counts are different in a 5 μm to a 15 μm thick section. Finally these criteria would have probably led to the diagnosis of AD in at least 5% of the nondemented individuals between 55 to 64 years of age[137] and in only 1:12 centenarians, three of whom were clinically demented: one SDAT, one multi-infarct dementia and one mixed dementia.[140]

Terry et al.[27] excluded from their normal group, cases with more than three neocortical SP and any NFT per mm^2 above age 70, and included only specimens with no neocortical SP below this age. These criteria which should be widened especially in old age would exclude 16% of a nonselected sample of nondemented individuals of age 55 to 64 studied by Ulrich[137] and all of 12 centenarians in institutions studied by Hauw et al.,[140] 9 of whom were not considered demented.

Tierney et al.[20] have established neuropathologic criteria for AD and compared them to clinical diagnosis obtained with the NINCDS criteria. Their criteria were mainly concerned by the regional extension of the changes rather than by their density in a given region. The three sets of inclusion criteria were one or more NFT and/or SP/x25 microscopic field: (1) in the hippocampus, irrespective of neocortical findings, (2) in both neocortex and hippocampus, and (3) in the neocortex irrespective of hippocampal findings. Three sets of vascular exclusion criteria were applied to exclude cases from pure AD. The "accurace" i.e. the percentage of agreement between clinical and pathologic data was calculated between clinical diagnosis and each of the nine possible sets of neuropathologic criteria. The highest agreement rate, i.e. 88% accuracy, was obtained with the first inclusion criteria combined with the following exclusion criteria: "one or more ischemic lesions that totaled 50 ml or more of brain tissue in the neocortex, subcortical white matter, and/or hippocampus". According to those inclusion criteria, all of the 9 nondemented centenarians[140] would have been diagnosed as affected by SDAT.

In conclusion, the technical procedures used to identify SP and NFT have to be precisely checked for they can influence markedly the density of these changes. Indeed, (1) changes are irregularly distributed in the neocortex, especially the NFT which are virtually absent in the calcarine cortex and rare in the premotor cortex. Marked variation in the number of changes is noticed from one cortical region to another.[222,329] (2) Section thickness has an effect on the density of the changes. (3) Various staining procedures reveal a variable number of lesions in contiguous slides. (4) Changes have a laminar distribution in the neocortex. The counting of the changes should thus be performed in columns from the pial surface to the white matter. Moreover, there are several reported cases which are intellectually normal and show neocortical SP,[27] or clinically demented with an exceptionally low number of such changes.[20,23,26]

It seems thus that the diagnosis of Alzheimer disease can not be afforded by neuropathology alone, but by a combination of clinical and neuropathologic criteria, the approach adopted originally by Alzheimer[1] himself. It seems worthless to define quantitative criteria of changes necessary to establish a postmortem histologic diagnosis of AD unless one obtains a preliminary consensus between neuropathologists on the conditions (specimen localization, section thickness, staining and counting methods) under which a specific cognitive impairment can be linked to AD.

SOME HYPOTHESES ABOUT ALZHEIMER DISEASE ETIOLOGY

Until recently, age was the only defined risk factor for AD. The annual incidence rate increases from 2.4 cases/100,000 from 40 to 60 to 127 cases/100,000 after 60.[8] A few other risk factors have been recently suggested.

Suspected for a long time, a genetic contribution to the etiology of AD has received strong support in the past few years. In some reports, familial cases have been estimated to account for as many as a third[330] or even 43% of cases.[331] It has even been suggested that at least 80% of the cases would be familial if average lifespan would be longer.[332,333] The conventional genetic approach to AD is impeded by heterogeneity in diagnosis, the lack of specific antemortem marker and the late onset of the disease.[334]

The familial forms of AD with multiple affected individuals are, on the whole, rare. Some 50 families have been described.[334,335] In some pedigrees, the disease appears to segregate as an autosomal dominant disorder. In these families, the age of onset is usually early (45 to 60) and constant within the kinship. The frequency of this kind of transmission is difficult to assess. Genetic cases may appear sporadic if other members of the family died before they developed the disease. On the contrary, familial cases may appear genetic if they cluster for other reasons, for example environmental.[336] Because of their rarity, the affected families represent a biased sample of AD. The early (and sometimes very early) onset of disease in most families with multiple affected individuals argues for heterogeneity of familial and non-familial cases. The explanations used in studies of familial aggregation among the relatives of AD cases [See below], do not fit easily with the data from the pedigree studies of large families.

In the more common non-familial (sporadic ?) cases, the data consistent with the genetic hypothesis come from the observation of familial aggregation among the pooled relatives of groups of AD cases. They have shown an increased risk of dementia in first degree relatives of probands with AD, that is consistent with autosomal dominant genetic transmission.[334] One of the best known works is that of Heston and colleagues, whose probands were obtained from the files of Minnesota State Hospital.[337] In all of 25 families where a secondary case had come to autopsy, the diagnosis of AD was confirmed. This study showed that there was a higher familial risk in early onset versus late onset probands. In the early onset group, the risk to other first degree family members approached 50% by age 90. There was significant intrafamilial correlation in age of onset but secondary cases appeared at ages older than index cases. This has been related to greater severity of the disease in those index cases that come first to the attention of the observer[337] or to high attrition from competing risks in older patients (which induces bias toward early onset in any observed population as compared to the theoretical distribution of the disease) which would be most evident in institutionalized patients, and to the phenomenon of regression toward the mean: when one initial sample comes from the tail of a distribution, subsequent sampling may be expected to show more typical values.[334] A recent case control study has confirmed that cumulative lifetime risk for developing AD type dementia was greater among relatives of AD probands and reached 50%, which was consistent

with an autosomal dominant mode of transmission, although the lifetime risk was similar in early onset of dementia, than among relatives of late onset probands. This raises the possibility that age at onset of dementia in AD may be genetically determined.[335] Some limitations of these studies should be considered. Selection bias (higher rate of inclusion of AD patients with one or more relative affected in a case control study based on a hospital series) and awareness bias (relative reporting dementia among AD family members being more aware of dementia syndromes than the relative of controls) can occur. In addition, most reported dementing illness lack precise diagnosis.[338]

The simultaneous mapping of the familial Alzheimer disease[339] and amyloid protein (Goldgaber et al., 1987) genes to the long arm of chromosome 21 has suggested that these genes may be identical. This fitted well with the increased incidence of Alzheimer changes—and particularly of amyloid deposit—in aged Down syndrome (trisomy 21). Refinement of the mapping of the amyloid protein and familial AD genes has not confirmed their identity. The regional localization of the amyloid precursor gene by both physical and genetic mapping shows that it is located at a distance from the locus q11-21 for the genetic defect responsible for AD in some families.[340] It has been estimated that the two loci are about 7.5 c Morgans apart. This localization close to the AD locus could be a coincidence. Other genes, which are candidates for AD, such as the Supra-oxyde-dismutase gene, the neurofilament gene, the tau gene, the choline acetyl transferase gene have been localized to a chromosome 21.[335] The amyloid gene is more closely linked to the 21q 22 region associated with Down syndrome. In the latter, increased level of mRNA for amyloid in the brain[340] suggests that the deposition is due to dosage related increase in the gene product. However, more evidence for the need of triplication of A4 locus to develop AD is needed. Studies of partial trisomies 21 (translocations) may give an answer to this question.[336] In AD, the mechanism of the accumulation of amyloid is unclear. No clear evidence for gene duplication at the amyloid locus could be afforded.[340–342]

Twin studies suggest that environmental factors play a role in AD. The largest involved 22 twin pairs. In 4 cases, the diagnosis was confirmed at autopsy. Seven monozygotic pairs were concordant for AD, 10 were discordant (concordance rate: 41%). Two dizygotic pairs were concordant for AD, 3 were discordant (concordance rate: 40%). Although the difficulties already mentioned for the other genetic studies have to be kept in mind, this study supports the belief that, etiologically, AD cannot be entirely accounted for by a single autosomal dominant gene.[33]

An hypothesis suggests that the accumulation of aluminum in the brain is the cause of neurofibrillary tangles and dementia. The amyloid core of SP contains aluminosilicates.[239] However, the neurofibrillary changes in aluminum intoxicated animals are composed of 10 nm diameter filaments, which ultrastructurally resemble normal neurofilaments and thus are different from the PHF of AD.

A third hypothesis postulates that AD is caused by an infectious agent, possibly an unconventional agent or prion. However, no scrapie-associated fibers (characteristic of unconventional infections, kuru, Creutzfeldt-Jakob disease, the Gerstmann-Straussler-Scheinker syndrome in human and scrapie in animal) have been seen in AD. In addition, the proteins making the amyloid fibers seen in these disorders are different from the A4 protein found in AD.

Another hypothesis would be that AD is due to an accelerated aging process. Indeed, age is the highest risk factor for AD.[343] However, in a few studies, the prevalence of dementia in the eldest old (over 90) seems to reach a plateau.[344,345] In addition, as repeatedly mentioned, neuronal atrophy and loss, plaques, tangles, amyloid angiopathy, granulovacuolar degeneration and Hirano bodies are found, with a density increasing with age in the brain of non-demented people. However, they do not reach such a density as in AD and cases difficult to classify as AD or "normal aging" are, on the whole, rare. Despite lessening severity among the elderly in SDAT, significant differences in the density of lesions are always detectable between old AD brain and age matched controls.[37] This is still the case in centenarians.[140] It has been proposed that a

threshold value for these changes[15] or for some of them, such as neuronal atrophy and loss must be exceeded before dementia appears. This would explain why easily recognizable lesions (positive changes such as plaques and tangles) are usually less marked in late onset AD than in early onset cases. Since the majority of aged people, even the old ones, do not reach these threshold values,[140] aging alone is not likely the cause of AD. On the other hand, some of the changes due to age, such as lipofuscin storage, are not linked to dementia. Some constituents of the aging process would thus contribute to the development of dementia of the Alzheimer type. Other factors (genetic and/or environmental) would be needed to develop the disease.[70,150]

REFERENCES

1. Alzheimer, A.: Uber eine eigerartige Erkankung der Hirnrinde. Allgemeine Zeitscher. Psychiatr. Gerichtlisch. Med., 64:109, 1987.
2. Katzman, R.: Overview: demography, definitions and problems. In *The Neurology of Aging*. Edited by R. Katzman, R. Terry. Philadelphia, F.A. Davis Co, 1983.
3. Cummings, J.L., and Benson, D.F.: *Dementia: A Clinical Approach*. Boston, Butterworths, 1983.
4. Katzman, R., Lasker, B., and Berstein, N.: Advances in the diagnosis of dementia: accuracy of diagnosis and consequences of misdiagnosis of disorders causing dementia. In: *Aging and the Brain*. Edited by R.D. Terry. New York, Raven Press, 1988.
5. American Psychiatric Association, Task Force on Nomenclature and Statistics: *Diagnostic and Statistical Manual of Mental Disorders*, (3 ed.), 111. Washington DC, 1980.
6. McKahn, G., et al.: Clinical diagnosis of Alzheimer's disease: a report of the NINCDS-ADRDA work group under the auspices of the Department of Health and Human Services Task Force on Alzheimer's Disease. Neurology, 34:939, 1984.
7. Jorm, A.F., and Henderson, A.S.: Possible improvement to the diagnostic criteria for dementia in DSM-III. Br. J. Psych., 147:394, 1985.
8. Rocca, W.A., Amaducci, L.A., and Schoenberg, B.S.: Epidemiology of clinically diagnosed Alzheimer's disease. Ann. Neurol., 19:415, 1986.
9. Joachim, C.L., Morris, J.H., and Selkoe, D.J.: Clinically diagnosed Alzheimer's disease: autopsy results in 150 cases. Ann. Neurol., 24:50, 1988.
10. Morris, J.C., et al.: Validation of clinical diagnostic criteria for Alzheimer's disease. Ann. Neurol., 24:17, 1988.
11. Delay, J., and Brion, S.: *Les démences tardives*. Paris, Masson, 1962.
12. Terry, R.D.: Alzheimer's disease. In: *Textbook of Neuropathology*. Edited by R.L. Davis, D.M. Robertson. Baltimore, Williams & Wilkins, 1985.
13. Constantinidis, J.: Is Alzheimer's disease a major form of senile dementia? Clinical, anatomical and genetic data. In: *Alzheimer's Disease: Senile Dementia*

and Related Disorders. Edited by R. Katzman, R.D. Terry, K.L. Bick. New York, Raven Press, 1978.

14. Roth, M., and Wischik, C.M.: The heterogeneity of Alzheimer's disease and its implications for scientific investigations of the disorder. In: Recent Advances in Psychogeriatrics. Edited by T. Arie. Edinburgh, Churchill Livingstone, 1985.

15. Roth, M.: The association of clinical and neurological findings and its bearing on the classification and etiology of Alzheimer's disease. Br. Med. J., 42:42, 1986.

16. Selnes, O.A., et al.: Language dysfunction in early- and late-onset possible Alzheimer's disease. Neurology, 38:1053, 1988.

17. Amaducci, L., Rocca, W.A., Schoenberg, B.S.: Origin of a distinction between Alzheimer's disease and senile dementia. How history can clarify nosology. Neurology, 36:1497, 1986.

18. Terry, R.D.: Aging, senile dementia and Alzheimer's disease. In: Alzheimer's Disease: Senile Dementia and Related Disorders, 7:11. 1978. Edited by R. Katzman, R.D. Terry, and K.L. Bick. New York, Raven Press, 1978.

19. Galen, R.S., and Gambino, S.R.: Beyond Normality: the Predictive Value and Efficiency of Medical Diagnoses. New York, John Wiley and Sons, 1975.

20. Tierney, M.C., et al.: The NINCDS-ADRDA work group criteria for the clinical diagnosis of probable Alzheimer's disease: a clinico-pathologic study of 57 cases. Neurology, 38:359, 1988.

21. Adolfsson, R., et al.: Prevalence of dementia disorders in institutionalized Swedish old people. Acta Psychiat. Scand., 631:225, 1981.

22. Tomlinson, B.E., Blessed, G., and Roth, M.: Observations on the brain of non-demented old people. J. Neurol. Sci., 7:331, 1968.

23. Tomlinson, B.E., Blessed, G., Roth, M.: Observations on the brain of demented old people. J. Neurol. Sci., 11:205, 1970.

24. Berg, L., et al.: Mild senile dementia of the Alzheimer type: research diagnostic criteria, recruitment, and description of a study population. J. Neurol. Neurosurg. Psychiat., 45:962, 1982.

25. Mountjoy C.Q., et al.: Cortical neuronal counts in normal elderly controls and demented patients. Neurobiol. Aging, 4:1, 1983.

26. Suldava, R., et al.: Accuracy of clinical diagnosis in primary degenerative dementia: correlation with neuropathological findings. J. Neurol. Neurosurg. Psych., 46:9, 1983.

27. Terry, R.D., de Teresa, R., and Hansen, L.A.: Neocortical cell counts in normal human adult ageing. Ann. Neurol., 21:530, 1987.

28. Tomlinson, B.E., and Corsellis, J.A.N.: Ageing and the dementias. In: Greenfield's Neuropathology. Edited by J. Humes Adams, J.A.N. Corsellis, L.W. Duchen. London, Edward Arnold, 1984.

29. Miller, A.K.H., and Corsellis, J.A.N.: Evidence for a secular increase in human brain weight during the past century. Ann. Human. Biol., 4:253, 1977.

30. Miller, A.K.H., Alston, R.L., and Corsellis, J.A.N.: Variations with age in the volumes of gray and white matter in the cerebral hemispheres of man: measurements with an image analyser. Neuropathol. Appl. Neurobiol., 6:119, 1980.

31. Dekaban, A.S., and Sadowsky, D.: Changes in brain weight during the span of human life: relation of brain weight to body height and body weight. Ann. Neurol., 4:345, 1978.

32. Davis, P.J.M., and Wright, E.A.: A new method for measuring cranial capacity volume and its application to the assessment of cerebral atrophy at autopsy. Neuropathol. Appl. Neurobiol., 3:34, 1977.

33. Kemper, T.: Neuroanatomical and neuropathological changes in normal aging and in dementia. In: Clinical Neurology of Aging. Edited by L.M. Albert. New York, Oxford University Press, 1984.

34. Jacoby, R.J., and Levy, R.: Computed tomography in the elderly II: Senile dementia: diagnosis and functional impairment. Br. J. Psychiat., 136:256, 1980.

35. Creasey, H., et al.: Quantitative computed tomography in dementia of the Alzheimer type. Neurology, 36:1563, 1986.

36. Hubbard, B.M., and Anderson, J.M.: A quantitative study of cerebral atrophy in old age and senile dementia. J. Neurol. Sci., 50:135, 1981.

37. Hansen, L.A., et al.: Neocortical morphometry, lesion counts, and choline acetyltransferase levels in the age spectrum of Alzheimer's disease. Neurology, 38:48, 1988.

38. Duyckaerts, C., et al.: Cortical atrophy in senile dementia of the Alzheimer type is mainly due to a decrease in cortical length. Acta Neuropathol. (Berl) 66:72, 1985.

39. Rakic, P.: Specification of cerebral cortical areas. Science, 241:170, 1988.

40. Morel, F., Wildi, E.: Contribution à la connaissance des différentes altérations cérébrales du grand âge. Arch. Suisse Neurol. Psych., 76:174, 1955.

41. Brody, H.: Organization of cerebral cortex. III. A study of aging in the human cerebral cortex. J. Comp. Neurol., 102:511, 1955.

42. Brody, H.: Cell counts in cerebral cortex and brainstem in Alzheimer's disease. In: Senile Dementia and Related Disorders, 7:345, 1978. Edited by R. Katzman, R.D. Terry, K.L. Bick. New York, Raven Press, 1978.

43. Creasey, H., Rapoport, S.I.: The aging human brain. Ann. Neurol., 17:2, 1985.

44. Terry, R.D, and Hansen, L.A.: Some morphometric aspects of Alzheimer disease and of normal aging. In: Aging and the Brain. Edited by R.D. Terry. New York, Raven Press, 1988.

45. Konigsmark, B., and Murphy, E.A.: Volume of ventral cochlear nucleus in man: its relationship to neuronal population and age. J. Neuropath. Exp. Neurol., 31:304, 1972.

46. Vijayashankar, N., and Brody, H.: The neuronal population of the nuclei of the trochlear nerve and the locus coeruleus in the human. Anat. Rec., 172:421, 1973.

47. Vijayashankar, N., and Brody, H.: A study of aging in the human abducens nucleus. J. Comp. Neurol., 173:433, 1977.

48. Monagle, R.D., and Brody, H.: The effects of age upon the main nucleus of the inferior olive in the human. J. Comp. Neurol., 155:61, 1974.

49. Hanley, T.C.: Neuronal fall-out in the ageing brain: a critical review of the quantitative data. Age and Ageing, 3:133, 1974.

50. Maleci, O.: Contributo all conoscenza della variazioni quantitative delle cellule nervose nelle senescenza. Arch. Ital. Anat., 33:883, 1934.

51. Vijayashankar, N., and Brody, H.: A quantitative study of the pigmented neurons in the nuclei coeruleus and subcoeruleus in man as related to aging. J. Neuropath. Exp. Neurol., 38:490, 1979.

52. Tomonago, M.: On the morphological changes in

locus coeruleus in the senile brain. Jap. J. Geriatr., 16:545. 1979.

53. Tomlinson, B.E., Irving, D., and Blessed, G.: Cell loss in the locus ceruleus in senile dementia of Alzheimer type. J. Neurol. Sci., 4:419, 1981.

54. McGeer, P.L., McGeer, E.G., and Suzuki, P.S.: Aging and extrapyramidal function. Arch. Neurol., 34:33, 1977.

55. Mann, D.M.A., and Yates, P.O.: The effects of ageing on the pigmented nerve cells of the human locus coeruleus and substantia nigra. Acta Neuropathol. (Berl), 47:93, 1979.

56. Hall, T.C., Miller, A.K.H., and Corsellis, J.A.N.: Variation in human Purkinje cell population according to age and sex. Neuropath. Appl. Neurobiol., 1:267, 1975.

57. Brody, H., and Vijayashankar, N.: Anatomical changes in the nervous system. In: Handbook of the Biology of Aging. Edited by C.E. Finch, L. Hayflick. New York, Van Nostrand, 1977.

58. Bugiani, O., et al.: Nerve cell loss with aging in the putamen. Euro. Neurobiol., 17:286, 1978.

59. Pesce, C., and Reale, A.: Aging and the nerve cell population of the putamen: a morphometric study. Clin. Neuropath., 6:16, 1987.

60. Herzog, A.G., and Kemper, T.L.: Amygdaloid changes in aging and dementia. Arch. Neuro., 37:625, 1980.

61. Ball, M.J., and Lo, R.: Neuronal loss, neurofibrillary tangles and granulovacuolar degeneration in the hippocampus with ageing brain and senile dementia. Acta Neuropath., 37:111, 1977.

62. Dam, A.M.: The density of neurons in the human hippocampus. Neuropath. Appl. Neurobiol., 5:249, 1979.

63. Burns, B.D.: The Mammalian Cerebral Cortex. London. Edward Arnold, 1958.

64. Leboucq, G.: Le rapport entre lipoides et la surface de l'hémisphère cérébral chez l'homme et les singes. Mem. Acad. Roy. Med. Belg., 10:55, 1929.

65. Hauw, J., Duyckaerts, C., Partridge, M.: Neuropathological aspects of brain aging and SDAT. In: Modern Trends in Aging Research. Edited by Y. Courtois, et al. London, INSERM-EURAGE/John Libbey Eurotext, 1986.

66. Haug, H., et al.: The significance of morphometric procedures in the investigation of age changes in cytoarchitectonic structures of human brain. J. Hirnforsch., 25:353, 1984.

67. Meyer-Ruge, W., Ulrich, J., and Abdel-Al, S.: Stereologic findings in normal brain aging and Alzheimer's disease. In: Senile Dementia: Outlook for the Future. New York, A. Liss, 1984.

68. Henderson, G., Tomlinson, B.E., and Gibson, P.H.: Cell counts in human cerebral cortex in normal adults throughout life using an image analysing machine. J. Neurol. Sci., 46:113, 1980.

69. Braak, H., and Braak, E.: Ratio of pyramidal cells versus non-pyramidal cells in the human frontal isocortex and changes in ratio with ageing and Alzheimer's disease. Prog. Brain Res., 70:185, 1986.

70. Hauw, J-J., Duyckaerts, C., and Delaère, P.: How do we distinguish aged-related changes from those due to disease processes (physiology, morphology)? Dahlem Workshop on the aetiology of dementia of Alzheimer type. (In press).

71. Terry, R.D., et al.: Some morphometric aspects of the brain in senile dementia of the Alzheimer type. Ann. Neurol., 10:184, 1981.

72. Mountjoy, C.Q.: Correlations between neuropathological and neurochemical changes. Brit. Med. Bull., 42:81, 1986.

73. Mann, D.M.A., Yates, P.O., and Marcyniuk, B.: Some morphometric observations on the cerebral cortex and hippocampus in presenile Alzheimer's disease, senile dementia of Alzheimer type and Down's syndrome in middle age. J. Neurol. Sci., 69:139, 1985.

74. Doebler, J.A., et al.: Neuronal RNA in relation to neuronal loss and neurofibrillary pathology in the hippocampus in Alzheimer's disease. J. Neuropath. Exp. Neurol., 46:28, 1987.

75. Hyman, B.T., et al.: Memory-related neural systems are disrupted at multiple levels by Alzheimer's disease. In: Proceedings of the International Symposium on Alzheimer's Disease. Kuopio, 1988.

76. Mann, D.M.A.: Neuropathology and Neurochemical Aspects of Alzheimer's Disease. In: Psychopharmacology of the Aging Nervous System, In: Handbook of Psychopharmacology, 20:1, 1988. Edited by L.L. Iversen, S.D. Iversen, and S.H. Snyder. New York, Plenum Press.

77. Hyman, B.T., et al.: Alzheimer's disease: cell specific pathology isolates the hippocampal formation. Science, 225:1168, 1984.

78. Whitehouse, P.J., et al.: Alzheimer's disease: evidence for selective loss cholinergic neurons in the nucleus basalis. Ann. Neurol., 10:122, 1981.

79. Hohman, C., Antuono, P., and Coyle J.T.: Basal forebrain cholinergic neurons and Alzheimer's disease. In: Psychopharmacology of the Aging Nervous System. Edited by L.L. Iversen, S.D. Iversen, S.H. Snyder. Handbook of Psychopharmacology, 20:69, 1988, Plenum Press, New York.

80. Doucette, R., et al.: Cell loss from the nucleus basalis of Meynert in Alzheimer's disease. Can. J. Neurol. Sci., 13:435, 1986.

81. Etienne, P., et al.: Nucleus basalis neuronal loss and neuritic plaques in advanced Alzheimer's disease. Can. J. Physiol. Pharmacol., 64:318, 1986.

82. Marcyniuk, Mann D.M.A., and Yates, P.O.: The topography of cell loss from locus coeruleus in Alzheimer's disease. J. Neurol. Sci., 76:335, 1986.

83. Yamamoto, T., and Hirano, A.: Nucleus raphe dorsalis in Alzheimer's disease: neurofibrillary tangles and loss of large neurons. Ann. Neurol., 17:573, 1985.

84. Zweig, R.M., et al.: The neuropathology of aminergic nuclei in Alzheimer's disease. Ann. Neurol., 24:233, 1988.

85. Esiri, M.M., and Wilcock, G.K.: The olfactory bulb in Alzheimer's disease. J. Neurol. Neurosurg. Psych., 47:56, 1984.

86. Mann, D.M.A., Yates, P.O., and Marcyniuk, B.: Changes in Alzheimer's disease in the magnocellular neurons of the supraoptic and paraventricular nuclei of the hypothalamus and their relationship to the noradrenergic deficy. Clin. Neuropathol., 4:127, 1985.

87. Swaab, D.F., Fliers, E., and Partiman, T.S.: The suprachiasmatic nucleus of the human brain in relation to sex, age and senile dementia. Brain Res., 342:37, 1985.

88. Hinton, D.R., et al.: Optic-nerve degeneration in Alzheimer's disease. N. Engl. J. Med., 315:485, 1986.

89. Blanks, J.C., and Blanks, H.I.: Retinal defects in Alzheimer's patients. In: Proceedings of the International

Symposium on Alzheimer's Disease, June 12–15, 1988, Kuopio, 133, 1988.

90. Rossnor, M.N., et al.: Neurochemical characteristic of early and late onset types of Alzheimer's disease. Br. Med. J., *288*:961, 1984.

91. Escourolle, R., Poirier, J.: *Manual of Basic Neuropathology.* 2nd. Ed., Philadelphia, W.B. Saunders Co., 1977.

92. Williams, R.S., Ferrante, R.J., and Caviness, V.S.: The Golgi rapid method in clinical neuropathology: the morphologic consequences of suboptimal fixation. J. Neuropath. Exp. Neuro., *37*:13, 1978.

93. Braak, H., and Braak, E.: Golgi preparation as a tool in Neuropathology with particular reference to investigations of the human telencephalic cortex. Prog. Neurobiol., *25*:93, 1985.

94. Kowall, N.W., and Kosik, K.S.: Axonal disruption and aberrant localization of Tau protein characterize the neuropil pathology of Alzheimer's disease. Ann. Neurol., *22*:93, 1985.

95. Brion, J.P., et al.: Neurofibrillary tangles in Alzheimer's disease: an immunohistochemical study. J. Submicrosc. Cytol., *17*:89, 1985.

96. Braak, H., et al.: Occurrence of neuropil threads in the senile human brain and in Alzheimer's disease: a third location of paired helical filaments outside neurofibrillary tangles and neuritic plaques. Neurosc. Letters, *65*:351, 1986.

97. Braak, H., and Braak, E.: Neuropil threads occur in dendrites of tangle-bearing nerve cells. Neuropath. Appl. Neurobiol., *14*:39, 1988.

98. Duyckaerts, C., et al.: Fiber disorganization in the neocortex of patients with senile dementia of the Alzheimer type. Neuropathol. Appl. Neurobiol., *15*:233, 1989.

99. Davies, C.A., et al.: A quantitative morpometric analysis of the neuronal and the synaptic content of frontal and temporal cortex in patients with Alzheimer's disease. J. Neurol. Sci., *78*:151, 1987.

100. Flood, D.G., et al.: Dendritic extent in human dentate gyrus granule cells in normal aging and senile dementia. Brain Res., *402*:205, 1987.

101. Arendt, T., et al.: Dendritic changes in the basal nucleus of Meynert and in the diagonal band in Alzheimer disease. A quantitative Golgi investigation. Neurosci., *19*:1265, 1986.

102. Geddes, J.W., et al.: Plasticity of hippocampal circuitry in Alzheimer's disease. Science, *230*:1179, 1985.

103. Represa, A., et al.: Is senile dementia of the Alzheimer type associated with hippocampal reactive synaptogenesis? Compte. Rendus Acad. Sci., *306*:575, 1988.

104. Represa, A., et al.: Is senile dementia of the Alzheimer type associated with hippocampal plasticity? Brain Res. *457*:355, 1988.

105. Kirshner, D.A., Abraham, C., and Selkoe, D.J.: Structure of Alzheimer paired helical filaments by x-ray diffraction (abstract). Trans. Am. Soc. Neurochem., *16*:142, 1985.

106. Crowther, R.A., and Wischik, C.M.: Image reconstruction of the Alzheimer paired helical filament. EMBO J., *4*:3661, 1985.

107. Hirano, A.: Neurons, Astrocytes, and Ependyma. In: *Textbook of Neuropathology.* Edited by R.L. Davis, D.M. Robertson. Baltimore, Williams & Wilkins, 1985.

108. Kidd, M.: Alzheimer's disease. An electron microscopic study. Brain, *87*:307, 1964.

109. Wisniewski, H.M., Merz, P.A., and Iqbal, K.: Ultrastructure of paired helical filaments of Alzheimer's neurofibrillary tangle. J. Neuropath. Exp. Neuro., *43*:643, 1984.

110. Wischik, C.M., et al.: Subunit structure of paired helical filaments in Alzheimer's disease. J. Cell Biol., *100*:1905, 1985.

111. Wen, G.Y., et al.: Coexistence of two types of paired helical filaments in Alzheimer's diseased brains. J. Neuropathol. Exp. Neurol., *45*:337, 1986.

112. Selkoe, D.J., Ihara, Y., and Salazar, F.J.: Alzheimer's disease: insolubility of partially purified paired helical filaments in sodium dodecyl suflate and urea. Science, *215*:1243, 1982.

113. Selkoe, D.J., et al.: *Biochemical and immunocytochemical studies of Alzheimer's Disease.* Edited by R. Katzman. New York, Cold Spring Harbor Laboratory, 1983.

114. Rubenstein, R., et al.: Paired helical filaments associated with Alzheimer's disease are readily soluble structure. Brain Res., *372*:80, 1986.

115. Hussey S., et al.: Solubility of neurofibrillary tangles and ultrastructure of paired helical filaments in sodium dodecylsulfate. Acta Neuropathol., *75*:494, 1988.

116. Perry, G., et al.: Paired helical filaments from Alzheimer disease patients contain cytoskeletal components. Proc. Natl. Acad. Sci. (USA), *82*:3916, 1986.

117. Anderton, B.H. et al.: Monoclonal antibodies show that neurofibrillary tangles and neurofilaments share antigenic determinants. Nature, *298*:84, 1982.

118. Sternberger, N.H., Sternberger, L.A., and Ulrich, J.: Aberrant neurofilament phosphorylation in Alzheimer disease. Proc. Natl. Acad. Sci. (USA), *82*:4274, 1985.

119. Grundke-Iqbal, I., et al.: Abnormal phosphorylation of the microtubule-association protein (tau) in Alzheimer cytoskeletal pathology. Proc. Natl. Acad. Sci. (USA), *83*:4913, 1986.

120. Nikina, N., and Ihara, Y.: One of the antigenic determinants of paired helical filaments is related to tau protein. J. Biochem., *99*:1541, 1986.

121. Flament-Durand, J., and Couck, A.M.: Spongiform alterations in brain biopsies of presenile dementia. Acta Neuropathol. (Berl), *46*:159, 1979.

122. Gray, E.G., Spongiform encephalopathy: a neurocytologist's viewpoint with a note on Alzheimer's disease. Neuropath. appl. Neurobiol., *12*:149, 1986.

123. Selkoe, D.J.: Deciphering Alzheimer's disease: the pace quickens. TINS *10*:181, 1987.

124. Mori, I., Kondo, J., and Ihara, Y.: Ubiquitin is a component of paired helical filaments in Alzheimer's disease. Science *235*:1641, 1987.

125. Perry, G., et al.: Ubiquitin is detected in neurofibrillary tangles and senile neurites of Alzheimer disease brains. Proc. Natl. Acad. Sci. (USA), *84*:3033, 1987.

126. Brion, J.P., van den Bosch de Aguilar, and Flament-Durand, J.: Senile dementia of the Alzheimer type: morphological and immunocytochemical studies. In: *Senile Dementia of the Alzheimer Type: Early Diagnosis, Neuropathology and Animal Models.* Edited by R.J. Joynt, A. Weindl. Berlin, Springer-Verlag, 1985.

127. Persuy, et al.: Anti-PHF antibodies: an immunohistochemical marker of the lesions of the Alzheimer's disease. Characterization and comparison with Bodian's silver impregnation. Virchows Arch. (A), *407*:13, 1985.

128. Delacourte, A., and Defossez, A.: Alzheimer's disease: tau proteins, the promoting factors of microtu-

bule assembly are major components of paired helical filaments. J. Neurol. Sci., 76:173. 1986.

129. Gambetti, P., et al.: Composition of paired helical filaments of Alzheimer's disease as determined by specific probes. In: *Banbury Report 27: Molecular Neuropathology of Aging*. Edited by P. Davies, C.E. Finch. New York, Cold Spring Harbor Laboratory, 1987.

130. Duyckaerts, C., et al.: Quantitative assessment of the density of neurofibrillary tangles and senile plaques in senile dementia of the Alzheimer type. Comparison of immunocytochemistry with a specific antibody and Bodian's protargol method. Acta Neuropathol. (Berl), 73:167, 1987.

131. Wolozin, B.L., et al.: A neuronal antigen in the brains of Alzheimer patients. Science, 232:648, 1986.

132. Wolozin B., and Davies, P.: Alzheimer-related neuronal protein A68: specificity and distribution. Ann. Neurol., 22:251, 1987.

133. Davies, P., et al.: A new protein in Alzheimer's disease. In: *Molecular Neuropathology of Aging*. Banbury Report, 27:459, 1987. New York, Cold Spring Harbor Laboratory, 1987.

134. Emory, C.R., et al.: Ganglioside monoclonal antibody (A2B5) labels Alzheimer neurofibrillary tangles. Neurology, 37:768, 1987.

135. Mesulam, M.M., and Moran, M.A.: Cholinesterases within neurofibrillary tangles related to age and Alzheimer's disease. Ann. Neurol., 22:223, 1987.

136. Mann, D., Tucker, C.M., and Yates, P.E.: The topographic distribution of senile plaques and neurofibrillary tangles in the brain of non-demented persons of different ages. Neuropathol. Appl. Neurobiol., 13:123, 1987.

137. Ulrich, J.: Senile plaques and neurofibrillary tangles of the Alzheimer type in non demented individuals at presenile age. Gerontology, 28:86, 1982.

138. Matsuyama, M., and Nakamura, S.: Senile changes in the brain in the Japanese: incidence of Alzheimer's neurofibrillary changes and senile plaque. In: *Alzheimer's Disease: Senile Dementia and Related Disorders*, (Aging Vol. 7). Edited by R. Katzman, R.D. Terry, K.L. Blick. New York, Raven Press, 1978.

139. Miller, F.D., et al.: A descriptive study of neuritic plaques and neurofibrillary tangles in an autopsy population. Am. J. Epidemiol., 120:331, 1984.

140. Hauw, J.J., et al.: Étude neuropathologique de 12 centenaires. La fréquence de la démence sénile de type Alzheimer n'est pas particulièrement élévée dans ce groupe de personnes tres âgées. Rev. Neurol. (Paris), 142:107, 1986.

141. Kawasaki, H., et al.: Neurofibrillary tangles in human upper cervical ganglia. Morphological study with immunohistochemistry and electron microscopy. Acta Neuropathol. (Berl), 75:156, 1987.

142. Van den Bosch de Aguilar, P., and Goemaere-Vanneste, J.: Paired helical filaments in spinal ganglion neurons of elderly rats. Virchows Arch. Cell Pathol, 47:217, 1984.

143. Bancher, C., et al.: Neurofibrillary tangles in Alzheimer's disease and progressive supranuclear palsy; antigenic similarities and differences. Acta Neuropathol. (Berl), 74:39, 1987.

144. Tabaton, M., et al.: Influence of neuronal location on antigenic properties of neurofibrillary tangles. Ann. Neurol., 23:604, 1988.

145. Wisniewski, H.M., et al.: Neurofibrillary changes in advanced hydrocephalus: a clinicopathological study. J. Neuropathol. Exp. Neurol, 46:340, 1987.

146. Kato, T., et al.: Neurofibrillary tangle formation in the Nuclei Basalis of Meynert ipsilateral to a massive cerebral infarct. Ann. Neurol. 23:620, 1988.

147. Nicklowitz, W.J., and Mandybur, T.I.: Neurofibrillary changes following childhood lead encephalopathy. J. Neuropathol. Exp. Neurol., 34:445, 1975.

148. Harada, K., et al.: Alzheimer's tangles in sudanophilic leukodystrophy. Neurology, 38:55, 1988.

149. Terry, R.D., et al.: Senile dementia of the Alzheimer type without neocortical neurofibrillary tangles. J. Neuropath. Exp. Neurol., 46:262, 1987.

150. Wisnievski, H.M., et al.: Alzheimer's disease, a cerebral form of amyloidosis. In: *Immunology and Alzheimer's Disease*. Edited by P. Pouplard-Barthelaix, J. Emile, Y. Christen. Berlin, Springer-Verlag, 1988.

151. Wilcock, G.K., and Esiri, M.M.: Plaques, tangles and dementia. A quantitative study. J. Neurol. Sci., 56:343, 1982.

152. Duyckaerts, C., et al.: Does amyloid precede paired helical filaments in the senile plaque? A study of 15 cases with graded intellectual status in aging and Alzheimer disease. Neuroscience Let., 91:354, 1988.

153. Saper, C.B.: Chemical Neuroanatomy of Alzheimer's disease. In: *Psychopharmacology of the Aging Nervous System*. In: *Handbook of Psychopharmacology*, 20:131, 1988. Edited by L.L. Iversen, S.D. Iversen, and S.H. Snyder. Plenum Press, New York.

154. Ball, M.J., and Nutall, K.: Topographic distribution of neurofibrillary tangles and granulo-vacuolar degeneration in hippocampal cortex of aging and demented patients. A quantitative study. Acta Neuropathol., 42:73, 1978.

155. Ohm, H., and Braak, H.: Olfactory bulb changes in Alzheimer's disease. Acta Neuropathol (Berl), 73:365, 1987.

156. Pearson, R.C.A., et al.: Anatomical correlates of the distribution of the pathological changes in the neocortex in Alzheimer disease. Proc. Natl. Acad. Sci. (USA), 82:4531, 1985.

157. Morrison, J.H., et al.: A monoclonal antibody to nonphosphorylated neurofilament protein marks the vulnerable cortical neurons in Alzheimer's disease. Brain Res., 416:331, 1987.

158. Wisniewski, H.M., Terry, R.D.: Reexamination of the pathogenesis of the plaque. In: *Progress in Neuropathology*. Edited by H.M. Zimmerman. New York, Grune & Straton, 1973.

159. Mann, D.M.A., et al.: The progression of the pathological changes of Alzheimer's disease in frontal and temporal neocortex examined both at biopsy and autopsy. Neuropath. Appl. Neurobiol., 14:177, 1988.

160. Probst, A., et al.: Neuritic plaques in senile dementia of the Alzheimer type: A Golgi analysis in the hippocampal region. Brain Res., 268:249, 1983.

161. Braunmuhl von A.: Alterskrankung des Zentralnervensystems. Senile involution. Senile demenz. Alzheimersche Krankheit. In: *Handbuch der Speziellen Pathologischen Anatomie und Histologie*. Edited by W. Scholtz. XIII/IA:337, 1957. Berlin, Springer.

162. Schecter, R., et al.: Fibrous astrocytes in senile dementia of the Alzheimer type. J. Neuropath. Exp Neurol., 40:95, 1981.

163. Flament-Durand, J., Couck, A.M., and Brion, J.P.: New morphological data observed in human brains with senile dementia of the Alzheimer type (SDAT). In: *Aging of the Brain and Senile Dementia: The Inventory of EEC Potentialities*. Eurage Meeting. Edited by D.L. Knook, G. Calder, L. Amaducci, 1983.

164. Probst, A., et al.: A special type of senile plaque, possibly an initial stage. Acta Neuropathol. (Berl), 74:133, 1987.

165. Struble, R.G., et al.: Cholinergic innervation in neuritic plaques. Science 216:413, 1982.

166. Perry, E.K.: The cholinergic hypothesis-ten years on. Br. Med. Bull. 42:63, 1986.

167. Price, D.L., et al.: Neuropathological, neurochemical, and behavioral studies of the aging non-human primate. In: *Behavior and Pathology of Aging in Rhesus Monkeys.* Edited by R.T. Davis, C.W. Leathers. New York, Alan R. Liss, 1982.

168. Walker, et al.: Multiple transmitter systems contribute neurites to individual senile plaques. J. Neuropath. Exp. Neurol., 47:138, 1988.

169. Cervera, P., et al.: Tyrosine-hydroxylase immunoreactivity in senile plaques is not related to the density of tyrosine hydroxylase positive fibers in patients with Alzheimer type dementia. Neurosci. Lett., 110:210, 1990.

170. Glenner, G.G., and Wong, C.W.: Alzheimer's disease: initial report of the purification and characterization of a novel cerebrovascular amyloid protein. Bioch. Biophys. Res. Com., 120:884, 1984.

171. Kang, J., et al.: The precursor of Alzheimer's disease amyloid A4 protein resembles a cell-surface receptor. Nature, 325:733, 1987.

172. Masters, C.L., and Beyreuther, K.: The molecular pathology of the amyloid A4 precursor of Alzheimer's disease. In: *Proceedings of the International Symposium on Alzheimer's Disease.* Kuopio, 1988.

173. Carrell, R.W.: Alzheimer disease. Enter a protease inhibitor. Nature, 331:478, 1988.

174. Hardy, J.: Molecular biology and Alzheimer's disease: more questions than answers. TINS, 11:293, 1988.

175. Masters, C.L., Beyreuther, K.: Amyloidogenic A4 protein submit: clues to the pathogenesis of the neurofibrillary tangle, Alzheimer plaque, and congophilic angiopathy. In: *Aging and the Brain.* Edited by R.D. Terry. New York, Raven Press, 1988.

176. Coria, F., et al.: Isolation and characterization of amyloid P component form Alzheimer's disease and other types of cerebral amyloidosis. Lab Invest., 58:454, 1988.

177. Glenner, G.G.: On primal cases in Alzheimer's disease. Neurobiol. Aging, 7:506, 1986.

178. Wisniewski, H.M., et al.: AD/SDAT, plaques, tangles and BBB changes. Neurobiol. Aging, 7:504, 1986.

179. Goldagaber, D., et al.: Characterization and chromosome localization of a cDNA encoding brain amyloid of Alzheimer's disease. Science, 235:877, 1987.

180. Tanzi, R.E., et al.: Amyloid B protein gene: mRNA distribution, and genetic linkage near the Alzheimer locus. Science, 235:880, 1987.

181. Miyakawa, T., et al.: The interrelationship between senile plaques and blood vessels in Alzheimer's disease and senile dementia. Morphological mechanism of senile plaque production. Virchows Arch. Abt. B Cell Pathol., 40:181, 1982.

182. Mountjoy, C.Q., Tomlinson, B.E., and Gibson, P.H.: Amyloid and senile plaques and cerebral blood vessels. A semi-quantitative investigation of a possible relationship. J. Neuro. Sci., 57:89, 1982.

183. Hauw, J.J., et al.: Maladie d'Alzheimer, amyloide, microglie et astrocytes. Rev. Neurol. (Paris), 144:155, 1988.

184. Rogers, J., and Morrison, J.H.: Quantitative morphology and regional and laminar distribution of senile plaques in Alzheimer's disease. J. Neurosci., 5:2801, 1985.

185. Duyckaerts, C., et al.: Laminar distribution of neocortical senile plaques in senile dementia of the Alzheimer type. Acta Neuropathol. (Berl), 70:249, 1986.

186. Lewis, D.A., et al.: Laminar and regional distributions of neurofibrillary tangles and neuritic plaques in Alzheimer's disease: a quantitative study of visual and auditory cortices. J. Neurosci., 7:1799, 1987.

187. Kosik, K.S., Rogers, J., and Kowall, N.W.: Senile plaques are located between apical dendritic clusters. J. Neuropath. Exp. Neurol., 46:1, 1987.

188. Rudelli, R.D., Ambler, M.W., and Wisniewski, H.M.: Morphology and distribution of Alzheimer (neuritic) plaque and amyloid plaques in striatum and diencephalon. Acta Neuropathol. (Berl) 64:273, 1984.

189. Arendt, T., Taubert, G., Bigl, V., et al.: Amyloid deposition in the nucleus basalis of Meynert complex: a topographic marker for degenerating cell clusters in Alzheimer's disease. Acta Neuropathol. (Berl), 75:226, 1987.

190. Blessed, G., Tomlinson, B.E., and Roth, M.: The association between quantitative measures of dementia and of senile changes in the cerebral grey matter of elderly subjects. Br. J. Psychiat., 114:797, 1968.

191. Katzman, R., et al.: Clinical, pathological, and neurochemical changes in dementia: a subgroup with preserved mental status and numerous neocortical plaques. Ann. Neurol., 23:138, 1988.

192. Okazaki, H., et al.: Primary cerebral amyloid angiopathy. Mayo Clin. Proc., 54:22, 1979.

193. Chamouard, J.M., et al.: Accès ischémiquies transitoires au cours d'une angiopathie amyloide. Rev. Neurol. (Paris), 144:596, 1988.

194. Castano, E.M., and Frangione, B.: Human amyloidosis, Alzheimer disease and related disorders. Lab. Invest., 58:122, 1988.

195. Glenner, G.G., Henry, J.H., and Fujihara, S.: Congophilic angiopathy in the pathogenesis of Alzheimer's degeneration. Ann. Path., 1:120, 1981.

196. Vinters, H.V.: Cerebral amyloid angiopathy. A critical review. Stroke, 18:311, 1987.

197. Davies, L., et al.: A4 amyloid protein deposition and the diagnosis of Alzheimer's disease: prevalence in aged brains determined by immunocytochemistry compared with conventional neuropathologic techniques. Neurology (in press).

198. Rosenblum, W.I., and Haider, A.: Negative correlations between parenchymal amyloid and vascular amyloid in the hippocampus. Am. J. Pathol., 130:532, 1988.

199. Joachim, C.L., et al.: Tau epitopes are incorporated into a range of lesions in Alzheimer's disease. J. Neuropath. Exp. Neurol., 46:611, 1987.

200. Tomlinson, B.E., and Kitchener, D.: Granulo-vacuolar degeneration of hippocampal pyramidal cells. J. Pathol., 106:165, 1972.

201. Ball, M.J., and Lo, R.: Granulovacuolar degeneration in the ageing brain and in the senile dementia. J. Neuropath. Exp. Neurol., 36:474, 1977.

202. Sumpter, P.Q., et al.: An ultrastructural analysis of the effects of accumulation of neurofibrillary tangles in pyramidal cells of the cerebral cortex in Alzheimer's disease. Neuropathol. Appl. Neurobiol., 12:305, 1986.

203. Galloway, P.G., Perry, G., and Gambetti, P.: A study

of actin binding proteins in Hirano bodies. J. Neuropathol. Exp. Neurol., 45:355, 1986.

204. Galloway, P.G., et al.: Hirano bodies contain tau protein. Brain Res., 403:337, 1987.

205. Gibson, P.H., and Tomlinson, B.E.: Numbers of Hirano bodies in the hippocampus of normal and demented people with Alzheimer's disease. J. Neurol. Sci., 33:199, 1977.

206. Brion, S., Masse, G., and Plas, J.: Histopathologie de la spongiose dans la maladie de Creutzfeldt-Jakob et dans les démences séniles et préseniles. In: *Virus non conventionnels et affections du système nerveux central.* Edited by L. Court, F. Cathala. Paris, Masson, 1983.

207. Probst, A., et al.: Senile dementia of the Alzheimer type: Astroglial reaction to extracellular neurofibrillary tangles in the hippocampus. Acta Neuropath. (Berl), 57:75, 1982.

208. Brun, A., and Englund, E.: A white matter disorder in dementia of the Alzheimer type: a pathoanatomical study. Ann. Neurol., 19:253, 1986.

209. Hachinski, V.C., Potter, P. and Merskey, H.: Leuko-Araiosis. Arch. Neurol., 44:21, 1987.

210. Durand-Fardel, M.: *Traité clinique et pratique des maladies des vieillards.* Paris, Germer Bailliere, 1854.

211. Hauw, J.J.: Leukoaraiosis: The brain interstitial atrophy ("l'atrophie interstitielle du cerveau") of Durand-Fardel. Arch. Neurol., 45:140, 1988.

212. Inzitari, D., et al.: Vascular risk factors and leukoaraiosis. Arch. Neurol., 44:42, 1987.

213. Naeser, M.A., et al.: Decrease computerized tomography numbers in patients with presenile dementia. Arch. Neurol., 37:401, 1980.

214. Albert, M., et al.: CT density numbers in patients with senile dementia of the Alzheimer type. Arch. Neurol., 41:1264, 1984.

215. Ichimya, Y., et al.: A computed tomography study of Alzheimer's disease by regional volumetric and parenchymal density measurements. J. Neurol., 233:164, 1986.

216. Awad, I.A., et al.: Incidental subcortical lesions identified on Magnetic Resonance Imaging in the elderly. II. Postmortem pathological correlations. Stroke, 17:1090, 1986.

217. Mishkin, M.: A memory system in the monkey. Phil. Trans. R. Soc. (London), 298:85, 1982.

218. Scoville, W.B., and Milner, B.R.: Loss of recent memory after bilateral hippocampal lesions. J. Neurol. Neurosurg. Psychiat., 20:11, 1957.

219. Duyckaerts, C., et al.: Bilateral and limited amygdalohippocampal lesions causing a pure amnesic syndrome. Ann. Neurol., 18:314, 1985.

220. Hooper, M.W., and Vogel, F.S.: The limbid system in Alzheimer's disease. Am J. Path., 85:1, 1976.

221. Brun, A., and Englund, E.: Regional pattern of degeneration in Alzheimer's disease: neuronal loss and histopathological grading. Histopathology, 5:549, 1981.

222. Morrison, J.H., Lewis, D.A., and Campbell, M.J.: Distributions of neurofibrillary tangles and nonphosphorylated neurofilament protein. Immunoreactive neurons in cerebral cortex: implications for loss of corticocortical circuits in Alzheimer's disease. In: *Molecular Neuropathology of Aging.* Edited by P. Davies, C.E. Finch. Banbury Report, 27:109, 1987. New York, Cold Spring Harbor Laboratory, 1987.

223. Appel, S.H.: A unifying hypothesis for the cause of amyotrophic lateral sclerosis. Parkinsonism and Alzheimer's disease. Ann. Neurol., 10:499, 1981.

224. Mesulam, M.M.: Alzheimer plaques and cortical cholinergic innervation. Neuroscience, 17:277, 1986.

225. Arendt, T., and Bigl, V.: Alzheimer plaques and cortical cholinergic innervation. Neuroscience, 17:277, 1986.

226. German, D.C., White, C., and Sparkman, D.R.: Alzheimer's disease: neurofibrillary tangles in nuclei that project to the cerebral cortex. Neuroscience, 21:305, 1987.

227. Palmer, A., et al.: Excitatory amino acid-releasing and cholinergic neurones in Alzheimer's disease. Neurosci. Lett., 66:199, 1986.

228. Bell, M.A., and Ball, M.J.: Morphometric comparison of hippocampal microvasculature in ageing and demented people: diameters and densities. Acta Neuropathol. (Berl), 53:299, 1981.

229. Brierley, J.B., and Graham, D.I.: Hypoxia and vascular disorders of the central nervous system. In Greenfield's Neuropathology. Edited by J. Humes Adams, J.A.N. Corsellis, L.W. Duchen. London, Edward Arnold, 1984.

230. Moragos, W.F., et al.: Glutamate dysfunction in Alzheimer's disease: a hypothesis. TINS, 10:65, 1987.

231. Hyman, B.T., et al.: Alzheimer's disease: glutamate depletion in the hippocampal perforant pathway zone. Ann. Neurol., 22:37, 1987.

232. Alafussof, I., et al.: Blood-brain barrier in Alzheimer dementia and in non-demented elderly. An immunocytochemical study. Acta Neuropathol., 73:160, 1987.

233. Mooradian, A.D.: Effects of aging on the blood-brain barrier. Neurobiol. Ageing, 9:31, 1988.

234. Gajdusek, D.C.: Hypothesis: interference with axonal transport of neurofilaments as common mechanism in certain diseases of the central nervous system. N. Engl. J. Med., 312:714, 1985.

235. Rapoport, S.I.: Brain evolution and Alzheimer's disease. Rev. Neurol. (Paris), 144:79, 1988.

236. Mann, D.M.A.: The neuropathology of Alzheimer disease: a review with pathogenetic, etiological and therapeutic considerations. Mech. Ageing Developm., 31:213, 1985.

237. Wisniewski, A.M., et al.: Alzheimer's disease, a cerebral form of amyloidosis. In: *Immunology and Alzheimer's disease.* Edited by A. Pouplard-Barthelaix, J. Emile, Y. Christen. Berlin, Springer-Verlag, 1988.

238. Hardy, J.A., et al.: An integrative hypothesis concerning the pathogenesis and progression of Alzheimer's disease. Neurobiol. Ageing, 7:489, 1986.

239. Candy, J.M., et al.: Aluminosilicates and senile plaques formation in Alzheimer's disease. Lancet, 1:354, 1986.

240. Drachman, D.A.: How normal aging relates to dementia: a critique and classification. In: *Aging of the Brain.* Edited by D. Samuel, et al. New York, Raven Press, 1983.

241. Davies, P., and Maloney, A.J.F.: Selective loss of cholinergic neurons in Alzheimer's disease. Lancet 2:1403, 1976.

242. Bowen, D.M., et al.: Neurotransmitter enzymes and indices of hypoxia in senile dementia and other abiotrophies. Brain 99:459, 1976.

243. Perry, E.K., et al.: Necropsy evidence of central cholinergic deficits in senile dementia. Lancet 1:189, 1977.

244. Nordberg, A., et al.: Change in nicotinic receptor subtypes in temporal cortex of Alzheimer brains. Neurosci. Lett., 86:317, 1988.

245. Rossor, M.: Neurochemical studies in dementia. In: *Psychopharmacology of the Aging Nervous System.* In: *Handbook of Psychopharmacology, 20*:107, 1988. Edited by L.L. Iversen, S.D. Iversen, S.H. Snyder. Plenum Press, New York.

246. Whitehouse, P.J., et al.: Reductions in 3H nicotinic acetylcholine binding in Alzheimer's disease and Parkinson's disease: an autoradiographic study. Neurology, *38*:720, 1988.

247. Rylett, E.G., Ball, M.J., and Colhoun, E.H.: Evidence for high affinity choline transport in synaptosomes prepared from hippocampus and neocortex of patients with Alzheimer's disease. Brain Res., *289*:169, 1983.

248. Sims, N.R., et al.: Presynaptic cholinergic dysfunction in patients with dementia. J. Neurochem., *40*:503, 1983.

249. Neary, D., et al.: Alzheimer's disease: a correlative study. J. Neurol. Neurosurg. Psychiat., *49*:229, 1986.

250. Lewis, P.R., and Shute, C.C.D.: The cholinergic limbic system: projection to the hippocampal formation, medical cortex, nuclei of the ascending cholinergic reticular system and the subfornical organ and the subfornical organ and supraoptic crest. Brain, *90*:521, 1967.

251. Berger, B. and Gaspar, P.: Subcortical neuronal projection to the cerebral cortex. Their role in SDAT. In: *Histopathology of the Aging Brain* (Interdisciplinary topics in Gerontology. Basel, Karger, 59, 1988.

252. Johnston, M.V., McKinney, M., and Coyle, J.T.: Neocortical cholinergic innervation: a description of extrinsic and intrinsic components in the rat. Exp. Brain Res., *43*:159, 1981.

253. Lamour, Y., et al.: Basal forebrain neurons projecting to the rat frontoparietal cortex: electrophysiological and pharmacological properties. Brain Res., *362*:122, 1986.

254. Drachman, D.A., and Leavitt, J.: Human memory and the cholinergic system: a relationship to aging? Arch. Neurol., *30*:113, 1974.

255. Arendt, T., et al.: Neuronal loss in different parts of the nucleus basalis is related to neuritic plaque formation in cortical target areas in Alzheimer's disease. Neuroscience, *14*:1, 1985.

256. Perry, R.H., et al.: Extensive loss of choline acetyl transferase activity is not related to neuronal loss in nucleus of Meynert in Alzheimer's disease. Neurosci. Lett., *33*:311, 1982.

257. Cross, A.J., et al.: Reduced DBH activity in Alzheimer's disease. Br Med. J., *282*:93, 1981.

258. Berger, B., Escourolle, R., and Moune, M.A.: Axones catécholaminergiques du cortex cérébral humain. Observation, en histofluorescence, de biopsies cérébrales dont 2 cas de maladie d'Alzheimer. Rev. Neurol., *132*:183, 1976.

259. Berger, B., et al.: Catecholaminergic innervation of the human cerebral cortex in presenile and senile dementia. Histochemical and biochemical studies. In: *Enzymes and Neurotransmitters in Mental Disease.* Edited by E. Usdin, T.L. Sourkes, M.B.H. Youdim. Chichester, John Wiley & Sons, 1980.

260. Cross, A.J., et al.: Studies on neurotransmitter receptor systems in neocortex and hippocampus in senile dementia of the Alzheimer type. J Neurol. Sci., *74*:109, 1984.

261. Bondareff, W., et al.: Loss of neurones of origin of adrenergic projection to cerebral cortex (nucleus locus caeruleus) in senile dementia. Neurology, *32*:164, 1982.

262. Iversen, L.L., et al.: Loss of pigmented dopamine B hydroxylase positive cells from locus caeruleus in senile dementia of Alzheimer type. Neurosci. Lett., *39*:95, 1983.

263. Mann, D.M.A., Yates, P.O., and Hawkes, J.: The pathology of the human locus caeruleus. Clin. Neuropathol., *2*:1, 1983.

264. Ishii, T.: Distribution of Alzheimer's neurofibrillary changes in the brain stem and hypothalamus of senile dementia. Acta Neuropathol., *6*:181, 1966.

265. Felten, D.L., and Sladek, J.R.: Monoamine distribution in primate brain. V. Monoaminergic nuclei: anatomy, pathways and local organization. Brain Res. Bull., *10*:171, 1983.

266. Curcio, C.A., and Kemper, T.: Nucleus raphe dorsalis in dementia of Alzheimer type: neurofibrillary changes and neuronal packing density. J. Neuropath. Exp. Neurol., *43*:359, 1984.

267. Gottfries, C.G., Roos, B.E., and Winblad, B.: Monoamine and monoamine metabolites in the human brain post mortem in senile dementia. Aktuelle Gerontol., *6*:429, 1976.

268. Adolfsson, R., et al.: Changes in brain catecholamines in patients with dementia of Alzheimer type. Br. J. Psychiat., *135*:216, 1979.

269. Gottfries, C.G., et al.: Biochemical changes in dementia disorders of Alzheimer type (AD/SDAT). Neurobiol. Aging, *4*:261, 1983.

270. Arai, H., Kosaka, K., and Iizuka, R.: Changes of biogenic amines and their metabolites in postmortem brains from patients with Alzheimer type dementia. J. Neurochem, *43*:388, 1984.

271. Hirano, A., and Zimmerman, H.M.: Alzheimer's neurofibrillary changes. A topographical study. Arch. Neurol., *7*:227, 1962.

272. Mann, D.M.A., Yates, P.O., and Marcyniuk, B.: Dopaminergic neurotransmitter systems in Alzheimer's disease and in Down's syndrome at middle age. J. Neurol. Neurosurg. Psychiatry, *50*:341, 1987.

273. Porrino, L.J., and Goldman-Rakic, P.S.: Brainstem innervation of prefrontal and anterior cingulate cortex in the rhesus monkey revealed by retrograde transport of HRP. J. Comp. Neurol., *205*:63, 1982.

274. Arendt, T.: Correlation between cortical plaque count and neuronal loss in nucleus basalis in Alzheimer's disease. Neuroscience Lett., *48*:81, 1984.

275. Rossor, M.N., et al.: Neuropeptides and dementia. In: *Peptides and Neurological Diseases* (Progress in brain research. vol 66). Edited by P.C. Emson, M. Rossor, M. Tohyama. Amsterdam, Elsevier, 1986.

276. Yates, C.M., et al.: Thyrotropin releasing hormone, luteinizing hormone-releasing hormone and substance P immunoreactivity in post-mortem brain from cases of Alzheimer type dementia and Down's syndrome. Brain Res., *258*:445, 1983.

277. Biggins, J.A., et al.: Postmortem levels of thyrotropin releasing hormone and neurotensin in the amygdala in Alzheimer's disease, schizophrenia and depression. J. Neurol. Sci., *58*:117, 1983.

278. Ferrier, I.N., et al.: Neuropeptides in Alzheimer type dementia. J. Neurol. Sci., *62*:159, 1983.

279. Yates, C.M., et al.: Neurotension immunoreactivity is increased in Down's syndrome but not in Alzheimer type dementia. J. Neurol Sci., *67*:327, 1985.

280. Perry, R., et al.: Neuropeptides in Alzheimer's disease, depression and schizophrenia. A post mortem

analysis of vasoactive intestinal polypeptide and cholecystokinin in cerebral cortex. J. Neurol. Sci., 51:465, 1981.

281. Rossor, M.N., et al.: Normal concentrations of cholecystokinin-like immunoreactivity with reduced choline acetyltransferase activity in senile dementia of the Alzheimer type. Life Sci., 29:405, 1981.

282. Crystal, H.A., and Davies, P.: Cortical substance P-like immunoreactivity in cases of Alzheimer's disease and senile dementia of the Alzheimer type. J. Neurochem., 38:1781, 1982.

283. Rossor, M.N., et al.: Reduced cortical CAT activity is not accompanied in vasoactive intestinal polypeptides. Brain Res., 201:249, 1980.

284. Davies, P., Katzman, R., and Terry, R.D.: Reduced somatostatin immunoreactivity in cases of Alzheimer's disease and Alzheimer senile dementia. Nature, 288:279, 1980.

285. Lowe, S.L., et al.: Gamma-aminobutyric acid concentration in brain tissue at two stages of Alzheimer's disease. Brain, 111:785, 1988.

286. Gaspar, P., et al.: Subpopulations of somatostatin-immunoreactive neurons display different vulnerability in senile dementia of the Alzheimer type. Brain Res., 490:1, 1989.

287. Roberts, G.W., et al.: Localization of neuronal tangles in somatostatin neurones in Alzheimer's disease. Nature, 314:92, 1985.

288. Vincent, S.R., et al.: Neuropeptide coexistence in human cortical neurones. Nature, 298:65, 1982.

289. Allen, J.M., et al.: Elevation of neuropeptide Y (NPY) in substantia innominata in Alzheimer's type dementia. J. Neurol. Sci., 64:325, 1984.

290. Dawbarn, D., et al.: Decreased somatostatin immunoreactivity but not neuropeptide Y immunoreactivity in cerebral cortex in senile dementia of Alzheimer type. Neurosci. Lett., 70:154, 1986.

291. Foster, N.L., et al.: Brain choline acetyltransferase activity and neuropeptide Y concentrations in Alzheimer's disease. Neurosci. Lett., 63:71, 1986.

292. Chan-Palay, V., et al.: Distribution of altered hippocampal neurones and axons immunoreactive with antisera against neuropeptide Y in Alzheimer type dementia. J. Comp. Neurol., 248:376, 1986.

293. Chan-Palay, V., et al.: Cortical neurones immunoreactive with antisera against neuropeptides Y are altered in Alzheimer type dementia. J. Comp. Neurol., 238:390, 1985.

294. Nakamura, S., and Vincent, S.R.: Somatostatin and neuropeptide Y immunoreactive neurones in the neocortex in senile dementia of Alzheimer type. Brain Res., 370:11, 1986.

295. Bissette, G., et al.: Corticotropin-releasing factor-like immunoreactivity in senile dementia of the Alzheimer type. JAMA, 254:3067, 1985.

296. De Souza, E.B., et al.: Alzheimer's disease: reciprocal changes in cortico-tropin-releasing factor (CRF)-like immunoreactivity and CRF receptors in cerebral cortex. Nature, 319:593, 1986.

297. Bowen, D.M., et al.: "Classical" neurotransmitters in Alzheimer disease. In: Aging and the Brain (Aging vol 32). Edited by R.D. Terry. New York, Raven Press, 1988.

298. Rossor, M.N., et al.: A post-mortem study of the cholinergic and GABA systems in senile dementia. Brain, 105:313, 1982.

299. Hardy, J.A., et al.: Region specific loss of glutamate innervation in Alzheimer's disease. Neurosci. Lett., 73:77, 1987.

300. Cowburn, R., et al.: Presynaptic and postsynaptic glutaminergic function in Alzheimer's disease. Neurosci. Lett., 66:109, 1988.

301. Smith, C.C.T., et al.: Amino acid release from biopsy samples of temporal neocortex from patients with Alzheimer's disease. Brain Res., 264:138, 1983.

302. Bertrand, I., and Koffas, D.: Cas d'idiotie mongolienne adulte avec nombreuses plaques séniles et concretions calcaires pallidales. Rev. Neurol. (Paris), 78:338, 1946.

303. Solitaire, G.B., and Lamarche, J.B.: Alzheimer's disease and senile dementia as seen in mongoloids. Am. J. Ment. Defic., 70:840, 1966.

304. Ball, M.J., Schapiro, M.B., and Rapaport, S.I.: Neuropathological relationship between Down syndrome and senile dementia of the Alzheimer type. In: The Neurobiology of Down syndrome. Edited by C.J. Epstein. New York, Raven Press, 1986.

305. Wisniewski, H.M., Rabe, A., and Wisniewski, E.: Neuropathology and dementia in people with Down's syndrome. In: Molecular Neuropathology of Aging (Banbury Report vol. 27). Edited by P. Davies, C.E. Finch. Cold Spring Harbor Laboratory, 1987.

306. Berr, C., et al.: Absence of familial association between dementia of Alzheimer type and Down syndrome. Am. J. Clin. Genet., (in press), 1988.

307. Kirkpatrick, J.B., Hicks, P.J.: Nucleus Basalis in Down's syndrome, (abstract). J. Neuropathol. Exp. Neurol., 43:307, 1984.

308. Allsop, D., et al.: Isolated senile plaque cores in Alzheimer's disease and Down's syndrome show differences in morphology. J. Neurol. Neurosurg. Psych., 49:886, 1986.

309. Szumanska, G., et al.: Lectin histochemistry of plaques and tangles in Alzheimer disease. Acta Neuropath. (Berl), 73:1, 1987.

310. Sylvester, P.E.: Ageing in the mentally retarded. In: Scientific Studies in Mental Retardation. Edited by J. Dobbing, et al.: London, Royal Society of Medicine, 1984.

311. Pollack, M., and Hornabrook, R.W.: The prevalence, natural history and dementia of Parkinson's disease. Brain, 89:429, 1966.

312. Celesia, G.G., and Wanamaker, W.M.: Psychiatric disturbances in Parkinson's disease. Dis Nervous System, 33:577, 1972.

313. Leverens, J., and Sumi, S.M.: Parkinson's disease in patients with Alzheimer's disease. Arch. Neurol., 43:662, 1986.

314. Hakim, A.M., and Mathieson, G.: Dementia in Parkinson disease: a neuropathologic study. Neurology, 29:1209, 1979.

315. Boller, F., et al.: Parkinson's disease, dementia and Alzheimer disease: clinico-pathological correlations. Ann. Neurol., 7:329, 1980.

316. Gaspar, P., and Gray, F.: Dementia in idiopathic Parkinson's disease: a neuropathological study on 32 cases. Acta Neuropathol. (Berl), 64:43, 1984.

317. Dubois, B., et al.: Démence et maladie de Parkinson: corrélations biochimiques et anatomo-cliniques. Rev. Neurol. (Paris), 141:184, 1985.

318. Ruberg, M., and Agid, Y.: Dementia in Parkinson's Disease. In: Psychopharmacology of the Aging Nervous System. (Handbook of Psychopharmacology, Vol 2). Edited by L.L. Iversen, S.D. Iversen, and S.H. Snyder. New York, Plenum Press, 1988.

319. Jellinger, K., and Grisold, W.: Cerebral atrophy in Parkinson syndrome. Exp. Brain Res., 26(5):1982.

320. Forno, L.S., and Alvord, E.C.: The pathology of Par-

kinsonism. In: *Recent Advances in Parkinson's Disease.* Edited by F. McDowell, C. Markham. Philadelphia, F.A. Davis Co., 1971.

321. Kawasaki, H., Shimada, H., and Tomonaga, M.: Morphological study on the Lewy bodies in the sympathetic ganglia of the aged persons. Jpn. J. Geriat., *25*:282, 1988.

322. Forno, L.S.: Pathology of Parkinsonism: A preliminary report of 24 cases. J. Neuros., *24*:266, 1966.

323. Martilla, R.J., et al.: Parkinson's disease in a nationwide chart. Neurology, *38*:1271, 1988.

324. Terry, R.D., and Katzman, R.: Senile dementia of the Alzheimer type. Ann. Neurol., *14*:497, 1983.

325. Jellinger, K.: Neuropathological aspects of dementias resulting from abnormal blood and cerebrospinal fluid dynamics. Acta Neurol. Belg., *76*:83, 1976.

326. Buhl, L., and Bojsen-Moller, M.: Frequency of Alzheimer's disease in a post-mortem study of psychiatric patients. Dan. Med. Bull., *35*:288, 1988.

327. Khachaturian, Z.S., et al.: Diagnosis of Alzheimer's disease. Arch. Neurol., *42*:1097, 1985.

328. Gambetti, P., Autilio-Gambetti, L., and Papasozomenos, S.C.: Bodian's silver method stains neurofilament polypeptides. Science, *213*:1521, 1981.

329. Esiri, M.M., Pearson, R.C.A., and Powell, T.P.S.: The cortex of the primary auditory area in Alzheimer's disease. Brain Res., *366*:385, 1986.

330. Nee, L.E., et al.: Dementia of the Alzheimer type: clinical and family studies of 22 twin pairs. Neurology, *37*:359, 1987.

331. Fitch, N., Becker, R., and Heller, A.: The inheritance of Alzheimer's disease: a new interpretation. Ann. Neurol., *23*:14, 1988.

332. Brietner, J.C.S., and Folstein, M.F.: Familial nature of Alzheimer's disease. N. Engl. J. Med., *311*:192, 1984.

333. Alperovitch, A., and Berr, C.: Familial aggregation of dementia of Alzheimer type: analysis from an epidemiological point of view. In: *Genetics and Alzheimer's Disease.* Edited by P.M. Sinet, Y. Lamour, Y. Christen. Berlin, Springer-Verlag, (in press), 1988.

334. Breitner, J.C.S.: Alzheimer's disease: genetic theories of etiology. In: *Psychopharmacology of the Aging Nervous System* (*Handbook of Psychopharmacology* vol 20). Edited by L.L. Iverson, S.D. Iversen, S.H. Snyder. New York, Plenum Press, 1988.

335. Huff, F.J., et al.: Risk of dementia in relatives of patients with Alzheimer's disease. Neurology, *38*:786, 1988.

336. Hardy, J.A., Owen, M.J., and Goate, A.N.: The molecular genetics of Alzheimer's disease. In: *Proceedings of the International Symposium on Alzheimer's Disease.* Kuopio, 1988.

337. Heston, L.H.: Dementia of the Alzheimer type. A perspective from family studies. In: *Biological Aspects of Alzheimer's Disease* (Banbury Report, Vol 15). Edited by R. Katzman. Cold Spring Harbor Laboratory, 1983.

338. Amaducci, L., Lippi, A., and Fratiglioni, L.: What risk factors are known? In: *Etiology of Dementia of Alzheimer Type.* Edited by A.S. Henderson, J.H. Henderson. Dahlem Konferenzen. Chichester, John Wiley & Sons Limited. (In press)

339. St. George-Hyslop, P.H., et al.: The genetic defect causing familial Alzheimer's disease maps on chromosome 21. Science, *235*:885, 1987.

340. Tanzi, R.E., et al.: The genetic defect in familial Alzheimer's disese is not tightly linked to the amyloid beta protein gene. Nature, *329*:156, 1987.

341. Van Broeckhoven, C., et al.: Failure of familial Alzheimer's disease to segregate with the A4-amyloid gene in several European families. Nature, *329*:153, 1987.

342. Warren, A.C., et al.: Beta-amyloid gene is not present in three copies in autopsy-validated Alzheimer's disease. Genomics, *1*:307, 1987.

343. Henderson, A.S.: The risk factors for Alzheimer's disease: a review and a hypothesis. Acta Psych. Scand. (In press).

344. Hagnell, O., Lanke, J., Rorsman, B., et al.: Does the incidence of age psychosis decrease? Neuropsychobiol., *7*:201, 1981.

345. Heeren, T.J., and Lagaay, A.M.: Prevalence of dementia in the "oldest old" in a dutch population: preliminary result. In: *Proceedings of the International Symposium on Alzheimer's Disease,* (abstract). Kuopio, 1988.

346. Wisniewski, H.M., et al.: Current hypotheses of Alzheimer disease etiology. In: *Fifth Paulo Foundation International Symposium Pathobiology of Alzheimer's Disease.* Hanasaari, 1988.

5

Spinocerebellar System Degenerations

JOO HO SUNG and
RONALD C. KIM

SPINOCEREBELLAR SYSTEM DEGENERATIONS (ATROPHIES) OF ADULT ONSET

This group of degenerative disorders is characterized clinically by ataxia or incoordination of movement and pathologically by progressive degeneration of the spinocerebellar system, including the cerebellum and its afferent and efferent pathways. The system may be affected selectively or together with other functionally unrelated neuronal systems. Due to lack of knowledge concerning their etiology, attempts have been made to classify these disorders according to clinical, pathological or genetic features, or varying combinations thereof.[1-5]

Since progressive ataxia is the salient clinical feature common to all spinocerebellar degenerations, clinical classifications have been based on variations in the associated clinical features such as peripheral neuropathy, motor and sensory abnormalities referable to the spinal cord, ocular findings, extrapyramidal disturbances, and dementia.[6]

Pathologically, these disorders are characterized by non-specific degeneration of spinocerebellar neurons progressing to cell loss, with atrophy of the affected nuclei and their fiber tracts. Pathologic classifications have been based largely on the distribution of the lesions in various portions of the spinocerebellar projection systems, together with lesions in other systems. Morphologic abnormalities have been observed in the cerebellum and its afferent and efferent neurons and fibers within the spinal cord and brain stem, in all possible combinations. Pathologically, three main forms are recognized, namely, spinal, cerebellar cortical and olivopontocerebellar;[7-9] spinocerebellar degeneration has also been described in association with degenerations of other systems.

Friedreich's ataxia, which represents the *spinal form*, was the first to be described, and is the best known among spinocerebellar disorders. The disease is usually inherited as an autosomal recessive trait and begins before the age of 25 years.[10] The major clinical features are ataxia of gait, absent tendon reflexes, dysarthria, pyramidal tract signs, loss of position and vibration sense, kyphoscoliosis, cardiac dysfunction, and pes cavus. The course is inexorably progressive, and most are chairbound by the age of 44 years.[10] The pathologic changes are generally limited to the spinal cord, with progressive degeneration of the dorsal columns, dorsal nucleus of Clarke and spinocerebellar and pyramidal tracts.[9] The dorsal spinal ganglia and peripheral nerves are also affected.[11] This disorder of the young is beyond the scope of this chapter and for details, readers are referred to several excellent reviews such as those by Harding,[10] Eadie,[12] and Barbeau.[13,14]

Spinocerebellar disorders of adult onset were first grouped together by Marie under the heading of "hereditary cerebellar ataxia," to be distinguished from Friedreich's ataxia.[7] The term 'Marie's ataxia' is still in clinical use today.[6] The cases that Marie originally collected were, however, shown later to be clinically as well as pathologically heterogeneous,[7,9] and the use of the term "hereditary cerebellar ataxia" to designate a specific form of disease is now considered to be unjustified.[7]

Cerebello-olivary degeneration, which represents the *cerebellar form*, is characterized by primary degeneration of the cerebellar cortex with secondary or trans-synaptic degeneration of the inferior olivary nuclei. Pathologically, this disorder closely resembles that form of cerebellar cortical atrophy associated with chronic alcoholism,[15] but the latter, as well as other cerebellar disorders associated with known causes, such as anoxia, various intoxications and carcinomas, is not included in this chapter.

Olivo-ponto-cerebellar degeneration is characterized by primary degeneration of neurons of the nuclei basis pontis and inferior olivary nuclei, and secondary degeneration of the cerebellar cortex. Pathologic changes are, however, not limited to the brain stem nuclei and cerebellum but also frequently involve the spinal cord, substantia nigra or striatonigral system. When combined with degeneration within other systems, the condition is referred to as multiple system degeneration (atrophy).[16,17]

Combined spinocerebellar and other system degenerations include dentatorubropallidoluysian degeneration and Machado-Joseph disease. Olivo-ponto-cerebellar degeneration with involvement of other systems belongs to this category but is discussed separately, following traditional methods of classification.

There still remains, however, considerable nosologic confusion because of the occurrence of complex clinical and pathologic variations or intermediate forms, even among individuals within the same family.[8,18,19]

CEREBELLO-OLIVARY DEGENERATION (ATROPHY)

This is a degenerative disorder of middle or later life with primary cerebellar cortical degeneration and retrograde degeneration of the inferior olivary nuclei. Both familial and sporadic cases of the disorder have been described. Holmes[20] was the first to report an afflicted family, and many familial cases have since been reported.[21-26] In the majority of families, the disorder is inherited as an autosomal dominant trait. Weiner and Konigsmark[2] divided the hereditary diseases of the cerebellar parenchyma into two types, autosomal dominant and autosomal recessive lateonset cerebellar atrophy. Marie, Foix, and Alajouanine[27] described in detail sporadic cases of cerebello-olivary degeneration occurring in later life under the heading of "delayed cerebellar atrophy, predominantly cortical."[28] In contrast to the frequent reports of familial cases, sporadic cases are less frequently described, either because of their rare occurrence or the lesser degree of interest on the part of investigators.[9,29]

Clinically, the disorder starts insidiously between the fourth and sixth decades of life with unsteady or ataxic gait and speech difficulty, which slowly progress for many years to old age. Nystagmus may develop late in the course.

Pathologic findings are generally limited to the cerebellum and inferior olivary nuclei; the spinal cord is usually preserved. The cerebellum is grossly shrunken with gaping fissures and sulci, particularly along the superior surface near the midline (Fig. 5–1). Histologically, there is severe loss of Purkinje cells within the archi- and paleocerebellum and the remaining

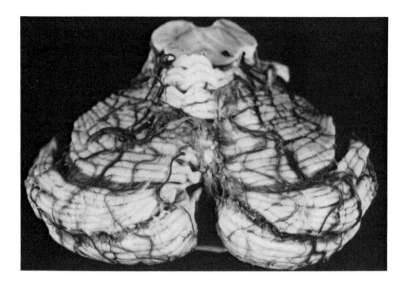

Fig. 5–1. Cerebellum shows severe atrophy with marked gaping of fissures.

superior surface, but granule cell loss, in contrast, is relatively mild (Fig. 5–2). Associated with Purkinje cell loss is marked proliferation of Bergmann astrocytes. There are also striking clusters of axon terminals (basket fibers) of stellate cells ("empty baskets") (Fig. 5–3) and occasional torpedo-like swellings of Purkinje cell axons within the granule cell layer, best appreciated in sections to which silver stains (such as that of Bielschowsky) have been applied. These changes are generally less severe in the neocerebellum and along the inferior surface. The deep cerebellar nuclei usually show mild gliosis in response to degeneration of Purkinje cell axon terminals, but their neurons are generally spared (Fig. 5–4).

In the inferior olivary nuclei there is severe loss of neurons, particularly within the dorsal lamellae and accessory olivary nuclei (Fig. 5–5), which correspond topographically to the cortical degeneration observed along the superior surface and within the paleocerebellum. The inferior olivary nuclei are not affected in the recessive form of cerebellar cortical degeneration.[2]

OLIVO-PONTO-CEREBELLAR DEGENERATION (ATROPHY)

Olivo-ponto-cerebellar degeneration or atrophy (OPCA) is a progressive degenerative disorder of middle or later life that is charac-

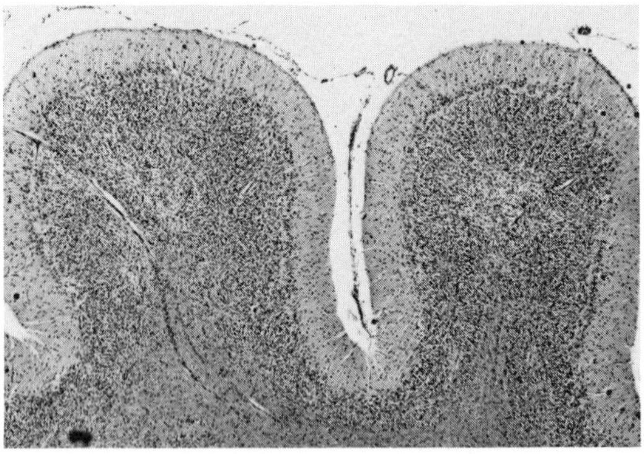

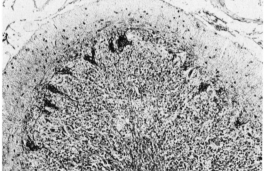

Fig. 5–2. Cerebellar folia show total loss of Purkinje cells, Bergmann astrocytosis and relative preservation of internal granular cells. Luxol fast blue-PAS stain; ×50.

Fig. 5–3. Cerebellar cortex with striking clusters of basket fiber terminals ("empty baskets") in place of lost Purkinje cells. Bielschowsky's silver stain; × 120.

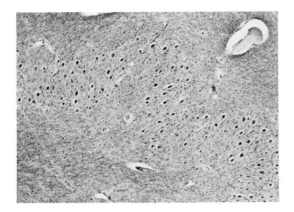

Fig. 5–4. Dentate nucleus shows mild gliosis but good preservation of neurons. Luxol fast blue-PAS stain; ×50.

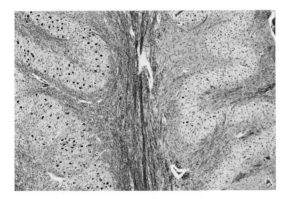

Fig. 5–5. Inferior olivary nucleus shows severe loss of neurons and mild gliosis in the dorsal lamella (right) and relative preservation of neurons in the ventral lamella (left). Luxol fast blue-PAS stain; ×50.

terized pathologically by degeneration of neurons within the nuclei pontis, inferior olivary nuclei and cerebellar cortex. The disorder was first established as a clinicopathologic entity by Dejerine and Thomas[30] although both sporadic and familial cases had been described earlier by others.[9,28,31–33] Berciano[34] in his review of 117 anatomically proven cases of OPCA from the literature found 54 to be familial and 63 to be sporadic. OPCA rarely occurs in "pure" form, i.e. with lesions limited to the medulla, pons, and cerebellum; it is almost always associated with lesions in other structures that may or may not be related to the spinocerebellar system.

The constant clinical features are ataxia of gait and dysarthria, as in other spinocerebellar degenerations, beginning between the third and fifth decades of life; the clinical onset is generally earlier in familial than in sporadic cases. Both sexes are affected about equally. Clinical evidence of cerebellar dysfunction is frequently associated with parkinsonian symptoms, dementia, urinary incontinence, pyramidal signs, and amyotrophy.

The disorder is steadily progressive, lasting for 6 and 15 years on the average in sporadic and familial cases, respectively,[34] and death occurs usually as a result of intercurrent infection. For further clinical details, readers are referred to the reviews by Eadie.[31–33]

Pathologically, there is no essential difference between the hereditary and sporadic forms of OPCA.[9,28,35] The main gross findings are atrophy of the basis pontis, inferior olives, and cerebellum (Fig. 5–6). Histologically, neuronal loss affects the pontine, inferior olivary and arcuate nuclei, and the cerebellar cortex. The three nuclei are believed to originate from a single group of nerve cells, the cell bands of Essick,[36] all of which are affected in OPCA.[37,38] A severe diffuse loss of neurons within the pontine nuclei, together with degeneration of the fiber tracts emanating therefrom (Fig. 5–7), accounts for gross atrophy of the basis pontis and middle cerebellar peduncles (Fig. 5–8). Similarly, the inferior olivary and arcuate nuclei lose most of their neurons and undergo diffuse astrogliosis (Fig. 5–9). The hilus of the inferior olivary nucleus and the inferior cerebellar peduncles become rarefied or atrophic. In the cerebellum, there is a variable loss of Purkinje cells accompanied by Bergmann astrocytosis, more so in the lateral lobes or neocerebellum than in the paleocerebellum. Loss of nerve cells within the Purkinje cell layer is, however, considerably less severe than that observed within the pontine and inferior olivary nuclei, and is believed to be the result of anterograde trans-synaptic degeneration. As is readily demonstrated in sections to which Bielschowsky's silver staining has been applied, there are striking clusters of basket fibers in place of the lost Purkinje cells and frequent torpedo-like swellings of Purkinje cell axons within the granule cell layer (Fig. 5–10). The granule cells are less severely affected

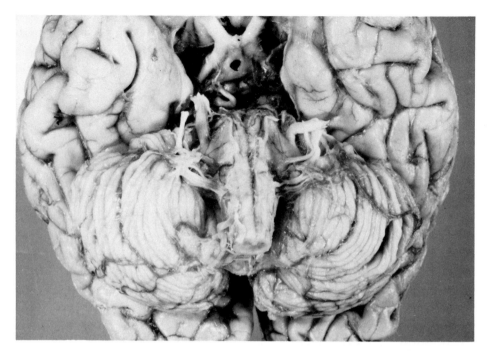

Fig. 5–6. Atrophic pons with shrunken ventral surface, cerebellar atrophy with widening of sulci, and atrophy of the inferior olives.

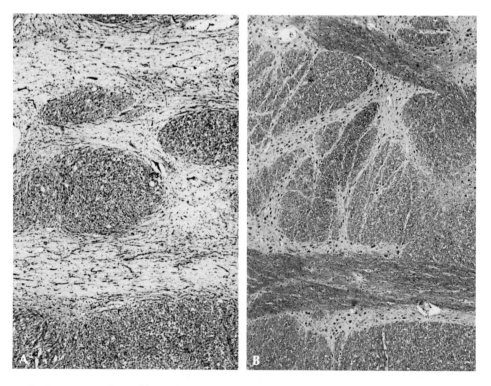

Fig. 5–7. Basis pontis with total loss of neurons and degeneration of transverse fibers in OPCA (A) and normal basis pontis for control (B). Luxol fast blue-PAS stain; ×50.

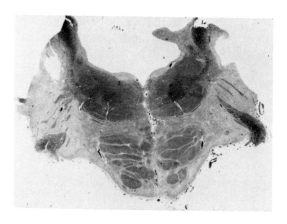

Fig. 5–8. Pons shows severe degeneration of the transverse fibers of the basis pontis and middle cerebellar peduncles but preservation of the corticospinal tracts, superior cerebellar peduncles and tegmentum of pons. Luxol fast blue-PAS stain; ×4.

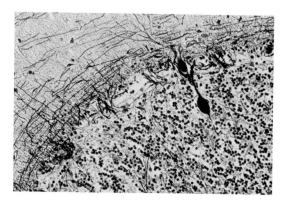

Fig. 5–10. Cerebellar cortex shows severe loss of Purkinje cells, clusters of basket fibers ("empty baskets") and a torpedo-like swelling of a Purkinje cell axon. Bielschowsky's silver stain; ×300.

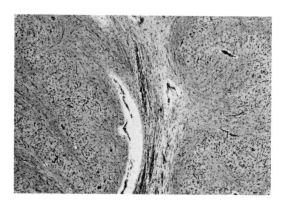

Fig. 5–9. Inferior olivary nucleus with total loss of neurons and diffuse gliosis in both ventral (left) and dorsal (right) lamellae and rarefaction of the fibers in the hilus. Luxol fast blue-PAS stain; ×50 (compare with Fig. 5–5).

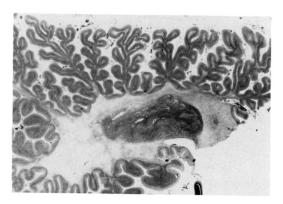

Fig. 5–11. Cerebellum shows severe degeneration of the white matter and relative preservation of the dentate nucleus and its fibers. Luxol fast blue-PAS stain; ×4.

than the Purkinje cells. The cerebellar cortical changes have been studied electron microscopically.[39] The cerebellar white matter is often degenerated to a severe degree disproportionate to the milder cortical degeneration, possibly due to the "dying back" of pontocerebellar and olivo-cerebellar fibers (Fig. 5–11). The dentate nucleus often shows a mild astrogliosis in response to degeneration of Purkinje cell axon terminals, but its neurons, along with the fibers within the superior cerebellar peduncles, are usually preserved (Fig. 5–12).

As mentioned earlier, a "pure" form of

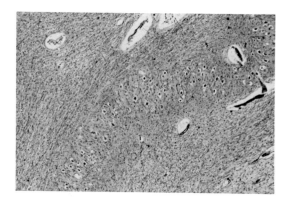

Fig. 5–12. Dentate nucleus shows good preservation of the neurons but with mild gliosis. Luxol fast blue-PAS stain; ×50.

OPCA, without associated damage to structures other than the pons, medulla, and cerebellum, is rarely seen. Among the other structures, the spinal cord appears most frequently to be affected. The dorsal columns, spinocerebellar tracts, cell columns of Clarke, pyramidal tracts and anterior horn cells may all show degeneration (Fig. 5–13). OPCA is also frequently associated with nigral or striatonigral degeneration.[17,35,40–42] Combined systems degeneration is commonly associated with degeneration of neurons of the dorsal vagal nuclei and intermediolateral cell columns. Loss of autonomic neurons seems to account for clinical autonomic failure.[16,42–46] Graham and Oppenheimer[16] proposed the term "multiple system atrophy" for combined OPCA and striatonigral degeneration, and suggested that the two conditions are different manifestations of the same basic disease.[17] A clinical syndrome named after Shy and Drager[47] is now generally recognized to be orthostatic hypotension associated with degeneration of multiple systems, including autonomic neurons.[16,17,42] In support of the concept of multisystem atrophy, the incidence of combined OPCA and striatonigral degeneration among the cases reported in the literature as OPCA,[28,35,48] as striatonigral degeneration,[49,50] or as some other form of neurodegenerative disease[16,42,44] is fairly high.

In the author's (JHS) experience, combined OPCA and striatonigral degeneration is seen more commonly than either disorder alone. Of 13 cases examined personally in the last 27 years, 9 showed combined systems degeneration, 2 showed OPCA with nigral degeneration, and 2 showed pure striatonigral degeneration. Degenerative changes affect one or the other system more severely, or may affect both systems equally, thus accounting for the variability in clinical presentation that may be seen. Clinical manifestations reflecting degeneration of one system may overshadow those of degeneration of the other.

Because of genetic, clinical and pathologic variations, there has been considerable nosologic confusion. Greenfield[9] divided OPCA into a familial (Menzel) type and a sporadic (Dejerine-Thomas) type. Eadie[31,–33] also listed "variants" of the hereditary and sporadic types. Konigsmark and Weiner[1] further divided OPCA into 5 types according to the combination of genetic, clinical, and pathologic features. They are as follows: OPCA I, Menzel (dominant) type; OPCA II, Fickler-Winkler (recessive) type; OPCA III, dominant with retinal degeneration; OPCA IV, Schut-Haymaker (dominant) type; OPCA V, dominant with dementia, ophthalmoplegia and extrapyramidal signs. They considered that some or all of the sporadic cases may belong to the recessively transmitted OPCA II.

These classifications, undertaken without regard for etiology, have obvious limitations and do not adequately cover all intermediate or overlapping forms, but the present state of our knowledge does not allow more precise (e.g. etiologic) categorization. A molecular marker or markers, if found, would be of great value in sorting out this group of disorders.

DENTATORUBRO-PALLIDOLUYSIAN ATROPHY

This is a rare progressive disorder that was first described by Titica and van Bogaert,[51] but Smith et al.[52] subsequently referred to it as combined dentatorubral and pallidoluysian degeneration, which they regarded as a form of cerebellar ataxia.[53] Further sporadic[54] and familial cases[55–57] have been reported mostly from Japan. Iizuka et al.,[56] in their review of 16 reported cases and 4 of their own, divided the disorder into three clinical types: (1) the ataxochoreoathetoid type, (2) the pseudo-Huntington type, and (3) the myoclonus-epilepsy type.

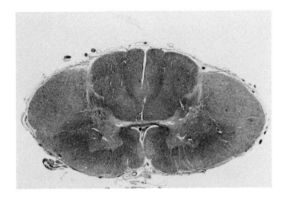

Fig. 5–13. Cervical spinal cord shows degeneration (pallor) of the spinocerebellar and pyramidal tracts (marked) and dorsal columns (mild). Luxol fast blue-PAS stain; ×8.

Type 1 is usually sporadic, while types 2 and 3 are mostly familial; types 2 and 3 may in fact occur within the same family. The disorder begins between the second and fifth decades of life and progresses slowly for more than 10 years in the majority of cases.

Pathologically, the three types are essentially similar, the constant finding in all being degeneration of the dentatorubral and pallidoluysian systems. Neurons of the dentate nuclei are severely lost, the superior cerebellar peduncles are degenerated and the red nuclei are mildly atrophic. All of the changes are accompanied by mild gliosis. There is marked neuronal loss and gliosis within the globus pallidus (particularly in its lateral segment) and subthalamic nucleus (corpus Luysii) and degeneration of the lenticular and subthalamic fasciculi. The dentatorubral system is generally more severely affected than the pallidoluysian system. Also commonly affected are the long fiber tracts of the spinal cord, cerebellar cortex, inferior olives, substantia nigra, fastigiovestibular system and tegmentum of the midbrain and pons. This disorder, by virtue of the presence of degenerative lesions involving two or more systems, resembles combined olivoponto-cerebellar and striatonigral degeneration and may be regarded as a form of multisystem atrophy. The relationship, if any, between the two disorders or to other forms of spinocerebellar degeneration is not known.

Degeneration of the dentate nuclei and their efferent fiber systems (superior cerebellar peduncles) is not uncommon in Friedreich's ataxia[58] and in olivo-ponto-cerebellar atrophy.[34] We are not aware, however, of the existence of any degenerative disorder that affects the dentatorubral system selectively.[59] Dyssynergia cerebellaris myoclonica[60] or the Ramsay Hunt syndrome,[9] which is characterized by myoclonic epilepsy and cerebellar ataxia,[61] presumably represents primary atrophy of the dentate system or dentatorubral degeneration, but pathologic examination has so far also shown evidence of damage to structures outside of the dentatorubral system.[59]

MACHADO-JOSEPH DISEASE

"Machado disease"[62] and "Joseph disease",[63] initially described in families of Por-

tuguese ancestry, are now regarded as a single hereditary disorder with variable phenotypic expression, and the disorder is currently referred to as Machado-Joseph disease.[64,65] The disorder has also been described under other names, such as nigro-spino-dentatal degeneration with nuclear ophthalmoplegia,[66] Azorean disease,[67] and autosomal dominant striatonigral degeneration.[68] The disease has also been reported in non-Portuguese ethnic groups including black[69,70] and Japanese families.[71,72]

Machado-Joseph disease is inherited as an autosomal dominant trait and begins most often between the ages of 20 and 40.[65] The constant clinical feature is an ataxia of gait, which progresses to incoordination of the limbs and dysarthria. The progressive ataxia is variably followed by a host of other manifestations, including spasticity, loss of vibratory sense, amyotrophy, progressive external ophthalmoplegia, and fasciculations. On the basis of the predominating clinical features the disorder has been divided into three main types:[65,73] Type 1, with a spastic ataxia ("Joseph" phenotype); type 2, with normoreflexic ataxia; and type 3, with amyotrophic polyneuropathy and fasciculations ("Machado" phenotype). Progressive external ophthalmoplegia may occur early in the course. The clinical phenotypes may vary between different families or among members of the same family. The age of onset varies according to the type; the onset is between 10 and 30 years in type 1, between 20 and 40 years in type 2, and after 40 to 50 years in type 3.[65] The phenotypes are, however, not fixed; type 1 can change with time to type 2 or 3 and type 2 to type 3.[65]

In pathologic reports,[65–68,71,74,75] certain lesions are constant while others are variable as would be expected on the basis of differences in clinical presentation. Like all other degenerative disorders, the characteristic pathologic condition is loss of neurons and gliosis along with degeneration of their efferent fibers. The structures that are constantly affected are the dentate nuclei and superior cerebellar peduncles, substantia nigra, cell columns of Clarke and spinocerebellar tracts, and anterior horns of the spinal cord. The structures that are variably involved include the pontine nuclei,[66,74,75] cranial nerve nuclei,[67,74,75] putamen,[68] pyramidal tracts,[67] pallido-luysian system,[75] and gracile tracts.[67] By virtue of the involvement of the spinocerebellar, extrapyramidal and motor systems, the disorder may be regarded as a form of multiple system atrophy, for which the term "ataxic multisystem degeneration" has been proposed.[65] In this respect, Machado-Joseph disease resembles olivo-ponto-cerebellar atrophy and dentatorubro-pallidoluysian atrophy. Goto et al.[76] described, in a Japanese family, 4 cases of a dominantly inherited disorder that clinically resembled Machado-Joseph disease, but autopsy examination of 1 case revealed dentatorubral-pallidoluysian degeneration. The 4 patients in this family and the 2 in Azorean families reported by Sachdev et al.[75] appear to provide a pathologic link between dentatorubro-pallidoluysian atrophy and Machado-Joseph disease.

REFERENCES

1. Konigsmark, B.W. and Weiner, L.P.: The olivopontocerebellar atrophies: A review. Medicine 49:227, 1970.
2. Weiner, L.P. and Konigsmark, B.W.: Hereditary disease of the cerebellar parenchyma. Birth Defects 7:192, 1971.
3. Kondo, K. and Sobue, I.: Genetic and clinical patterns of heritable cerebellar ataxias in adults. I Genetic analyses. J. Med. Genet. 17:416, 1980.
4. Kondo, K., Hirota, K. and Katagiri, T.: Genetic and clinical patterns of heritable cerebellar ataxias in adults. II Clinical manifestations. J. Med. Genetics 18:276, 1981.
5. Hardin, A.E.: Classification of the hereditary ataxias and paraplegias. Lancet 1:1151, 1983.
6. Harding, A.E.: The clinical features and classification of the late onset autosomal dominant cerebellar ataxias. A study of 11 families, including descendants of 'The Drew family of Walworth'. Brain 105:1, 1982.
7. Holmes, G.: An attempt to classify cerebellar disease, with a note on Marie's hereditary cerebellar ataxia. Brain 30:545, 1907b.
8. Schut, J.W. and Haymaker, W.: Hereditary ataxia: A pathologic study of five cases of common ancestry. J. Neuropath. Clin. Neurol. 1:183, 1951.
9. Greenfield, J.G.: The Spinocerebellar Degenerations. Oxford, Blackwell Scientific Publications, 1954.
10. Harding, A.E.: Friedreich's ataxia: A clinical and genetic study of 90 families with an analysis of early diagnostic criteria and intrafamilial clustering of clinical features. Brain 104:589, 1981.
11. Hughes, J.T., Brownell, B. and Hewer, R.L.: The peripheral sensory pathway in Friedreich's ataxia. An examination by light and electron microscopy of the posterior nerve roots, posterior root ganglia, and peripheral sensory nerves in cases of Friedreich's ataxia. Brain 91:803, 1968.
12. Eadie, M.J.: Cerebello-olivary atrophy (Holmes type). In: Handbook of Clinical Neurology (Eds.) Vinken, P.J.,

Bruyn, G.W. and DeJong, J.M.B.V., vol. 21, New York, American Elsevier, 1975, pp. 403–414.
13. Barbeau, A.: Friedreich's ataxia 1980. An overview of the physiopathology. Canad. J. Neurol. Sci. 7:455, 1980.
14. Barbeau, A.: Friedreich's disease 1982: Etiologic hypotheses. A personai analysis. Canad. J. Neurol. Sci. 9:243–263, 1982.
15. Victor, M., Adams, R.D. and Mancall, E.L.: A restricted form of cerebellar cortical degeneration occurring in alcoholic patients. Arch. Neurol. 1:579, 1959.
16. Graham, J.G. and Oppenheimer, D.R.: Orthostatic hypotension and nicotine sensitivity in a case of multiple system atrophy. J. Neurol. Neurosurg. Psychiat. 32:28, 1969.
17. Oppenheimer, D.: Neuropathology and neurochemistry of autonomic failure. A. Neuropathology of autonomic failure. In: Autonomic Failure. A Textbook of Clinical Disorders of the Autonomic Nervous System (Ed. Bannister, R.), New York, Oxford University Press, 1988, pp. 451–463.
18. Schut, J.W.: Hereditary ataxia. Clinical study through six generations. Arch. Neurol. Psychiat. 63:535, 1950.
19. Koeppen, A.H., Hans, M.B., Shepherd, D.I. et al.: Adult-onset hereditary ataxia in Scotland. Arch. Neurol. 34:611, 1977.
20. Holmes, G.: A form of familial degeneration of the cerebellum. Brain 30:466, 1907a.
21. Akelaitis, A.J.: Hereditary form of primary parenchymatous atrophy of the cerebellar cortex associated with mental deterioration. The Am. J. Psychiat. 94:1115, 1938.
22. Hall, B., Noad, K.B. and Latham, O.: Familial cortical cerebellar atrophy. Brain 64:178, 1941.
23. Weber, F.P. and Greenfield, J.G.: Cerebello-olivary degeneration: An example of heredo-familial incidence. Brain 65:220, 1942.
24. Richter, R.: A clinico-pathologic study of parenchymatous cortical cerebellar atrophy: Report of a familial case. J. Nerv. Mental Dis. 91:37, 1940.
25. Richter, R.B.: Late cortical cerebellar atrophy. A form of hereditary cerebellar ataxia. Am. J. Human Genet 2:1, 1950.
26. Hoffman, P.M., Stuart, W.H., Earle, K.M. et al.: Hereditary late-onset cerebellar degeneration. Neurology (Minneapolis) 21:771, 1971.
27. Marie, P., Foix, C. et Alajouanine, T.: De l'atrophie cérébelleuse tardive a prédominance corticale. (Atrophie parenchymateuse primitive des lamelles du Cervelet, atrophie paléocérébelleuse primitive). Revue Neurologique 29:849 and 1082, 1922.
28. Critchley, M. and Greenfield, J.G.: Olivo-ponto-cerebellar atrophy. Brain 71:343, 1948.
29. Baloh, R.W., Yee, R.D. and Honrubia, V.: Late cortical cerebellar atrophy. Clinical and oculographic features. Brain 109:159, 1986.
30. Déjérine, J. et Thomas, A.: L'atrophie olivo-ponto-cérébelleuse. Nouvelle Iconographie de la Salpêtrière 13:330, 1900.
31. Eadie, M.J.: Olivo-ponto-cerebellar atrophy (Dejerine-Thomas type). In: Handbook of Clinical Neurology (Eds.) Vinken, P.J., Bruyn, G.W. and DeJong, J.M.B.V., vol. 21, New York, American Elsevier, 1975a, pp. 415–431.
32. Eadie, M.J.: Olivo-ponto-cerebellar atrophy (Menzel type). In: Handbook of Clinical Neurology (Eds.) Vinken, P.J., Bruyn, G.W. and DeJong, J.M.B.V., vol. 21, New York, American Elsevier, 1975b, pp. 433–449.

33. Eadie, M.J. Olivo-ponto-cerebellar atrophy (variants). In: *Handbook of Clinical Neurology* (Eds.) Vinken, P.J., Bruyn, G.W. and DeJong, J.M.B.V., vol. 21, New York, American Elsevier, 1975c, pp. 451–457.

34. Berciano, J.: Olivopontocerebellar atrophy. A review of 117 cases. J Neurol. Sci. *53*:253, 1982.

35. Jellinger, K. und Tarnowska-Dziduszko, E.: Die ZNS-Veranderungen bei den olivo-ponto-cerebellaren Atrophien. Zeitschrift fur Neurologie *199*:192, 1971.

36. Essick, C.R.: The development of the nuclei pontis and the nucleus arcuatus in man. Am. J. Anat. *13*:25, 1912.

37. Winkler, C.: A case of olivo-pontine cerebellar atrophy and our conceptions of Neo- and Palaio-cerebellum. Schweizer Archiv fur Neurologie und Psychiatrie *13*:684, 1923.

38. Hassin, G.B. and Harris, T.H.: Olivopontocerebellar atrophy. Arch. Neurol. Psychiat. *35*:43, 1936.

39. Petito, C.K., Hart, M.N., Porro, R.S. et al.: Ultrastructural studies of olivopontocerebellar atrophy. J. Neuropath. Exp. Neurol. *32*:503, 1973.

40. Scherer, H.-J.: Extrapyramidale Storungen bei der olivopontocerebellaren Atrophie. Ein Beitrag zum Problem des lokalen vorzeitigen Alterns. Zeitschrift fur die gesamte Neurologie und Psychiatrie *145*:406, 1933.

41. Rosenhagen, H.: Die primare Atrophie des Bruckenfusses und der unteren Oliven (dargestellt nach klinischen und anatomischen Beobachtungen). Archiv fur Psychiatrie und Nervenkrankheiten *116*:163, 1943.

42. Sung, J.H., Mastri, A.R. and Segal, E.: Pathology of Shy-Drager syndrome. J. Neuropath. Exp Neurol. *38*:353, 1979.

43. Johnson, R.H., Lee, G.D.J., Oppenheimer, D.R. et al.: Autonomic failure with orthostatic hypotension due to intermediolateral column degeneration. A report of two cases with autopsies. Q. J. Med. *35*:276, 1966.

44. Schwarz, G.A.: The orthostatic hypotension syndrome of Shy-Drager. A clinicopathologic report. Arch. Neurol. *16*:123, 1967.

45. Bannister, R. and Oppenheimer, D.R.: Degenerative diseases of the nervous system associated with autonomic failure. Brain *95*:457, 1972.

46. Oppenheimer, D.R.: Lateral horn cells in progressive autonomic failure. J. Neurol. Sci. *46*:393, 1980.

47. Shy, G.M. and Drager, G.A.: A neurological syndrome associated with orthostatic hypotension. A clinical-pathologic study. Arch. Neurol. *2*:511, 1960.

48. Lambie, C.G., Latham, O. and McDonald, G.L.: Olivo-ponto-cerebellar atrophy (Marie's ataxia). Med. J. Australia *2*:626, 1947.

49. Adams, R.D., van Bogaert, L. and Vander Eecken, H.: Striato-nigral degeneration. J. Neuropath. Exp. Neurol. *23*:584, 1964.

50. Takei, Y. and Mirra, S.S.: Striatonigral degeneration: A form of multiple system atrophy with clinical parkinsonism. In: *Progress in Neuropathology* (Ed.) Zimmerman, H.M., vol. 2, New York, Grune & Stratton, 1973, pp. 217–251.

51. Titica, J. and van Bogaert, L.: Heredo-degenerative hemiballismus. A contribution to the question of primary atrophy of the corpus Luysii. Brain *69*:251, 1946.

52. Smith, J.K., Gonda, V.E. and Malamud, N.: Unusual form of cerebellar ataxia. Combined dentato-rubral and pallido-Luysian degeneration. Neurology (Minneapolis) *8*:205, 1958.

53. Smith, J.K.: Dentatorubropallidoluysian atrophy. In: *Handbook of Clinical Neurology* (Eds.) Vinken, P.J., Bruyn, G.W. and DeJong, J.M.B.V., vol. 21, New York, American Elsevier, 1975, pp. 519–534.

54. Neumann, M.A. Combined degeneration of globus pallidus and dentate nucleus and their projections. Neurology (Minneapolis) *9*:430, 1959.

55. Naito, H. and Oyanagi, S.: Familial myoclonus epilepsy and choreoathetosis: Hereditary dentatorubral-pallidoluysian atrophy. Neurology (Minneapolis) *32*:798, 1982.

56. Iizuka, R., Hirayama, K. and Maehara, K.: Dentato-rubro-pallido-luysian atrophy: a clinico-pathological study. J. Neurol. Neurosurg. Psychiat. *47*:1288, 1984.

57. Takahashi, H., Ohama, E., Naito, H., et al.: Hereditary dentatorubral-pallidoluysian atrophy: Clinical and pathologic variants in a family. Neurology (Minneapolis) *38*:1065, 1988.

58. Oppenheimer, D.R.: Brain lesions in Friedreich's ataxia. Can. J. Neurol. Sci. *6*:173, 1979.

59. Bird, T.D. and Shaw, C.M.: Progressive myoclonus and epilepsy with dentatorubral degeneration: a clinico-pathological study of the Ramsay Hunt syndrome. J. Neurol. Neurosurg. Psychiat. *41*:140, 1978.

60. Hunt, J.R.: Dyssynergia cerebellaris myoclonica—primary atrophy of the dentate system: A contribution to the pathology and symptomatology of the cerebellum. Brain *44*:490, 1921.

61. Gilbert, G.J.: Dyssynergia cerebellaris myoclonica. In: *Handbook of Clinical Neurology* (Eds.) Vinken, P.J., Bruyn, G.W. and DeJong, J.M.B.V., vol. 21, New York, American Elsevier, pp. 509–518, 1975.

62. Nakano, K.K., Dawson, D.M. and Spence, A.: Machado disease. A hereditary ataxia in Portuguese emigrants to Massachusetts. Neurology (Minneapolis) *22*:49, 1972.

63. Rosenberg, R.N., Nyhan, W.L., Coutinho, P. et al.: Joseph's disease: An autosomal dominant neurological disease in the Portuguese of the United States and the Azores Islands. Adv. Neurol. *21*:33, 1978.

64. Lima, L. and Coutinho, P.: Clinical criteria for diagnosis of Machado-Joseph disease: Report of a non-Azorean Portuguese family. Neurology (Minneapolis) *30*:319, 1980.

65. Barbeau, A., Roy, M., Cunha, L. et al.: The natural history of Machado-Joseph disease. An analysis of 138 personally examined cases. Canad. J. Neurol. Sci. *11*:510, 1984.

66. Woods, B.T. and Schaumburg, H.H.: Nigro-spino-dentatal degeneration with nuclear ophthalmoplegia. A unique and partially treatable clinicopathological entity. J. Neurol. Sci. *17*:149, 1972.

67. Romanul, F.C.A., Fowler, H.L., Radvany, J., et al.: Azorean disease of the nervous system. N. Engl. J. Med. *296*:1505, 1977.

68. Rosenberg, R.N., Nyhan, W.L., Bay, C. et al.: Autosomal dominant striatonigral degeneration. A clinical, pathologic, and biochemical study of a new genetic disorder. Neurology (Minneapolis) *26*:703, 1976.

69. Healton, E.B., Brust, J.C.M., Kerr, D.L., et al.: Presumably Azorean disease in a presumably non-Portuguese family. Neurology (Minneapolis) *30*:1084, 1980.

70. Cooper, J.A., Nakada, T., Knight, R.T. et al.: Autosomal dominant motor system degeneration in a black family. Ann. Neurol. *14*:585, 1983.

71. Sakai, T., Ohta, M. and Ishino, H.: Joseph disease in a non-Portuguese family. Neurology (Minneapolis) *33*:74, 1983.

72. Kitamura, J., Kubuki, Y., Tsuruta, K., et al.: A new family with Joseph disease in Japan. Homovanillic acid, magnetic resonance, and sleep apnea studies. Arch. Neurol. *46*:425, 1989.

73. Coutinho, P. and Andrade, C.: Autosomal dominant system degeneration in Portuguese families of the Azores Islands. A new genetic disorder involving cerebellar, pyramidal, extrapyramidal and spinal cord motor functions. Neurology (Minneapolis) 28:703, 1978.

74. Woods, B.T. and Schaumburg, H.H.: Nigrospinodentatal degeneration with nuclear ophthalmoplegia. In: *Handbook of Clinical Neurology* (Eds.) Vinken, P.J., Bruyn, G.W. and DeJong, J.M.B.V., vol. 22, New York, American Elsevier, 1975, pp. 157–176.

75. Sachdev, H.S., Forno, L.S. and Kane, C.A.: Joseph disease: A multisystem degenerative disorder of the nervous system. Neurology (Minneapolis) 32:192, 1982.

76. Goto, I., Tobimatsu, S., Ohta, M., et al.: Dentatorubropallidoluysian degeneration: Clinical, neuro-ophthalmologic, biochemical, and pathologic studies on autosomal dominant form. Neurology (Minneapolis) 32:1395, 1982.

6

Motor System Degenerations

RONALD C. KIM and
JOO HO SUNG

The motor system includes the giant pyramidal (Betz) cells of the motor cortex (upper motor neurons) and the motor neurons of the spinal anterior horns and brain stem motor nuclei (lower motor neurons) and their associated fiber tracts. It is affected in a variety of sporadic or familial degenerative disorders of the central nervous system. In one group of disorders motor neurons are selectively affected, while in others they are affected together with other neuronal systems. Disorders with selective motor system degeneration include amyotrophic lateral sclerosis, spinal and bulbar muscular atrophy, and primary lateral sclerosis, which are traditionally grouped together under the heading of motor neuron disease (MND). No specific etiology has been established for any form of MND and it is, therefore, uncertain as to whether these disorders represent the same condition, with genetic, clinical, and pathologic variations, or separate and distinct disease entities. Guamanian amyotrophic lateral sclerosis is a unique form

of MND. Other varieties of MND include familial amyotrophic lateral sclerosis, Strümpell's familial spastic paraplegia and certain types of multiple system degeneration. Among the latter, involvement of the motor system predominates clinically over that of other systems in some forms, whereas signs and symptoms of motor dysfunction are less striking and become manifest later in the course of illness in others.

AMYOTROPHIC LATERAL SCLEROSIS (ALS)

The classical or sporadic form of ALS is a disease of the upper and lower motor neuron systems that typically becomes manifest in middle or late life and affects men more commonly than women. Onset of illness is usually heralded by steadily progressive weakness and muscle atrophy, especially of the hands, reflecting cervical spinal cord involvement. Muscle fasciculations are often seen. Hyperactive reflexes and Babinski responses appear almost invariably at some stage of illness, but may be preempted as signs of lower motor neuron dysfunction become predominant. Bulbar signs, notably those of hypoglossal nucleus involvement, may be encountered. Objective signs of sensory dysfunction are notably lacking. Ultimately, there may be complete paralysis of the limbs and, if there is bulbar involvement, the patient may progress to a "locked-in" state, with inability to swallow or breathe. The course is typically one of relentless progression to death within 5 years or so, although wide variations in length of survival have been observed. In most instances the disease is fairly symmetrical, but the rate of development may differ on the two sides.

Grossly visible alterations within the CNS are usually fairly subtle. The external surface of the brain is occasionally characterized by atrophy that is limited to the precentral gyrus (motor cortex). In coronal section there may rarely be evidence of softening or sclerosis of those portions of the white matter (e.g., the posterior limb of the internal capsule) through which the pyramidal or corticospinal tract fibers pass. In such instances there may also be shrinkage and sclerosis of the corresponding

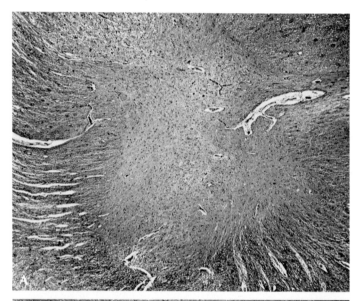

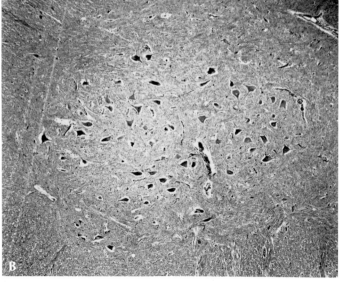

Fig. 6–1. Third lumbar spinal anterior horn. Note the severe neuronal loss and astrogliosis in ALS (A) as compared to the normal population of anterior horn cells in an unaffected subject (B). Hematoxylin-eosin stain; ×50.

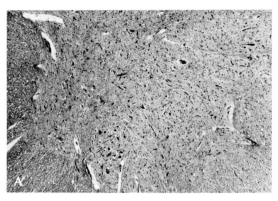
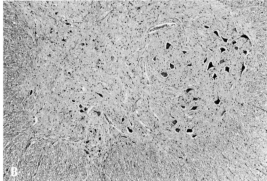

Fig. 6–2. Second sacral anterior horn. Note the severe loss of motor neurons and good preservation of Onuf's nucleus in ALS (A) as compared to that of an unaffected individual (B). Hematoxylin-eosin stain; ×50.

portions of the cerebral peduncles, basis pontis, and medullary pyramids. These alterations extend into the spinal cord, where the lateral corticospinal tracts are situated. With advanced disease the ventral spinal roots are notably thinned in contrast to the well-preserved dorsal spinal roots. Generalized muscle atrophy is usually striking.

Microscopically, the hallmarks of the disease are loss of lower motor neurons, particularly within the spinal anterior horns and the hypoglossal nuclei, and degeneration of the corticospinal tracts. Within the spinal cord, such nerve cell loss is most readily appreciated at the cervical and lumbar enlargements (Fig. 6–1), and has been shown to affect large motor neurons selectively.[1,2] Not all spinal levels are equally severely involved.[3] The intermediolateral horn cells (preganglionic autonomic neurons) in the thoracic segments are generally spared. In the sacral cord, neurons of Onuf's nucleus (which is believed to innervate the striated musculature of the vesical and rectal sphincters) are also spared (Fig. 6–2).[4–7] Cell loss tends to be focal and asymmetrical during the earlier stages,[8] and is regularly accompanied by a proliferation of hypertrophied astrocytes. The rate of progression of the pathologic process may show considerable variation from one case to the next. Although the manner in which the cells degenerate is not well defined, the process has been described as one of simple atrophy and pigmentary degeneration (lipofuscinosis). With rapid progression, neuronophagia may be observed. Central chrom-

atolysis, however, is seldom if ever encountered.[3,9] Immunocytochemically, an abnormal (excessive) accumulation of phosphorylated neurofilaments has been demonstrated within neuronal perikarya.[10,11] In those subjects with a relatively short clinical course and in whom the loss of nerve cells is not complete, axonal or dendritic swellings (spheroids) filled with 10 nm filaments can be identified in up to 60% of cases in silver-stained sections.[12–15] In some instances, residual neurons are seen to contain eosinophilic intracytoplasmic inclusions (Bunina bodies) (Fig. 6–3). These structures, which are not specific for ALS, are distributed predominantly within motor neurons, although they may also be seen at other sites.[16] Ultrastructurally, their appearance is somewhat variable, although they typically contain an

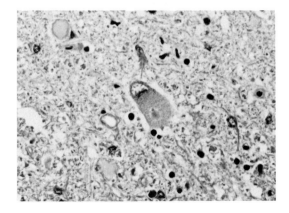

Fig. 6–3. Anterior horn cell with a rounded cytoplasmic inclusion (Bunina) body in ALS. Hematoxylin-eosin stain; ×480.

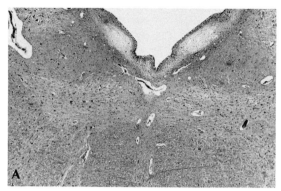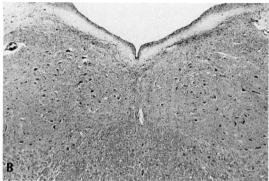

Fig. 6–4.   Hypoglossal nuclei. Note the severe neuronal loss and atrophy in ALS (A) as compared to the intact neurons in an unaffected individual (B). Hematoxylin-eosin stain; ×50.

admixture of filaments and other organelles or organelle fragments.[17] The significance of these bodies is uncertain at the present time.

Within the brain stem, the hypoglossal nucleus (Fig. 6–4) is affected most often, followed, in descending order of frequency, by the nucleus ambiguus, the motor nucleus of the trigeminal nerve and the facial nerve nucleus.[18] Those nuclei that are responsible for the regulation of eye movements are selectively spared, although, on at least one occasion, clinical ophthalmoplegia with nerve cell loss within the oculomotor, trochlear, and abducens nerve nuclei has been described.[19]

Morphometric studies have shown that, within the ventral spinal and cranial nerve roots, there is a selective reduction in the number of large myelinated axons and a decrease in transverse fascicular area.[2,20–25] An identical pattern of nerve fiber loss has been described in the peripheral nervous system, including the phrenic nerve.[26]

The morphologic alterations observed in skeletal muscle are those of neurogenic atrophy, and may be characterized by small or large group atrophy, fiber type grouping, fiber hypertrophy, fiber splitting or target-fiber formation. Muscle biopsy, in conjunction with electrophysiologic findings, is often used either to confirm the diagnosis of lower motor neuron disease or to provide an indication of its severity, although the prognosis cannot be judged on the basis of biopsy findings alone.[27,28]

In typical cases of ALS there is obvious morphologic evidence of upper motor neuron dis-

ease, although the extent of such involvement may show considerable variation. Loss of myelinated axons is particularly striking within the lateral corticospinal tracts (Fig. 6–5), with frequent involvement of the uncrossed ventral pyramidal tract fibers as well. This is accompanied by a variably intense proliferation of lipid-laden macrophages and reactive astrocytes. Fiber loss, which is frequently asymmetrical in the earlier stages of illness,[29] is seen to best advantage in sections stained either for myelin or with the Marchi method for degenerating myelin.[30,31] The tendency for damage to predominate distally has given rise to the notion of a proximally progressing, "dying-back" type of pathologic process.[32] Quantitative studies have shown that the large myelinated fibers appear to be affected preferentially.[33]

As seen in myelin-stained preparations, corticospinal tract involvement may extend upward into the medullary pyramids, the basis pontis, the cerebral peduncles, the posterior limb of the internal capsule, or the corona radiata. The large pyramidal (Betz) cells within the primary motor cortex are said to be affected in the majority of instances, even when there is relatively little loss of myelinated fibers within the corticospinal tracts.[3,34] Whether or not these cells are lost, however, is difficult to judge with certainty, as it is possible that they have undergone shrinkage, rendering them indistinguishable from other pyramidal neurons. A variety of degenerative changes have been described, including intracytoplasmic lipopigment accumulation, central chromatolysis and, using the Golgi impregnation technique, striking alterations in the dendritic arbor.[35,36] There is also an interesting recent account of a distinctive pattern of clustering of GFAP-immunoreactive astroglial cells, presumably in response to loss of nerve cells.[37]

Although ALS is generally thought of as being a purely motor system disorder, there is some pathologic evidence to suggest that other parts of the nervous system may also be affected. Averback and Crocker,[38] for example, claim that there is frequently a significant loss of neurons within the nucleus dorsalis of Clarke, a finding that would be consistent with the loss of myelinated fibers that has occasionally been described within the spinocerebellar tracts.[18,29,39,40] Other ascending and descending tracts, such as the vestibulospinal, rubrospinal, and spinothalamic tracts, are also said to be affected at times.[18,40] Interestingly, despite the lack of sensory signs and symptoms in ALS, Kawamura et al.[2] have described a significant loss of nerve cells in the L5 dorsal root ganglion and a loss of large dorsal root axons. In addition, Dyck et al.[41] and Bradley et al.[26] have reported a loss of myelinated fibers in the peroneal and sural nerves, respectively. Intracranially, Brownell et al.[3] found evidence of nerve cell loss within the thalamus (particularly the ventral nuclear complex), striatum, globus pallidus, and subthalamic nucleus in some of their cases. Discrete bundles of degenerating fibers have also been identified in Marchi preparations of the corpus callosum.[3,30,31]

The etiology of ALS has not been determined, although a number of possible contributing factors have been suggested. A detailed account is beyond the scope of this discussion, but is provided in several comprehensive reviews.[42,43] Only a few of the possibilities will be highlighted here.

Gowers[44] promoted the concept of abiotrophy or premature aging as an important factor in the development, not only of ALS, but of other neurologic disorders as well. In keeping with this idea, it has been shown that there is a progressive reduction in the number of spinal anterior horn cells and motor units with increasing age.[45,46] Calne et al.[47] have suggested that motor neuron disease may be the result of an abiotrophic interaction between aging and the environment, in which subclinical injury sustained earlier in life (e.g., viral infection or an exogenous toxin) predisposes the aging individual to the development of clinical disease.

Among the exogenous toxins that have been considered as being of possible etiologic sig-

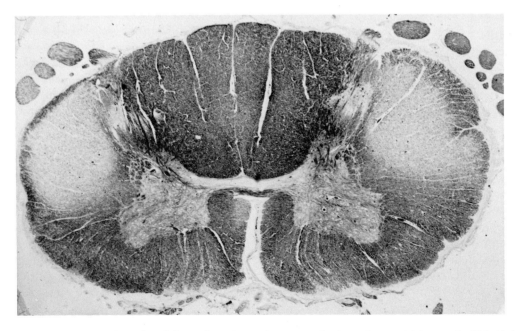

Fig. 6–5. Cervical spinal cord with loss of myelinated axons in the lateral pyramidal tracts in ALS. Mahon stain; ×12.

nificance, heavy metals have received the most attention. Lead and mercury intoxication, in particular, are said to be capable of giving rise to a clinical syndrome that closely resembles motor neuron disease.[48-52] The frequency with which a history of exposure to lead is obtained among patients with ALS is significantly higher than that of the general population.[53,54] Elevated blood levels of lead have also been documented in subjects with ALS.[55,56] The relevance of these findings to the pathogenesis of the disease, however, remains in question.

Several groups of investigators have detected a significant increase in the frequency with which a history of prior traumatic injury to the spine was elicited, relative to controls.[57,58]

Among the possible infectious causes, more has been written of the strong clinical resemblance between ALS and the progressive muscle weakness that may develop years after an episode of acute anterior poliomyelitis.[59,60] Poskanzer et al.[61] elicited a prior history of polio in a significantly higher proportion of ALS patients than among controls. The absence of clinical or pathologic evidence of upper motor neuron involvement, however, has led most investigators to question the possibility of an etiologic relationship between the two disorders.

According to an interesting hypothesis proposed by Weiner,[62] loss of motor neurons in ALS may be a consequence of loss of androgen receptors. Androgen receptors have been demonstrated, in laboratory animals, on nerve cells within the hypoglossal, glossopharyngeal, facial, and trigeminal nerve nuclei and within the spinal anterior horns; in contrast, they are sparsely distributed on nerve cells within the oculomotor, trochlear and abducens nerve nuclei, sites that are typically spared in ALS.[63] Experimentally, it has been shown repeatedly that androgen depletion will adversely affect the morphology of adult mammalian CNS neurons.[64,65] On the basis of these observations, and taking into account the preponderance of males among those afflicted with ALS (except in the postmenopausal period, during which the sex incidence appears roughly to be equal), Weiner has suggested that the age-related reduction of testosterone levels, in combination with a loss of androgen receptors,

may be of importance in the pathogenesis of the disease.

SPINAL (AND BULBAR) MUSCULAR ATROPHY (SMA) OF ADULT ONSET

Spinal muscular atrophy with onset in infancy (Werdnig-Hoffmann disease) or in childhood or adolescence (Kugelberg-Welander syndrome) is well established.[66,67] There has, however, been considerable nosologic confusion regarding SMA of adult onset. The confusion stems from its clinical similarity to SMA of juvenile onset on the one hand, and ALS without evidence of pyramidal tract involvement on the other. The main clinical feature is slowly progressive proximal limb weakness, often affecting bulbar muscles, but without pyramidal tract signs. The disease, which usually begins after the third decade of life,[66] is slowly progressive, but, although it is incapacitating, life expectancy is often not shortened. Adult-onset SMA accounts for 5 to 20% of cases in most large series of cases of motor neuron disease.[3,18,34] The majority are hereditary, although the pattern of inheritance may be autosomal recessive,[67] autosomal dominant[68] or X-linked recessive.[69-71] The main pathologic feature is degeneration and loss of neurons from the spinal anterior horns (Fig. 6–6) and often from the bulbar motor nuclei as well, much as in ALS. There is, however, no evidence of pyramidal tract degeneration, even though the course of illness may be quite protracted (Fig. 6–7). It is presently unclear whether or not SMA of adult onset and SMA of infantile or juvenile onset represent variations of a single disease entity.

PRIMARY LATERAL SCLEROSIS

Several published reports have appeared recently of pathologically documented cases that fulfill the criteria for the diagnosis of *primary lateral sclerosis*, namely, loss of myelinated fibers within the corticospinal tracts without evidence of loss of cranial nerve motor neurons or spinal anterior horn cells.[72-74] Younger et al. believe that the condition represents a syndrome the diagnosis of which is possible during life, provided that a careful clinical inves-

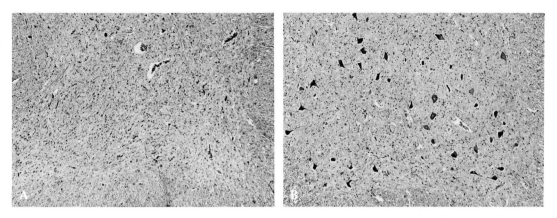

Fig. 6-6. Lumbar spinal anterior horn. Nearly complete loss of motor neurons in SMA (A) as compared to the normal population of motor neurons in an unaffected individual (B). Hematoxylin-eosin stain; ×50.

tigation is undertaken to rule out other possible causes.

AMYOTROPHIC LATERAL SCLEROSIS IN GUAM

A peculiar form of motor neuron disease has been recognized for nearly a century among the indigenous Chamorro population on the island of Guam.[75] This disorder, when first studied intensively, was observed with extraordinarily high frequency, and, together with the parkinsonism-dementia complex, was at one time responsible for nearby 25% of deaths among adult Chamorros.[76] Although few subjects with motor neuron disease developed signs and symptoms of the parkinsonism-dementia complex, some 15% of those with parkinsonism-dementia showed evidence of lower motor neuron disease during the course of illness, and it is currently believed that the two conditions represent different parts of the spectrum of the same disease. Clinically, motor neuron disease on Guam is indistinguishable from the classical form of ALS, although the mean age of onset is slightly earlier. The mean duration of illness from onset to death is about 4 to 6 years.

Neuropathologically, there is a loss of motor neurons from the spinal anterior horns and the hypoglossal nuclei, together with a loss of myelinated axons within the pyramidal tracts. In addition, however, there is widespread neurofibrillary degeneration within the cerebral cortex (especially the orbital gyri), hippocampus (especially Sommer's sector and the subiculum), hypothalamus, basal ganglia (especially the amygdala), substantia nigra, locus ceruleus, brain stem reticular formation, cranial nerve nuclei and cerebellar dentate nucleus, and, occasionally, within residual spinal anterior horn cells.[76,77]

Efforts to establish the etiology of the disease proved fruitless for many years. Despite the familial clustering of cases, no definite pattern of inheritance was evident. The sharply declining incidence of the disease in Guam in recent years[78] and the high frequency among Chamorros who had emigrated earlier[79] have strongly suggested the importance of environmental factors in the causation of the disorder. Spencer et al.[80] have recently produced signs of motor neuron, extrapyramidal and behavioral dysfunction in cynomolgus monkeys by feeding them β-N-methylamino-L-alanine (L-BMAA), a nonprotein amino acid derivative of the seed of the false sago palm, *Cycas circinalis.* (The cycad seed was once a major source of carbohydrate for the Chamorro population.) Pathologically, there was evidence of damage to the perikarya of Betz cells and large spinal anterior horn cells and to the neurites of cells within the pars compacta of the substantia nigra. These authors have suggested, on the basis of these observations, that cycad ingestion may be the environmental agent responsible for the development of motor neuron disease, not only on Guam, but at other sites in the western Pacific, including the Kepi region of New Guinea[81] and the Kii peninsula in

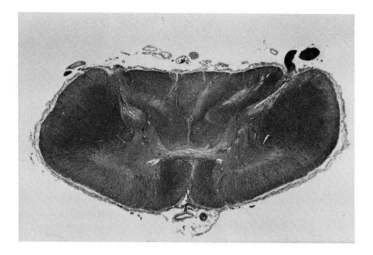

Fig. 6–7. Cervical spinal cord. Preservation of lateral pyramidal tracts in a 59-year-old man with SMA for more than 12 years. Luxol fast blue-PAS stain; ×9.

southern Japan.[82] In a more general sense, these findings also provide support for the notion that other forms of motor neuron disease, such as the classical form of ALS, may also be environmentally induced.

FAMILIAL AMYOTROPHIC LATERAL SCLEROSIS

It has been estimated that some 5 to 10% of cases of ALS are familial. Familial ALS, which is the most clearly defined form of familial motor neuron disease, is clinically indistinguishable from classic ALS.[83–88] Mulder et al.[87] have suggested, however, on the basis of an extensive review of the Mayo Clinic experience, that onset of illness tends to be slightly earlier, male-to-female ratio closer to unity and survival somewhat shorter. The disorder is transmitted in autosomal dominant fashion. Pathologically two groups of familial ALS have been described.[89] In one group, pathologic changes are limited to the spinal anterior horn and brain stem motor nuclei and pyramidal tracts, as in the sporadic form. In the other, pathologic changes affect not only the lower and upper neurons, but also the dorsal columns and spinocerebellar system.[84,85,90] Unlike sporadic ALS, however, both large and small lower motor neurons are affected, and some of those that remain are distended by hyaline intracytoplasmic inclusion bodies[85,91] that may be surrounded by peripheral "haloes" in such a manner as to impart a resemblance to the Lewy inclusion bodies of Parkinson's disease (Fig. 6–8). Also frequent is central chromatol-

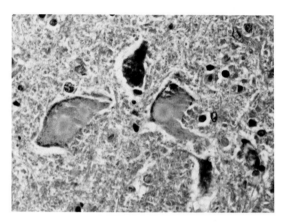

Fig. 6–8. Hypoglossal nucleus in familial ALS. Two nerve cells harboring hyaline cytoplasmic inclusions. Hematoxylin-eosin stain; ×480.

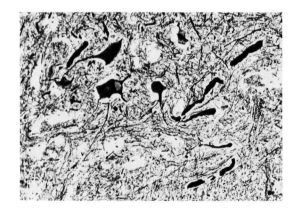

Fig. 6–9. Lumbar anterior horn with swollen axons in familial ALS. Bielschowsky's silver stain; × 120.

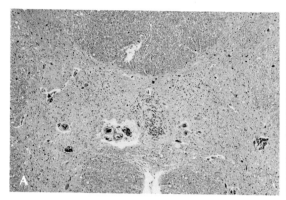
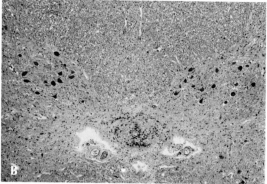

Fig. 6–10. Spinal cord (T11) showing severe neuronal loss in the dorsal nuclei of Clarke in familial ALS (A) as compared with normal nuclei in an unaffected subject (B). Hematoxylin-eosin stain; ×50.

ysis and frequent axonal swelling of spinal motor neurons (Fig. 6–9). In the more common form, there is a severe nerve cell loss within the nucleus dorsalis of Clarke (Fig. 6–10), with a corresponding loss of myelinated fibers within the dorsal spinocerebellar tracts. Another characteristic finding is loss of myelinated fibers within the middle-root zones of the dorsal columns. The relationship between the familial and classical forms of ALS is unclear at the present time.

STRÜMPELL'S FAMILIAL SPASTIC PARAPLEGIA

This is a rare hereditary disorder characterized clinically by slowly progressive spastic weakness affecting predominantly the lower extremities.[92] Impairment of deep sensation and spastic paresis of the upper extremities occur late in the course. Cerebellar signs, amyotrophy, and mental retardation are not observed in typical cases. Affected patients often live a normal life span in spite of progressively worsening disability. This disorder is inherited as an autosomal dominant trait in most and in autosomal recessive fashion in few affected families.[93,94] Two clinical forms have been suggested on the basis of onset before or after the age of 35 years.[93]

There have only been a few detailed autopsy studies.[92,95] Pathologically, there is bilateral degeneration of the pyramidal tracts and of the gracile fasciculi that is more pronounced distally (Fig. 6–11), suggesting a "dying back" process affecting long tract axons. Betz cells,

Fig. 6–11. Thoracic spinal cord in familial spastic paraplegia showing degeneration of the lateral pyramidal and gracile tracts but preservation of Clarke's cell columns and ventral horns. Luxol fast blue-PAS stain; ×14.

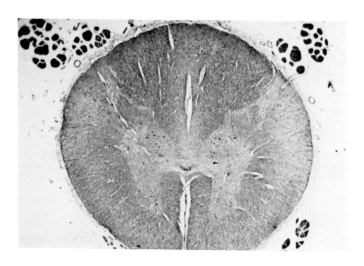

anterior horn cells, Clarke's cell columns or spinocerebellar tracts may also be involved.

MND ASSOCIATED WITH OTHER SYSTEM DEGENERATIONS

Lower and/or upper motor neurons may be affected to varying degrees in other system degenerations. Motor dysfunction may, however, be mild and delayed or overshadowed by involvement of other systems. Such conditions include olivopontocerebellar atrophy[96,97] and/or striatonigral degeneration,[98,99] Machado-Joseph disease,[100–102] pallido-luyso-nigral atrophy,[103,104] hereditary dentatorubral-pallidoluysian atrophy,[105] and possibly other disorders as well.[86,106,107]

REFERENCES

1. Tsukagoshi, H., Yanagisawa, N., Oguchi, K., et al.: Morphometric quantification of the cervical limb motor cells in controls and in amyotrophic lateral sclerosis. J. Neurol. Sci. 41:287, 1979.
2. Kawamura, Y., Dyck, P.J., Shimono, M., et al.: Morphometric comparison of the vulnerability of peripheral motor and sensory neurons in amyotrophic lateral sclerosis. J. Neuropath. Exp. Neurol. 40:667, 1981.
3. Brownell, B., Oppenheimer, D.R. and Hughes, J.T.: The central nervous system in motor neurone disease. J. Neurol. Neurosurg. Psychiat. 33:338, 1970.
4. Mannen, T., Iwata, M., Toyokura, Y., et al.: Preservation of a certain motoneurone group of the sacral cord in amyotrophic lateral sclerosis: its clinical significance. J. Neurol. Neurosurg. Psychiat. 40:464, 1977.
5. Sung, J.H.: Autonomic neurons of the sacral spinal cord in amyotrophic lateral sclerosis, anterior poliomyelitis and "neuronal intranuclear hyaline inclusion disease": Distribution of sacral autonomic neurons. Acta Neuropathologica (Berlin) 56:233, 1982.
6. Konno, H., Yamamoto, T., Iwasaki, Y. et al.: Shy-Drager syndrome and amyotrophic lateral sclerosis. Cytoarchitectonic and morphometric studies of sacral autonomic neurons. J. Neurol. Sci. 73:193, 1986.
7. Gibson, S.J., Polak, J.M., Katagiri, T., et al.: A comparison of the distributions of eight peptides in spinal cord from normal controls and cases of motor neurone disease with special reference to Onuf's nucleus. Brain Res. 474:255, 1988.
8. Swash, M., Leader, M., Brown, A. et al.: Focal loss of anterior horn cells in the cervical cord in motor neuron disease. Brain 109:939, 1986.
9. Sobue, G., Hashizume, Y., Sahashi, K., et al.: Amyotrophic lateral sclerosis. Lack of central chromatolytic response of motor neurocytons corresponding to active axonal degeneration. Arch. Neurol. 40:306, 1983.
10. Munoz, D.G., Greene, C., Perl, D.P. et al.: Accumulation of phosphorylated neurofilaments in anterior

11. Manetto, V., Sternberger, N.H., Perry, G., et al.: Phosphorylation of neurofilaments is altered in amyotrophic lateral sclerosis. J. Neuropath. Exp. Neurol. 47:642, 1988.
12. Carpenter, S.: Proximal axonal enlargement in motor neuron disease. Neurology (Minneapolis) 18:841, 1968.
13. Delisle, M.B. and Carpenter, S.: Neurofibrillary axonal swellings and amyotrophic lateral sclerosis. J. Neurol. Sci. 63:241, 1984.
14. Hirano, A., Donnenfeld, H., Sasaki, S. et al.: Fine structural observations of neurofilamentous changes in amyotrophic lateral sclerosis. J. Neuropath. Exp. Neurol. 43:461, 1984.
15. Sasaki, S., Kamei, H., Yamane, K. et al.: Swelling of neuronal processes in motor neuron disease. Neurology (Minneapolis) 38:1114, 1988.
16. Tomonaga, M.: Selective appearance of Bunina bodies in amyotrophic lateral sclerosis. A study of the distribution in midbrain and sacral cord. J. Neurol. 223:259, 1980.
17. Tomonaga, M., Saito, M., Yoshimura, M., et al.: Ultrastructure of the Bunina bodies in anterior horn cells of amyotrophic lateral sclerosis. Acta Neuropathologica (Berlin) 42:81, 1978.
18. Malamud, N.: Neuromuscular system disease. In: Pathology of the Nervous System (Ed.) Minckler, J., vol. 1, New York, McGraw-Hill, 1968, pp. 712–725.
19. Harvey, D.G., Torack, R.M. and Rosenbaum, H.E.: Amyotrophic lateral sclerosis with ophthalmoplegia. A clinicopathologic study. Arch. Neurol. 36:615, 1979.
20. Hanyu, N., Oguchi, K., Yanagisawa, N. et al.: Degeneration and regeneration of ventral root motor fibers in amyotrophic lateral sclerosis. Morphometric studies of cervical ventral roots. J. Neurol. Sci. 55:99, 1982.
21. Sobue, G., Matsuoka, Y., Mukai, E., et al.: Pathology of myelinated fibers in cervical and lumbar ventral spinal roots in amyotrophic lateral sclerosis. J. Neurol. Sci. 50:413, 1981a.
22. Sobue, G., Matsuoka, Y., Mukai, E., et al.: Spinal and cranial motor nerve roots in amyotrophic lateral sclerosis and X-linked recessive bulbospinal muscular atrophy: Morphometric and teased-fiber study. Acta Neuropathologica (Berlin) 55:227, 1981b.
23. Tandan, R. and Bradley, W.G.: Amyotrophic lateral sclerosis: Part 1. Clinical features, pathology, and ethical issues in management. Ann. Neurol. 18:271, 1985a.
24. Kondo, A., Nagara, H., Sato, Y., et al.: A morphometric study of myelinated fibers in lumbar ventral roots and hypoglossal nerves in motor neuron diseases. Clin. Neuropath. 5:217, 1986.
25. Atsumi, T. and Miyatake, T.: Morphometry of the degenerative process in the hypoglossal nerves in amyotrophic lateral sclerosis. Acta Neuropathologica (Berlin) 73:25, 1987.
26. Bradley, W.G., Good, P., Rasool, C.G. et al.: Morphometric and biochemical studies of peripheral nerves in amyotrophic lateral sclerosis. Ann. Neurol. 14:267, 1983.
27. Patten, B.M., Zito, G. and Harati, Y.: Histologic findings in motor neuron disease. Relation to clinically determined activity, duration, and severity of disease. Arch. Neurol. 36:560, 1979.
28. Froes, M.M.Q., Kristmundsdottir, F., Mahon, M. et

al.: Muscle morphometry in motor neuron disease. Neuropath. Appl. Neurobiol. *13*:405, 1987.

29. Swash, M., Scholtz, C.L., Vowles, G. et al.: Selective and asymmetric vulnerability of corticospinal and spinocerebellar tracts in motor neuron disease. J. Neurol. Neurosurg. Psychiat. *51*:785, 1988.

30. Smith, M.C.: Nerve fibre degeneration in the brain in amyotrophic lateral sclerosis. J. Neurol. Neurosurg. Psychiat. *23*:269, 1960.

31. Hughes, J.T.: Pathology of amyotrophic lateral sclerosis. Adv. Neurol. *36*:61, 1982.

32. Cavanagh, J.B.: The 'dying back' process. A common denominator in many naturally occurring and toxic neuropathies. Arch. Pathol. Lab. Med. *103*:659, 1979.

33. Sobue, G., Hashizume, Y., Mitsuma, T. et al.: Size-dependent myelinated fiber loss in the corticospinal tract in Shy-Drager syndrome and amyotrophic lateral sclerosis. Neurology (Minneapolis) *37*:529, 1987.

34. Lawyer, T., Jr. and Netsky, M.G. Amyotrophic lateral sclerosis. A clinicoanatomic study of fifty-three cases. Arch. Neurol. Psychiat. *69*:171, 1953.

35. Hammer, R.P., Jr., Tomiyasu, U. and Scheibel, A.B.: Degeneration of the human Betz cell due to amyotrophic lateral sclerosis. Exp. Neurol. *63*:336, 1979.

36. Udaka, F., Kameyama, M. and Tomonaga, M.: Degeneration of Betz cells in motor neuron disease. A Golgi study. Acta Neuropathologica (Berlin) *70*:289, 1986.

37. Kamo, H., Haebara, H., Akiguchi, I., et al.: A distinctive distribution of reactive astroglia in the precentral cortex in amyotrophic lateral sclerosis. Acta Neuropathologica (Berlin) *74*:33, 1987.

38. Averback, P. and Crocker, P.: Regular involvement of Clarke's nucleus in sporadic amyotrophic lateral sclerosis. Arch. Neurol. *39*:155, 1982.

39. Holmes, G.: The pathology of amyotrophic lateral sclerosis. Rev. Neurol. Psychiat. (Edinburgh) *7*:693, 1909.

40. Bonduelle, M.: Amyotrophic lateral sclerosis. In: *Handbook of Clinical Neurology* (Eds.) Vinken, P.J., Bruyn, G.W. and DeJong, J.M.B.V., vol. 22, New York, American Elsevier, 1975, pp. 281–338.

41. Dyck, P.J., Stevens, J.C., Mulder, D.W. et al: Frequency of nerve fiber degeneration of peripheral motor and sensory neurons in amyotrophic lateral sclerosis. Morphometry of deep and superficial peroneal nerves. Neurology (Minneapolis) *25*:781, 1975.

42. Tandan, R. and Bradley, W.G. Amyotrophic lateral sclerosis: Part 2. Etiopathogenesis. Ann. Neurol. *18*:419, 1985b.

43. Mitsumoto, H., Hanson, M.R. and Chad, D.A.: Amyotrophic lateral sclerosis. Recent advances in pathogenesis and therapeutic trials. Arch. Neurol. *45*:189, 1988.

44. Gowers, W.R.: A lecture on abiotrophy. Lancet *1*:1003, 1902.

45. McComas, A.J., Upton, A.R.M. and Sica, R.E.P.: Motoneurone disease and ageing. Lancet *2*:1477, 1973.

46. Tomlinson, B.E. and Irving, D.: The numbers of limb motor neurons in the human lumbosacral cord throughout life. J. Neurol. Sci. *34*:213, 1977.

47. Calne, D.B., Eisen, A., McGeer, E. et al.: Alzheimer's disease, Parkinson's disease, and motoneurone disease: Abiotropic interaction between ageing and environment? Lancet *2*:1067, 1986.

48. Boothby, J.A., deJesus, P.V. and Rowland, L.P.: Re-

versible forms of motor neuron disease. Arch. Neurol. *31*:18, 1974.

49. Barber, T.E.: Inorganic mercury intoxication reminiscent of amyotrophic lateral sclerosis. J. Occupat. Med. *20*:667, 1978.

50. Conradi, S., Ronnevi, L.-O. and Norris, F.H.: Motor neuron disease and toxic metals. Adv. Neurol. *36*:201, 1982.

51. Adams, C.R., Ziegler, D.K. and Lin, J.T.: Mercury intoxication simulating amyotrophic lateral sclerosis. JAMA *250*:642, 1983.

52. Mitchell, J.D.: Heavy metals and trace elements in amyotrophic lateral sclerosis. Neurol. Clin. *5*:43, 1987.

53. Campbell, A.M.G., Williams, E.R. and Barltrop, D.: Motor neurone disease and exposure to lead. J. Neurol. Neurosurg. Psychiat. *33*:877, 1970.

54. Felmus, M.T., Patten, B.M. and Swanke, L.: Antecedent events in amyotrophic lateral sclerosis. Neurology (Minneapolis) *26*:167, 1976.

55. Conradi, S., Ronnevi, L.-O., Nise, G. et al.: Abnormal distribution of lead in amyotrophic lateral sclerosis. Reestimation of lead in the cerebrospinal fluid. J. Neurol. Sci. *48*:413, 1980.

56. Ronnevi, L.-O., Conradi, S. and Nise, G.: Further studies on the erythrocyte uptake of lead in vitro in amyotrophic lateral sclerosis (ALS) patients and controls. Abnormal eythrocyte fragility in ALS. J. Neurol. Sci. *57*:143, 1982.

57. Murros, K. and Fogelholm, R.: Amyotrophic lateral sclerosis in Middle-Finland: an epidemiological study. Acta Neurologica Scandinavica *67*:41, 1983.

58. Gallagher, J.P. and Sanders, M.: Trauma and amyotrophic lateral sclerosis: A report of 78 patients. Acta Neurologica Scandinavica *75*:145, 1987.

59. Mulder, D.W., Rosenbaum, R.A. and Layton, D.D., Jr.: Late progression of poliomyelitis or forme fruste amyotrophic lateral sclerosis? Mayo Clin. Proceed. *47*:756, 1972.

60. Dalakas, M.C., Elder, G., Hallett, M., et al.: A long-term follow-up study of patients with post-poliomyelitis neuromuscular symptoms. N. Engl. J. Med. *314*:959, 1986.

61. Poskanzer, D.C., Cantor, H.M. and Kaplan, G.S. The frequency of preceding poliomyelitis in amyotrophic lateral sclerosis. In: *Motor Neuron Diseases: Research on Amyotrophic Lateral Sclerosis and Related Disorders* (Eds.) Norris, F.H., Jr. and Kurland, L.T., New York, Grune & Stratton, 1969, pp. 286–290.

62. Weiner, L.P. Possible role of androgen receptors in amyotrophic lateral sclerosis. A hypothesis. Arch. Neurol. *37*:129, 1980.

63. Sar, M. and Stumpf, W.E. Androgen concentration in motor neurons of cranial nerves and spinal cord. Science *197*:77, 1977.

64. DeVoogd, T.J.: Androgens can affect the morphology of mammalian CNS neurons in adulthood. Trends Neurosci. *10*:341, 1987.

65. Leedy, M.G., Beattie, M.S. and Bresnahan, J.C.: Testosterone-induced plasticity of synaptic inputs to adult mammalian motoneurons. Brain Res. *424*:386, 1987.

66. Emery, A.E.H.: The nosology of the spinal muscular atrophies. J. Med. Genet. *8*:481, 1971.

67. Pearn, J.H., Hudgson, P. and Walton, J.N.: A clinical and genetic study of spinal muscular atrophy of adult onset. The autosomal recessive form as a discrete disease entity. Brain *101*:591, 1978.

68. Jansen, P.H.P., Joosten, E.M.G., Jaspar, H.H.J., et al.:

A rapidly progressive autosomal dominant scapulo-humeral form of spinal muscular atrophy. Ann. Neurol. *20*:538, 1986.

69. Kennedy, W.R., Alter, M. and Sung, J.H.: Progressive proximal spinal and bulbar muscular atrophy of late onset. A sex-linked recessive trait. Neurology (Minneapolis) *18*:671, 1968.

70. Harding, A.E., Thomas, P.K., Baraitser, M., et al.: X-linked recessive bulbospinal neuronopathy: a report of ten cases. J. Neurol. Neurosurg. Psychiat. *45*:1012, 1982.

71. Barkhaus, P.E., Kennedy, W.R., Stern, L.Z. et al.: Hereditary proximal spinal and bulbar motor neuron disease of late onset. A report of six cases. Arch. Neurol. *39*:112, 1982.

72. Fisher, C.M.: Pure spastic paralysis of corticospinal origin. Canad. J. Neurol. Sci. *4*:251, 1977.

73. Beal, M.F. and Richardson, E.P., Jr.: Primary lateral sclerosis. A case report. Arch. Neurol. *38*:630, 1981.

74. Younger, D.S., Chou, S., Hays, A.P., et al.: Primary lateral sclerosis. A clinical diagnosis reemerges. Arch. Neurol. *45*:1304, 1988.

75. Hirano, A., Kurland, L.T., Krooth, R.S. et al.: Parkinsonism-dementia complex, an endemic disease on the island of Guam. I. Clinical features. Brain *84*:642, 1961a.

76. Kurland, L.T. and Brody, J.A.: Amyotrophic lateral sclerosis. Guam type. In: *Handbook of Clinical Neurology* (Eds.) Vinken, P.J., Bruyn, G.W. and DeJong, J.M.B.V., vol. 22, New York, American Elsevier, 1975, pp. 339–347.

77. Hirano, A., Malamud, N. and Kurland, L.T.: Parkinsonism-dementia complex, an endemic disease on the island of Guam. II. Pathological features. Brain *84*:662, 1961b.

78. Garruto, R.M., Yanagihara, R. and Gajdusek, D.C.: Disappearance of high-incidence amyotrophic lateral sclerosis and parkinsonism-dementia on Guam. Neurology (Minneapolis) *35*:193, 1985.

79. Garruto, R.M., Gajdusek, D.C. and Chen, K.-M.: Amyotrophic lateral sclerosis among Chamorro migrants from Guam. Ann. Neurol. *8*:612, 1980.

80. Spencer, P.S., Nunn, P.B., Hugon, J., et al.: Guam amyotrophic lateral sclerosis-parkinsonism-dementia linked to a plant excitant neurotoxin. Science *237*:517, 1987.

81. Gajdusek, D.C. and Salazar, A.M.: Amyotrophic lateral sclerosis and parkinsonian syndromes in high incidence among the Auyu and Jakai people of West New Guinea. Neurology (Minneapolis) *32*:107, 1982.

82. Shiraki, H. and Yase, Y. Amyotrophic lateral sclerosis in Japan. In: *Handbook of Clinical Neurology* (Eds.) Vinken, P.J., Bruyn, G.W. and DeJong, J.M.B.V., vol. 22, New York, American Elsevier, 1975, pp. 353–419.

83. Kurland, L.T. and Mulder, D.W.: Epidemiologic investigations of amyotrophic lateral sclerosis. 2. Familial aggregations indicative of dominant inheritance. Neurology (Minneapolis) *5*:182, 1955 (Part I) and 249 (Part II).

84. Engel, W.K., Kurland, L.T. and Klatzo, I.: An inherited disease similar to amyotrophic lateral sclerosis with a pattern of posterior column involvement. An intermediate form? Brain *82*:203, 1959.

85. Hirano, A., Kurland, L.T. and Sayre, G.P.: Familial amyotrophic lateral sclerosis. A subgroup characterized by posterior and spinocerebellar tract involvement and hyaline inclusions in the anterior horn cells. Arch. Neurol. *16*:232, 1967.

86. Hudson, A.J. Amyotrophic lateral sclerosis and its association with dementia, parkinsonism and other neurological disorders: A review, Brain *104*:217, 1981.

87. Mulder, D.W., Kurland, L.T., Offord, K.P. et al.: Familial adult motor neuron disease: Amyotrophic lateral sclerosis. Neurology (Minneapolis) *36*:511, 1986.

88. Kato, T., Hirano, A. and Kurland, L.T.: Asymmetric involvement of the spinal cord involving both large and small anterior horn cells in a case of familial amyotrophic lateral sclerosis. Clin. Neuropath. *6*:67, 1987.

89. Horton, W.A., Eldridge, R. and Brody, J.A.: Familial motor neuron disease. Evidence for at least three different types. Neurology (Minneapolis) *26*:460, 1976.

90. Tanaka, J., Nakamura, H., Tabuchi, Y. et al.: Familial amyotrophic lateral sclerosis: Features of multisystem degeneration. Acta Neuropathologica (Berlin) *64*:22, 1984.

91. Takahashi, K., Nakamura, H. and Okada E.: Hereditary amyotrophic lateral sclerosis. Histochemical and electron microscopic study of hyaline inclusions in motor neurons. Arch. Neurol. *27*:292, 1972.

92. Behan, W.M.H. and Maia, M.: Strümpell's familial spastic paraplegia: genetics and neuropathology. J. Neurol. Neurosurg. Psychiat. *37*:8, 1974.

93. Harding, A.E.: Hereditary "pure" spastic paraplegia: a clinical and genetic study of 22 families. J. Neurol. Neurosurg. Psychiat. *44*:871, 1981.

94. Boustany, R.-M.N., Fleischnick, E., Alper, C.A., et al.: The autosomal dominant form of "pure" familial spastic paraplegia: Clinical findings and linkage analysis of a large pedigree. Neurology (Minneapolis) *37*:910, 1987.

95. Holmes, G.L. and Shaywitz, B.A.: Strümpell's pure familial spastic paraplegia: case study and review of the literature. J. Neurol. Neurosurg. Psychiat. *40*:1003, 1977.

96. Landis, D.M.D., Rosenberg, R.N., Landis, S.C., et al.: Olivopontocerebellar degeneration. Clinical and ultrastructural abnormalities. Arch. Neurol. *31*:295, 1974.

97. Berciano, J. Olivopontocerebellar atrophy. J. Neurol. Sci. *53*:253, 1982.

98. Takei, Y. and Mirra, S.S.: Striatonigral degeneration: A form of multiple system atrophy with clinical parkinsonism. In: *Progress in Neuropathology,* (Ed.) Zimmerman, H.M., vol. 2, New York, Grune & Stratton, 1973, pp. 217–251.

99. Sung, J.H., Mastri, A.R. and Segal, E.: Pathology of Shy-Drager syndrome. J. Neuropath. Exp. Neurol. *38*:353, 1979.

100. Nakano, K.K., Dawson, D.M. and Spence, A.: Machado disease. A hereditary ataxia in Portuguese emigrants to Massachusetts. Neurology (Minneapolis) *22*:49, 1972.

101. Rosenberg, R.N., Nyhan, W.L., Bay, C. et al.: Autosomal dominant striatonigral degeneration. A clinical, pathologic, and biochemical study of a new genetic disorder. Neurology (Minneapolis) *26*:703, 1976.

102. Sakai, T., Ohta, M. and Ishino, H.: Joseph disease in a non-Portuguese family. Neurology (Minneapolis) *33*:74, 1983.

103. Gray, F., De Baecque, C., Serdaru, M. et al.: Pallido-luyso-nigral atrophy and amyotrophic lateral sclerosis. Acta Neuropathologica (Berlin) Suppl. VII 348, 1981.

104. Gray, F., Eizenbaum, J.F., Gherardi, R., et al.: Luyso-

pallido-nigral atrophy and amyotrophic lateral sclerosis. Acta Neuropathologica (Berlin) *66*:78, 1985.

105. Takahashi, H., Ohama, E., Naito, H., et al.: Hereditary dentatorubral-pallidoluysian atrophy: Clinical and pathologic variants in a family. Neurology (Minneapolis) *38*:1065, 1988.

106. Frank, G., and Vuia, O.: Chorea Huntington-Amyotrophische Lateralsklerose-Spastische Spinalparalyse. Zur Kombination von Systemerkrankungen. Zeitschrift fur Neurologie *205*:207, 1973.

107. Rosenberg, R.N.: Amyotrophy in multisystem genetic diseases. In: *Advances in Neurology. Human Motor Neuron Diseases.* (Ed.) Rowland, L.P. vol. 36, New York, Raven Press, 1982, pp. 149–158.

CHAPTER 7

Huntington's Disease

RONALD C. KIM and
JOO HO SUNG

Huntington's disease is a relatively rare dementing disorder in which involuntary (choreiform) movements are a prominent feature. The condition is transmitted in autosomal dominant fashion, with nearly complete penetrance. Although its distribution is worldwide, circumstantial evidence suggests that the disease may have been exported from a locus in northwestern Europe by Dutch and English seafarers.[1]

Reports prior to the first complete clinical description[2] failed to distinguish between Huntington's disease and other forms of chorea. Onset of illness in the classic adult form typically occurs in the fourth decade although the range is wide, extending from infancy to extreme old age. What most commonly draws the patient's attention to the disease is the development of choreiform movements, often in association with characteristic grimacing movements of the face. The development of mental symptoms is usually heralded by the appearance of emotional disturbances, irrita-

bility, and personality changes that eventually progress to a state of apathy and frank dementia. At times the personality changes may precede the movement disorder. The course of illness is one of relentless progression, culminating in death within 15 years or so of onset, most often as a result of intercurrent cardiopulmonary disease. Two well recognized variants are the childhood form (which is characterized by tremor, rigidity, seizures, the absence of choreiform movements, and a more rapidly progressive course) and the rigid or akinetic form (which is characterized by clinical features and a rate of progression that is intermediate between those of the classic and childhood forms). Among the 25% or so in whom the disease is of late onset (after the age of 50) there is a preponderance of maternal transmission.[3,4] There is a suggestion that late-onset disease progresses more slowly than that which begins in middle adult life.[5]

Recently, using restriction endonucleases to analyze DNA polymorphisms in lymphoblastoid cell lines, researchers have identified a genetic linkage marker (D4S10) for Huntington's disease at the G8 locus on chromosome 4.[6,7] In addition to providing a basis for presymptomatic (and even prenatal) inheritance testing, this exciting development hopefully will lead to precise identification of the abnormal gene and its gene products.

Macroscopically, the brain usually looks normal externally although it is often small, weighing 1100 g or less after fixation. As seen in coronal section the degree of convolutional atrophy varies but can be considerable, particularly frontally and temporally, where thinning of the cortical ribbon may be associated with reductions in cortical volume of up to 20%.[8] More striking, especially in those subjects with advanced disease, is the presence of marked shrinkage and yellow-brown discoloration of the striatum (Fig. 7–1). This is most readily appreciated rostrally, where the medial border of the head of the caudate nucleus, which constitutes the ventrolateral margin of the lateral ventricle, is either concave or flat-

tened rather than convex, resulting in a corresponding degree of rostral ventricular enlargement. The configuration of the ventricle can be detected during life with the aid of imaging techniques such as computed tomography or magnetic resonance, and, when observed postmortem, is considered to be so characteristic that the diagnosis of Huntington's disease may be made with confidence on the basis of macroscopic appearances alone, although, on rare occasion, Pick's disease must also be considered in the differential diagnosis. Either the caudate nucleus or putamen may be preferentially affected, more commonly the former. The cerebral white matter is correspondingly reduced in bulk. Recently, Vonsattel et al.,[9] recognizing that the severity of the gross abnormalities might vary according to the rapidity of progression and duration of the illness, have, on the basis of examination of a large number of cases, proposed a grading system for the pathologic findings (see below). According to this system, brains showing grade 0 morphology would be grossly indistinguisha-

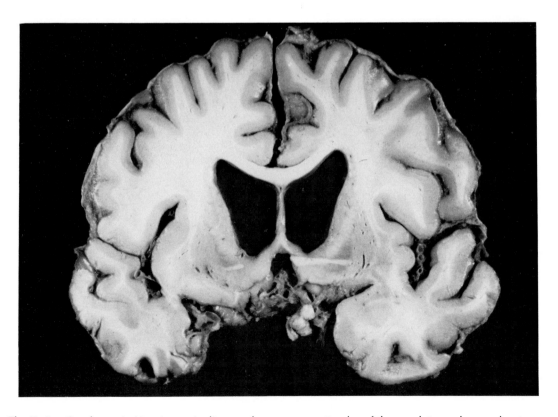

Fig. 7–1.   Cerebrum in Huntington's disease shows severe atrophy of the caudate nucleus and putamen, resulting in flattening of the caudate eminence of the ventricular surface.

ble from normal, whereas those showing grade 4 morphology would be characterized by severe atrophy of the caudate nucleus and putamen.

Microscopically, in the advanced stages of illness, the most dramatic finding, first described by Dunlap[10] and confirmed repeatedly since, is nerve cell loss and astrocytosis within the striatum (Fig. 7–2). Initially it was felt that the predominating population of small neurons was affected preferentially, with relative sparing of the larger nerve cells.[11,12] Although most observers have expressed the view that the caudate nucleus is more severely affected, a few have stated that the putamen is more heavily damaged. A recent detailed study by Vonsattel and colleagues[9] of 163 autopsied cases has led to the suggestion that the clinical and pathologic severity of Huntington's disease are closely correlated, and that they can be graded. The scale that they have proposed is as follows:

Grade 0: No discernible gross or microscopic abnormality, despite the presence of substantial clinical evidence of disease;

Grade 1: No discernible gross atrophy of the striatum, with moderate astrocytosis and only a subtle loss of nerve cells;

Grade 2: Grossly appreciable atrophy of the head of the caudate nucleus, with preservation of its medial convexity, and perceptible nerve cell loss and astrocytosis affecting the caudate more severely than the putamen;

Grade 3: Grossly apparent atrophy of the head of the caudate nucleus, with flattening of its medial border, and nerve cell loss that is severe within the caudate and moderate within the putamen;

Grade 4: Severe gross atrophy of the head of the caudate nucleus (with concavity of its medial border) and putamen, and, microscopically, severe nerve cell loss throughout both of these structures, together with slight to moderate astrocytosis within the nucleus accumbens.

Topographically, at least in the earlier stages of illness, the loss of nerve cells within the striatum is not uniform. Within the caudate nucleus, there appears to be a medial-to-lateral progression of nerve cell loss,[9,12] whereas, within the putamen, there is a dorsoventral gradient.[9,14,15]

Evidence is also accumulating to suggest that not all populations of striatal nerve cells are equally severely affected. Examination of Golgi-stained material has recently shown that, of the five or more neostriatal cell types that can be identified using this method,[16,17]

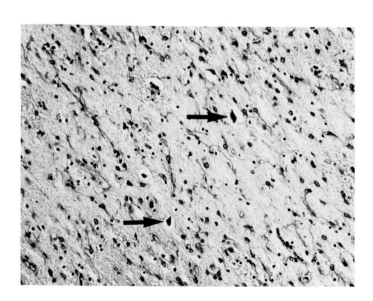

Fig. 7–2. Caudate nucleus in Huntington's disease shows severe nerve cell loss and astrocytosis, with a few persisting large neurons (arrows). Hematoxylin and eosin stain; × 270.

medium-sized spiny neurons, which are present in greatest abundance and which constitute a major source of striatal efferents, appear to be affected earliest and most severely in Huntington's disease.[18]

The chemoarchitecture of the mammalian neostriatum is such that it is a mosaic of two interdigitating compartments: (a) an acetylcholinesterase (AChE)-poor *patch compartment* that contains relatively high concentrations of opiate receptors, enkephalin, substance P and dynorphin and widely distributed, often discrete clusters of nerve cells that receive input from prelimbic cortex and project to the pars compacta of the substantia nigra, and (b) an intervening AChE-enriched *matrix compartment* that exhibits relatively high concentrations of nicotinamide adenine dinucleotide phosphate (NADPH) diaphorase, somatostatin (SS) and neuropeptide Y (NPY) activity and receives sensorimotor cortical input and projects to the pars reticularis of the substantia nigra.[19-21] In Huntington's disease it has been shown that, although the volume of the AChE-rich matrix zone is reduced, the large aspiny AChE-bearing neurons and the medium-sized aspiny neurons in which NADPH diaphorase, SS and NPY appear to be co-localized are selectively spared.[22-27] In contrast, although the volume of the AChE-poor patch zone is within the range of normal, the spiny GABA-, enkephalin-, substance P- and dynorphin-bearing neurons contained therein are all strikingly reduced in number.[24,28,29]

The results of neuropathologic evaluation of other parts of the nervous system have been more variable. The nucleus accumbens appears relatively to be spared, for reasons that are not understood.[9,26,30] Vonsattel et al. observed astrocytosis only in cases of grade 4 severity, and Bots and Bruyn described indentation of some of the neuronal nuclei (see below). Bruyn,[31] Gebbink,[32] Forno and Jose,[13] and Roos[33] among others, have described a loss of large neurons within the globus pallidus, particularly in the lateral pallidal segment, together with a reduction in the concentration of striatopallidal fibers. The findings in the thalamus have been inconstant, although Dom et al.[34] claim to have demonstrated a loss of small nerve cells within its ventrolateral portion. Bruyn[35] reported loss of nerve cells

within the supraoptic, ventromedial, and lateral nuclei of the hypothalamus. Lange et al.[12] described a 25% nerve cell loss within the subthalamic nucleus. In the pars reticularis of the substantia nigra, it has been stated that mild neuronal loss,[8,36] astrocytosis,[13] and loss of striatonigral fibers[32] can often be appreciated. Other sites within the brain stem, e.g., the superior and inferior olivary, lateral vestibular, dorsal vagal, and hypoglossal nuclei, may also be affected.[33,36] Although significant cerebellar involvement is seen in only a minority of cases, at times there may be striking loss of Purkinje cells[37,38] or dentate nucleus neurons;[31] the Purkinje cell loss is said to be more striking in (but not limited to) cases of earlier (juvenile) onset.[31,36] The cerebral cortex has proven to be more difficult to evaluate, although there seems to be general agreement that, particularly in those with severe dementia, there is a loss of nerve cells that preferentially affects specific layers, especially the third and less often the fifth and sixth.[13,31,33,36] Morphometric studies have shown a significant reduction in cross-sectional area not only of cerebral cortex, but of cerebral white matter, thalamus, and striatum.[39] The basis for the cerebral cortical abnormalities is unclear at the present time. One group of investigators has not been able to demonstrate either a reduction in cortical choline acetyltransferase activity or a loss of nerve cells from the nucleus basalis of Meynert.[40]

Electron microscopy of cerebral cortical and neostriatal tissue from subjects with Huntington's disease has demonstrated findings of a rather nonspecific nature, e.g., lipofuscin accumulation within neurons and glial cells and degeneration of presynaptic terminals.[41-43] Interestingly, Bots and Bruyn,[30] Roos et al.,[44] and Roos[33] have described the presence of neuronal nuclear membrane indentations within the nucleus accumbens, caudate nucleus, and frontal cortex, a finding that has so far not been observed in association with any other neurologic disorder. The significance of this finding, however, is unclear at the present time.

The results of biochemical investigations in Huntington's disease have been reviewed recently by Bird[45] and by Beal and Martin[46] and are in general agreement with the neuropathologic, histochemical and immunocytochemical findings already described. They will be summarized only briefly here. Most dramatic has been the demonstration of reduced levels of the neurotransmitter GABA[47] and of its synthesizing enzyme, glutamic acid decarboxylase (GAD).[48] Bird and Iversen[49,50] and McGeer and McGeer[51] have shown that GAD activity is decreased within the striatum, globus pallidus, and substantia nigra, but not within the cerebral cortex. They have also demonstrated significantly reduced levels of choline acetyltransferase activity within these same sites, although tyrosine hydroxylase activity is within the range of normal. Interestingly, neuroreceptor binding sites for GABA appear to be present in normal concentrations,[52,53] whereas those for acetylcholine are decreased within the striatum.[54,55] Cross and Rossor[56] found that type 1 dopamine receptors, as determined by 3H-piflutixol binding, were reduced in the striatum, globus pallidus and substantia nigra, whereas type 2 receptors, as determined by 3H-spiperone binding, were reduced in the putamen but normal in the substantia nigra. Taken together, the major biochemical findings as outlined above suggest that, in Huntington's disease, there is degeneration of the striatal GABA-containing interneurons and that, in contrast to Parkinson's disease, there is a relative deficiency of cholinergic as opposed to dopaminergic tone.[57]

Recently, attention has been directed toward the development of several possible experimental models of Huntington's disease. Intrastriatal injection of the neuroexcitatory amino acids kainic acid (a seaweed derivative), ibotenic acid (a mushroom toxin) or quinolinic acid (an endogenous tryptophan metabolite) has been shown to produce lesions that closely resemble those seen in Huntington's disease.[58-62] Of the three agents, however, only quinolinic acid destroys GABA- and substance P-containing neurons, while selectively sparing those bearing SS, NPY and NADPH diaphorase.[63-65] It thus appears that the quinolinic acid model most closely mimics the human disease. Quinolinic acid is believed to exert its effects upon the N-methyl-D-aspartate (NMDA) subgroup of glutamate receptors, and its neurotoxic effects can be blocked by NMDA receptor antagonists.[60] The recent

demonstration that striatal NMDA receptor binding is severely reduced in Huntington's disease[66] is of particular interest in this regard. What role if any is played by endogenous quinolinic acid in the pathogenesis of Huntington's disease, however, must await further studies.

REFERENCES

1. Bruyn, G.W. and Went, L.N.: Hungtington's chorea. In: Handbook of Clinical Neurology. Edited by P.J. Vinken, G.W. Bruyn, and H.L. Klawans. Amsterdam, North-Holland, 1986, vol. 49, pp. 267–313.
2. Huntington, G.: On chorea. Med. Surg. Reporter, Philadelphia, 26:317, 1872.
3. Myers, R.H., et al.: Maternal transmission in Huntington's disease. Lancet, 1:208, 1983.
4. Hall, J.G. and Te-Juatco, L.: Association between age of onset and parental inheritance in Huntington's chorea. Am. J. Med. Genet., 16:289, 1983.
5. Myers, R.H., et al.: Late onset of Huntington's disease. J. Neurol. Neurosurg. Psychiatry, 48:530, 1985.
6. Gusella, J.F., et al.: A polymorphic DNA marker genetically linked to Huntington's disease. Nature, 306:234, 1983.
7. Gilliam, T.C., Gusella, J.F. and Lehrach, H.: Molecular strategies to investigate Huntington's disease. Adv. Neurol., 48:17, 1988.
8. Bruyn, G.W., Bots, G.Th.A.M. and Dom, R.: Huntington's chorea: Current neuropathological status. Adv. Neurol., 23:83, 1979.
9. Vonsattel, J.-P., et al.: Neuropathological classification of Huntington's disease. J. Neuropathol. Exp. Neurol., 44:559, 1985.
10. Dunlap, C.B.: Pathologic changes in Huntington's chorea with special references to corpus striatum. Arch. Neurol. Psychiat. 18:867, 1927.
11. Dom, R., Baro, F. and Brucher, J.M.: A cytometric study of the putamen in different types of Huntington's chorea. Adv. Neurol. 1:369, 1973.
12. Lange, H., Thorner, G., Hope, A. et al.: Morphometric studies of the neuropathological changes in choreatic diseases. J. Neurol. Sci., 28:401, 1976.
13. Forno, L.S. and Jose, C.: Huntington's chorea: A pathological study. Adv. Neurol., 1:453, 1973.
14. McCaughey, W.T.E.: The pathologic spectrum of Huntington's chorea. J. Nerv. Ment. Dis., 133:91, 1961.
15. Roos, R.A.C., Pruyt, J.F.M., de Vries, J. et al.: Neuronal distribution in the putamen in Huntington's disease. J. Neurol. Neurosurg. Psychiat. 48:422, 1985.
16. DiFiglia, M., Pasik, P. and Pasik, T.: A Golgi study of neuronal types in the neostriatum of monkeys. Brain Res., 114:245, 1976.
17. Graveland, G.A., Williams, R.S. and DiFiglia, M.: A Golgi study of the human neostriatum: Neurons and afferent fibers. J. Comp. Neurol. 234:317, 1985.
18. Graveland, G.A., Williams, R.S. and DiFiglia, M.: Evidence for degenerative and regenerative changes in neostriatal spiny neurons in Huntington's disease. Science, 227:770, 1985.
19. Graybiel, A.M. and Ragsdale, C.W., Jr.: Biochemical anatomy of the striatum. In: Chemical Neuroanatomy. Edited by P.C. Emson. New York, Raven Press, 1983, pp. 427–504.
20. Gerfen, C.R.: The neostriatal mosaic: Compartmental-

ization of corticostriatal input and striatonigral output systems. Nature, *311*:461, 1984.

21. Gerfen, C.R.: The neostriatal mosaic. I. Compartmental organization of projections from the striatum to the substantia nigra in the rat. J. Comp. Neurol. *236*:454, 1985.

22. Ferrante, R.J., et al.: Selective sparing of a class of striatal neurons in Huntington's disease. Science, *230*:561, 1985.

23. Ferrante, R.J., et al.: Sparing of acetylcholinesterase-containing striatal neurons in Huntington's disease. Brain Res., *411*:162, 1987.

24. Ferrante, R.J., et al.: Morphologic and histochemical characteristics of a spared subset of striatal neurons in Huntington's disease. J. Neuropathol. Exp. Neurol. *46*:12, 1987.

25. Kowall, N.W., et al.: Neuropeptide Y, somatostatin, and reduced nicotinamide adenine dinucleotide phosphate diaphorase in the human striatum: A combined immunocytochemical and enzyme histochemical study. Neuroscience, *20*:817, 1987.

26. Kowall, N.W., Ferrante, R.J. and Martin, J.B.: Patterns of cell loss in Huntington's disease. Trends Neurosci., *10*:24, 1987.

27. Beal, M.F., et al.: Somatostatin and neuropeptide Y concentrations in pathologically graded cases of Huntington's disease. Ann. Neurol., *23*:562, 1988.

28. Martin, J.B.: Huntington's disease: New approaches to an old problem. Neurology, *34*:1059, 1984.

29. Ferrante, R.J., et al.: Topography of enkephalin, substance P and acetylcholinesterase staining in Huntington's disease striatum. Neurosci. Letters, *71*:283, 1986.

30. Bots, G.Th.A.M. and Bruyn, G.W.: Neuropathological changes of the nucleus accumbens in Huntington's chorea. Acta Neuropathol. (Berl.), *55*:21, 1981.

31. Bruyn, G.W.: Huntington's chorea: Historical, clinical and laboratory synopsis. In: *Handbook of Clinical Neurology.* Edited by P.J. Vinken and G.W. Bruyn. Amsterdam, North-Holland, 1968. vol. 6, pp. 298–378.

32. Gebbink, Th.B.: Huntington's chorea: Fibre changes in the basal ganglia. In: *Handbook of Clinical Neurology.* Edited by P.J. Vinken, and G.W. Bruyn. Amsterdam, North-Holland, 1968, vol. 6, pp. 399–408.

33. Roos, R.A.C.: Neuropathology of Huntington's chorea. In: *Handbook of Clinical Neurology.* Edited by P.J. Vinken, G.W. Bruyn, and H.L. Klawans. Amsterdam, North-Holland, 1986, vol. 49, pp. 315–326.

34. Dom, R., Malfroid, M. and Baro, F.: Neuropathology of Huntington's chorea: Studies of the ventrobasal complex of the thalamus. Neurology, *26*:64, 1976.

35. Bruyn, G.W.: Neuropathological changes in Huntington's chorea. Adv. Neurol., *1*:399, 1973.

36. Bird, E.D.: The brain in Huntington's chorea. Psychol. Med., *8*:357, 1978.

37. Rodda, R.A.: Cerebellar atrophy in Huntington's disease. J. Neurol. Sci., *50*:147, 1981.

38. Jeste, D.V., Barban, L. and Parisi, J.: Reduced Purkinje cell density in Huntington's disease. Exp. Neurol., *85*:78, 1984.

39. de la Monte, S.M., Vonsattel, J.-P. and Richardson, E.P., Jr.: Morphometric demonstration of atrophic changes in the cerebral cortex, white matter, and neostriatum in Huntington's disease. J. Neuropathol. Exp. Neurol., *47*:516, 1988.

40. Clark, A.W., et al.: The nucleus basalis in Huntington's disease. Neurology, *33*:1262, 1983.

41. Tellez-Nagel, I., Johnson, A.B. and Terry, R.D.: Studies on brain biopsies of patients with Huntington's chorea. J. Neuropathol. Exp. Neurol. 33:308, 1974.

42. Roizin, L., Stellar, S. and Liu, J.C.: Neuronal nuclear-cytoplasmic changes in Huntington's chorea: Electron microscope investigations. Adv. Neurol. 23:95, 1979.

43. Forno, L. and Norville, R.L.: Ultrastructure of the neostriatum in Huntington's and Parkinson's disease. Adv. Neurol., *23*:123, 1979.

44. Roos, R.A.C., Bots, G.Th.A.M. and Hermans, J.: Quantitative analysis of morphological features in Huntington's disease. Acta Neurol. Scand., *73*:131, 1986.

45. Bird, E.D.: Huntington's chorea: Etiology and pathogenesis. In: *Handbook of Clinical Neurology.* Edited by P.J. Vinken, G.W. Bruyn, and H.L. Klawans. Amsterdam, Elsevier, 1986, vol. 49, pp. 255–265.

46. Beal, M.F. and Martin, J.B.: Neuropeptides in neurological disease. Ann. Neurol., *20*:547, 1986.

47. Perry, T.L., Hansen, S. and Kloster, M.: Huntington's chorea: Deficiency of gamma-aminobutyric acid in brain. N. Engl. J. Med., *288*:337, 1973.

48. Bird, E.D., Mackay, A.V.P., Rayner, C.N. and Iversen, L.L.: Reduced glutamic-acid-decarboxylase activity of post-mortem brain in Huntington's chorea. Lancet, *1*:1090, 1973.

49. Bird, E.D. and Iversen, L.L.: Huntington's chorea: Postmortem measurement of glutamic acid decarboxylase, choline acetyltransferase and dopamine in basal ganglia. Brain, *97*:457, 1974.

50. Bird, E.D. and Iversen, L.L.: Neurochemical findings in Huntington's chorea. In: *Essays in Neurochemistry and Neuropharmacology.* Edited by M.B.H. Youdim, W. Lovenberg, D.F. Sharman, and J.R. Laguado, Jr. London, John Wiley, 1977, pp. 177–195.

51. McGeer, P.L. and McGeer, E.G.: Enzymes associated with the metabolism of catecholamines, acetylcholine and GABA in human controls and patients with Parkinson's disease and Huntington's chorea. J. Neurochem. *26*:65, 1976.

52. Enna, S.J., et al.: Huntington's chorea: Changes in neurotransmitter receptors in the brain. N. Engl. J. Med., *294*:1305, 1976.

53. Cross, A.J. and Waddington, J.L.: Substantia nigra gamma-aminobutyric acid receptors in Huntington's disease. J. Neurochem. 37:321, 1981.

54. Hiley, C.R. and Bird, E.D.: Decreased muscarinic receptor concentration in post-mortem brain in Huntington's chorea. Brain Res., *80*:355, 1974.

55. Wastek, G.J. and Yamamura, H.I.: Biochemical characterization of the muscarinic cholinergic receptor in human brain: Alterations in Huntington's disease. Mol. Pharmacol., *14*:768, 1978.

56. Cross, A. and Rossor, M.: Dopamine D-1 and D-2 receptors in Huntington's disease. Eur. J. Pharmacol., *88*:223, 1983.

57. Spokes, E.G.S.: Neurochemical alterations in Huntington's chorea: A study of post-mortem brain tissues. Brain, *103*:179, 1980.

58. Coyle, J.T. and Schwarcz, R.: Lesion of striatal neurones with kainic acid provides a model for Huntington's chorea. Nature, *263*:244, 1976.

59. McGeer, E.G. and McGeer, P.L.: Duplication of biochemical changes of Huntington's chorea by intrastriatal injections of glutamic and kainic acids. Nature, *263*:517, 1976.

60. Schwarcz, R., Whetsell, W.O., Jr. and Mangano, R.M.: Quinolinic acid: An endogenous metabolite that produces axon-sparing lesions in rat brain. Science, *219*:316, 1983.

61. Schwarcz, R., et al.: Excitotoxic models for neurodegenerative diseases. Life Sci., *35*:19, 1984.

62. Whetsell, W.O., Jr., Kohler, C. and Schwarcz, R.: Quinolinic acid: A glia-derived excitotoxin in the mammalian central nervous system. In: *The Biochemical Pathology of Astrocytes.* Edited by M.D. Norenberg, L. Hertz, and A. Schousboe. New York, Alan R. Liss, 1988, pp. 191–202.

63. Beal, M.F., et al.: Excitotoxin lesions do not mimic the alteration of somatostatin in Huntington's disease. Brain Res., *361*:135, 1985.

64. Beal, M.F., et al.: Replication of the neurochemical characteristics of Huntington's disease by quinolinic acid. Nature, *321*:168, 1986.

65. Ellison, D.W., et al.: Amino acid neurotransmitter abnormalities in Huntington's disease and the quinolinic acid animal model of Huntington's disease. Brain, *110*:1657, 1987.

66. Young, A.B., et al.: NMDA receptor losses in putamen from patients with Huntington's disease. Science, *241*:981, 1988.

8

Parkinson's Disease and Parkinsonian Syndromes

FRANCOISE GRAY,
JACQUES POIRIER and
FRANCESCO SCARAVILLI

Parkinsonian syndromes are characterized clinically by the association of extrapyramidal hypertonia, akinesia, and involuntary tremor. These signs have been correlated with a lesion of the nigrostriatal dopaminergic system, in particular with depletion of dopamine in the striatum which, in the majority of cases, is secondary to severe nerve cell loss in the substantia nigra (SN).[1]

In addition to the idiopathic form (Parkinson's disease, paralysis agitans), clinically similar syndromes are seen in association with lesions of the SN due to other causes. On the other hand, involvement of the SN and a parkinsonian syndrome may occur in other degenerative diseases.

PARKINSON'S DISEASE

Parkinson's disease (PD) affects both sexes at a rate of approximately 1 in 400 individuals, usually in the later middle age (mean 55 + or − 11 years). The disease is most prevalent in octogenerians, in fact, 75 to 88% are in their seventh or eighth decade of life.[2] No causative agents are known; because of the localization of the lesions, of the involvement of nerve cells and its possible occurrence in families, PD is included in the group of degenerative illnesses.

HISTORY

The evolution of our knowledge of the pathologic changes in this disease developed over several stages. In his Essay on the Shaking Palsy (Fig. 8–1), Parkinson[3] suggested that the lesion is localized to the upper cervical cord and lower medulla. Subsequently, other authors suggested the possibility of the involvement of the basal ganglia and in particular of the pallidum[4–8] and noted the characteristic lesions of the SN (Figs. 8–2 and 8–3).[9–18] The essential role of the changes of the SN (Fig. 8–4), and in particular of the degeneration of the dopaminergic cells, in the pro-

179

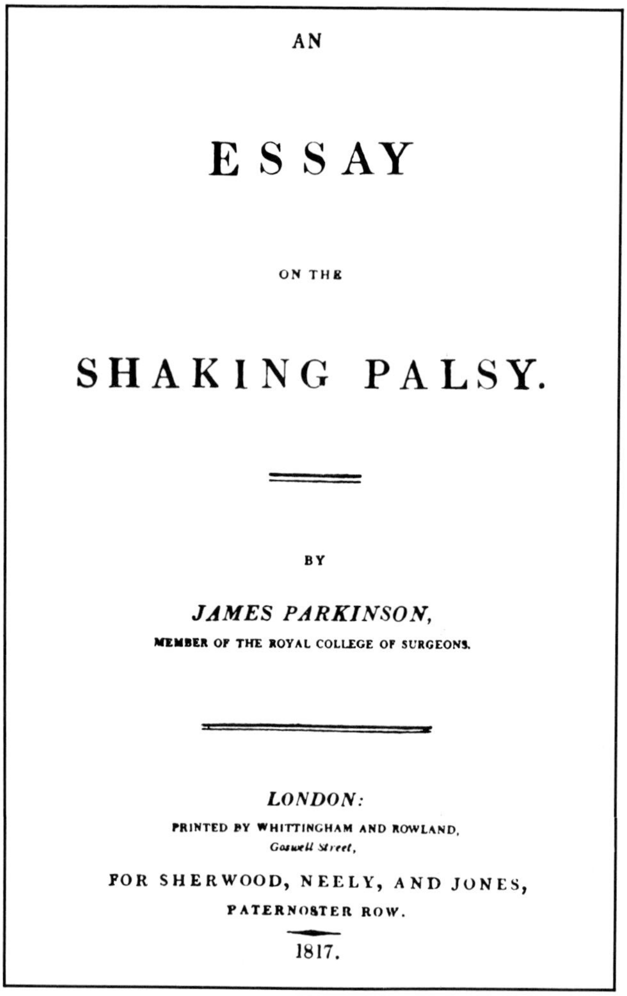

AN

ESSAY

ON THE

SHAKING PALSY.

BY

JAMES PARKINSON,
MEMBER OF THE ROYAL COLLEGE OF SURGEONS.

LONDON:
PRINTED BY WHITTINGHAM AND ROWLAND,
Goswell Street,

FOR SHERWOOD, NEELY, AND JONES,
PATERNOSTER ROW.

1817.

Fig. 8–1. Title page of the initial description of the disease by Sir James Parkinson.

duction of the extrapyramidal symptoms, has been proven by the demonstration of low levels of dopamine in the striatum of patients with Parkinson's disease,[1] by the improvement of the motor symptoms after treatment with L-dopa and, more recently, by the appearance of a parkinsonian syndrome after intoxication with N-methyl-4-4phenyl-1,2,3,4,6-tetrahydrophyridine (MPTP).[19] This drug is known to produce degneration of the dopaminergic neurons of the nigrostriatal pathway.

However, the fact that pathologic changes are not limited exclusively to the SN is in keeping with the existence of symptoms other than extrapyramidal, in particular with those due to autonomic failure or with a disorder of higher cerebral functions, which, on occasion, may be severe. Histologic examination has confirmed the presence of lesions morphologically similar to those of the SN in pigmented and non-pig-

mented nuclei in the brainstem.[17,18,20] Moreover, biochemical investigations by Javoy-Agid et al.[21] have shown that, in addition to the striatum, other dopaminergic as well as nondopaminergic pathways are affected by the disease.

Neuropathologic studies in the last few years have aimed at clarifying the anatomic substratum of the dementia associated with PD[22] and at defining the ultrastructure and the immunocytochemical properties of the Lewy bodies (Fig. 8–5). PD is characterized by the involvement of a selected group of nuclei in which neuronal loss of variable severity and specific inclusions are observed.

The lesions of the pigmented nuclei of the brainstem represent a constant feature. On macroscopic examination, the SN appears pale in all cases; the loss of pigment is usually bilateral and symmetrical and is most severe in

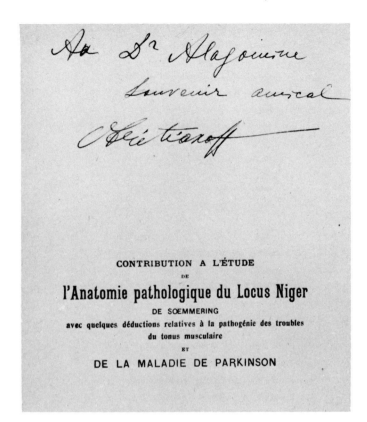

Fig. 8–2. Title page of the thesis of Tretiakoff dedicated to Professor Alajouanine.

the middle part of the zona compacta, while the medial and lateral areas are relatively spared. The pathologic condition consists of selective nerve cell loss of variable intensity, while residual melanin pigment may be seen in the neuropil or contained in macrophages. Astrocytic and microglial proliferation is also present but is usually mild. Lewy bodies are observed in the majority of the cases. A most discrete cell loss and the presence of Lewy bodies are also observed in the nucleus paranigralis. This nucleus situated in the ventral part of the ventral tegmental area is considered as the origin of the meso-cortico-limbic pathway in rodents and possibly in primates.[21] Similar lesions may be found also in the locus cereuleus, the principal source of noradrenergic innervation of the central nervous system, and in the dorsal nucleus of the vagus.[18,23] In addition, Lewy bodies have been frequently observed in the nucleus parabrachialis pigmentosus, nucleus tegmenti pedunculo-pontinus, and nucleus subceruleus.[20,24,25] Abnormalities morphologically comparable to those described in the pigmented nuclei are found in

the cells of the sympathetic ganglia which are known to contain neuromelanin. Although the presence in the ganglia of Lewy bodies had been previously described by Herzog,[26] Wohlwill,[27] and Hechst and Nussbaum,[28] the high rate of involvement of the sympathetic system in PD has been emphasized by Den Hartog Jager and Bethlem.[20] Lewy bodies have been found in two thirds of the cases.[29] Other abnormalities include cell loss and the presence of nodules of Nageotte.

Non-pigmented nuclei in various regions of the CNS may also be involved in the disease. When Lewy bodies cannot be found, the severity of the lesion is difficult to appreciate since there is no free pigment and the glial reaction is discrete. In these circumstances, morphometric studies may be necessary to evaluate the amount of cell loss. Abnormalities of the nucleus basalis of Meynert, the principal site of origin of neocortical noradrenergic innervation, have been known for a long time. It is in this nucleus that Lewy[5] described for the first time the intracellular inclusions which bear his name. Lesions of the substantia in-

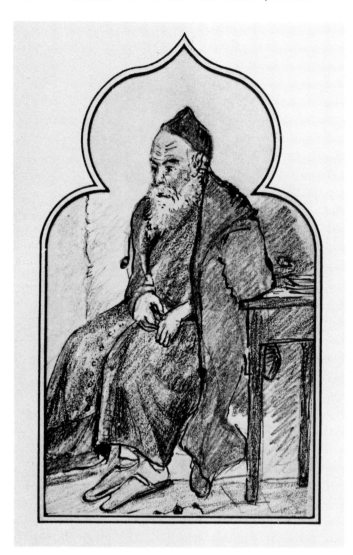

Fig. 8–3. Drawing representing "a Jew from Tetouan with Parkinson's disease" made by Charcot during a travel to Morocco.

nominata have been also reported.[11,15,30] Neuronal loss is present in nearly all cases; it varies in severity and is associated with a glial reaction and, in numerous instances, with Lewy bodies.[22,30–37]

Lewy bodies have been consistently observed in the hypothalamus and particularly in the mammillary bodies and lateral and posterior hypothalamic nuclei.[38] Using morphometric methods, additional changes have been detected in the nerve cells of the supraoptic and paraventricular nuclei. They consist of a decrease of the nucleolar volume and of intracytoplasmic RNA which suggest a decrease in functional activity, possibly secondary to a re-

duction of the noradrenergic input from the locus ceruleus.[39]

Lesions have also been described in the reticular substance of the mesencephalon and pons,[18,40] in particular in the griseum centrale mesencephali, nucleus supratrochlearis, centralis superior and processus griseus pontis supralemniscallis[24,25] and, more recently, in the nucleus of Darkschewitsch.[41] The amount of nerve cell loss has also been determined in the dorsal nucleus of the raphe and in the nucleus of Edinger-Westphal. The former is, with the central superior nucleus, the origin of the ascending serotoninergic pathway;[25] the latter is probably cholinergic.[41]

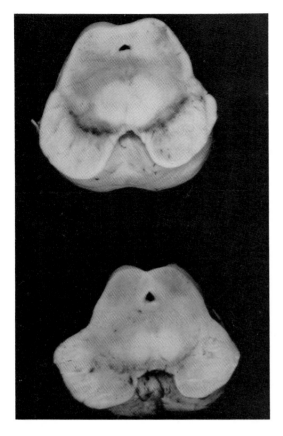

Fig. 8–4. Parkinson's disease: macroscopic aspect. Horizontal section of the cerebral peduncle through the decussation of the superior cerebellar peduncles: depigmentation of the substantia nigra (below), compared with a normal substantia nigra.

Lewy bodies and nerve cell loss have been frequently observed in the intermediolateral tract of the thoracic cord;[18,24] usually associated with dysautonomia[42] and on rare occasions, in the anterior horn of the spinal cord.

The cerebral cortex is usually normal. Senile plaques and neurofibrillary tangles, in variable amounts, are observed in greater number than could be accounted for by the co-existence of senile dementia of Alzheimer type.[43,44] In rare cases of progressive dementia, most of them observed in Japan, eosinophilic inclusions resembling Lewy bodies, have been reported in cortical neurons, mainly in the amygdaloparahippocampal region in association with senile changes.[45–47]

Pathologic changes in the nucleus lenticularis are described as nonspecific. In the putamen, which represents the terminal part of the nigrostriatal pathway and shows severe depletion of dopamine, the rare morphologic changes observed are similar to those seen in old patients. On the other hand, Bugiani et al.[48] observed nerve cell loss in the striatum, involving predominantly large neurons. Mild cell loss, with a proportional degree of glial proliferation, increase of lipofuscin, status cribrosus, and mineralization of the vessel walls have been reported in the globus pallidus, which, in the rat, contains dopaminergic fibers representing collaterals of the nigrostriatal pathway.[49] However, these changes are non-

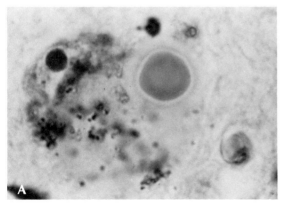
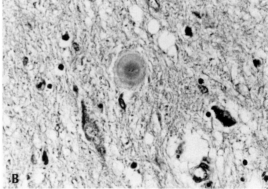

Fig. 8–5. Lewy inclusion bodies, colH and E. A, Substantia Nigra, Lewy body in a pigmented nerve cell perikaryon, × 500. B, Dorsal Vagal Nucleus, Lewy body in a nerve cell process. × 250

specific and could be attributed either to aging or vascular pathologic condition. The density of nerve and glial cells and the nerve/glia ratio in Parkinsonian patients are similar to those of normal controls of the same age.[5,51]

CLINICOPATHOLOGIC CORRELATIONS

Many other areas of the nervous system may be involved in Parkinson's disease. The multiplicity and complexity of neurologic signs found in patients with PD suggest that on one hand, the extrapyramidal signs can be related to the lesions of the striatonigral pathways and to the possible involvement of the direct dopaminergic input to the motor areas of the cortex as recently shown in the monkey.[52] On the other, the anatomic background of the autonomic and intellectual impairment seems more complex.

Signs of autonomic failure occur frequently in PD and consist of postural (orthostatic) hypotension,[53] impairment of peripheral vasodilatation and/or inability to sweat.[54−56] Terminal autonomic and respiratory failure, hypothermia and severe hypotension are often observed in the absence of any underlying visceral abnormality.[18] These signs have been interpreted as due to lesions of the dorsal nucleus of the vagus,[18,23] of the hypothalamus,[38] of the intermediolateral columns of the cord[42] and/or of the sympathetic ganglia;[29] moreover, the uneven distribution and association of the abnormalities explain the variable clinical presentation. The nucleus of Edinger-Westphal, from which the cholinergic parasympathetic preganglionic fibers innervating the ciliary ganglion originate, may also be affected.[25,41] Patients with orthostatic hypotension and progressive autonomic failure, who suffer from Shy-Drager disease,[57] are separated by Bannister and Oppenheimer[58] into two groups; in the first are those with evidence of multiple system atrophy [see below]; the second group, the first case of which was reported by Fichefet et al.,[59] comprises cases in which Lewy inclusion bodies, identical in appearance to those seen in PD, are present in the pigmented nuclei. Reviewing 10 cases of the latter group, Oppenheimer observed severe neuronal loss in the intermediolateral col-

umn in all cases in which the spinal cord could be examined, while the cell density in the same region was normal in parkinsonian patients without autonomic failure.

Mental disease in PD is reported with increasing though varying frequency.[60] The reason for this difference resides in the difficulty in assessing the dementia in these patients, once the slow mentation, typical of the disease, and the appearance of episodes of confusion and depression related to medication have been taken into consideration.[60] In addition to the biochemical defect, due to the disease or induced by treatment, various anatomic abnormalities may be held responsible for the appearance of the dementia in PD. Clinical examination[22] has not shown a correlation between dementia and the severity of the changes in the SN. Oyanagi et al.[61] have reported the case of a patient suffering from severe dementia and showing lesions limited to the SN. It is suggested that the nucleus paranigralis and the dopaminergic meso-cortico-limbic pathway may have also been involved.[62] The presence of more severe lesions of the locus ceruleus in demented parkinsonian patients may be compared with the low levels of cortical noradrenaline and the changes of noradrenergic fibers found in Alzheimer's disease.[63,64] The presence of larger numbers of Lewy bodies in the substantia reticularis of the pons and medulla of demented than in the nondemented parkinsonians led Fujimura and Umbach[40] to postulate that involvement of the ascending activating system may play a role in the deterioration of the mental functions in PD. A correlation has also been established between the severity of the lesions, the low levels of choline-acetyl-transferase (CAT) in the nucleus basalis of Meynert and the dementia.[22,31] The increasing incidence of cortical lesions typical of senile dementia of the Alzheimer type is interpreted as due to the longer survival of patients with PD. These abnormalities are more frequent in these patients than in age matched controls.[43,44] Large numbers of atypical Lewy bodies (cortical Lewy bodies, see below) have been observed in the cortex, with or without the other features associated with senile dementia.[65] The difficulty in establishing a correlation between the severity of each of these anatomic changes[25,36,65] and the degree of dementia presumably is caused by the presence of several lesions.[22,66]

LEWY BODIES

SPECIFICITY

Lewy bodies can be seen in every case of PD. However, since they have been subsequently described in other pathologic conditions, their pathognomonic significance is disputed. Lewy bodies have been observed in the brains of aged individuals.[67,68] In a study of 50 brains of old people which contained Lewy bodies, Forno[69] found that their distribution was similar to that observed in PD and that their presence was associated with neuronal loss in the SN. Furthermore, 22% of the patients had mild parkinsonian signs. The author concluded that such brains should be regarded as showing pre-clinical or sub-clinical PD. The presence of Lewy bodies in pathologic conditions involving the SN, such as postencephalitic parkinsonism,[68,70] OPCA,[71,72] PSP[73] is interpreted by the majority of the authors as due to the coexistence of the two diseases; indeed, in such cases the distribution of Lewy bodies is similar to that of PD. Lewy bodies in the SN and in the cortex have been observed in cases of Hallervorden-Spatz disease[74] and infantile neuro-axonal dystrophy.[75] Similar conclusions apply to the observation of Lewy bodies in cases of progressive dementia with flexor quadriparesis described by Okasaki et al.[76] and in a 24-year-old man with a 10-year history of SSPE.[77] However, these associations occur only in rare instances and the general consensus is that Lewy bodies are the hallmark of PD.

MORPHOLOGIC FEATURES

Lewy bodies are intraneuronal inclusions present in perikaryon or in the cell processes, in the brainstem, sympathetic ganglia, or in the cortex. Lewy bodies in the SN[78] are in the perikaryon, thus displacing the nucleus and melanin pigment towards the cell border. Lewy bodies are round or oval and consist of an intensely acidophilic core surrounded by a peripheral rim which is weakly or not stained by any histologic method. The central core is usually homogeneous, but it may contain an area either more densely stained or of a different color and surrounded by concentric layers making the body resemble a target. Their numbers vary: they are usually single in an affected neuron, but multiple bodies may be observed. In the nucleus basalis of Meynert and dorsal nucleus of the vagus,[5] locus ceruleus,[79] hypothalamus[38] and, above all, in the sympathetic ganglia,[29] in addition to typical intracytoplasmic bodies, the cell processes of some neurons may be the site of hyaline and acidophilic inclusions which are more elongated and show indistinct edges. These are called "intraneuritic Lewy bodies"[46] and are functionally indistinguishable from the intraperikaryal inclusions.[20,29] In the rare cases of progressive dementia in which cortical Lewy bodies are numerous (diffuse Lewy body disease), the inclusions within the perikarya (cerebral Lewy bodies) show irregular borders and are less eosinophilic; in addition, they do not show either the central core or a well-defined halo.[46,65] The central core of the bodies is composed of proteins and does not contain nucleic acids, lipids, mucopolysaccharides, amyloid, iron, or lead.[17,18,68,80] The presence of sphingomyelins, suggested by Den Hartog and Jager,[81] could not be confirmed by other investigators. Microprobe analysis has identified the presence of calcium, sulfur, and phosphate in Lewy bodies.[82]

Electron microscopic examination[29,83,84,85] has revealed that Lewy bodies consist of filaments 8 to 10 nm wide, intermingled with granular material and dense core vesicles. The filaments are arranged haphazardly in the core and are radially oriented in the outer zone. The difference in appearance between the bodies in the perikaryon and those in the cell processes are due to the variable proportions of filamentous and granular material. The presence of both types of Lewy bodies in the same region, as well as the existence of forms of transition between the two indicate that they represent the same type of lesion.[29,46,86,87] Immunocytochemical studies,[88] have shown that several monoclonal and polyclonal antibodies to neurofilaments can label Lewy bodies, either diffusely or at their periphery. These structures are not visualized by antibodies directed against the neurofibrillary tangles seen in Alzheimer's disease.[85] Nakashima and Ikuta[89] found that

Lewy bodies react positively to an antibody to tyrosine hydroxylase and Hirsch et al.[90] have raised two monoclonal antibodies that visualize the bodies but not neurofilaments.

Investigations of the pathogenesis of PD, based on its morphologic features, have followed three directions.

1. A defect of the metabolism of neuromelanin has been suggested by the pathology of the pigmented nuclei in the brainstem, such as the SN and locus ceruleus.[91,92] In addition, ultrastructural observations have shown that filaments at the periphery of the Lewy bodies are in direct continuity with the surrounding melanin. Duffy and Tennyson[83] described elongated structures intermingled with modified melanin and similar in size to the filaments forming the Lewy bodies. The hypothesis that these filaments are the precursors of Lewy bodies has not been confirmed.[84] According to Graham,[93] the presence of neuromelanin represents a process of auto-oxidation of catecholamines which also release toxic products which cause the death of nerve cells.

2. A primary disturbance of the metabolism of monoamines could also explain the distribution of the Lewy bodies which are situated predominantly within monoaminergic neurons[24] as well as the degeneration of several monoaminergic systems as shown by neurochemical studies.[94] Dense core vesicles, similar to those containing monoamines, are often present in Lewy bodies. Nakashima and Ikuta[89] have shown that Lewy bodies contain thyrosine hydroxylase.

3. The observation that the filaments contained in Lewy bodies and neurofilaments share the same antigenic properties has suggested that a primary abnormality of the cytoskeleton may play a role and that there could be similarities between PD on one hand and Alzheimer's disease.[85] The simultaneous appearnce of these equally common diseases in the same patient seems to occur with a higher frequency than could result from coincidence.[43] Also commonly observed is the presence, in the same nucleus, of Lewy bodies and neurofibrillary degeneration (NFD). Paired helical filaments (PHF), which are a component of NFD, have been found by Forno et al.[95] in intra-axonal Lewy bodies and Okama and Ikuta[25] have demonstrated that Lewy bodies

and NFD seen in post-encephalitic parkinsonism and Alzheimer's disease share the same sites of predilection. However, although a common abnormality of the neurofilaments could be at the origin of both Lewy bodies and NFD, their ultrastructural appearance and antigenic structure indicate a different mechanism of formation.

In conclusion, at present none of these pathogenetic hypotheses, which are not mutually exclusive, is, on its own, completely satisfactory. The study of an animal model of chronic parkinsonian syndrome after MPTP poisoning in primates[96] could provide valuable insights into the pathogenetic mechanisms of the disease. MPTP, which shows an affinity for myelin,[97] produces lesions which closely resemble those of PD and involve, in addition to the SN, the locus ceruleus. Intraneuronal eosinophilic inclusions have been observed on occasion in the SN, locus ceruleus, dorsal motor nucleus of the vagus and basal nucleus of Meynert.[98]

DEGENERATIVE DISEASE WITH PARKINSONIAN SYMPTOMS

Under the term "degenerative diseases" are described illnesses of the central nervous system which are due to nerve cell degeneration and are not produced by any known inflammatory, toxic, metabolic, or vascular factor. Such diseases have common characteristic features which justify their grouping inasmuch as they appear in families and have a genetic basis.

DEGENERATIVE DISEASES INVOLVING THE GREY NUCLEI

MULTIPLE SYSTEM DEGENERATION

This term (MSD) emphasizes the frequent association, in some cases of dysautonomia, between the lesions characteristic of striatonigral degeneration and those of olivo-pontocerebellar atrophy (OPCA).[99–104] It is suggested that the two syndromes may be variants of the same disease. The occurrence of abnormalities in the putamen and/or in the SN in cases of OPCA is known[105–107] and in the one of the cases reported by Adams et al.[103,104] striatonigral degeneration was associated with lesions typical of OPCA. Other studies have confirmed the association of the two diseases.[42,72,108-110] The heterogeneous group of OPCA has been subdivided and among the cases showing these lesions only a few, mainly sporadic forms of the type described by Dejerine and Thomas,[111] could be included in the group of MSD.[112]

MSD are sporadic diseases that appear usually in the fourth-sixth decades with various degree of extrapyramidal, cerebellar, and/or autonomic disturbance. The clinical findings, at least in the initial stages of the illness, may be only those of a parkinsonian syndrome. The diagnosis of MSD may be suspected in cases in which treatment with DOPA fails to produce any clinical improvement or when the presence of other symptoms complicates the clinical presentation. However, the effect of treatment with DOPA is not an absolute criterion to establish the differential diagnosis with PD.[113] On morphologic examination, lesions are invariably present in the zona compacta of the SN, while the pars reticulata is normal.[109] Histologic changes are particularly severe in the middle third of the lateral region and consist of nerve cell loss of various intensity with free pigment and mild glial proliferation. Neurofibrillary tangles are not a feature and Lewy bodies are only occasionally seen. Similar abnormalities are usually seen also in the locus ceruleus and less frequently in the dorsal nucleus of the vagus.[104,114-117] Lesions of the striatum occur frequently and have been found by Gray et al.[118] in 20 of 22 cases. Their localization and microscopic features are characteristic of the disease.[72,104,107,114-117] The lesions are bilateral and most often symmetrical and are localized at, or most severe in, the posterolateral and superior regions of the putamen; in some cases they extend to the whole nucleus, which appears wasted and may also involve the caudate and the outer pallidum. Macroscopically, the putamen appears severely atrophic, shows grey-green discoloration and sometimes contains lacunar spaces. Microscopically, in extremely severe cases, the neuronal loss involves both large and small cells; when the changes are milder, small cells are predominantly affected; cell loss is accompanied by intense glial proliferation, hyperpla-

sia of the capillary endothelium and dilated perivascular spaces. Aggregates of dark brown pigment are also seen in the remaining nerve cells, astrocytes and/or macrophages. The pigment consists, among other components, of a blood pigment containing iron, lipofuscin, and neuromelanin. According to Borit et al.,[115] the latter could be the result of the polymerization of dopamine present in the axonal terminals of the nigrostriatal pathway. This finding would suggest that the abnormalities observed in the SN are secondary to the degeneration of the striatum. Furthermore, the degeneration of the striopallidal fibers explains the atrophy and gliosis observed in the pallidum in the presence of normal nerve cells.

The olivo-ponto-cerebellar system is frequently involved though the severity of its changes varies considerably.[118] Lesions of the pontine nuclei and pontocerebellar fibers are among the commonest findings, but they vary from neuronal loss localized to the anterolateral regions of the pons or myelin pallor of the median part of the middle cerebellar peduncles, to complete cell loss leading to macroscopic atrophy of the basis pontis and of the middle cerebellar peduncles. In the latter event, the total myelin loss of these pathways contrasts with the normal appearance of the corticospinal tracts. Changes in the cerebellar cortex occur less frequently and are less severe; they consist of widespread involvement of the Purkinje cells which is secondary to the loss of cells in the pons. The relative sparing of Purkinje cells explains the normal appearance of the ribbon of the dentate nucleus upon which they establish synaptic contacts. In some cases abnormalities are also observed in the inferior olives and olivocerebellar pathways, but their distribution and severity depend on the extent of the involvement of the cerebellar cortex.

Lesions of the lateral horns of the spinal cord are frequently observed. Oppenheimer[119] showed nerve cell loss in the intermediolateral nucleus in 18 cases of multiple system atrophy and established a correlation between the severity of the loss and the clinical appearance of autonomic failure. In their study of 15 cases, Gray et al.[120] could confirm the invariable involvement of the lateral horns; however, since they could not find any correlation between the extent of cell loss and autonomic failure, they concluded that changes in other regions (i.e. dorsal nucleus of the vagus, sympathetic ganglia) are necessary to produce this syndrome.

On the basis of the distribution of the lesions and their severity, various syndromes have been described: involvement of the striatonigral pathway is manifested clinically as a parkinsonian syndrome; lesions of the pontocerebellar system manifest themselves with ataxia; there are also cases in which abnormalities are found in the striatum, SN, pons and cerebellum, the arteries and lateral horns of the spinal cord, the latter being usually associated with dysautonomia. The rather frequent and stereotyped association between all these lesions, in the absence of any known etiopathogenetic mechanism are the characteristic features of multiple system degeneration.[121]

IDIOPATHIC POSTURAL HYPOTENSION (SHY-DRAGER DISEASE)

This disease is a progressive condition appearing during the second half of life and producing autonomic disturbances (in particular hypotension, as well as impotence, incontinence, inability to sweat) and extrapyramidal signs.[57] Pathologic studies have shown that cases are separable into one group showing the features of Parkinson's disease and another displaying multiple system atrophy.[121]

IDIOPATHIC PALLIDAL DEGENERATION

It was first described in 1917 by Hunt,[122] van Bogaert reported a series of cases, emphasized the frequent involvement of the subthalamic nucleus and the association with cerebellar atrophy.[123] Subsequent publications have stressed the association between the lesions of the globus pallidus and the subthalamic nucleus on one hand, changes in the dentate nucleus and its afferent fibers, the so-called dentato-rubro-pallido-luysian atrophy and degeneration of motor neurons.[124–130] Most of the cases are familial and the disease appears before the end of the third decade; the clinical

presentation varies considerably from one case to another.[125,131] A large number of cases presenting clinically as juvenile Parkinson's disease seem to correspond to this condition.[131] Morphologically, Jellinger[124,125] proposed a division into pure pallidal atrophy, pallido-luysian atrophy, pallidal atrophy associated with changes in the SN and/or striatum and pallidal atrophy associated with other forms of system degeneration. The lesion in the globus pallidus consists of neuronal loss, most severe in the outer half, while the inner segment shows myelin pallor, which may extend to the ansa lenticularis, and glial proliferation. The subthalamic nucleus often shows a considerable degree of involvement that may lead to macroscopic atrophy, extreme nerve cell loss and dense glial proliferation.[130,132] In the SN the nerve cell loss is particularly accentuated in the pars reticularis and is associated with free pigment and a mild degree of gliosis. Neurofibrillary tangles or Lewy bodies have never been observed. The presence of other system degenerations, in addition to the lesions typical of the disease, suggests some overlap with the dentatorubral and spinocerebellar atrophies.[130,131]

Cases of pallido-nigro-luysian atrophy clinically manifest during the presenium.[133–135] These cases have clinicopathologic characteristics similar to those described in progressive supranuclear palsy, although they differ from the latter by the striking involvement of the globus pallidus, the subthalamic nucleus and the small number of neurofibrillary tangles. They also differ from the atrophy of the pallidum and may be authentic forms of the disease of Steele, Richardson, and Olzewski.[136]

PROGRESSIVE SUPRANUCLEAR PALSY

This disease, which is not uncommon, appears after the sixth decade of life and, in its typical form, has clinically severe akinesia, hypertonia, dystonia and, infrequently, tremor. Hypertonia lacks the plasticity of parkinsonian rigidity and extends to involve the muscles of the neck. Additional neurologic signs are commonly present and include a paralysis of vertical eye movements which has given the syndrome its name.[137] However, the clinical presentation may vary considerably and some cases may present as parkinsonian syndromes. Numerous clinicopathologic investigations[136,138] have revealed that some nuclei of the brain are constantly and severely affected: the SN shows widespread nerve cell loss, marked glial proliferation. Biochemical studies[139] have confirmed the involvement of the dopaminergic nigrostriatal system and have shown that the mesocortical and meso-limbic systems are unaffected. The superior colliculi, pretectal region, periaqueductal grey matter, reticular formations of the mesencephalon (in particular those near the midline) and, to lesser extent, the reticular formation of the pons are the site of such severe nerve cell loss and reactive glial proliferation that the mesencephalon or the basis pontis may appear atrophic at naked eye. In these areas neurofibrillary tangles are numerous. Abnormalities of the globus pallidus, though invariably present, vary in intensity and localization: in some cases both cell loss and gliosis are more severe in the inner segment and tangles are scanty. The distribution and severity of these lesions would explain the partial or complete lack of response of the patients to treatment with L-Dopa. Severe nerve cell loss with a comparable amount of glial proliferation and numerous neurofibrillary tangles are also observed in the subthalamic nucleus, while other nuclei, such as the dentate nucleus, locus ceruleus, oculomotor and pontine nuclei, reticular formations of the medulla, inferior olives, striatum and thalamus are less frequently and less severely affected, with predominance of tangles over nerve cell loss and gliosis. The cerebellar cortex and the anterior horns of the spinal cord are rarely involved. The presence and the density of neurofibrillary tangles in the medial temporal regions must be evaluated bearing in mind the often advanced age of the patients.

The various combinations of these lesions explain the multiplicity of the clinical presentations.[136,137] The distribution of the lesions does not follow the pattern of multiple system degenerations, although some cases seem to suggest it.[133,140-144] The localization of the pathologic changes, the frequent findings of atrophy of the pons, and the presence of neurofibrillary tangles are reminiscent of postencephalitic parkinsonism and have lead some authors to suggest a viral etiology for this syndrome.[145] However, attempts to transmit the disease to experimental animals by injecting pathologic material has failed. Ultrastructural studies have shown that neurofibrillary tangles in progressive supranuclear palsy differ morphologically from those observed in postencephalitic parkinsonism Steele-Richardson-Olzewski syndrome.[146-148] Hallervorden-Spatz disease[149] described in 1922 as a familial disease with onset between 7 and 9 years and progressive evolution leading to death before the end of the third decade. Clinically, this condition is characterized by progressive dementia, bradykinesia, rigidity, dysarthria accompanied, in some cases, by choreic or athetoid movements and a slight degree of pyramidal signs. Cases with late onset can present with a parkinsonian syndrome.[150] Macroscopically, the characteristic feature is a rusty-brown discoloration of the globus pallidus and SN. Histologically, these nuclei show neuronal loss and a great increase of iron pigment and of round bodies derived from swollen axons. The latter changes, also known as spheroids, may be found in a variety of pathologic conditions.[151] but are particularly numerous and widespread in neuroaxonal dystrophy (Seitelberger's disease). In view of the morphologic similarities between the two conditions and of the existence of forms of transition, some authors consider Hallervorden-Spatz disease as a juvenile form of neuroaxonal dystrophy localized to the deep grey nuclei.[152] Numerous Lewy bodies have been observed in the cortex and/or SN of some cases.[74]

CORTICO-SUBCORTICAL DEGENERATION PRODUCING DEMENTIA

Pick's Disease [See Chap. 3]. An extrapyramidal syndrome is seen only occasionally in Pick's disease, in spite of the frequent occurrence of subcortical changes.[153] Escourolle[154] reported evidence of a true parkinsonian syndrome in 20 of 192 cases of Pick's disease. The caudate nucleus and the putamen are the most frequently involved while the lesions in the globus pallidus are more discrete and appear to be non-specific.[155-156] Abnormalities of the SN such as neuronal loss and glial proliferation are often seen.

Alzheimer's Disease [See Chap. 4]. Extrapyramidal signs are sometimes observed in patients suffering from Alzheimer's disease or senile dementia and they occur in late stages of the illness. Plastic rigidity develops progressively and predominates in the forelimbs; akinesia may also be severe while tremor is only occasionally present. It has already been mentioned that these symptoms may be due to the simultaneous occurrence of dementia and Parkinson's disease. Nevertheless, lesions typical of Alzheimer's disease may be found not only in the cortex, but also in the subcortical nuclei such as the nucleus basalis of Meynert and locus ceruleus. Involvement of the SN by the pathologic process is frequently described and varies in intensity. In the most severely affected cases, the area appears devoid of pigment and histologically shows, in addition to a variable degree of neuronal loss, free pigment and reactive gliosis, neurofibrillary tangles, and senile plaques. The latter changes may be observed also in the reticular nuclei of the mesencephalon.

Parkinson-Dementia Complex of Guam. The disease was endemic among the Chamorro population in Guam, one of the Mariana islands. It develops insidiously during the fifth or sixth decade and has a progressive evolution leading to death after approximately 4 years. The most typical clinical features are dementia, parkinsonian syndrome and involvement of the lower motor neurons.[157-158] The pathologic condition in the central nervous system was described by Hirano et al.[157-158] and consists of cortical atrophy, particularly in the frontotemporal lobes, associated with loss of pigmentation of the SN and locus ceruleus. On histologic examination, changes are more widespread and extend to the cerebral cortex, hippocampus, amygdala, hypothalamus, globus pallidus, thalamus, SN and tegmentum. They consist of nerve cell loss, glial proliferation, presence of neurofibrillary tangles, and granulovacuolar degeneration (GVD). Similar alterations, but without GVD, are also described in the anterior horns of the spinal cord, particularly in the corticospinal tract degeneration, and in the nucleus of the hypoglossus. Ultrastructurally, the tangles resemble those seen in Alzheimer's disease and in postencephalitic parkinsonism.[159]

CEREBELLAR AND SPINO-CEREBELLAR DEGENERATIONS

Olivo-ponto-cerebellar Atrophy. In addition to the sporadic forms of OPCA, Dejerine-Thomas type, belonging to the group of multiple system atrophy, in which the SN is invariably involved, this area may be also affected in other varieties of OPCA in which, consequently, a parkinsonian syndrome may develop. Reviewing 117 cases from the literature, Berciano[110] observed that 46% of the familial cases of OPCA, Menzel type, showed changes in the SN. In cases of OPCA with autosomal dominant inheritance and presenting severe reduction of the saccadic movements and peripheral neuropathy, the SN is invariably affected.[160-162] Because of the complex clinical presentations, parkinsonian signs are not always easily recognizable; nevertheless, the patient described by Alajouanine et al. showed an expressionless facies.[163] A case of OPCA due to glutamate dehydrogenase deficiency has been reported.[164]

Machado-Joseph Disease. Machado-Joseph disease is an autosomal dominant ataxia described in Portuguese and American families which may be a mutation of the same gene responsible for the autosomal dominant OPCA, Schut-Weier type.[165] The disease is characterized by progressive cerebellar ataxia, pyramidal signs and progressive external ophthalmoplegia with variable degrees of extrapyramidal and peripheral signs. The main pathologic findings consist of nerve cell loss and gliosis in the substantia nigra, dentate, pontine and cranial nerve nuclei, anterior horns, Clarke's columns and posterior root ganglia with consequent loss of fibers of the superior and middle cerebellar peduncles and spino-cerebellar tracts.[166]

Cerebello-Olivary Atrophy. Familial cases of cerebello-olivary degeneration presenting clinically as a Parkinsonian syndrome which included abnormalities of the SN have been reported.[167–169]

Amyotrophic Lateral Sclerosis [See Chap. 3]. The association between amyotrophic lateral sclerosis (ALS) and parkinsonian syndrome is usually considered to be a coincidence except in cases of syndrome of Guam.[170] However, the possibility that this association is not fortuitous has been reported by the presentation of ALS and parkinsonian syndrome in the same patient or in members of the same family.[171–173] In two non-familial cases, suffering also from progressive dementia, neuropathologic examination revealed degenerative changes in the upper and lower motor nerve cells, cell loss in the cortex, mild gliosis, and spongiform changes in the external cortical layers, which correlated with the dementia. The cell loss and gliosis in the SN without neurofibrillary tangles or Lewy bodies were considered part of the same degenerative process.[174]

OTHER PARKINSONIAN SYNDROMES

A common cause of secondary parkinsonism is drug intoxication, which is responsible for 90% of the cases.[2] Treatment with neuroleptic drugs produces extrapyramidal syndromes which disappear after the drug is either withdrawn or its dosage is reduced. As for the pathogenetic mechanisms producing the syndrome, central depletion of catecholamines (reserpine, tetrabenzanine) or a block of the postsynaptic dopaminergic receptors of the striatum (phenothiazines, butyrophenones) seem to be the most likely possibilities. The morphologic basis is poorly understood and the neuropathologic reports give conflicting description. In the majority of the cases, cerebral abnormalities, observed after prolonged periods or treatment, are nonspecific and seem to be related to the age of the patients or to the events immediately preceding death.[175] Cases of irreversible parkinsonian syndromes have been observed after intoxication with MPTP, derived from meperidine;[19,176] in these cases, neuropathologic examination has revealed a selective neuronal loss in the SN with one occasional eosinophilic inclusion in the cytoplasm of nerve cells resembling Lewy bodies.

Similar lesions have been produced in animals [See above].

Postencephalitic Parkinsonism. Cases of parkinsonian syndromes, often having oculocephalogyric crises, have appeared several years after an attack of encephalitis lethargica.[177–178] The encephalitis was observed in an epidemic form in Europe between 1915 and 1926, but sporadic cases were reported as late as 1935. Some of the rare cases described after 1940[179] are questionable. The organism responsible for the illness, most probably a virus, has not been isolated with the limited techniques available at the time of the epidemic and the pathogenesis of the delayed extrapyramidal symptoms has not been explained. Parkinsonian syndromes, usually of short duration, may supervene during an encephalitic episode of known etiology. Irreversible syndromes, appearing at variable times after such an episode, are rare and differ clinically from the postencephalitic parkinsonism which follows encephalitis lethargica. There are no pathologic descriptions of the acute phases, but the possibility of a simultaneous occurrence of encephalitis and idiopathic parkinsonism cannot be ruled out.[180] Unlike in idiopathic parkinsonism, morphologic lesions, although ubiquitous, are not localized in functionally related areas and predominate in the upper part of the brainstem. The original reports of lesions of the SN in postencephalitic parkinsonism have been known since von Economo.[10,15,16,181–184] Although in most cases the whole SN appears uniformly pale, on occasion its involvement may be asymmetrical. Nerve cell loss is usually severe, sometimes complete and reactive glial proliferation is usually proportional to the cell loss. Extracellular melanin pigment may be observed, although it may not be present in severe and/or old cases. The number of neurofibrillary tangles vary considerably, but they are nearly always found in these cases, while perivascular infiltrates of mononuclear cells are only occasionally seen. The reticular formation of the midbrain may be so severely affected by the pathologic process that the resulting atrophy of the tegmentum may become macroscopically evident. Severe neuronal loss and intense gliosis are observed; numerous intraneuronal neurofibrillary tangles are also seen, mainly in the midline structures. The abnormalities described in the midbrain may be present, although irregularly, also in other nuclei of the brainstem:[185] their severity and localization vary from case to case and they may be asymmetrical. The locus ceruleus and, to lesser extent, the dorsal nucleus of the vagus, may show neuronal loss with presence of free melanin, reactive gliosis and presence of neurofibrillary tangles. The reticular formation of the pons and medulla, the nuclei of the cranial nerves (oculomotor, XII) may be especially involved while the cerebellum and spinal cord are usually unaffected. Morphologic changes may be seen also more cranially: numerous neurofibrillary tangles have been observed in the hypothalamus, where they are associated with moderate nerve cell loss and reactive gliosis.[186] The basal ganglia, in particular the globus pallidus, may be normal or be the site either of nonspecific changes or, in some cases, of neurofibrillary tangles, typical of the disease. The existence of such lesions in the globus pallidus is known.[70,187] Neurofibrillary tangles are sometimes seen in the nucleus basalis of Meynert. When they are numerous, their presence is usually associated with moderate nerve cell loss, foci of gliosis and an occasional inflammatory infiltrate in the Ammon's horn.[186] The remainder of the cortex is usually normal.

Neurofibrillary changes in postencephalitic parkinsonism were described for the first time by Feynes[187] and subsequently by Hallervorden[12-13] and von Braunmuhl.[155] On light microscopy, they consist of interweaving bundles of abnormal filaments within the nerve cell cytoplasm. The filaments are weakly impregnated by silver methods and are positive with Congo red for amyloid. In the brainstem the cells which show these changes are ballooned with displacement by the filaments of the normal components of the cell; on the other hand, cells in the cortex tend to assume a more fusiform shape which is underlined by the bundles of fibrils. In both cases, at a later stage, the fibrillary material may be the only remaining component of the cell. Ultrastructurally, the abnormal fibrillary material consists of paired helical filaments 10 nm wide[188] arranged in bundles. Straight filaments, 15 nm wide, similar to those present in progressive

supranuclear palsy, have been described in postencephalitic parkinsonism, but only in the locus ceruleus.[186] Immunocytochemical studies have shown that these abnormal filaments share the same antigenic properties of normal filaments but, in addition, are also visualized by the antibodies to the filaments found in Alzheimer's disease.[85]

Such lesions may be present in the brainstem of postencephalitic parkinsonism, idiopathic Parkinson's disease, Alzheimer's disease, senile dementia, progressive supranuclear palsy, dementia pugilistica, Parkinson-dementia complex of Guam, Down syndrome and in some cases of lead poisoning in children or SSPE and may represent a nonspecific reaction of some nerve cells to multiple insults.

Lesions similar to those found in postencephalitic parkinsonism have been described in the SN in cases of Creutzfeldt-Jakob disease (C-J), a transmissible form of dementia presumed to be due to a slow virus. Although extrapyramidal signs are frequently observed during the dementing stage, a true parkinsonian syndrome develops only rarely. In 1968, Van Rossum[189] described three cases of C-J disease with slow evolution in which the SN was the commonest site of lesions and presented with hypokinesia, rigidity and, on occasion, tremor, and dysarthria. A sub-cortical form in C-J disease involves mainly striatum and thalamus; lesions of the SN are uncommon and have been described.[18] Features include loss of nerve cells, free pigment, gliosis, and spongiform changes.

Parkinsonian Syndromes Secondary to Carbon Monoxide Poisoning. Parkinsonian syndromes[190] are among the variety of extrapyramidal manifestations of carbon monoxide poisoning and are characterized by the severity of hypertonia, akinesia; and tremor and abnormal movements. Necrotic lesions result from anoesia and involve most frequently the anterodorsal regions of the medial globus pallidus and the adjacent areas of the internal capsule. Their localization, whether in isolation or in association with lesions of the white matter, correlates with the extrapyramidal symptoms. Changes have been described, though infrequently, also in SN[124] and consist of mild nerve cell loss, presence of free pigment and reactive glial proliferation.[18] In a study of 22 cases of carbon monoxide poisoning, Lapresle and Fardeau[191] found changes of the globus pallidus in 17 instances, while only 1 case showed a circumscribed area of necrosis in the SN.

Parkinsonian Syndromes Following Manganese Poisoning. They are well known and have been described by Edsall and Drinker.[192] Pathologic reports note severe neuronal loss and glial proliferation in the globus pallidus, most marked in its medial part.[193,194] In the cases described by Canavan et al.[195] the changes in the globus pallidus were associated with more widespread lesions, mainly in the cortex. In all the cases in which the SN has been examined, it has been reported as normal. Experimental studies in monkeys of the effect of manganese[196] have confirmed the predominant involvement of the globus pallidus and the absence of abnormalities in the substantia nigra.

Arteriosclerotic Parkinsonism. In the past, stress has been often laid on vascular lesions as a cause of parkinsonism.[7,9,184,197] Following comprehensive review of the arteriosclerotic parkinsonian syndromes,[198] vascular pathology has been widely considered as one of the causes of parkinsonism or, by some authors, even the cause of Parkinson's disease. This view has subsequently been criticized by Eadie and Sutherland,[199] Schwan and England,[200] and Escourolle et al.[18] and, at present, the role of vascular lesions in the etiology of parkinsonian syndromes is considered with skepticism. While in rare instances unilateral infarction of the SN is followed by parkinsonian syndrome,[200,201] in many cases the presence of "etat crible" or of areas of disintegration of the basal ganglia in aged subjects is not associated with signs of parkinsonism. Indeed, numerous cases considered to be suffering from arteriosclerotic parkinsonism have the clinical features of pseudobulbar palsy and show morphologic appearances of lacunar lesions in the deep grey nuclei. Furthermore, the frequent association in the same brain of degenerative changes of the SN and Lewy bodies and variously distributed areas of ischemia or hemorrhage suggests that the two types of lesion may often co-exist in the same aged individual.[18,25]

Parkinsonian Syndromes and Syphilis. Involvement of the mesencephalon in syphilitic infection, either in isolation or during the evolution of paretic dementia, has been reported in rare instances, but its etiology is debatable.[18]

Parkinsonian Syndromes and Tumors. The occurrence of various types of parkinsonian syndromes in patients with cerebral tumors is a well known, though rare, event. Extrapyramidal signs have been reported in 10 of 474 cases by Sciarra and Sprofkin[202] and 21 of the 1500 patients described by Tolosa et al.[203] presented parkinsonian syndrome. Direct involvement of the SN by a space occupying lesion (tuberculoma),[204,205] lymphoma,[205] localized in the cerebral peduncle, has been only occasionally observed. While tumors situated at the base may sometimes produce a parkinsonian syndrome,[206] tumors which infiltrate extensively the grey nuclei usually fail to produce it.[18] In the great majority of the cases symptoms are produced by tumors of the midline (parasagittal meningiomas, frontal, septal, intraventricular or suprasellar tumors) or by temporal tumors not infiltrating the grey nuclei.[205] The pathogenetic mechanism at the root of these syndromes is poorly understood and probably is not the same in every case. Destruction of the nerve cells of the SN by the tumor is observed only on rare occasions.[205] The disappearance of the syndrome following removal of the tumor indicates that either indirect compression or stretching of the grey nuclei (by the mass or by the intermediary of the temporal herniation) be the cause of the symptoms. A specific involvement of the nerve cells of the SN or their dopaminergic fibers directed to the striatum was suggested by biochemical studies in a case of craniopharyngioma[207] and by the improvement obtained by treatment with Dopa in another case.[208] Other possible mechanisms have been proposed, such as changes in the extrapyramidal centers in the frontal cortex[209] or an association with a parkinsonian syndrome due to another cause.[210]

Post-traumatic Parkinsonian Syndromes. Once cases of Parkinson's disease following head injury or cerebral herniation have been excluded, parkinsonian syndromes directly related to brain trauma are rare.[200,211]

Morphologic studies of three cases revealed hemorrhagic lesions within the SN secondary to uncal herniation.[212] Parkinsonian syndromes, uncomplicated or associated with progressive dementia (dementia pugilistica), have been described after repeated head injuries. This condition may occur years after the last trauma and affects amateur as well as professional boxers who have been dazed or knocked out on many occasions. Neuropathologic examination by Corsellis et al.[213] has shown nerve cell loss and free pigment in the SN, scarring and neuronal loss in the cerebellum and changes in the midline structures such as enlargement of the cavum and fenestration of the leaves of the intraventricular septum and atrophy of the fornix or the corpus callosum. Numerous neurofibrillary tangles without senile plaques were present throughout the cerebral cortex (particularly the medial temporal regions) and the brainstem.

REFERENCES

1. Hornykiewicz, O.: Dopamine and extrapyramidal motor function and dysfunction. Neurotransmitters. Research Publications: Assoc. Res. Nerv. Mental Dis., 50:390, 1972.
2. Derouesne, C.: Mouvements involontaires. In: *Pratique neurologique.* Paris, Flammarion, 1982.
3. Parkinson, J.: *Essay on the Shaking Palsy.* London, Willingham et Rowland, 1817.
4. Jelgersma, G.: Neue anatomosche Befunde bei Paralysis agitans und bei chronischer Chorea. Neurol. Zb1, 27:995, 1908.
5. Lewy, F.H.: Paralysis agitans. I. Pathologische Anatomie. In: *Handbuch des neurologie,* Bd III. Edited by M. Lewandowsky. Berlin, Springer, 1912.
6. Vogt, C. et al.: Zur Lehre der Erkrankungen des striaren Systems. J. Psychol. Neurol. (Lpz), 25(3):627, 1920.
7. Lhermitte, J., Cornil, L.: Recherches anatomiques sur la maladie de Parkinson. Rev. Neurol. (Paris), 28:625, 1921.
8. Bielschowsky, M.: Weitere Bemerkungen zur normalen und pathologischen Histologie des striaren Systems. J. Psychol. Neurol., 27:233, 1922.
9. Brissaud, E.: Lecons sur les maladies nerveuses (23eme leçon: *Nature et pathogenie de la maladie de Parkinson*). Paris, Masson, pp. 488–501, 1895 .
10. Tretiakoff, C.: Contribution a l'etude de l'anatomie pathologique du locus niger de Soemmering avec quelques deductions relatives a la pathogenie des troubles du tonus musculaire et de la maladie de Parkinson. Thèse Medicine, University of Paris, 1919.
11. Foix, C., and Nicolesco, J.: *Les noyaux gris centraux et la region mesencephalo-sous-optique.* Masson, Paris, 1925.
12. Hallervorden, J.: Zur Pathogenese des post-encephalitischen Parkinsonismus. Klin. Wschr., 12:692, 1933.
13. Hallervorden, J.: Anatomische Untersuchungen zur Pathogenese des post-encephalitischen Parkinsonismus. Dtsch Z Nervenheilk, 136:68, 1935.
14. Hallervorden, J.: Paralysis agitans. In: *Handbuch der speziellen pathologischen Anatomine und Histologie des Nervensystems.* (Ed) W. Scholz. Berlin, Springer, 1957.
15. Hassler, R.: Zur Pathologie der Paralysis agitans und des post-encephalitischen Parkinsonismus. J. Psychol. Neurol. (Lpz), 48:387, 1938.
16. Klaur, R.: Parkinsonische Krankheit (Paralysis agitans usw). Arch. Psychiat. Nervenk., 140:251, 1940.
17. Greenfield, J.G., and Bosanquet, F.D.: The brainstem lesions in parkinsonism. J. Neurol. Neurosurg. Psychiat., 16:213, 1953.
18. Escourolle, R., de Recondo, J., and Gray, F.: Etude anatomo-pathologique des syndromes parkinsoniens, In: *Monamines, noyaux gris centraux et syndrome de Parkinson.* (Eds.) J. Ajuriaguerra, and G. Gauthier. Geneve, George et Cie S.A., 1971.
19. Davis, G.C., et al.: Chronic parkinsonism secondary to intravenous injection of meperidine analogues. Psychiat. Res. 1:249, 1979.
20. Den Hartog Jager, W.A., and Bethlem, J.: The distribution of Lewy bodies in the central and autonomic nervous system in idiopathic paralysis agitans. J. Neurol. Neurosurg. Psychiat., 23:283, 1960.
21. Javoy-Agid, F., et al.: Biochemical neuropathology of Parkinson's disease. Adv. Neurol, 40:189, 1984.
22. Gaspar, P., and Gray, F.: Dementia in idiopathic Parkinson's disease, A neuropathological study of 32 cases. Acta Neuropathol. (Berl), 64:43, 1984.
23. Eadie, M.J., and Sutherland, J.M.: Arteriosclerosis in Parkinsonism. J. Neurol. Neurosurg. Psychiat., 27:237, 1964.
24. Ohama, E., and Ikuta, F.: Parkinson's disease: distribution of Lewy bodies and monoamine neuron system. Acta. Neuropathol. (Berl), 34:311, 1976.
25. Jellinger, K.: Overview of morphological changes in Parkinson's disease. Adv. Neurol. 45:1, 1986.
26. Wolhill, F.: Zur pathologischen Anatomie des peripherischen Sympathicus. Dtsch Z Nervenheilk, 107:124, 1929.
27. Herzog, E.: Histopathologische veranderungen im Sympathicus und ihre Bedeutung. Dtsch z Nervenheilk, 107:75, 1928.
28. Hechst, B., and Nussbaum, L.: Bietrage zur Histopathologie des sympatischen Ganglien. Arch. Psychiat. Nervenk, 85:556, 1931.
29. Forno, L.S., and Norville, R.L.: Ultrastructure of Lewy bodies in the stellate ganglion. Acta Neuropathol. (Berl), 34:183, 1976.
30. Buttlar-Brentano von, K.: Das Parkinson-Syndrom in Lichte des lebensgeschichtlichen Veranderungen des Nucleus basalis. J. Hirnforsch, 2:56, 1955.
31. Whitehouse, P.J., et al.: Basal forebrain neurons in the dementia of Parkinson's disease. Ann. Neurol., 13:243, 1983.
32. Forno, L.S., and Alvord, Jr., E.C.: Depigmentation in the Nerve Cells of the substantia Nigra and Locus Ceruleus in Parkinsonism. Adv. Neurol., 5:195, 1974.
33. Candy, J.M., et al.: Pathological changes in the nucleus of Meynert in Alzheimer's and Parkinson's disease. J. Neurol. Sci., 54:277, 1983.
34. Arendt, T., Bigl, V., Arendt A., et al.: Loss of neurons in the nucleus basalis of Meynert in Alzheimer's disease, paralysis agitans and Korsakoff's disease. Acta Neuropathol., (Berl), 61:101, 1983.
35. Forno, L.S., and Alvord, Jr., E.C.: The Pathology of

Parkinsonism. Some New Observations and Correlations (Part I). In: *Recent Advances In Parkinson's Disease.* (Eds) R. Mc Dowell, and M. Markham. Philadelphia, F.A. Davis Co., 1971.

36. Tagliavini, F., Pilleri, G., and Bouras, C., Constantinidis, J.: The basal nucleus of Meynert in idiopathic Parkinson's disease. Acta Neurol. Scand., *69*:20, 1984.

37. Nakano, I., and Hirano, A.: Parkinson's disease: neuron loss in the nucleus basalis without concomitant Alzheimer's disease. Ann. Neurol., *15*:415, 1984.

38. Lanston, J.W., and Forno, L.S.: The hypothalamus in Parkinson disease. Ann. Neurol., *3*:129, 1978.

39. Mann, D.M.A., and Yates, P.O.: Pathological basis for neurotransmitter changes in Parkinson's disease. Neuropathol. Appl. Neurobiol., *9*:3, 1983.

40. Fujimura, H., and Umbach, I.: Role de la substance reticulee dans la demence de la maladie de Parkinson. Rev. Neurol. (Paris), *143*:108, 1987.

41. Hunter, S.: The rostral mensencephalon in Parkinson's and Alzheimer's disease. Acta Neuropathol. (Berl), *68*:53, 1985.

42. Oppenheimer, D.R.: Neuropathology of progressive autonomic failure. In: *Autonomic Failure.* (Ed) R. Bannister. Oxford, Oxford University Press, 1983.

43. Hakim, A.H., and Mathieson, G.: Dementia in Parkinson's disease: A neuropathologic study. Neurology, *29*:1209, 1979.

44. Boller, F., Mizutani, T., Roessmann, U., et al.: Parkinson disease, dementia, and Alzheimer disease: clinicopathological correlations. Ann. Neurol., *7*:329, 1980.

45. Forno, L.S., and Langston, J.W.: The amygdala-parahippocampal region. A predilection site for Lewy bodies. (Abstract) J. Neuropathol. Exp. Neurol., *47*:354, 1988.

46. Yoshimura, M.: Cortical changes in Parkinsonian brain: a contribution to the delineation of "diffuse Lewy body disease". J. Neurol., *229*:17, 1983.

47. Sima, A.A.F., et al.: Lewy body dementia without Alzheimer changes. Can. J. Neurol. Sci., *13*:490, 1986.

48. Bugiani, O., et al.: Loss of striatal neurons in Parkinson's disease: a cytometric study. Eur. Neurol., *19*:339, 1980.

49. Lindvall, O., and Bjorklund, A.: Depaminergic innervation of the globus pallidus by collaterals from the nigrostriatal pathway. Brain Res., *172*:169, 1979.

50. Sabuncu, N.: Quantitative Untersuchungen am menschlichen Pallidum. Falle ohne extrapyramidale Bewegungssterungen. Dtsch Z Nervenhielk, *195*:57, 1969a.

51. Sabuncu, N.: Quantitative Untersuchungen am Pallidum beim Parkinsonsyndrom. Dtsch Z Nervenhielk, *196*:40, 1969b.

52. Berger, B., et al.: Major dopamine innervation of the cortical motor areas in the Cynomolgus monkey. A radioautographic study with comparative assessment of serotonergic afferents. Neuroscience Letters, *72*:121, 1986.

53. Gross, M., Bannister, R., and Godwin-Austen, R.: Orthostatic hypotension in Parkinson's disease. Lancet *I*:174, 1972.

54. Appenzeller, O., and Goss, J.E.: Autonomic deficits in Parkinson's syndrome. Arch. Neurol., *24*:50, 1971.

55. Turkka, J.T., and Myllyla, V.V.: Sweating dysfunction in Parkinson's disease. Eur. Neurol., *26*:1, 1987.

56. Gubbay, S.S., and Barwick, D.D.: Two cases of acci-

dental hypothermia in Parkinson's disease with unusual EEG findings. J. Neurol. Neurosurg. Psychiat., *29*:459, 1966.

57. Shy, G.M., and Drager, G.A.: A neurological syndrome associated with orthostatic hypotension; A clinical-pathologic study. Arch. Neurol. (Chic), *2*:511, 1960.

58. Bannister, R., and Oppenheimer, D.R.: Degenerative disease of the nervous system associated with autonomic failure. Brain, *95*:457, 1972.

59. Fichefet, J.P., et al.: Etude anatomo-clinique d'un cas d'hypotension orthostatique idiopathique. Acta Cardiol. (Brux), *20*:332, 1965.

60. Benson, D.F.: Parkinsonian dementia: cortical or subcortical? Adv. Neurol. *40*:235, 1984.

61. Oyanagi, K., Nakashima, S., Ikuta, F., et al.: An autopsy case of dementia and parkinsonism with severe degeneration exclusively in the substantia nigra. Acta Neuropathol. (Berl), *70*:190, 1986.

62. Torack, R.M., and Morris, J.C.: The association of vertical tegmental area histopathology with adult dementia. Arch. Neurol., *45*:497, 1988.

63. Berger, B., Escourolle, R., and Moyne, M.A.: Axones cathecholaminergiques du cortex cerebral humain. Observation en histofluorescence de biopsies cerebrales dont 2 cas de maladie d'Alzheimer. Rev. Neurol. (Paris), *132*:183, 1976.

64. Berger, B., Escourolle, R., and Moyne, M.A.: Axones cathecholaminergic innervation of the human cerebral cortex in presenile and senile dementia. Histochemical and biochemical studies. In Enzymes and neurotransmitters in mental disease. Edited by E. Usdin, B.H. Youdim. New York, Wiley 1980.

65. Kosaka, K., Yoshimura, M., Ikeda, K., et al.: Diffuse type of Lewy body disease: progressive dementia with abundant cortical Lewy bodies and senile changes of varying degree. A new disease? Clin. Neuropath., *3*:185, 1984.

66. Chui, H.C., et al.: Pathologic correlates of dementia in Parkinson's disease. Arch Neurol., *43*:991, 1986.

67. Beheim-Schwartzbach, D.: Uber Zelleibveranderungen im Nucleus coeruleus beim Parkinson-Symptomen. J. Nerv. Ment. Dis., *116*:169, 1952.

68. Lipkin, L.E.: Cytoplasmic inclusions in ganglion cells, associated with parkinsonian states. A neurocellular change studied in 53 cases and 206 controls. Am. J. Pathol., *35*:1117, 1959.

69. Forno, L.S.: Concentric hyalin intraneuronal inclusions of Lewy type in the brain of elderly persons (50 incidental cases): relationships to parkinsonism. J. Am. Ger. Soc., *17*:557, 1969.

70. Denny-Brown, D.: *The Basal Ganglia and Their Relation to Disorders of Movements.* Oxford, Oxford University Press, 1962.

71. Sigwald, J., Lapresle, J., Raverdy, P., et al.: Atrophie cerebelleuse familiale avec association de lesions nigeriennes et spinales. Presse. Med., *72*:557, 1964.

72. Jellinger, K., and Danielczyk, W.: "Striato-nigrale Degeneration." Acta Neuropathol. (Berl), *10*:242, 1968.

73. Mori, H., Yoshimura, M., Tomonaga, M., et al.: Progressive supranuclear palsy with Lewy bodies. Acta Neuropathol. (Berl), *71*:344, 1986.

74. Antoine, J.C., et al.: Maladie de Hallervorden-Spatz avec corps de Lewy. Rev. Neurol. (Paris), *141*:806, 1985.

75. Defendini, R., Markesberg, W.R., Mastri, A.R., et al.: Hallervorden Spatz disease and infantile neuroaxonal dystrophy: ultrastructural observations, ana-

tomical pathology and nosology. J. Neurol. Sci., 20:7, 1973.

76. Okasaki, H., Lipkin, L.E., and Aronson, S.M.: Diffuse intracytoplasic ganglionic inclusions (Lewy type) associated with progressive dementia and quadripareses in flexion. J. Neuropathol. Exp. Neurol., 20:237, 1961.

77. Cobb, W.A., Marshall, J., and Scaravilli, F.: Long term survival in subacute sclerosing panencephalitis. J. Neurol. Neurosurg. Psychiat., 47:176, 1984.

78. Kosaka, K.: Lewy bodies in cerebral cortex. Report of three cases. Acta Neuropathol. (Berl), 42:127, 1978.

79. Forno, L.S., and Norville, R.L.: Ultrastructural studies of the human locus coeruleus (in middle-aged and older persons with and without parkinsonism). Excerpta Medica, 2:459, 1975.

80. Bethlem, J., and Den Hartog Jager, W.A.: The incidence and characteristics of Lewy bodies in idiopathic paralysis agitans (Parkinson's disease). J. Neurol. Neurosurg. Psychiat., 23:74, 1960.

81. Den Hartog Jager, W.A.: Sphingomyelin in Lewy inclusion bodies in Parkinson's disease. Arch Neurol., 21:615, 1969.

82. Kimula, Y., Utsuyama, M., Yoshimura, M., et al.: Element analysis of Lewy and adrenal bodies in Parkinson's disease by electron probe microanalysis. Acta Neuropathol., 50:233, 1983.

83. Duffy, P.E., and Tennyson, V.J.: Phase and electron microscopic observations of Lewy bodies in idiopathic paralysis agitans (Parkinson's disease). J. Neuropathol. Exp. Neurol., 24:398, 1965.

84. Roy, S., and Wolman, L.: Ultrastructural observations in Parkinsonism. J. Pathol., 99:39, 1969.

85. Yen, S.H., Dickson, D.W.., Peterson, C., et al.: Cytoskeletal abnormalities in Neuropathology. Prog. Neuropath., 6:63, 1986.

86. Yagishita, S., et al.: Atypical senile dementia with widespread Lewy type inclusion in the cerebral cortex. Acta Neuropathol. (Berl), 49:187, 1980.

87. Alvord, Jr., E.C., and Forno, L.S.: Pathology. In: Handbook of Parkinson's Disease. (Ed) W.C. Koller. New York, Marcel Dekker, Inc., 1987.

88. Goldman, J.E., Yen, S.H., Chiu, F.C., et al.: Lewy bodies of Parkinson's disease contain neurofilament antigens. Science, 221:1082, 1983.

89. Nakashima, S., and Ikuta, F.: Tyrosine hydroxylase protein in Lewy bodies of Parkinsonian and senile brains. J. Neurol. Sci., 66:91, 1984.

90. Hirsch, E., et al.: Monoclonal antibodies raised against Lewy bodies in brains from subject with Parkinson's disease. Brain Res., 345:374, 1985.

91. Mann, D.M.A., and Yates, P.O.: Possible role of neuromelanin in the pathogenesis of Parkinson's disease. Mech. Ageing Dev., 21:193, 1983.

92. Forno, L.S.: The Lewy body in Parkinson's disease. Advances in Neurology, 45:35, 1986.

93. Graham, D.G.: On the origin and significance of neuromelanin. Arch. Pathol. Lab. Med., 103:359, 1979.

94. Agid, Y., Javoy-Aged, F., and Ruberg, M.: Biochemistry of neurotransmitters in Parkinson's disease. In: Movement Disorders. 2-Neurology. (Eds) C.D. Marsden, and S. Fahn. London, Butterworths, 1987.

95. Forno, L.S., Barbour, P.J., and Norville, R.L.: Presenile dementia with Lewy bodies and neurofibrillary tangles. Arch. Neurol., 35:818, 1978.

96. Burns, R.S., et al.: A primate model of Parkinsonism: selective destruction of dopaminergic neurons in the pars compacta of the substantia nigra by N-methyl-

4-phenyl-1,2,3,6-tetrahydropyridine. Proc. Natl. Acad. Sci. USA, 80:4546, 1983.

97. Lynden, A., Bondersson, U., Larsson, B.S., et al.: Melanin affinity of 1-methyl 4-phenyl-1,2,5,6 tetrahydropyridine, an inducer of chronic Parkinsonism in human. Acta Pharmacol. Toxicol., 53:429, 1983.

98. Forno, L.S., and Norville, R.L.: Locus coeruleus lesion and eosinophilic inclusions in MPTP-induced Parkinsonism in the squirrel monkey X. International Congress of Neuropathology, Stockholm. Abstract No. 430, 1975.

99. Graham, J.G., and Oppenheimer, D.R.: Orthostatic hypotension and nicotine sensitivity in a case of multiple system atrophy. J. Neurol. Neurosurg. Psychiat., 32:28, 1969.

100. Johnson, R.H., Lee, G. de J., Oppenheimer, D.R., and Spalding, J.M.K.: Autonomic failure with orthostatic hypotension due to intermedio-lateral column degeneration. A report of two cases with autopsies. Quart. J. Med., 35:276, 1966.

101. Nick, J.. et al.: Hypotension orthostatique idiopathique avec syndrome neurologique complexe a predominance extra-pyramidale. Etude anatomo-clinique d'un cas. Rev. Neurol. (Paris), 116:213, 1967.

102. Schwartz, G.A.: The orthostatic hypotension syndrome of Shy-Drager. A clinicopathologic report. Arch. Neurol. (Chic), 69:450, 1953.

103. Adams, R.D., van Bogaert, L., and Vander Eecken, H.: Degenerescences nigro-striees et cerebello-nigro-striees. Psychiat. Neurol., 142:219, 1961.

104. Adams, R.D., van Bogaert, L., and Vander Eecken, H.: Striato-nigral degeneration. J. Neuropathol. Exp. Neurol., 23:584, 1964.

105. Scherer, H.J.: Extrapyramidale Storungen bei der olivopontocerebellaren Atrophie. Ein Beitrag zum Problem des lokalen vorzeitigen Alterns. Z. Ges. Neurol. Psychiat., 145:406, 1933.

106. Welte, E.: Die Atrophie des Systems des Brueckenfusses und der unteren Oliven. Arch. Psychiat. Nervenkr., 109:649, 1939.

107. Rosenhagen, H.: Die primare Atrophie des Brueckenfusses und der unteren Oliven (dargestellt nach klinischen und anatomischen Beobachtungen). Arch. Psychiat. Nervenkr., 116:163, 1943.

108. Jellinger, K., and Tarowska-Dziduszko, E.: Die ZNS-Veranderungen bei den olivo-ponto-cerebellaren Atrophien. Z. Neurol., 199:192, 1971.

109. Takei, V., and Mirra, S.S.: Striatonigral Degeneration: A Form of Multiple System Atrophy with Clinical Parkinsonism. Progress in Neuropathology, 2:217, 1973.

110. Berciano, J.: Olivopontocerebellar Atrophy. A review of 177 cases. J. Neuro. Sci., 53:253, 1982.

111. Dejerine, J., and Thomas, A.: L'atrophie olivo-ponto-cerebelleuse. Nouv. Iconogr. Salpet., 13:330, 1900.

112. Duvoisin, R.C., and Plaitakis, A.: The Olivopontocerebellar Atrophies. New York, Raven Press, 1984.

113. Feve, J.R., et al.: Degenerescence striato-nigrique. Etude clinique et anatomique d'un cas ayant reagi tres favorablement a la L-Dopa. Rev. Neurol. (Paris), 133:271, 1977.

114. Koeppen, A.H., Barron, K.D., and Cox, J.F.: Striatonigral Degeneration. Acta Neuropath. (Berl), 19:10, 1971.

115. Borit, A., Rubinstein, L.J., and Urich, H.: The Striatonigral Degenerations: Putaminal Pigments and Nosology. Brain, 98:101, 1975.

116. Boudin, G., Guillard, A., Mikol, J., et al.: Degeneresc-

ence striato-nigrique. A propos del l'etude clinique, therapeutique et anatomique de 2 cas. Rev. Neurol., (Paris), *132*:137, 1976.

117. Michael, D., et al.: Degenerescence striato-nigrique. A propos de deux observations anatomo-cliniques. Rev. Neurol. (Paris), *132*:3, 1976.

118. Gray, F., Vincent, D., and Hauw, J.J.: Multiple system atrophy (MSA). A clinico-pathological study of 23 cases. (in preparation).

119. Oppenheimer, D.R.: Lateral horn cells in progressive autonomic failure. J. Neurol. Sci., *46*:393, 1980.

120. Gray, F., Vincent, D., and Hauw, J.J.: Quantitative study of lateral horn cells in 15 cases of multiple system atrophy. Acta Neuropathol. (Berl), *75*:513, 1988.

121. Oppenheimer, D.R.: Diseases of the basal ganglia, cerebellum and motor neurons. In: *Greenfield's Neuropathology.* (Eds) J.H. Adams, J.A.N. Corsellis, L.W. Duchen. London, Edward Arnold, 1984.

122. Hunt, J.R.: Progressive atrophy of the globus pallidus (primary atrophy of the pallidal system). A system disease of the paralysis agitans type, characterized by atrophy of the motor cells of the corpus striatum. Brain, *40*:58, 97.

123. Bogaert, L. Van: Aspects cliniques et apthologiques des atrophies pallidales et pallido-luysiennes progressives. J. Neurol. Neurosurg. Psychiat., *9*:125, 1946.

124. Jellinger, K.: Progressive Pallidumatrophie. J. Neurol. Sci., *6*:19, 1968.

125. Jellinger, K.: Neuroaxonal dystrophy: its natural history and related disorders. Prog. Neuropath. *2*:129, 1973.

126. Smith, J.K.: Dentato-rubro-pallido-lysian atrophy. In: *Handbook of Clinical Neurology.* Edited by P.J. Vinken, G.W. Bruyn. Amsterdam, North Holland, 1975.

127. Naito, H., and Oyanagi, S.: Familial myoclonus epilepsy and choreoathetosis: Hereditary dentatorubral-pallidoluysian atrophy. Neurology (Ny), *32*:798, 1982.

128. Gray, F., de Baecque, C., Serdaru, M., et al.: Pallido-luyso-nigral atrophy and amyotrophic lateral sclerosis. Acta Neuropathol. (Berl), *Suppl VI11*:348, 1981.

129. Serratrice, G.T., Toga, M., and Pelissier, J.F.: Chronic spinal muscular atrophy and pallidonigral degeneration. Report of a case. Neurology, *33*:306, 1983.

130. Gray, F., et al.: Luyso-pallido-nigral atrophy and amyotrophic lateral sclerosis. Acta Neuropathol. (Berl), *66*:78, 1985.

131. Mayer, J.M., et al.: Familial juvenile parkinsonism with multiple systems degenerations. A clinicopathological study. J. Neurol. Sci., *72*:91, 1986.

132. Titeca, J., and Van Bogaert, L.: Heredodegenerative hemiballismus. A contribution to the question of primary atrophy of the corpus Luysii. Brain, *69*:251, 1946.

133. Contamin, F., Escourolle, R., Nick, J., et al.: Atrophie pallido-nigro-luysienne. Syndrome akinetique avec pallilalie, rigidite oppositionnelle et catatonie. Rev. Neurol. (Paris), *124*:107, 1971.

134. Takahashi, K., Nakashima, R., Takeo, T., et al.: Pallido-nigro-luysial atrophy associated with degeneration of the centrum medianum. A clinico-pathologic and electron-microscopic study. Acta Neuropathol. (Berl), *37*:81, 2977.

135. Kosaka, K., et al.: Pallidonigro-luysial atrophy with massive appearance of corporea amylacea in CNS. Acta Neuropathol. (Berl), *53*:169, 1981.

136. Dubas, F., Gray, F., and Escourolle, R.: Maladie de

Steele-Richardson-Olszewski sans opthalmoplegie six cas anatomo-cliniques. Rev. Neurol. (Paris), *139*:407, 1983.

137. Steele, J.C., Richardson, J.C., and Olszewski, J.: Progressive supranuclear palsy. Arch. Neurol., *10*:333, 1964.

138. Rouzaud, M., et al.: L'ophtalmoplegie supre-nucleaire progressive (Syndrome de Steele-Richardson-Olszewski). Nouvelle observations anatomo-clinque. Rev. Neurol. (Paris), *130*:143, 1974.

139. Ruberg, M., et al.: Dopaminergic and cholinergic lesions in progressive supranuclear palsy. Ann. Neurol., *18*:523, 1985.

140. Verhaart, W.Y.C.: degeneration of brain stem reticular formations, other parts of brain stem and cerebellum: example of heterogeneous degeneration of central nervous system. J. Neuropathol. Exp. Neurol., *17*:382, 1958.

141. Alvord, Jr., E.C., et al.: The Pathology of Parkinsonism: A Comparison of Degenerations in Cerebral Cortex and Brainstem. Advances in Neurol., 5:175, 1974.

142. Brusa, A.: Degenerescence plurisystematisee du nevraxe, de caractere sporadique a debut tardif et evolution prolongee. Rev. Neurol. (Paris), *104*:412, 1961.

143. Brusa, A., Bugiani, O., and Priori, A.: Les degenerescences plurisystematisees du nevraxe. Nouvelle contribution anatomo-clinique. Semin. Hop. Paris, 23:1574, 1967.

144. Weinmann, R.L.: Heterogenous system degeneration of the central nervous system associated with peripheral neuropathy. Neurology, *17*:597, 1967.

145. Chavany, J.A., Van Bogaert L., and Godlewski, S.: Sur un syndrome de rigidite a predominance axiale avec perturbation des automatismes oculo-palpebraux d'origine encephalitique. Press. Med., *50*:958, 1957.

146. Tellez-Nagel, J., and Wisniewski, H.M.: Ultrastructure of neurofibrillary tangles in Steele-Richardson-Olszewski syndrome. Arch. Neurol., *29*:324, 1973.

147. Alvord, Jr., E.C.: The Pathology of Parkinsonism. In: *Pathology of the Nervous System* (I). (Ed) J. Minckler. New York, McGraw-Hill, 1968.

148. Takauchi, S., Mitzuhara, T., and Miyoshi, K.: Unusual paired helical filaments in progressive supranuclear palsy. Acta Neuropathol. (Berl), *59*:225, 1983.

149. Hallervorden, J., and Spatz, H.: Eigenartige erkrankung im extrapyramidalen System mit besonderer Beteiligung des Globus pallidus und der Substantia nigra. Z. Neurol. Psychiat., *79*:254, 1922.

150. Jankovic, J., et al.: Late-onset Hallervorden-Spatz disease presenting as familial parkinsonism. Neurology, *35*:227, 1985.

151. Jellinger, K.: Neuroaxonal dystrophy: its natural history and related disorders. Prog. Neuropath. *2*:129, 1973.

152. Seitelberger, F., and Jellinger, K.: Neuroaxonal dystrophy and Hallervorden-Spatz disease. In: *Scientific Approaches to Clinical Neurology.* (Eds) E.S. Goldensohn, and S.H. Appel, Philadelphia, Lea & Febiger, 1977.

153. Winkelmann, N.W., and Book, M.H.: Asymptomatic extrapyramidal involvement in Pick's disease. A clinical pathological study of two cases. J. Neuropathol. Exp. Neurol., *8*:30, 1948.

154. Escourolle, R.: La maladie de Pick. *Etude critique*

d'ensemble et synthese anatomo-clinique. Foulon, Paris, These Medicine, University of Paris. 1956.

155. Braunmuhl, A. von: Encephalitis epidemica und Synaresislehre. Arch. Psychiat. Nervenkr., *181*:543, 1949.

156. Delay, J., Brion, S., and Escourolle, R.: Les lesions des noyaux gris et du tronc cerebral dans la maladie de Pick. Encephale, *49*:463, 1960.

157. Hirano, A., Dembitzer, H.M., Kurland, L.T., et al.: Parkinsonism-dementia complex, an endemic disease of the island of Guam. I. Clinical features. Brain, *84*:642, 1961.

158. Hirano, A., Malamud, N., and Kurkland, L.T.: Parkinsonism-dementia complex, an endemic disease of the island of Guam. II. Pathological features. Brain, *84*:662, 1961.

159. Hirano, A., Dembitzer, H.M., and Kurland, L.T.: The fine structure of some intraganglionic alterations: neurofibrillary tangles, granulovacuolar bodies and ''rod-like'' structures as seen in Guam amyotrophic lateral sclerosis and Parkinsonism-dementia complex. J. Neuropath. Exp. Neurol., *27*:167, 1968.

160. Wadia, N.H.: A variety of olivopontocerebellar atrophy distinguished by slow eye movements and peripheral neuropathy. In: *The Olivopontocerebellar Atrophies.* (Eds.) by R.C. Duvoisin, and A. Palitakis. New York, Raven Press, 1984.

161. Bonduelle, M., et al.: Atrophie olivo-ponto-cerebelleuse familiale avec myoclonies. Lew limites de lay dyssynergie cerebelleuse myoclonique (Syndrome de Ramsay-Hunt). Rev. Neurol. (Paris), *132*:113, 1976.

162. Rondot, P., de Recondo, J., Davous, P., et al.: Menzel's hereditary ataxia with slow eye movement and myoclonus. A clinico-pathological study. J. Neurol. Sci., *61*:65, 1983.

163. Alajouanine, T., et al.: A propos de l'association ''dyssynergia cerebellaris myoclonica'' de R. Hunt et heredo-degeneration spino-cerebelleuse type Friedreich. Etude clinique et electromyographique d'un cas. Rev. Neuro. (Paris)., *93*:577, 1955.

164. Rosenberg, R.N.: Joseph disease: an autosomal dominant motor system degeneration. Adv. Neuro., *41*:179, 1984.

165. Continho, P., Guimaraes, A., and Scaravilli, F.: The pathology of Machado-Joseph disease. Report of a possible homozygous case. Acta Neuropathol. (Berl) *58*:48, 1982.

166. Chokroverty, S., et al.: Pathology of olivopontocerebellar atrophy with glutamate dehydrogenase deficiency. Neurology (Cleveland), *34*:1451, 1984.

167. Guillain, G., Garcin, R., and Bertrand, I.: Sur un syndrome cerebelleux precede d'un etat hypertonique. Rev. Neurol. (Paris), *1*:565, 1931.

168. Bogaett, L. Van, and Borremans, P.: Sur une atrophie cerebelleuse corticale avec debut de sclerose axiale et atteinte des noyaux gris centraux. Troubles mentaux. Lipomatose symetrique. J. Belge. Neurol. Psychiat., *47*:249, 1947.

169. Carter, H.R., and Sukuvajana, C.: Familial cerebelloolivary degeneration with late development of rigidity and dementia. Neurology (Minn), *6*:876, 1956.

170. Legrand, R., Linquette, M., Delahousse, J., et al.: A propos d'un nouveau cas d'association d'une maladie de Parkinson et d'une sclerose latevale amyotrophique. Rev. Neuro. (Paris), *101*:191, 1959.

171. Bonduelle M., Bouygyes, P., Escourolle, R., et al.: Evolution simultanee chez un meme malade d'une maladie de Parkinson et d'une sclerose laterale amy-

otrophique. Discussion. Rev. Neurol. (Paris), *101*:63, 1959.

172. Bogaert, L. Van, and Radermecker, M.A.: Scleroses laterales amyotrophiques typiques et paralysies agitantes hereditaires dans une meme famille avec une forme de passage possible entre les deux affections. Mschr. Psychiat. Neuro., *127*:185, 1954.

173. Haberlandt, W.F.: Amyotrophische Lateralskerose. Stuttgart, Fischer, 1964.

174. Alvord, Jr., E.C.: Pathology of Parkinsonism. In: *Pathogenesis and Treatment of Parkinsonism.* (Ed) W.S. Fields. Springfield, Charles C Thomas, 1958.

175. Jellinger, K.: Neuropathologic finds after neuroleptic long-term therapy. Neurotoxicology, *114*:25, 1977.

176. Langston, J.W., Ballard, P., Tetrud, J.W. et al.: Chronic parkinsonism in humans due to a product of meperidine-analog synthesis. Science, *219*:979, 1983.

177. von Economo, C.: Encephalitis lethargica. Wiener Klinische Wochenschrift, *30*:581, 1971.

178. von Economo, C.: *Encephalitis lethargica. Its Sequelae and Treatment.* Oxford, Oxford University Press, 1931.

179. Howard, R.S., and Lees, A.J.: Encephalitis lethargica. A report of four recent cases. Brain, *110*:19. 1987.

180. Duvoisin, R.C., and Yahr, M.D.: Encephalitis and Parkinsonism. Arch. Neurol., *12*:227, 1965.

181. Marie, P., and Tretiakoff, C.: Anatomie pathologique de l'encephalite lethargique. Ann. Med., *1*:1, 1920.

182. Tretiakoff, C., and Bremer, F.: Encephalite lethargique avec syndrome parkinsonien et catatonie. Recherches tardives. Verification anatomique. Rev. Neurol. (Paris), *27*:772, 1920.

183. Foix, C.: Les lesions anatomiques de la maladie de Parkinson. Rev. Neurol. (Paris), *1*:566, 1921.

184. Lewy, F.H.: Zur pathologischen Anatomie der Paralysis agitans. Dtsch. Z. Nervenh., *50*:50, 1913.

185. Torvik, A., and Meen, D.: Distribution of the brain stem lesions in postencephalitic Parkinsonism. Acta. Neurol. Scan., *42*:415, 1966.

186. Ishii, T., and Nakamura, Y.: Distribution and ultrastructure of Alzheimer's neurofibrillary tangles in postencephalitic Parkinsonism of Economo type. Acta Neuropathol. (Berl), *55*:59, 1981.

187. Martin, J.P.: The globus pallidus in postencephalitic Parkinsonism. J. Neurol. Sci., *3*:566, 1965.

188. Wisniewski, H., Terry, R.D., and Hirano, A.: Neurofibrillary pathology. J. Neuropathol. Exp. Neuro., *29*:163, 1970.

189. Rossum, A. Van.: Spastic pseudo sclerosis (Creutzfeldt-Jakob disease). In: *Handbook of Clinical Neurology.* Edited by P.J. Vinken, G.W. Bruyn. Amsterdam, North Holland, 1968.

190. Desoille, H.: *Les troubles nerveux dus aux asphyxies aigues (et plus particulierement a l'asphyxie oxycarbonee).* These Medicine, University of Paris. Paris, Le Francois, 1932.

191. Lapresle, J., and Fardeau, M.: The central nervous system and carbon monoxide poisoning. II. Anatomical study of brain lesions following intoxication with carbon monoxide (22 cases). Prog. Brain Res., *24*:31, 1967.

192. Edsall, D.L., and Drinker, C.T.: *The Clinical Aspect of Chronic Manganese Poisoning.* Contribution of medical and biological research. Dedicated to Sir William Osler. New York, Paul B. Hoeber, 1919.

193. Stadler, H.: Zur Histopathologie des Gehirns bei Manganvergiftung. Z. Ges. Neurol. Psychiat., *154*:62, 1935.

194. Parnitzke, K.H., and Peiffer, J.: Zuf Klinik und pathologishen Anatomie der chronischen Braunsteinvergiftung. Arch. Psychiat. Nervenhilk, *192*:405, 1954.

195. Canavan, M.M., Cobb, S., and Drinker, C.K.: Chronic manganese poisoning. Report of a case with autopsy. Arch. Neuro. Psychiat. (Chic.), *32*:501, 1934.

196. Pentschew, A., Ebner, F.F., and Kovatch, R.M.: Experimental manganese encephalopathy in monkeys. J. Neuropathol. Exp. Neurol., *22*:488, 1963.

197. Souques, A.: Les syndromes Parkinsoniens. Rev. Neurol. (Paris)., *1*:534, 1921.

198. Alvord, Jr., E.C.: An Interpretation with Special Reverence to Other Changes in the Aging Brain. In: *The Pathology of Parkinsonism.* (Eds) R. McDowell, and M. Markham. Philadelphia, F.A. Davis Co., 1971.

199. Eadie, M.J., and Sutherland, J.M.: Arteriosclerosis in Parkinsonism. J. Neurol. Neurosurg. Psychiat., *27*:237, 1964.

200. Schwab, R.S., England, A.C.: Parkinson syndromes due to various specific causes. In: *Handbook in Clinical Neurology.* (Eds) P.J. Vinken, and G.W. Bruyn. Amsterdam, North Holland, 1968.

201. Hunter, R., Smith, J., Thomson, T., et al., Hemiparkinson with infarction of the ipsilateral substantia nigra. Neuropathol. Appl. Neurobiol., *4*:297, 1978.

202. Sciarra, D., and Sprofkin, B.E.: Symptoms and signs referable to the basal ganglia in brain tumors. Arch. Neurol. Psychiat. (Chic.), *69*:450, 1953.

203. Tolosa, E., Vilato, J., and Fuemayor, B.: Parkinsonisme tumoral. Neurochirurgie, *12*:555, 1966.

204. Blocq, P., and Marinesco, G.: Sur un cas de tremblement Parkinsonien hemiplegique symptomatique d'une tumeur du pedoncule cerebral. Rev. Neuro. (Paris), *2*:265, 1894.

205. Gherardi, R., et al.: Parkinsonian syndrome and central nervous system lymphoma involving the substantia nigra. A case report. Acta Neuropathol. (Berl), *65*:338, 1985.

206. Van Eck, J.H.: Parkinsonism as a misleading brain tumor syndrome. Psychiatr. Neurol. Neurochir., *64*:109, 1961.

207. Garcia de Ybenes, J., et al.: Biochemical findings in a case of Parkinsonism secondary to brain tumor. Ann. Neuro., *11*:313, 1982.

208. Lhermitte, F., Agid, Y., Serdaru, M., et al.: Syndrome Parkinsonien, tumeur frontale et L-Dopa. Rev. Neuro (Paris), *140*:138, 1984.

209. Coers, C., Kleyntjens, F., and Brihaye, J.: Syndrome Parkinsonien d'origine tumorale. Acta Neurol. Belg., *52*:737, 1952.

210. Grant, F.C.: The parkinsonian syndrome and brain tumor: a report of a case. Arch. Neurol. Psychiat. (Chic), *65*:784, 1951.

211. Grimberg, L.: Paralysis agitans and trauma. J. Nerv. Ment. Dis., *79*:14, 1934.

212. Lindenberg, R.: Die Schaedigungsmechanismen der Substantia nigra bei Hirntraumen und das Problem des posttraumatischen Parkinsonismus. Dtsch. Z. Nervenheilk., *185*:637, 1964.

213. Corsellis, J.A.N., Bruton, C.J., and Freeman-Browne, D.: The aftermath of boxing. Psychol. Med., *3*:270, 1973.

9

Nutritional Disorders and Alcoholism

SERGE DUCKETT and
SCOTT SCHOEDLER

The most important cause of ill health and death in the world today is malnutrition. Children and the elderly are primarily affected. The clinical and pathologic consequences of malnutrition were clearly described by physicians studying the victims of the famine during the Paris Commune of 1871, the Spanish Civil War (1936 to 1939), World War I, and World War II, particularly in concentration and prisoner-of-war camps. Parrot in 1887[1] published the first textbook on the effects of malnutrition on children. The important contributions of the German school of neuropathology to the field of nutritional disorders begins in 1881 with Karl Wernicke's description of a thiamine deficient encephalopathy and goes on to include the studies of Heilbronner, Bonnhaeffer, and Homen, to name a few.[2,3] Nobecourt in 1916[4] described the classic clinical picture of the undernourished of all ages. In 1935, Jackson[5] wrote the first comprehensive textbook on the effects of malnutrition on humans and animals. Spanish physicians described the effects of malnutrition on the civilian population during the Spanish Civil War. Grande and Peraita in 1941 wrote a monograph which described the effects of famine on 3000 patients in Madrid.[6] In 1947, Spillane[2] wrote a classic textbook on nutritional disorders of the human nervous system based largely on his personal experience as a neurologist in the British Army during World War II with access to prisoner-of-war victims of all warring nations.

Malnutrition is total or selective. Total starvation or marasmus sadly enough is often the result of man's actions, through concentration camps, war, or by his inactivity as in Ethiopia. Marasmus simply means no food and it maims or kills 10 million humans a year.[7,8] Selective malnutrition is caused by insufficient amounts of proteins, vitamins, or essential minerals in the diet.[9]

Nutritional disorders are common in older citizens living at home or in institutions. It may be caused by lack of appetite or proper food. Lack of appetite may be the result of a psychologic problem such as bereavement, loneliness, disinterest or disease. Lack of proper food is the result of dietary ignorance, poverty, geographic location, or seasonal deprivation. Recommended dietary allowances (RDA) have been proposed by the Food and Nutrition Board of the National Academy of Sciences.[10]

An adequate protein-calorie intake is essential for elderly citizens. An insufficient, unbalanced intake of proteins, carbohydrates, and lipids has a quicker and more serious consequence in young and older humans than in those age 15 to 55. An inadequate diet results in a reduction of physical activity and energy is drawn from their own tissues. Subcutaneous and muscle fats are used initially and this is evident by the emaciation of the patient. Proteins are required for gluconeogenesis. Once the source of fats is exhausted the patient is mentally and physically depressed coupled with hypotension, collapse, and death.

VITAMIN DEFICIENCIES[9]

Vitamin B deficiencies which can result in a pathologic condition of the peripheral and central nervous system are thiamine hydrochloride (B_1), nicotinic acid, riboflavin, and pantothenic acid (B_2 group); pyridoxine (B_6); cyanocobalamin and related compounds (B_{12}). The evidence that deficiencies in riboflavin, pantothenic acid, and pyridoxine results in a pathologic condition of the nervous system is largely based on experimental work.

Thiamine deficiency is associated with beriberi and Wernicke's encephalopathy. Beriberi is a disease of the peripheral nerves (dry beriberi) or of the heart (wet beriberi). The peripheral neuropathy is characterized by a sensation of pins and needles particularly in the feet and hands and in the lower limbs sometimes associated to motor problems, namely a foot drop. Retrobulbar neuritis occurs in some patients. The neuropathy appears to be caused by an accumulation of lactate and pyruvate in Schwann cells and neurons. It begins at the periphery with demyelination followed by axonal pathology (dying-back phenomenon). Wernicke's disease may be acute, subacute, or chronic. There are brainstem signs, convulsions, disturbances of consciousness, and

coma. The typical capillary lesions are situated in the grey matter around the third and fourth ventricles and the aqueduct with involvement of the mamillary bodies, the medial thalamic nuclei, the inferior colliculi, and the regions of the vestibular and dorsal vagal nuclei. The optic chiasma is sometimes involved.

Pellagra is caused by a deficiency of nicotinic acid. It has a classical triad of symptoms ("diarrhea, dermatitis, and dementia") that is gastrointestinal problems, a red erythema followed by well-demarcated pigmentation of the skin and neurologic signs, dementia, and distal polyneuropathy with corticospinal tract involvement. There are widespread involvements of the larger neurons of the cerebrum and demyelination of the posterior and lateral columns of the spinal cord and brainstem.

Vitamin B_{12} deficiency referred to as subacute combined degeneration of the spinal cord is usually associated with a macrocytic anemia. The disease also involves the cerebrum with manifestations of anxiety, depression, and hallucinations. There is progressive damage to the corticospinal tracts and posterior columns in the spinal cord and a polyneuropathy characterized by pins and needles sensation in the extremities and a glove and stocking impairment of sensation conveyed by the large myelinated fibers. Physiologic studies suggest that the neuropathy is of the "dying back" variety.

ETHYL ALCOHOL INTOXICATION

Detailed neuropathologic observations of the human nervous system following death due to alcoholic intoxication are rare and difficult to evaluate because of coexisting nutritional deficiencies and cardiovascular disease.[11] Similarly the definition of the manifestations of chronic alcohol intoxication was considered difficult for years because of associated health problems. With laboratory animals, however, these problems have been largely resolved by experimental work and extensive clinico-pathologic studies of humans.[12-40] It is now established that the habitual intake of ethyl alcohol can permanently injure the cerebrum and cerebellum [Fig. 9–1]. So-called alcoholic neuropathy is now as-

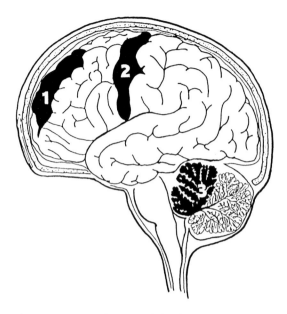

Fig. 9–1. Lateral view of the human brain. The black areas represent the parts of the CNS most affected by chronic ethyl alcohol intoxication, namely the superior frontal gyrus (1), the ascending frontal gyrus (2), and the superior portion of the vermis (3).

sumed to be the result of a nutritional deficiency. It is also established that Marchiafava-Bignami disease, cortical laminar astrocytosis of Morel, and central pontine myelinosis are caused by nutritional deficiencies and not directly by alcohol [See Chap. 3].

Alcoholism in the elderly carries with it a host of medical and social disabilities not seen in younger groups. The impact of alcoholism upon the elderly is grossly magnified by physical and psychologic problems inherent in advanced age. Alcohol has direct and indirect effects upon the elderly. The direct effect of alcohol in the human CNS is the destruction of neurons and atrophy of associated white matter in the cerebrum and cerebellum. Only recently, though, has the prevalance and the specific pathologic change in the brains of alcoholics been quantified. Much of the indirect impact is mediated through malnutrition. Since nutritional disorders are common in the elderly, alcohol presents an excess of empty calories and may lead to protein malnutrition and thiamine deficiency.[9]

THE EFFECT OF ALCOHOLIC INTOXICATION ON THE CEREBRUM

Predisposing Factors. Moderate intake, defined as 30 to 80 g per day of alcohol, translates into 3 to 8 glasses of wine or mixed drinks with 1 ounce of liquor.[12] There is no significant evidence that moderate alcohol consumption causes pathologic change in the brain. Neural tissue loss and an increase in pericerebral space and ventricular volume has been noted in the brains of humans who habitually drink more than the "moderate intake". Alcoholics have been grouped according to intake of more than 80 g of ethyl alcohol per day.[12]

The concept of predisposing factors toward developing brain damage from chronic alcohol use has been entertained. It has been noted that cortical shrinkage secondary to neurotoxic effects of alcohol is not uniformly seen among all alcoholics. Variations in the extent of CNS damage have been noted in individuals drinking similar amounts. In fact, there are no pathologic changes in the brains of a large number of alcoholics despite formidable drinking histories. Conversely, half to ⅔ of alcoholics suffer cortical shrinkage, many with relatively moderate alcohol abuse. Genetic predisposition and/or gender might also contribute toward developing brain atrophy. Lishman and Bergman[13,14] demonstrated that females develop at least equivalent pathologic changes with less severe drinking histories than do their male counterparts. This evidence is based on in vivo CT study of sulcal width and neuropsychologic testing.

Common medical problems associated with chronic alcoholism—liver cirrhosis, vitamin deficiency, and malnutrition—must also be considered when evaluating alcoholic neuropathology. Researchers have compensated for this potential interference by distinguishing alcoholics from those with cirrhosis and those with Wernicke's encephalopathy.[13,15–18] Observed increases in the severity of neuropathology among the groups might be taken to represent a measure of alcohol exposure. Particularly, it seem that alcoholics with Wernicke's develop cerebellar atrophy more frequently. In Torvik's study[16] the cirrhotic alcoholic subgroup showed a near equal incidence with and without cerebellar atrophy. Thus, he propends the mechanisms for liver cirrhosis and cerebellar atrophy are separate.

Alcohol and Aging. Advanced age has been correlated with cortical atrophy and ventricular dilatation; this pathologic condition overlaps with that of chronic alcoholism.[13] It is hypothesized that alcohol abuse accelerates the normal aging process in the brain.[13,19] Studies looking at the neuropathology of alcoholism in older age groups have difficulty differentiating the effects of age from those of alcohol abuse. This coincidence of aging is seen measuring different CNS parameters, brain weight, and Purkinje cell density, but probably represents a common end-point of many disease processes, neuronal death, and brain shrinkage.[13] There is rather convincing evidence, based on CT indices, that advanced age may make the brain more vulnerable to de novo exposure to alcohol. Lishman et al.[13] demonstrated that late onset alcoholics with comparatively short abuse histories develop equivalent cortical changes when compared to the early onset group of similar age. More to the point, older brains seem to catch up quickly, pathologically speaking, with less alcohol exposure.

Further evidence comparing alcoholic brain disorders to changes seen in aged brains comes from studying cerebral white matter water content.[20] It is reported that brain water content increases with age and with chronic alcohol use. This observation is based on pathologic and MRI studies and probably complements the data indicating brain shrinkage and ventricular dilatation in alcoholics and the elderly.[21,22]

Brain Weight and Alcoholism. The initial neuropathologic investigations of chronic al-

coholism centered on gross parameters of brain weight, volume, and ventricular volume. Previous CT studies of the brain repeatedly showed diffuse atrophy preferring the frontal lobe followed by the temporal, parietal, and occipital.[23] Overall brain weight is demonstrated to decrease 30 to 100 g in alcoholics compared to controls in all age groups except greater than 70 years.[12,13,16,17,20] Table 9–1 shows that brain weight is uniformly decreased (80 to 110 g) with advancing age. Thus, in the greater than 70 year age group it is difficult to hold alcohol abuse solely responsible for brain atrophy.[16]

A sensitive parameter for detecting brain shrinkage is the pericerebral space (PICS), the volume between the brain and the skull.[16,24] PICS determinations in alcoholics are consistent with the data of diminished brain weights, indicating that the alcoholic brain suffers a volume loss as well as mass loss.[12,17,20] Pathologic specimens were analyzed for % water content in control and alcoholic white matter.[20] The frontal lobe in alcoholics with Wernicke's syndrome contained significantly more water than in controls. Elevated water content was noted in all lobes of alcoholic samples, however, only the frontal lobe was significant. Data on this topic vary,[20,25–27] though, MRI examination of cortex and white matter free water content indicates a decrease during acute intoxication followed by an increase during withdrawal and abstinence.[20–22] This initial decrease of free water during intoxication may reflect an osmotic and/or diuretic phenomenon of ethyl alcohol. It is safe to infer that chronic, irreversible cerebral weight loss is not due to dehydration; consequently, cerebral shrinkage must be secondary to a loss of neural components. Supporting evidence for this

TABLE 9–1.   The Weight of the Brains of Normal Controls and Alcoholics According to Age.

Age groups	Alcoholics		Controls		Weight diff. (g)	P-values (t-test)
	No. of cases	Brain weight (g)	No. of cases	Brain weight (g)		
40–49	64	1436(±113)	39	1494(±108)	58	P=0.01
50–59	157	1423(±118)	111	1451(±116)	28	P=0.06
60–69	215	1384(±117)	236	1450(±122)	66	P<0.001
70–79	109	1372(±109)	200	1381(±108)	9	P>0.10
Total	545	1399(±116)	586	1430(±115)	31	P<0.001

From Torvik, A.: Acta. Med. Scand. *717*:47, 1987.

hypothesis comes from measuring the overall cerebral cross-sectional area of pathologic specimens in multiple coronal planes [Fig. 9–2]. Significantly, diminished cerebral area was determined in the alcoholic group and ranged from 3.8% (caudate, putamen, nucleus accumbens) to 9.4% (anterofrontal).[18] It is clear that cerebral mass and volume suffer quantitatively from alcoholism independent of the consequences of liver cirrhosis and nutritional factors. The data, at least grossly, support the idea that a pathologic condition of an alcoholic brain resembles an acceleration of the normal aging process.[13,19]

Grey and White Matter Changes in Alcoholics. Another area of interest in alcoholic intoxication has been the effect of the alcohol on the grey and white matter of the brain. De la Monte[18] noted a significant disparity of tissue loss in the grey and white matters of the alcoholic brain [Fig. 9–2]. Area of the cerebral cortex in alcoholic brains was 2.5 to 4.2% less than in controls. A small but significant decrease of grey matter was detected at all coronal levels. White matter in alcoholic samples suffered the greatest, with losses ranging from 6.1% in the occipital parietal (OCP) to 17.5% in the anterofrontal (AF). The ventricular volumes were 31.9 to 71% greater in the alcoholic group than in controls. It is interesting to note that the amount of ventricular enlargement nearly equals the degree of white matter dissolution. The author propends that ventricular enlargement compensates for the white matter atrophy and that a situation of hydrocephalus ex vacuo exists.[18] The white matter atrophy was noted in alcoholic neuropathology in other studies.[12,17,18,28] No pathognomonic lesion has been identified to account for white matter atrophy.[18,29] A unifying idea has been alluded to by many researchers, namely that axonal degeneration associated with neuronal cell

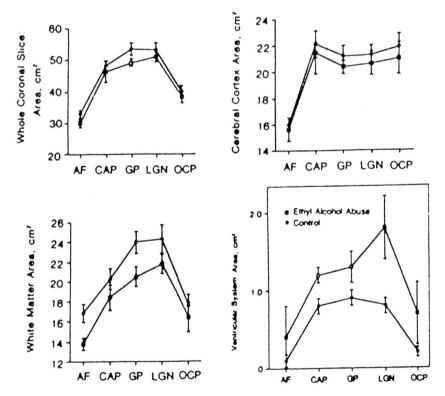

Fig. 9–2. Comparisons of the sizes of the grey and white matter, whole brain coronal sections and ventricles of alcoholic patients and normal controls. The measurements were done at five standardized levels: anterior frontal (AF); head of the caudate nucleus, putamen and nucleus accumbens (CAP); globus pallidus with amygdala (GP); hippocampus with lateral geniculate nucleus (LGN); parietal-occipital fissure (OCP). [de la Monte, S.M.: Arch. Neurol. 45:990, 1988]

TABLE 9–2. The Size of Large and Small Neurons in the Cerebral Cortex of Alcoholic Patients and Normal Controls. Values are expressed as mean area (SD)($\times 103$/mm^3). Alco + WE = alcoholics with Wernicke's encephalopathy; alco + cir = alcoholics with cirrhosis of the liver. *P < 0.05); **P < 0.001.

	Superior frontal cortex		Motor cortex	
	Large	Small	Large	Small
Control n = 22	8.7 (2.1)	18.0 (2.7)	8.5 (2.0)	18.7 (2.7)
Alcoholic n = 22	4.2** (3.0)	16.8 (7.6)	7.5 (2.6)	21.3 (6.3)
Alco + WE n = 4	3.7** (2.9)	15.0 (5.4)	7.3* (2.4)	21.2 (8.5)
Alco + cir n = 6	3.9** (3.7)	17.5 (11.1)	6.0* (1.9)	22.5* (6.1)

From Harper, C., et al.: J. Neurol. Sc. 92:81, 1989.

cell death in the cortex would primarily be manifested first as a pathologic condition of white matter.[17,18]

Different areas in the cerebral cortex were considered as well as cellular constituents and laminar populations. Actual cortical cell counts were performed on alcoholic brains with particular attention to the large (greater than 90 μm) cell populations.[15] Harper et al.[17] demonstrated significant neuronal dropout and a decrease in mean cellular area in the superior frontal gyrus of alcoholics.[15] In the motor cortex, only a decrease in the mean cellular area was detected, neuronal cell count did not differ significantly from controls. Conversely, glial cell concentration was elevated in the superior frontal gyrus of alcoholics.[17] It seems that alcohol preferentially targets the superior frontal gyrus in precipitating neuronal cell death and causes a reactive gliosis [Table 9–2 and Fig. 9–3]. Neuronal cell shrinkage is uniformly observed in the superior frontal gyrus and motor cortical regions, however, the author suggests that there may be a selective loss of the larger cells rather than a shrinkage of all neurons, since cell area was expressed as a mean.[17]

The loss of the small neurons in Alzheimer's disease and in aging does not have the same topographic and morphologic characteristics as that noted in the brain of alcoholics, however, that of the larger neurons are similar.[15,31,32] The data on neuronal cell drop out in advanced age vary. However, Harper et al.[5] demonstrated a significant age related loss of large (greater than 90 μm) cortical neurons throughout the superior frontal gyrus. Others

have agreed on a yearly fallout of 0.8 to 1.0%.[15,33–35] The observation that large cortical neurons are at risk probably reflects a high metabolic rate or some innate fragility common to highly specialized, irreplaceable cells. More specific determination of cortical atrophy in alcoholics attempts to localize cell loss to a particular cortical lamina. The superior frontal cortex of alcoholic brain specimens was arbitrarily partitioned into three layers roughly corresponding to laminae I to VI. Nearly equivalent neuron loss (20%) was detected in all regions.[15]

THE EFFECT OF ALCOHOLIC INTOXICATION ON THE CEREBELLUM

Cerebellar degeneration is the neuropathologic hallmark of alcoholism.[36] Atrophy of the cerebellar vermis has been the focus of much attention and is associated with a specific neurologic syndrome. There is a good correlation between the anatomic insult and functional impairment in the cerebellum of alcoholics. The somatic anatomy is projected upon the vermian cortex, with the anterior/superior vermis corresponding to the lower extremities. The selective impact of alcoholism on the anterosuperior vermis, therefore, results in difficulty standing and walking.

Cerebellar Degeneration. Alcohol induced ataxia is a grave problem to the elderly individual. Pre-existing deficits in sight, balance, and strength combined with a self-inflicted ataxia can have disastrous results. This

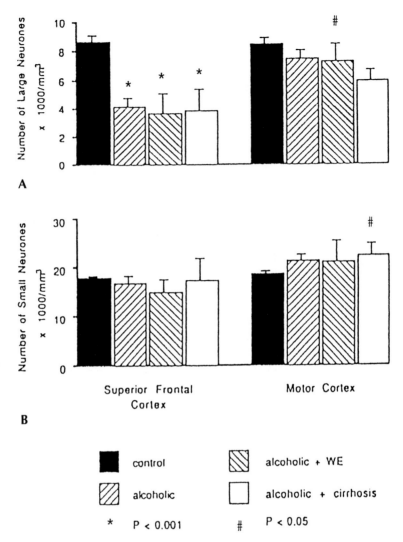

Fig. 9-3. The numbers of (A) large (> 90 μm²) and (B) small (41–90 μm²) neurons in the superior frontal and motor cortices. [Harper, C., et al. J. Neurol. Sc. 92:81, 1989]

is especially pertinent to individuals suffering from osteoporosis and those who live alone.

There is evidence that cerebellar atrophy is associated with aging. An age related atrophy in vermian cortex and Purkinje cells exists and is indistinguishable from that seen in alcoholism.[37-39] Torvik et al.[39] demonstrated an association between age and Purkinje cell density in the normal human vermis [Fig. 9–4]. Figure 9–5 illustrates the traditional division of the cerebellar vermis into three segments. There is a clear association between age and Purkinje cell density [Figure 9–4]. Thus, segment I, the superior vermis, is the most severely affected of the segments in the aging cerebellum. Most

of the pathologic changes occur after 70 years of age. The atrophy involves the granular, molecular, and Purkinje cell layer, which is identical to the change seen in alcoholism. Considerable individual variation in the degree of Purkinje cell loss can be appreciated in Figure 9–4. No atrophy of the cerebellar hemispheres is noted in the aging or alcoholic cerebellum.

It is generally agreed that the diagnosis of alcoholic cerebellar atrophy in patients over 70 years should be made carefully, particularly in light of the great variation with respect to age. It is also evident as seen above that the atrophic changes specific for the superior vermis might be due to physiologic aging.[37-39]

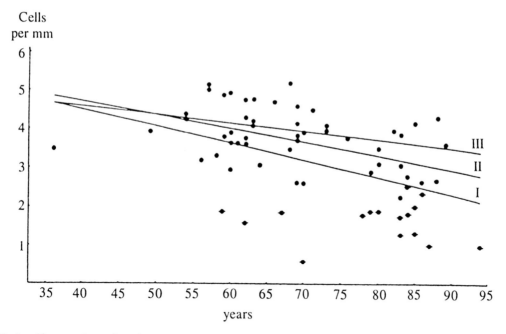

Fig. 9–4. The number of Purkinje cells per mm2 in the three segments of the vermis of normal aging patients. I—P<0.001; II—P<0.001; III—P<0.001. [Torvik, A., et al.: J. Neurol. Sc. 76:283, 1986]

Cerebellar Vermis and Alcoholism. Clinical observations suggest that cerebellar atrophy, particularly of the superior vermis, is common though variable among alcoholics. A recent study demonstrated superior vermal atrophy in 42% of alcoholics and 9% in controls.[38] Previously, a study of 8735 autopsy specimens (713 alcoholics) found histologic evidence of vermal atrophy in 26.8% of alcoholics and 1.7% in controls.[39] The true prevalence is probably at least 42% since, as the author points out, the latter study is based on a more rigid definition of atrophy.[28] It is interesting to note that superior vermal atrophy is detected in 1.7% and 9% in non-alcoholic controls. It is reasonable to assume that these few cases represent alcoholics in the denial phase. Also, the mean age of the control group in one study was 58 years.[38] The 9% prevalence of cerebellar atrophy in this control group, therefore, is generally consistent with the data on aging non-alcoholics in which 9% of individuals less than 70 years had cerebellar atrophy.[40]

It has been recognized for years that alcohol impacts primarily upon the superior vermis.[36] Recently, more specific examinations of the vermis in alcoholics have further localized and quantified the atrophy. For this purpose, a convenient parameter to evaluate is Purkinje cell concentration within the vermian cortex.[16,37,38] The vermis is divided anatomically into three segments; superior (I), posterior (II),

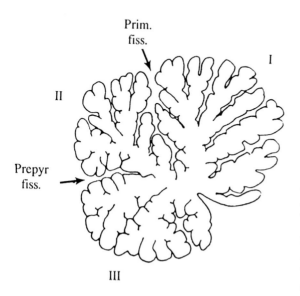

Fig. 9–5. This figure refers to Table 9–5. Sagittal section of the normal cerebellar vermis indicating the three segments, I, II, III. [Torvik, A., et al.: J. Neurol. Sc. 76:283, 1986]

TABLE 9–3. Purkinje Cell Densities/mm in the Three Segments of the Cerebellar Vermis of Alcoholic Patients and Normal Controls

	Controls (n = 36)	Alcoholics (n = 31)	Difference	P-values
Segment I*)	3.77(±0.98)	2.58(±1.34)	1.19	P<0.001
Segment II*)	4.08(±0.97)	3.21(±1.25)	0.87	P=0.01
Segment III*)	4.24(±0.73)	3.90(±0.84)	0.34	P<0.1
Ratio I:III	0.85(±0.19)	0.65(±0.29)	0.20	P=0.001

From Torvik, A., et al.: J. Neurol. Sc. 76:283, 1986.

and inferior (III) [Fig. 9–5]. The superior vermis in alcoholics has been shown to lose nearly 30% of its Purkinje cell population when compared to non-alcoholics[16,37,38] [Table 9–3]. The posterior segment suffers a less but significant decline, followed by the inferior segment.[16,38] These results are generally supported by data provided by Phillips et al.,[37] but vary somewhat with regard to the inferior segment (III). They found evidence for significant Purkinje cell attrition in the small lobes of the inferior segment without observing any change in segment II. Also, it was concluded that the small lobes anteriorly (A,B,C,I,J) [Fig. 9–6] in the vermis are at particular risk from alcohol abuse.[37]

Further histologic characterization of vermal atrophy in alcoholics comes from the examination of other cerebellar constituents. Determinations of histologic area from representative cortical segments shows that the alcoholic superior vermis is diminished by 26% (p< .05). The molecular layer in the cortex is predominantly responsible with a 39% (p<.05) area reduction, although the granular and medullary layers also contribute to the atrophy.[37] It is suggested that the molecular layer is the most sensitive indicator of alcohol abuse; it could be deduced that regions of high synaptic content manifest greater change than those of high cellular content.[37] This is reminiscent of the change seen in cerebral white matter in alcoholics. Additionally, the convexity of the vermian cortex is afflicted more than the depths of the sulci.[36,37,40]

CONCLUSION

Nutritional disorders and chronic alcohol intoxication are the major cause of ill health and death of elderly humans in the world. An important achievement of physicians during recent decades has been the clarification of the clinical manifestations caused by malnutrition distinct from those caused by chronic alcohol intoxication.

Recently, evidence has been presented that suggests that the physical vulnerability to the effects of alcohol may be an inherited trait.[41-43] Blum and his colleagues[44] have reported that at least one form of alcoholism may be caused by a gene location on the q22-q23 region of chromosome 11 which renders humans usually susceptible to the nefarious effects of alcohol.

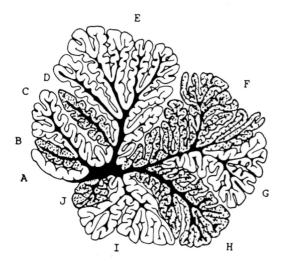

Fig. 9–6. Sagittal section of the cerebellar vermis of alcoholic patients. Areas A, B, C, I, J are the parts of the vermis with a depleted Purkinje cell population. [Phillips, S.C., et al.: Brain, *110*:301, 1987]

REFERENCES

1. Parrot, J.: Cliniques des Nouveaux-Nes. L Athrepsie. Paris, Masson, 1877.
2. Spillane, J.D.: Nutritional Disorders of the Nervous System. Edinburgh, E. & S. Livingstone Pub. Ltd., 1947.
3. Krucke, W.: Erkrankungen des peripheren Nervensystems. In: Handbuch der Speziellen Pathologischen Anatomie und Histologie (Vol. 5). Berlin, Springer Verlag, 1955.

4. Nobecourt, P.: Des hypotrophies et des cachexies des nourissons. Arch. Med. Eng., *19*:113;169;234;301. 1916.

5. Jackson, C.M.: *The Effects of Inanition and Malnutrition upon Growth and Structure.* Philadelphia, Blakiston, 1925.

6. Grande, F., and Peraita, M.: *Avitaminosis y Sistema Nervioso.* Madrid, Miguel Servet, 1941.

7. Duckett, S., and Winick, M.: Malnutrition and Brain Dysfunction. In: *Brain Dysfunction in Children: Etiology, Diagnosis.* Edited by P. Black. New York, Raven Press, 1981.

8. Young, V.R., and Scrimshaw, N.S.: The physiology of starvation. Sci. Am., *225*:114, 1971.

9. Gupta, K.L., Dworkin, B., and Gambert, S.R.: Common nutritional disorders in the elderly: Atypical manifestations. Geriatrics, *43(2)*:87, 1988.

10. Recommended Dietary Allowances. Food and Nutrition Board. National Academy of Sciences, Washington, DC, 1980.

11. Courville, C.B., and Myers, R.D.: Effects of extraneous poisons on the nervous system: alcohols. Bull. Los Angeles Neurol. Soc., *19*:66, 1954.

12. Harper, C., Kril, J., and Daly, J.: Does a "moderate" alcohol intake damage the brain? J. Neurol., Neurosurg., Psychiat., *51*:909, 1988.

13. Lishman, W.A., Jacobson, R.R., and Acker, C.: Brain damage in alcoholism: Current concepts. Acta Med. Scand. (suppl), *717*:5, 1987.

14. Bergman, H.: Brain dysfunction related to alcoholism: Some results from KARTAD project, In: *Neuropsychology of Alcoholism: Implications for Diagnosis and Treatment.* Edited by O.A. Parsons, N. Butters, F. Nathan, New York, Guilford Press, 1987.

15. Harper, C., and Kril, J.: Patterns of neuronal loss in the cerebral cortex in chronic alcoholic patients. J. Neurol. Sc., *92*:81, 1989.

16. Torvik, A.: Brain lesions in alcoholics: Neuropathological observations. Acta Med. Scand., *717*:47, 1987.

17. Harper, C., Kril, J., and Daly, J.: Are we drinking our neurons away? Br. Med. J., *294*:534, 1987.

18. de la Monte, S.M.: Disproportionate atrophy of cerebral white matter in chronic alcoholics. Arch. Neurol., *45*:990, 1988.

19. Wilkinson, D.A., and Carl, P.L.: Relationship of neuropsychological test performance to brain morphology in amnesic and non-amnesic chronic alcoholics. Acta Psychiat. Scand., *62(286)*:89, 1980.

20. Harper, C.G., Kril., J. and Daly, J.M.: Brain shrinkage in alcoholics is not caused by changes in hydration: A pathological study. J. Neurol., Neurosurg., Psychiat., *51*:124, 1988.

21. Beeson, J.A.E., et al.: Nuclear magnetic resonance observations in alcoholic cerebral disorder and the role of vasopressin. Lancet, *2*:923, 1981.

22. Smith, M.A., et al.: Brain water in chronic alcoholic patients measured by magnetic resonance imaging. Lancet, *1*:1273, 1985.

23. Cala, L.A.: Is CT scan a valid indicator of brain atrophy in alcoholism? Acta Med. Scand., *717*:27, 1987.

24. Harper, C., Kril, J., Raven, D., and Jones, N.: Intracranial cavity volumes: A new method and its potential applications. Neuropathol. Applied Neurobiol., *10*:25, 1984.

25. Lesch, P., Schmidt, E., and Schmidt, W.: Effects of chronic alcohol abuse on the structural lipids in the brain. Z Klin. Chem. Klin. Biochem., *10*:410, 1972.

26. Shaw, D.M., et al.: Electrolyte content of the brain in alcoholism. Br. J. Psychiat., *116*:185, 1970.

27. Shaw, D.M., Frizel, D., Camps, F.E., and White, S.: Brain electrolytesin depressive and alcoholic suicides. Br. J. Psychiat., *115*:69, 1969.

28. Harper, C.G., Kril, J.J., and Holloway, R.L.: Brain shrinkage in chronic alcoholics: A pathological study. Br. Med. J. Clin. Res., *290*:510, 1985.

29. Victor, M., and Adams, R.D.: The Alcoholic Dementias. In: *Handbook of Clinical Neurology* (vol. 2). Edited by P.J. Vinken, et al. Amsterdam, Elsevier Science Pub., 1985.

30. Palay, S.L., et al.: General morphology of neurons on neurolglia. In: *The Nervous System* (section 1). *Handbook of Physiology.* Edited by E.R. Kandel. Bethesda, Am. Physiolog. Soc., 1977.

31. Terry, R.D. et al.: Some morphometric aspects of the brain in senile dementia of the Alzheimer type. Ann. Neurol., *10*:184, 1981.

32. Terry, R.D., De Teresa, R., and Hansen, L.: Neocortical cell counts in normal human adult aging. Ann. Neurol., *21*:530, 1981.

33. Brody, H.: Organization of the cerebral cortex. III. A study of aging in the human cerebral cortex. J. Comp. Neurol., *102*:511, 1955.

34. Hubbard, B.M., and Beeson, J.A.E.: A quantitative study of cerebral atrophy in old age and senile dementia. J. Neurol., Sci., *50*:135, 1981.

35. Haug, H.: Are neurons of the human cerebral cortex really lost during aging? A morphometric examination. In: *Senile Dementia of the Alzheimer Type.* Edited by J. Traber, W. Grispen. Berlin, Springer-Verlag, 1985.

36. Victor, M., Adams, R.D., and Mancall, E.L.: A restricted form of cerebellar cortical degeneration occuring in alcoholic patients. Arch. Neurol. (Chic.), *1*:579, 1959.

37. Phillips, S.C., Harper, C.G., and Kril, J.: A quantitative histologic study of the cerebellar vermis in alcoholic patients. Brain, *110*:301, 1987.

38. Torvik, A., and Torp, S.: The prevalence of alcoholic cerebellar atrophy: A morphometric and histologic study of an autopsy material. J. Neurol. Sc., *75*:43, 1986.

39. Torvik, A., Lindbor, C.F., and Rodge, S.: Brain lesions in alcoholics: A neuropathological study with clinical correlations. J. Neurol. Sc., *76*:283, 1986.

40. Torvik, A., Torp, S., and Lindboe, C.F.: Atrophy of the cerebellar vermis in aging: a morphologic and histologic study. J. Neurol. Sc., *76*:283, 1986.

41. Devor, E.J., and Cloniger, C.R.: Genetics of alcoholism. Ann. Rev. Genet., *23*:19, 1989.

42. Tabakoff, B., and Hoffman, P.L.: Genetics and biological markers of risk for alcoholism. Pub. Health. Rep., *103*:690, 1988.

43. Gordis, E., Tabakoff, B., Goldman, D., and Berg, K.: Finding the gene(s) for alcoholism (editorial). JAMA, *263*:209A, 1990.

44. Blum, K., et al.: Allelic association of human dopamine D2 receptor gene in alcoholism. JAMA, *263*:2055, 1990.

10

Neoplasms Affecting the Nervous System of the Elderly

ELLSWORTH C. ALVORD, JR. and
CHENG-MEI SHAW

In this chapter we will consider those neoplasms that occur especially in the elderly: meningiomas, glioblastomas, and others. The first two not only are the most common, but also represent the extremes of degrees of malignancy. We will not have a simple explanation for the existence of these extremes but we will attempt to present some rational explanation for the different clinical behaviors of neoplasms of particular types. The central theme will focus on growth rates and will require not only reference to a theoretical model, but also recognition of the fact that at the present time there is no general theory of neoplasia that can explain the major effects of site and age on the clinical behaviors of specific histologic subtypes of neoplasms.

The theoretical model[1-64] begins with that of Collins et al.,[12] who made the simplest possible assumption that neoplasms grow exponentially from a single cell that divides into 2 cells, these into 4, these into 8, etc., all cells dividing

at a constant rate with no accompanying cell loss. If each cell were 10 μ on edge, 20 doublings would produce 1 mg, 30 doublings 1 g and 40 doublings 1 kg (Fig. 10–1). Most tumors are diagnosed when they are 2 to 3 cm in diameter, about 4 to 14 g, equivalent to about 34 doublings of 10-μ cells (Fig. 10–2). In the case of brain tumors, 36 doublings (about 64 g) are usually fatal.[1,13,31] If the doubling time is 1 month, this will take 3 years; if 1 year, then 36 years.

These last two examples only approach the extreme durations that have actually been measured and should serve to make obvious that children should have only rapidly growing tumors, whereas adults, especially older adults, may have either rapidly or slowly growing tumors depending on the age of onset of the tumor.[12] Meningiomas may approximate this pattern, many being slowly growing in elderly patients, but astrocytomas show the opposite pattern: young persons tend to have

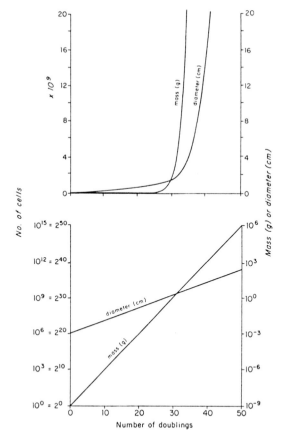

Fig. 10–1. The growth of 10-μ cells doubling at a constant rate without cell loss as visualized on arithmetric coordinates (above) or on semi-logarithmic coordinates (below). (From Alvord[1] reprinted from the Arch Neurol, *33*:73, 1976, copyright 1976, by the American Medical Association.)

slowly growing, low-grade astrocytomas and older persons rapidly growing, highly malignant ones (glioblastoma multiforme). Such examples should suffice to show that we do not have a general rule defining the behaviors of different neoplasms. There is no substitute for the Music Man's admonition, "Ya gotta know the territory!"

To return to the theoretical model, one can imagine a group of 100 brain tumor patients whose tumor cells are dividing at rates evenly distributed between 1 and 2 months, producing fatal or near-fatal tumors after 36 doublings, the first at 3 years and the last at 6 years (i.e., 36 to 72 months). If each of the tumors is excised completely, no recurrences should occur; but if only 1 cell is left behind in each

patient, recurrences should begin to appear after 3 years and all should have occurred by 6 years (Fig. 10–3A). Changing the distribution of growth rates by half (i.e., to 0.5 to 1 month doubling time) or by a factor of 2 (i.e., to 2 to 4 months) will shift the recurrences to 1.5 to 3 years or to 6 to 12 years (Fig. 10–3B), and similarly with further halving or doubling of the growth rate.

If, however, half of the 36 generations of the primary tumor were left behind, it would require only half the time for the recurrences to appear. This amount of tumor left behind, 2^{18} cells, is about 0.25 mg or cu mm, about a quarter the size of an ordinary pinhead, most likely grossly invisible. These recurrences would kill the patient at the same time as if they had begun from single cells doubling twice as fast (Fig. 10–4A). It is just the old grade school formula of "time times rate equals distance." Halving the "distance" between 18 generations and 36 generations (i.e., leaving 27 generations of the primary tumor behind) would result in fatal recurrences occurring at the same time as if 18 generations had been left behind but doubling twice as fast or as if a single cell had been left behind but doubling 4 times as fast (Fig. 10–4B). It may be noted that 2^{27} 10-μ cells are equivalent to about 0.1 g, 100 mg or cu mm, a relatively small amount that would be easily seen grossly as about 100 pinheads if in a solid sphere but might not be so easily seen if spread out in a membrane at the edges of an operative site.

This relationship between growth rates and amounts of tumor left behind illustrates one aspect of what might be analogous to Heisenberg's "Uncertainty Principle" (Fig. 10–5). This principle was, of course, developed 60 years ago to explain why one cannot define simultaneously both the position and the momentum of a subatomic particle, such as an electron.[21,24,64] In fact, Heisenberg[24] introduced the subject with the example of the position of a moving particle at different times, the rate being an average which might not actually exist at any particular moment. He went on to show that the product of the uncertainty of the position times the uncertainty of the momentum cannot be less than h/2π, h being Planck's constant (6.624×10^{-27} erg second or cm^2 sec^{-1}), which will not be incorporated into

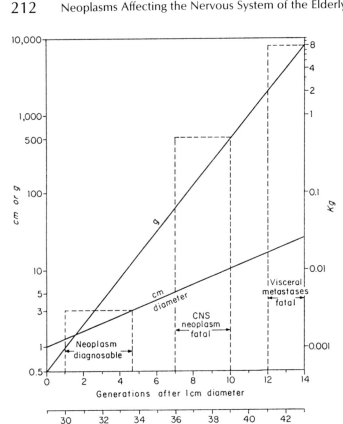

Fig. 10-2. The growth of a tumor after it has developed a diameter of 1 cm (equivalent to 29 doublings of the 10-μ cells shown in Fig. 10-1) with sizes indicated when the tumor is usually diagnosed and fatal. (From Alvord[1] reprinted from the Arch. Neurol, *33*:73, 1976, copyright 1976, by the American Medical Association.)

our analogy, since we will be dealing with much larger numbers! The basic analogy with cancer patients can still be recognized by the fact that both the growth rate and the amount of tumor left behind cannot be defined at any single point in time, e.g., at the time of operation. The growth rate could be defined by measurements of the tumor volume at 2 points in time, but this is rarely done preoperatively and not much more frequently postoperatively

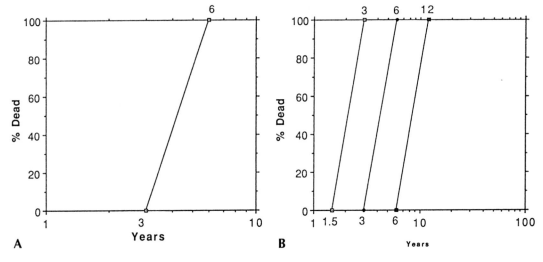

Fig. 10-3. Mortality curves (straight lines on this semi-logarithmic plot) for a theoretical recurrent brain tumor: A, 1 cell left behind doubling every 1 to 2 months, producing deaths after about 36 generations equivalent to 3 to 6 years; or B, doubling twice as fast or half as fast to kill at 1.5 to 3 years or 6 to 12 years.

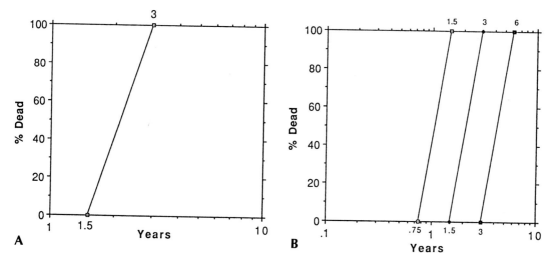

Fig. 10–4. Mortality curves for a theoretical recurrent brain tumor, as in Figure 10–3A but with 2^{18} cells (0.25 mg) left behind; A, doubling every 1 to 2 months to kill after 1.5 to 3 years; or B, doubling twice as fast or half as fast to kill after 0.75 to 1.5 years or 3 to 6 years.

with the tumor recurrence. The amount of tumor grossly remaining could also be estimated if it were non-infiltrating, such as a meningioma, but the measurement of any remaining microscopic invasion or infiltration, as in most gliomas, is certainly beyond current techniques.

Heisenberg's Uncertainty Principle

1) subatomic particles:

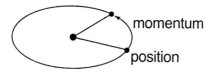

2) cancer:

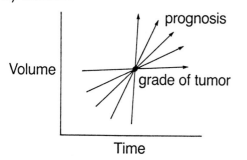

Fig. 10–5. An analogy between Heisenberg's "Uncertainty Principle" and the current practice of predicting the prognosis of cancer patients based only on the histologic grading of the tumor.

From this last point of view it may be helpful to point out the relationship between the volume of a sphere and of 0.5 cm and 1 cm shells surrounding it (Fig. 10–6). If the surgeon excises all the grossly visible glioma, for example, about 4 cm in diameter (about 33 g, equivalent to 35 generations), the 0.5 cm surrounding shell contains about 32 g (about 35 generations of cells). If all were tumor, only 1 doubling would remain for the patient; and if

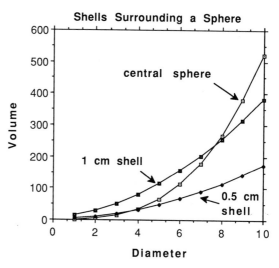

Fig. 10–6. Volumes of a central sphere and of the surrounding 0.5 and 1 cm shells. Note that the volumes of the 0.5 cm shell and of the 1 cm shell are greater than or equal to the central spheres up to diameters of about 4 cm and 8 cm, respectively.

only 6% of the cells were tumor, only 4 more doublings (i.e., to 12%, 24%, 48% and 96%) would remain for the patient. For a 1-cm surrounding shell the situation is much worse, the shell containing more volume than the central sphere up to about 8 cm in diameter. No wonder that gliomas are so rapidly recurrent and fatal.

Similarly with benign tumors, such as meningiomas or acoustic neurilemmomas, "subtotal" excisions that remove less than 90% of the tumor[60] permit recurrences to the original size within 1 to 3 doublings (Fig. 10–7) and "near total" excisions that remove 90 to 99% of the tumor[60] permit recurrences to the original size within 3.5 to 6.5 doublings. With slowly growing neoplasms with doubling times of the order of a year or so, as may occur especially in the elderly, these incomplete excisions can provide long periods of symptom-free survival and may be much safer than heroic attempts at complete excision which may interfere with the blood supply to the brain or spinal cord.

At this point in our theoretical considerations it becomes convenient to make a minor arithmetical change which will allow our double logarithmic graphs (Figs. 10–8 through 10–14) to be constructed more easily. The change is merely to use 36.5 rather than 36 doublings. While 36 has been an easy number to divide by 2 several times, the shift to 36.5 will be more convenient because $2^{36.5}$ doublings will produce 100 g of 10-μ cells and because 36.5 doublings every 10 days would require 365 days or 1 year. These numerical relationships make it possible to use parallel logarithmic scales based on multiples of 10. For example, as shown in Table 10–1, a single cell doubling at a constant rate every 1000

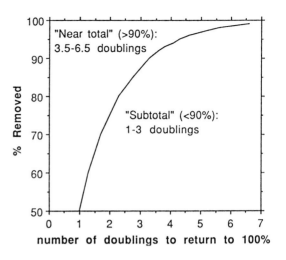

Fig. 10–7. Numbers of doublings required for a tumor to return to its original size following "subtotal" or "near-total" removals, defined as less than 90% or between 90 and 99%, respectively.[60]

days will produce 100 g of tumor in 100 years; doubling every 100 days, in 10 years, etc., the number of years being 1/10th the number of days. Furthermore, if half the number of generations ($2^{18.25}$ cells or about 0.3 mg) is left behind, the years required to produce 100 g are halved. If half again as much is left behind ($2^{27.38}$ cells or about 0.2 g), these times are halved again. Thus, the amount of tumor left behind, when measured in numbers of generations, has a major impact on recurrence time.

By contrast, as shown in Table 10–2, the amount of tumor to be produced has relatively little effect on the time required, a somewhat surprising answer until one realizes that it is a ratio of the exponents involved: 30 (the exponent to produce 1 g) is only 80% of 36.5 (the exponent to produce 100 g) and 43.5 (the ex-

TABLE 10–1.   Times to Produce 100 g of Tumor Related to Amounts of Tumor Left Behind and to Tumor Doubling Time

Tumor Doubling Time (days)	Years to 100 g of tumors if various amounts of tumors are left behind					
	2^0 1 cell	$2^{18.25}$ cells (0.3 mg)	$2^{27.38}$ cells (0.2 g)	$2^{31.94}$ cells (4 g)	$2^{34.22}$ cells (20 g)	$2^{35.36}$ cells (44 g)
1000	100	50	25	12.5	6.25	3.12
100	10	5	2.5	1.25	0.62	0.31
10	1	0.5	0.25	0.12	0.06	0.03
1	0.1	0.05	0.02	0.01	0.03	0.02

TABLE 10–2.   Times To Produce Various Amounts of Tumor Related to Tumor Doubling Time

Tumor doubling time (days)	Years to produce various amounts of tumor beginning with a single 10-micron cell				
	$2^{36.5}$ (100 g)	2^{30} (1 g)	$2^{33.5}$ (10 g)	2^{40} (1000 g)	$2^{43.5}$ (10,000 g)
1000	100	80	90	110	120
100	10	8	9	11	12
10	1	0.8	0.9	1.1	1.2
1	0.1	0.08	0.09	0.11	0.12

ponent to produce 10 kg) is only 120% of 36.5. As shown in Figures 10–1 and 10–2, it is the last few doublings that are responsible for major increases in mass.

To these gross aspects of growth rates can be added important cytokinetic features, especially mitotic or proliferative activities and cell losses.[5,20,26,43–63] Mitotic activity can be measured as a mitotic index (MI), the number of mitoses per 100 nuclei or, less quantitatively, the number per 10 high power fields. Proliferative activities are usually measured as a percentage of cells actively synthesizing DNA in preparation for mitosis. Such S-phase cells can be identified by flow cytometry of dissociated cells from fresh, fresh-frozen or paraffin-embedded tissue without any previous labeling or by a labeling procedure in vivo or in vitro utilizing a pulse of tritiated thymidine or bromodeoxyuridine (BrDU, also abbreviated as BrdUrd[5,20,62] or BUdR[26,27,63]). The various procedures yield slightly different percentages of S-phase cells or labeling indices (LI) but as a first approximation they can be considered essentially the same. The basic formulas have been presented by Steel,[55] as follows:

$$(1) \ Tp = \frac{\lambda Ts}{LI}$$

$$(2) \ \phi = 1 - \frac{Tp}{Td}$$

$$(3) \ \frac{Td}{Tc} = \frac{\log 2}{(1 - \phi) \log(GF + 1)}$$

where Tp = potential doubling time
Td = actual gross volume-doubling time
Tc = cell cycle time
Ts = time during which DNA is being synthesized

λ = a factor defining the timing of Ts within Tc and the age distribution of the cells
LI = labeling index
ϕ = cell loss factor, the proportion of newly formed cells that are lost
GF = growth fraction, the proportion of the total cells that are actually cycling.

When $\phi = 0$ and GF = 1, Td = Tp = Tc, as can be seen by appropriate simple substitutions in equations (2) and (3). When Tc = 1, 2, 4 or 5 days, Ts is approximately 0.5, 0.6, 0.83 or 1.0 days, respectively.[57] The value of λ varies from about 0.7 to 0.95 with an unlikely maximum of 1.4.[55] The value of λTs could, therefore, vary from 0.35 to 1.4 depending on Tc, but has been estimated at 0.22 or lower.[26,27,44,52,63]

Equations (1) and (2) can be combined, as follows:

$$(4) \ \phi = 1 - \frac{\lambda Ts}{LI \times Td}$$

$$or \ (5) \ 1 - \phi = \frac{\lambda Ts}{LI \times Td}.$$

If $1 - \phi = 1$ (i.e., if $\phi = 0$ so that there is no cell loss), then LI $\times$ Td = λTs. This relationship can be plotted as a series of oblique, equally spaced, parallel lines on double logarithmic graph paper for various arbitrary but progressively doubling values of λTs: 0.22, 0.44, 0.88 and 1.76 (Fig. 10–8).

If $1 - \phi = 0.5$ (i.e., if $\phi = 0.5$ so that 50% of the new cells are lost), then LI $\times$ Td = 2 λTs. If $1 - \phi = 0.25$ (i.e., if $\phi = 0.75$ with 75% of the new cells being lost), then LI $\times$ Td = 4λTs; and so on, progressively halving the "distance" to 100% cell loss and progressively

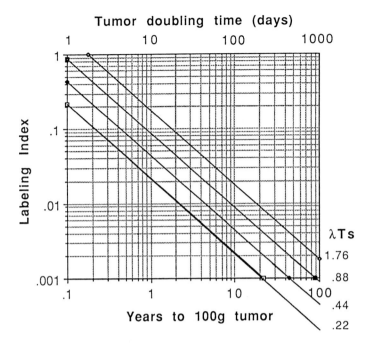

Fig. 10–8. A nomographic representation of the relationships defined by the equation $\phi = 1 - \dfrac{\lambda Ts}{LI \times Td}$ for various values of λTs when $\phi = 0$.

doubling the value of LI × Td. This relationship can also be expressed as a series of parallel lines starting with any one of the lines for λTs in Figure 10–8. Figure 10–9 is based on λTs = 0.22 since this uses the median estimates of earlier investigators[44,52,63] and since it fits the early results concerning gliomas.[26,27]

It may actually turn out, however, that the nomogram for λTs = 0.44 will be a better expression of the relationship when Tc = 1 to 2 days and the nomogram for λTs = 0.88 when Tc = 2 to 5 days, as may be characteristic of other tumors.[57,58] These nomograms can be easily constructed by eliminating the lowest

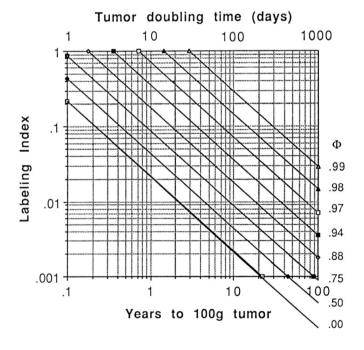

Fig. 10–9. Representations of the relationships defined by the equation $\phi = 1 - \dfrac{\lambda Ts}{LI \times Td}$ for various values of ϕ when $\lambda Ts = 0.22$.

one or two oblique lines in Figure 10–8 and re-labeling the remaining lines appropriately, as in Figure 10–9.

To see the effect of the growth fraction (GF) we can rewrite equation (3) as

$$(6) \quad Td = \frac{Tc \log 2}{(1 - \phi) \log(GF + 1)}$$

When Tc = 1 and $1 - \phi$ = 1, Td = $\frac{\log 2}{\log(GF + 1)}$. This is a variation on the formula for compound interest and is almost a straight line on double logarithmic graph paper (Fig. 10–10), to which parallel lines have been added, doubling Td as Tc doubles. Similarly, for Tc = 1 day, the effects of halving of $1 - \phi$ result in a doubling of Td (Fig. 10–11).

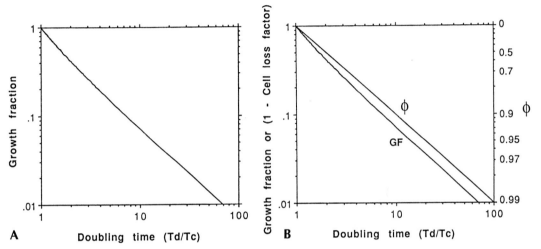

Fig. 10–10. The relationship between the tumor doubling time (Td) and the growth fraction (GF) as defined by the equation $Td = \frac{TC \log 2}{\log (1 + GF)}$ when Tc (the cell cycle time) = 1 day is almost a straight line on double logarithmic paper (A). The similar relationship defined by the equation $Td = \frac{Tc}{1 - \phi}$, where ϕ = the cell loss factor, is a straight line (B).

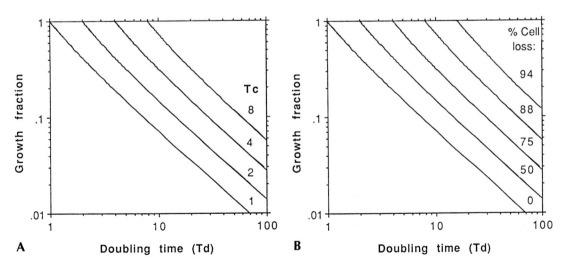

Fig. 10-11. Relationships between Td and GF, as in Figure 10–10, for various values of Tc (A) or cell loss factor (B).

TABLE 10–3.   Decreases in Growth Fraction (GF) To Produce Progressive Doubling of a Tumor's Doubling Time (Td); c.f. Figure 10–10

Td	GF
1	1.00
2	.41
4	.19
8	.09
16	.04
32	.02
64	.01
128	.005

Rather than superimpose both sets of lines from Figures 10–10 and 10–11 onto those of Figures 10–8 or 10–9, we find it less cluttering to calculate the values of GF corresponding to the progressive doubling of Td produced by the progressive halving of $1 - \phi$ in Figure 10–9, as shown in Table 10–3. By ignoring the slight curvature of the lines in Figures 10–10 and 10–11, we can now align the values of ϕ and GF that progressively double Td (Fig. 10–12).

Figure 10–12 now expresses all of the interactions between LI, ϕ and GF (all as decimals) as they combine to define Td (in days) and the times (in years) to produce 100 g of tumor beginning with a single 10-μ cell.

Since all of the oblique lines represent factors of 2, the scales of ϕ and GF can be raised together to represent increasing values of λTs. For example, a tumor with a labeling index (LI) of 0.1 (10%), a cell loss factor (ϕ) of 0 and a growth fraction (GF) of 1, on the assumption of λTs = 0.22 would have a doubling time (Td) of 2.2 days. One merely reads along the line for LI = 0.1 to the first oblique line representing either $\phi = 0$ or GF = 1. If the cell loss factor were 0.5 (50%) or if the growth fraction were 0.41 (41%), Td would double to 4.4 days, represented by the second oblique line. Theoretically, if ϕ and GF were as independent as Steel's equation (3) on page 215 suggests, one could slide the lines for ϕ and GF on each other as though their effects were additive (really multiplicative). However, since exit of cells from the cell cycle (decreasing GF) is one of the ways that cells can be lost (increasing ϕ), ϕ and GF are not completely independent variables and their combinations cannot be predicted for any particular type of tumor.

If 1 cell had been left behind, these 3 examples would represent tumors that would recur to 100 g in 0.22, 0.44 and 0.88 years, respectively. From Tables 10–1 and 10–2, however, we can alter the bottom scale to predict the time (in years) to produce any final amount of tumor beginning with any residual amount. The ratio of the actual survival time to the predicted survival time gives a retrospective estimate of the amount of tumor that must have been left behind (Fig. 10–13).

To give some sense of reality to Figure 10–12 we present Figure 10–14, which plots the

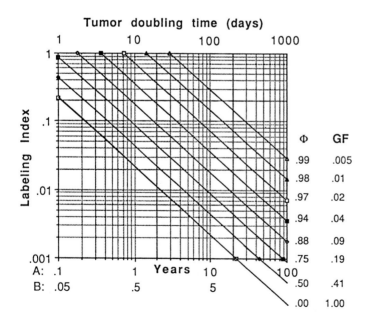

Fig. 10–12.   A nomographic representation of the relationships between LI, ϕ, GF, Td and the time to produce 100 g of tumor beginning with a single 10-μ cell (A) or 2 cells (B).[18,25]

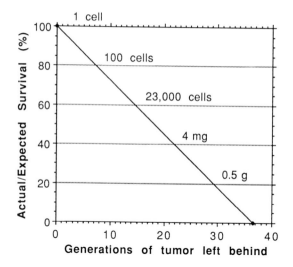

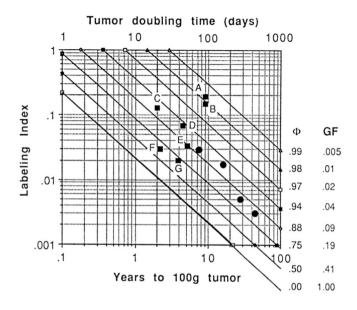

Fig. 10–13.   The amount of tumor left behind can be estimated from the ratio of actual to expected survival times, the expected survival time having been derived from Figure 10–12. One could construct similar graphs for total tumor masses of any desired amount with straight lines ending at 30 generations = 1 g, 40 generations = 1 kg, etc.

data summarized by Steel[55] (his Table 6.2) comparing thymidine labeling indices of 147 biopsied neoplasms and the doubling times measured in serial x rays of the lungs (as primary or metastatic lesions) and shows the extreme degree of variation among various types of tumors. Just how many of these variations can be attributed to differences in ϕ, GF or λTs remains for further studies since Steel's review

in 1977. There are already many, but few of them have measured Td in addition to one or more of the other factors. One example is shown in Figure 10–14: four meningiomas studied by Cho et al.,[10] who measured Td by serial scans of the head.

GF originally was estimated using prolonged labeling of cells throughout at least one cell cycle, those that failed to label being considered non-cycling (G_0) cells. The recent development of a monoclonal antibody (Ki-67) that reacts on fresh (frozen or unfixed) cells with a nuclear antigen present only in cycling cells[4,7,9,16–20,34,35,42] is now considered to provide a direct measurement of GF.

It is important to note that GF and LI are not the same, although some investigators[4,42] have treated them as the same. The confusion probably arises because of results obtained with completely resting cells which are stimulated by a mitogen and reach the same peak at the same time.[19] In a non-resting population of cells, however, the difference is readily apparent: the S-phase markers must be less than the total cycling cells identified by Ki-67. Another practical caution must be noted: lymphocytes infiltrating tumors are frequently "activated" immunologically, meaning that they are blast cells entering into the mitotic cycle. They can, therefore, be counted as "small cells" by either BrDU or Ki-67 techniques, thereby increasing the LI and/or GF. Although some investigators[29] have noted this as a potential problem,

Fig. 10–14.   Median tumor doubling times (Td) as measured by serial chest x–rays and labeling indices (LI) as measured by incorporation of tritiated thymidine for 147 human neoplasms summarized by Steel.[55] A = 23 undifferentiated bronchogenic carcinomas, B = 12 colo-rectal carcinomas, C = 14 childhood tumors, D = 23 squamous cell carcinomas of the head and neck, E = 25 melanomas, F = 28 lymphomas and G = 22 sarcomas. The solid circles represent 4 meningiomas in which Cho et al.[10] measured Td by serial CT scans preoperatively and LI by incorporation of BrDU.

appropriate corrections have not appeared in any of the published reports that we have found.

Rabinovitch[47] has reported that human diploid fibroblast-like cells have 2 components: cycling cells that show a probabilistic rate of transition from G_1 to S and a variable proportion of non-cycling cells, both of which change as the number of doublings increases. Thus, there is a progressive increase in the proportion of non-cycling cells with increasing age. He found no evidence that the non-cycling cells could revert to the cycling state. Whether neoplastic cells follow this pattern remains to be seen.

Some of the features of tumor growth that our theoretical considerations have revealed so far should be examined in more detail:

1. The amount of tumor required to kill a patient can vary tremendously, from 1 g to 10 kg, depending largely on the site (e.g., a primary in the larynx vs. metastases throughout the whole body), and the change in the time required to kill will vary only slightly, within 20% above or below the numbers shown at the bottom of the figures (Table 10–2). Between 10 g and 1 kg the time required will vary even less, only 10%.

2. Major changes in the time to recurrence follow relatively minor changes in the amount of tumor left behind (Table 10–1). Again we are dealing with exponents of 2, such that 20 doublings represent 1 mg, 30 doublings 1 g, and 40 doublings 1 kg. It is the progressive halving of the "distance" to failure as measured by exponents of 2, not mass, that progressively halves the time to recurrence.

3. Major changes in Td at the top scale of Figure 10–12 and consequently in the predicted time to failure at the bottom scale can be effected by relatively slight changes in the cell loss factor (ϕ) or in the growth fraction (GF) represented by the diagonal lines in Figure 10–12.

4. If we knew how to reduce the amount of tumor left behind, to reduce GF or to increase ϕ, we could achieve major improvements in results of treating patients with tumors.

The critical question connecting all of the above theory and reality is whether Td remains constant throughout the life of the tumor patient or whether it changes.[33,59] One can speculate that Td may either accelerate or decelerate but we really need more facts in humans before we can choose between the various possibilities. It should be noted that, unless LI, ϕ or GF change with time, Td will remain constant over time and the growth will remain exponential, still a straight line on semi-logarithmic paper because all of the factors only affect the slope which is still defined by Td. Only if LI, ϕ or GF change, will TD change; and if in the decelerating direction, it may be represented by Gompertzian growth, as seen in many experimental animals.[33] We should note, however, that a really discernible mathematical difference between simple exponential growth and Gompertzian growth can only occur after the point at which the tumor has reached a rather large fraction ($1/e = 0.368$) of its maximal potential;[55] in other words, the last two "simple" doublings may be markedly prolonged,[59] but we have yet to be persuaded that this occurs in other than exceptional human cases.

With this theoretical background, let us consider how some of the available results can be interpreted as approximating growth rates, recurrence rates and cure rates in particular types of brain tumors. Certain neoplasms affecting the nervous system are especially common in the elderly (glioblastoma multiforme, meningioma, metastatic carcinoma) and others are especially common in the young (medulloblastomas, ependymomas, craniopharyngiomas, cerebellar or optic gliomas, retinoblastomas, primitive neuroectodermal tumors), but exceptional examples may occur in either age direction so that we may not be able to ignore any of these. For example, about 1% of cerebellar astrocytomas (a typical tumor of childhood) occur in persons over 60 years of age,[65–73] Kepes et al.[69] reporting 3 cases over age 65. Many other neoplasms have a broad age range (pituitary adenoma, oligodendroglioma, acoustic neurilemmoma, malignant lymphoma). This review will, of course, concentrate on those neoplasms that occur most commonly in persons over 65 years of age, but will have to include others that occur frequently enough that they should be considered in the differential diagnosis.

GLIOMAS

HISTORIC[65-94]

Gliomas presumably develop from and mimic mature or immature glial cells that contribute their names to their classification by the simple addition of the suffix "-oma": astrocytes, oligodendroglia, and ependyma. Some classifications double the number by adding their immature ("-blast") forms. Some tumors contain neurons (mature ganglion cells or immature neuroblasts) or develop in certain characteristic locations (pineal, posterior pituitary) that also contribute their names to their classification (e.g., neuroblastoma, ganglioglioma, pinealoma,[97] infundibuloma). Others are so immature that they are identified only as "primitive neuroectodermal tumors," some of which are more classically recognized as medulloblastomas, especially when they arise in the cerebellum. Of all these primary tumors affecting the central nervous system (CNS), however, the astrocytomas comprise by far the majority, Burger and Vogel[76] having estimated about 60%. The most malignant astrocytoma, glioblastoma multiforme, is also the most common, about 50% of all astrocytomas, and has the poorest prognosis, especially in those over age 65 years.

The evolution of our understanding of the biology of brain tumors can be seen as a cyclic reevaluation by "lumpers" and "splitters."[67,74-94] Before World War I there were relatively few types of gliomas.[79,92] With the development of silver techniques by Hortega for differentiating various types of glia, Bailey and Cushing[74] recognized a tremendous increase in the number of cell types. This produced a corresponding increase in the number of types of tumors, since each tumor was thought to develop from or to produce essentially only one type of cell. The resulting complexity of the scheme of Bailey and Cushing[74] and the requirement for frozen sections and special modifications of fixation or staining for each of the silver impregnation techniques made the classification not generally applicable or, in view of the heterogeneity of cells seen in most tumors, not understandable by most pathologists.

Although several other simplifying proposals had been made, as by Ringertz,[87] it was the classification based on only a few cell types with 4 degrees of malignancy proposed by Kernohan et al.[81] and Kernohan and Sayre[80] that made a world-wide impression. In retrospect it was obviously their illustrations that must have made the impression since they presented only average and 3-year survival rates (Fig. 10–15), numbers that would not pass the simplest statistical analysis today. Indeed, it is somewhat ironic that the results published were not analyzed by Berkson and Gage,[75] statisticians also at the Mayo Clinic at the same time. What is not generally remembered is that Kernohan[80,81] regarded both grades 3 and 4 to be glioblastomas, thereby reducing the number of effective histologic grades to 3. What now becomes doubly ironic is that the newest analysis (Fig. 10–16) by Daumas-Duport et al.[78] from the same institution 4 decades later shows clearly that the 3 or 4 histologic grades of astrocytomas defined by Kernohan[80,81] are biologically only 2!

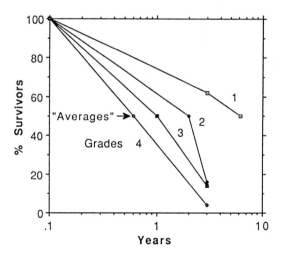

Fig. 10–15. The beginning of the argument favoring grading of astrocytomas (data from Kernohan et al.[81] and Kernohan and Sayre[80]): survival rates (uncorrected for duration of follow-up, amount of tumor left behind, site, size, treatment or clinical status) for astrocytomas of grades 1, 2, 3 and 4. Grades 3 and 4 with relatively little difference in prognosis were called glioblastoma multiforme. Although plotted at 50%, the figures given were for averages or means, not medians.

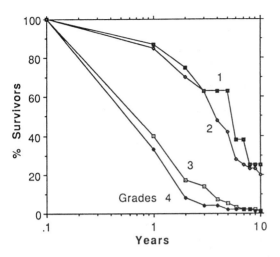

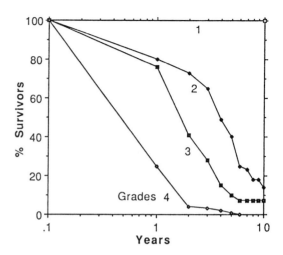

Fig. 10–16. A recent reconsideration of the grading of astrocytomas by the scheme of Kernohan[80,81] as reported by Daumas-Duport et al.:[78] 287 "ordinary" astrocytomas all subjected to postoperative x-irradiation and actuarially defined follow-up (still uncorrected for amount of tumor left behind, site, size and clinical status). There are really only 2 tiers: grades 1 and 2 and grades 3 and 4.

Fig. 10–17. A new histologic scheme (see Table 10–4) separates the same 287 "ordinary" astrocytomas shown in Figure 10–16 into 4 groups, but there were only 2 patients with grade 1 astrocytomas (data from Daumas-Duport et al.[78]).

As might be expected with cyclic reevaluations, this newest analysis by Daumas-Duport et al.[78] was accompanied by a new basis for classification of astrocytomas (Table 10–4 and Fig. 10–17)—and this after an interval of only about 5 years during which a consolidating simplification had independently been developed by two other groups of "lumper-splitters!"[77,87]

But we are getting ahead of our story.

The most widely used technique to classify tumors is by microscopic study of tissue sections stained with hematoxylin and eosin (H&E). Some pathologists maintain that if you cannot obtain agreement on H&E, you will not gain agreement with special stains; i.e., "don't confuse me with the facts." Human gliomas are traditionally classified according to the direction and level of differentiation of the tumor, but there is no consensus as to the details either using H&E or using special stains.[67,74–94]

Gliomas generally differentiate along ependymal, oligodendroglial or astrocytic directions but neuronal and microglial directions (even though these cells are not strictly glial) are also possible but rare. Tumors which show maturation along a single cell line are fairly easy to classify, but the common inclusion of other cell types introduces confusion since there are no accepted criteria as to how many other cells are required to change the diagnosis to a "mixed glioma."[95,96] Most tumors show only partial maturation, the undifferentiated cells being possibly small anaplastic cells, oligodendroglia, undifferentiated astrocytes or even lymphocytes! These last can now be identified by specific monoclonal antibodies and seen to be diffusely infiltrating throughout most tumors, but there is no agreement on how to differentiate the other cells and how to classify these potentially mixed gliomas. Many gliomas demonstrate multiple directions of differentiation. In these situations, it is difficult to evaluate both the direction and the level of differentiation. In spite of these difficulties, since the

TABLE 10–4.   A New Scheme for Classification of Astrocytomas (Daumas-Duport et al.[78])

Histologic feature	Potential score
Nuclear atypia	0–1
Mitosis	0–1
Endothelial proliferation	0–1
Necrosis	0–1
Total score for Grade I:	0
2:	1
3:	2
4:	3–4

most important reason for having a generally acceptable classification is to correlate with the prognosis, the following classification scheme currently seems the most appropriate to characterize the most common human gliomas: ependymoma, oligodendroglioma and astrocytoma.

EPENDYMOMA[98-106]

These tumors (Figs. 10–18 through 10–20) rarely occur in the elderly, only 2 of 25 patients of West et al.[106] being over age 65. They occur either intracranially, most commonly in the fourth ventricle, or intraspinally, most frequently in the filum terminale. They are commonly discrete masses, spherical or multilobulated when within a ventricle (Fig. 10–18) or elongated when within the spinal cord, but they may also infiltrate the adjacent neural tissue. Their histologic appearances are characteristic (Figs. 10–19 and 10–20): perivascular pseudo-rosettes mimicking choroid plexus or small ventricles (true rosettes with cilia and/or blephoroplasts, the basal bodies of cilia) and mucin formation (especially in myxopapillary forms in the cauda equina). Also included are so-called subependymomas or subependymal astrocytomas (Fig. 10–18B) which are recognized by clusters of nuclei separated by abundant fibrillary astrocytic stroma (Fig. 10–20B). Although subependymomas are frequently re-

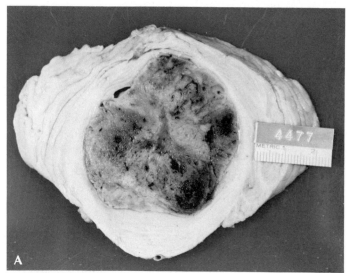

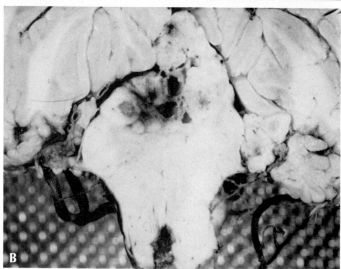

Fig. 10–18. Ependymoma (A, Np4477) and subependymoma (B, Np171) within the 4th ventricle.

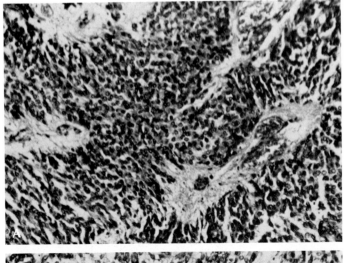

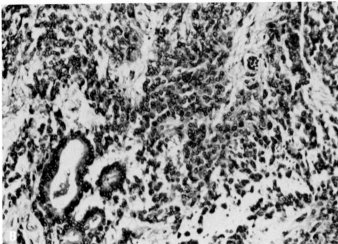

Fig. 10–19. Photomicrographs of ependymomas showing perivascular pseudorosettes (A, × 500) and true rosettes (B, × 500), both stained by H&E (S-59-207).

ported as hamartomas, non-growing masses incidentally found at autopsy near the obex of the fourth ventricle (Fig. 10–18B) or over the head of the caudate nucleus, they can grow more rapidly and become symptomatic. Furthermore, they appear to follow the same rule of other ependymomas in recurring locally no matter how completely the neurosurgeon thinks he removed them. Thus, local x-irradiation is necessary,[105] although a reasonable compromise now, as also suggested by Centeno et al.,[99] would be to follow the patient with the newer imaging techniques, such as magnetic resonance imaging (MRI) or computerized tomography (CT), at regular intervals and retreat as indicated at the time of recurrence.

Ependymomas are said to be distinguishable from astroblastomas[6] by having pointed rather than foot-like expansions of their processes radiating toward a blood vessel.[89] We have difficulty making this distinction and avoid the problem by the simple device of making astroblastomas so rare as to be practically non-existent!

There is a more important controversy that is still unresolved: whereas we believe that almost all ependymomas are histologically benign (although locally recurrent unless x-irradiated), others[100,103,104] believe that almost all are histologically malignant (requiring whole head and spine x-irradiation, chemotherapy and "staging" by examination of CSF for dissemination of tumor cells). Garrett and Simpson[101] report an intermediate position: only 3 of their 50 intracranial ependymomas

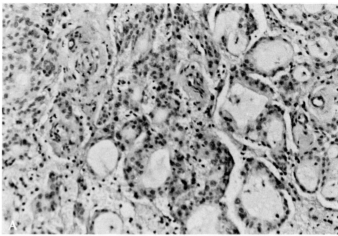
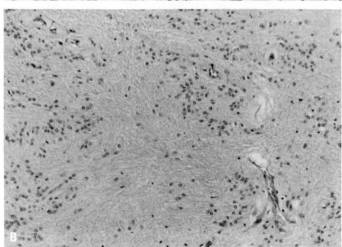

Fig. 10–20. Photomicrographs of a myxopapillary ependymoma (A, × 200, S-78-651) and of a subependymoma (B, × 200, Np1060), both stained by H&E. In the latter note the clusters of nuclei surrounded by densely fibrillary astrocytic matrix, which would be strongly positive for GFAP or by Holzer's stain (not shown).

were well differentiated (benign), whereas only 2 of their 41 spinal ependymomas were high grade (malignant).

OLIGODENDROGLIOMA[107–120]

These tumors (Figs. 10–21 through 10–24) can occur at any age. They are diffusely infiltrating neoplasms (Fig. 10–21) composed of a uniform population of cells with round to slightly oval nuclei, perinuclear halos and no cytoplasmic process formation (Figs. 10–22 and 10–23). Such a definition makes oligodendrogliomas a rather rare tumor. Once we recognize that the halos are an artifact and may, therefore, be absent and that the immature oligodendroglioblast may have oval nuclei and radiating cytoplasmic processes, the incidence of oligodendrogliomas increases considerably.

The observation by Choi and Kim[111] and Choi[110] that still-more-immature oligodendroglioblasts may contain glial fibrillary acidic protein (GFAP), usually considered a marker of astrocytes, makes the differentiation from astrocytes even more difficult. Although contamination with astrocytes is common, only Mørk et al.[118] have defined oligodendrogliomas as containing no more than 25% astrocytes, those with more being considered "mixed gliomas." Herpers and Budka[96] recognize "gliofibrillary oligodendrogliomas" and "transitional oligoastrocytomas" as subtypes of oligodendrogliomas.

The vasculature is generally composed of a delicate, but slightly thickened capillary network with frequent right-angle branching that contributes a pseudo-lobular pattern to the tumor (Fig. 10–23 A).

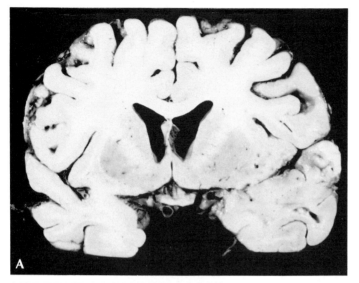

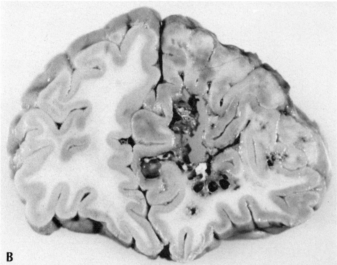

Fig. 10-21. Oligodendrogliomas of the left temporal pole (A, Np3778) or of the left frontal pole postoperatively (B, Np11125).

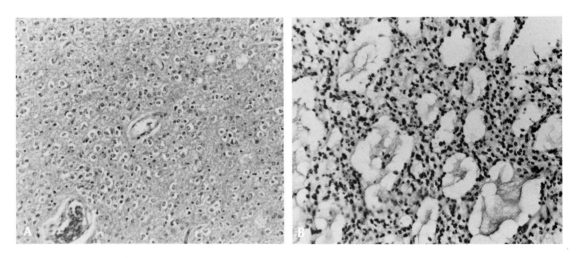

Fig. 10-22. Photomicrographs of oligodendrogliomas showing perinuclear halos (A, Np11504, × 200) and microcysts (B, Np4409, × 200, both stained by H&E).

226

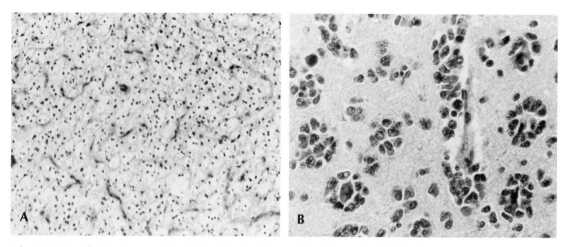

Fig. 10–23. Photomicrographs of oligodendrogliomas showing perinuclear halos and thick branching capillaries (A, S-4362-81, × 200) and marked satellitosis (B, Np15137, × 500, both stained by H&E).

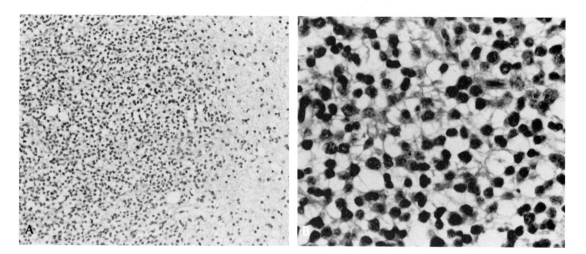

Fig. 10–24. Photomicrographs of an oligodendroglioma showing marked hypercellularity and few cytoplasmic processes (A, × 200; B, × 500; Np15137, both stained by H&E).

Oligodendrogliomas can vary in cellular density (Fig. 10–24) and nuclear pleomorphism and may have areas of microcysts (Fig. 10–22B) or necrosis. They frequently contain calcifications, especially in the cortex at the edge of the tumor. The extensive involvement of gray matter with marked perineuronal satellitosis frequently produces an encephaloid pachygyric pattern recognizable grossly (Fig. 10–21) and by MRI. Oligodendrogliomas are usually thought to be slow-growing tumors but their failure rates vary over a wide range (Fig. 10–25). Consideration of the various factors that have been analyzed in 3 different

medical centers[108,115–118] reveals that necrosis does not separate oligodendrogliomas prognostically (Figs. 10–26 and 10–27). This contrasts with the results in astrocytomas, as will be discussed in more detail below (c.f., Fig. 10–37). Microcystic oligodendrogliomas have a relatively good prognosis regardless of the degree of cell density or presence of necrosis (Figs. 10–26 and 10–27), at least as reported in one of the studies[117] but not in another[108] and not considered separately in the third.[116] Oligodendrogliomas with a high cell density or with a medium cell density and necrosis have a relatively poor prognosis (Figs. 10–26 and

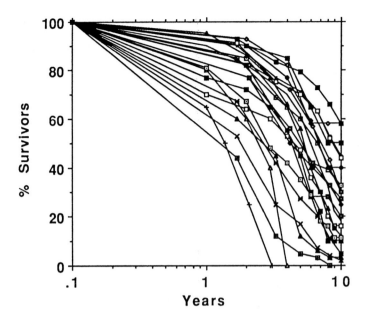

Fig. 10–25. Survival rates of patients with oligodendrogliomas of all types with various histologic characteristics.[107,108,116,118,119]

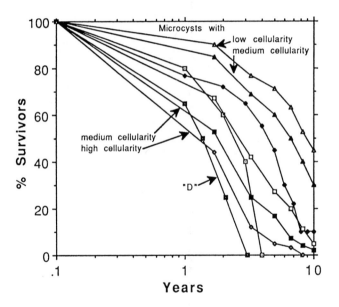

Fig. 10–26. Survival rates of patients with oligodendrogliomas showing areas of necrosis.[108,116,118] The worst have high to medium cellularity with "D" including endothelial proliferation and pleomorphism,[116] whereas the best have microcysts.

10–27). The remaining types of oligodendrogliomas have intermediate to relatively good prognoses.

Other good prognostic factors include the history of seizures only, on the average of about 5 years' duration in the pre-CT era,[117] and a normal neurologic functional status (see Table 10–5) on admission.[115] Each of these is associated with a median postoperative survival of about 5 years without considering the cellular subtype of oligodendroglioma. In contrast to ependymomas[105] and astrocytomas (see

below), Helseth and Mørk[113] could find no correlation of the prognosis of oligodendrogliomas with age, although Ludwig et al.[116] noted a preponderance of benign ones in the young and of malignant ones in older patients. With improvements in electroencephalographic techniques, and especially with CT and MRI, tumors in epileptic patients are being diagnosed more frequently at earlier times in their natural histories. Many of these in our experience are oligodendrogliomas.

The growth rates of oligodendrogliomas

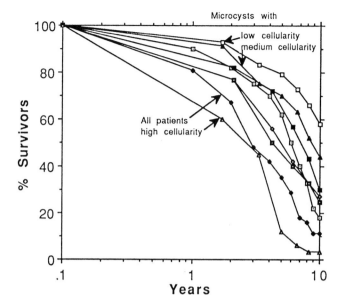

Fig. 10–27. Survival rates of patients with oligodendrogliomas showing no areas of necrosis.[108,116,118] Unlike astrocytomas (see Fig. 10–36 and 10–37), there is no difference in prognosis from those with areas of necrosis shown in Figure 10–26.

have been a problem for many decades with high mitotic rates observable in cases of prolonged survival. Although De Reuck et al.[112] did not consider their results significant, it is clear from their results that the mitotic activity was greater (median mitotic index = 6 to 9) in those who died within 1 to 26 months than in those surviving 12 to 40 or more months (median mitotic index = 2). Furthermore, Spaar et al.[50] report almost as wide a range of S-phase percentages (1 to 6.1%; median 3.4%) in oligodendrogliomas as in glioblastomas (1.1 to 17.1%; median = 4.5%). We obviously need

measurements of GF and ϕ to see how oligodendrogliomas really behave kinetically.

There is still controversy as to whether radiation therapy has any effect on oligodendrogliomas, controversial because of the lack of randomized trials. Such trials will be frustrating, however, since at least a decade of follow-up would be necessary to prove the point, as shown in Figure 10–28. In addition, the relatively good prognosis of what some investigators[107,115,119] included as oligodendrogliomas or mixed oligo-astrocytomas contrasts with what others[120] have called mixed tumors.

TABLE 10–5. The Karnofsky and WHO Performance Scales

	Karnofsky et al.[121]	WHO (Mork et al.[118])	
%			Status
100	Normal; no complaints; no evidence of disease	Normal	0
90	Able to carry on normal activity, minor signs or symptoms of disease		
80	Normal activity with effort, some signs or symptoms of disease	Normal activity with effort, some signs or symptoms of disease	1
70	Cares for self but unable to do active work or carry on normal activity	Cares for most personal needs but unable to work	2
60	Requires occasional assistance, able to care for most needs		
50	Requires considerable assistance and frequent medical care		
40	Disabled, requires special care and assistance, unable to care for self	Disabled, independent less than half the daytime	3
30	Severely disabled, hospitalization indicated	Completely disabled	4
20	Very sick, hospitalized, active support necessary		
10	Moribund		
0	Dead		

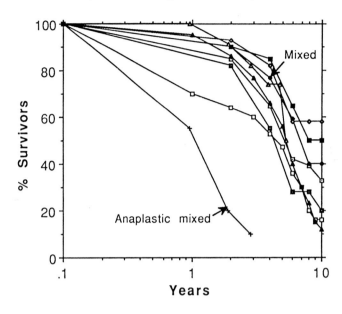

Fig. 10–28. Survival rates of patients with oligodendrogliomas or mixed gliomas without microcysts or necrosis.[107,119,120] The difference between the poor survivals of those with "mixed" and "anaplastic mixed" gliomas is difficult to reconcile with the good survivals of those with "anaplastic ologodendrogliomas" in the same report[120] which are hidden within the curves for best cases. The best results followed >4,500 cGy, but the patients were not randomly selected or corrected for site, size, clinical status or amount of tumor left behind.

Chemotherapy has been reported to decrease the size of some malignant oligodendrogliomas[109] but confirmation is obviously necessary.

ASTROCYTOMA[74–94,122–179]

These tumors can occur at any age but tend to be more malignant in the elderly. Astrocytomas account for over half of all primary tumors of the CNS.[76] They are diffusely infiltrating and have obvious fibrillary or gemistocytic differentiation of many if not most of their cells. We believe that they should first be classified grossly according to site (optic nerve or chiasm, cerebellum, spinal cord, etc.). What follows applies especially to supratentorial cerebral astrocytomas, which have been most extensively studied during the past decade or so. Their prognoses are infinitely varied, from almost vertical to almost horizontal (Fig. 10–29)!

Our approach will be to dissect apart certain sub-groups, but the reader must appreciate that there are no sharp subdivisions obvious in Figure 10–29. Even so, the real situation is not quite so bad as Figure 10–29 implies since they can be divided into 4 prognostic groups (Fig. 10–30) with relatively good correlation between histologic appearances (Fig. 10–31) and

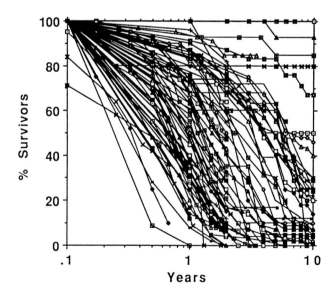

Fig. 10–29. Survival rates of patients with astrocytomas of all types with various histologic characteristics.

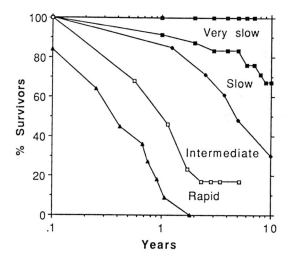

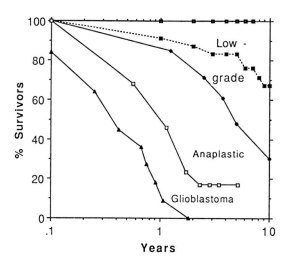

Fig. 10–30. The survival rates shown in Figure 10–29 can be divided into 4 groups representing patients with astrocytomas that recur as though they were neoplasms with very slow, slow, intermediate and rapid growth rates.

Fig. 10–31. The 4 groups shown in Figure 10–30 represent astrocytomas that can be classified as low-grade, anaplastic, or glioblastoma. The relatively few overlaps (not shown) occur in patients with anaplastic astrocytoma over 65 years of age[77] or with abnormal DNA by flow cytometry[134] and in patients with glioblastoma under age 45 years[77] (see Figs. 10–36, 10–39, and 10–40).

certain biologic features, such as age, neurologic status, mitotic activity and DNA characteristics.

To present our conclusion first, we suggest that these factors can be combined to yield a

relatively simple histologic classification which can be affected by a few biologic factors to yield a reasonably precise prognostic scale (Fig. 10–32). Such an eclectic approach requires that the reader be aware that limitations of language force some usages of words which others may have defined differently; thus, the reader must note the similarities and differences which we will try to point out as we progress through this analysis.

Let us begin with the histologic classification, which recognizes 3 basic tiers: high-grade (glioblastoma multiforme), intermediate-grade (anaplastic astrocytomas), and low-grade astrocytomas.

1. High-grade astrocytomas (glioblastoma multiforme) account for about half of all astrocytomas.[76] Although there is no need for the word *multiforme*, since there is no other type of glioblastoma, both grossly (Fig. 10–33) and microscopically (Figs. 10–34 and 10–35) the word *multiforme* is most appropriate since these tumors are characterized by hemorrhage, necrosis, and cyst formation as well as by moderate to high cellular density, many mitotic figures, and moderate to marked nuclear pleomorphism. They are most easily identified

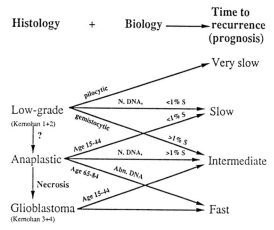

Fig. 10–32. The prognosis of patients with astrocytomas of 3 various histologic grades can be predicted more precisely if certain biologic features are taken into consideration (see text). The "?" indicates a subjective histologic division beyond which low-grade astrocytomas should not go. "1% S" includes not only % S-phase by flow cytometry but also % by labeling indices or number of mitoses per 10 high power fields.

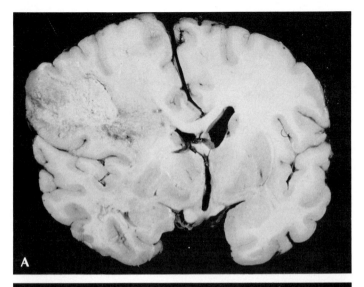

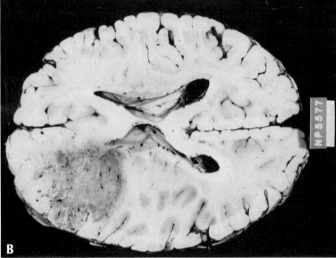

Fig. 10–33. Left central (A, VA-A-145-73) and left frontal (B, Np5577) glioblastomas.

by areas of necrosis with or without peri-necrotic nuclear palisading which appears to be due to increased local growth of tumor cells in the zone of increasing tissue hypoxia. Although Kernohan and Sayre[80] accepted necrosis in both of their grades 3 and 4, both of which they considered glioblastoma multiforme, they did not require it. More recently, however, necrosis in untreated astrocytomas has become the essential feature of glioblastomas.[76,77,85,86] It should be noted that Daumas-Duport et al.[78] suggest that equal weight can be given to endothelial proliferation (Fig. 10–35), which they found in only 6% of their grade 3 cases and in 82% of their grade 4 cases. In these latter cases they found endothelial pro-

liferation together with necrosis in 62% and each alone in about 20%.

Cohadon et al.[133] have also presented an even simpler scheme based on their observations that, if large amounts of material are available for study, (1) the presence of necrosis is always associated with neovascularization, nuclear pleomorphism, and abnormal cell density, (2) in the absence of necrosis, neovascularization is always associated with more than moderate nuclear pleomorphism and abnormal cell density, and (3) in the absence of necrosis or neovascularization, more than moderate nuclear pleomorphism is always associated with abnormal cell density. Thus, with small biopsy samples, the grading can be

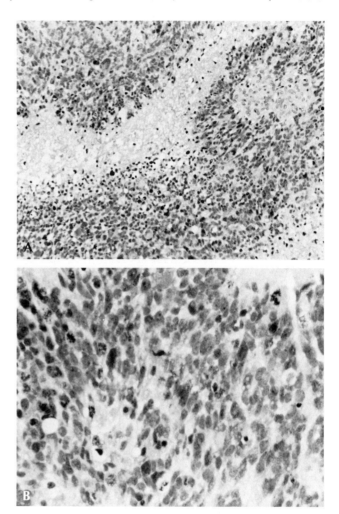

Fig. 10–34. Photomicrographs of a glioblastoma showing areas of necrosis (A, × 200) and mitoses and pleomorphism (B, × 500), both Np15287 stained by H&E.

based on the presence of the worst of any 1 of the 4 factors: (1) abnormal cell density with moderate nuclear abnormalities, (2) more than moderate nuclear pleomorphism, (3) neovascularization with endothelial proliferation, and (4) necrosis.

Glioblastomas have the worst prognosis (Fig. 10–36), worse than the worst of oligodendrogliomas (Fig. 10–37); therefore, one must be careful in distinguishing these two tumors, a distinction which cannot be based on the simple presence or absence of necrosis. This asymmetry in the classification will be discussed in more detail below. As with oligodendrogliomas, the neurologic status (Table 10–5) of patients with glioblastomas is an important determinant of the prognosis (Fig. 10–38).[85,133,168] In contrast to oligodendrogliomas, where the effect of age has been less well de-

fined,[116] there is a significant effect of age in glioblastomas:[77,85,133,135,168,173] the younger the age, the better the prognosis (Figs. 10–39 and 10–40).

2. Low-grade astrocytomas (Figs. 10–41 through 10–43) are at the other end of the scale. These have more than normal or "reactive" cellular density and more obvious maturation into mature fibrillary astrocytes than the more malignant astrocytomas. They have little or no nuclear atypia, little or no vascular proliferation (except in relation to cysts) and no necrosis. As might be expected, low-grade astrocytomas have a relatively good prognosis (Fig. 10–44). Shaw et al.[91] separated the new grades 1 and 2 of Daumas-Duport et al.[78] into 3 groups: pilocytic (with a good prognosis), gemistocytic (with a poor prognosis) and the others (with a good but intermediate progno-

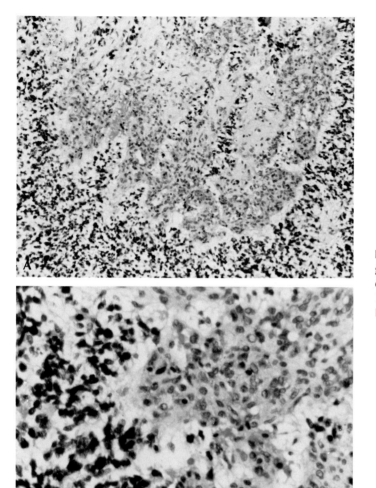

Fig. 10-35. Photomicrographs of a glioblastoma showing capillary endothelial proliferation (A, × 200; B, × 500), both Np4003 stained by H&E.

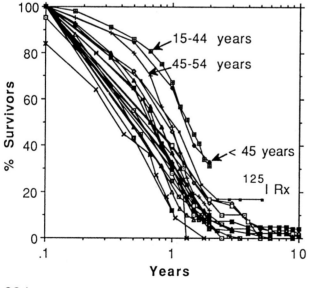

Fig. 10-36. Survival rates of patients with glioblastomas[77,78,86,127,129,134,145,169] subjected to various treatments, the best of which have lengthened the median survival to only about 1 year. Note that the two best survival curves occur in patients under age 45[77,129] and the next in those treated with ^{125}I implants.[145]

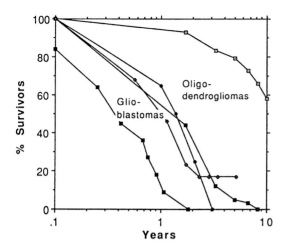

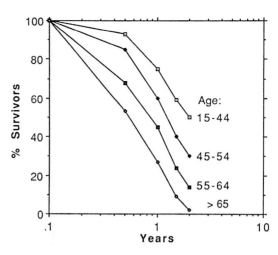

Fig. 10–37. A comparison of the survival rates of patients with glioblastomas (see Fig. 10–36) or oligodendrogliomas (see Fig. 10–25). There is practically no overlap.

Fig. 10–39. Survival rates of the same patients shown in Figure 10–38 with "malignant gliomas" according to age for comparison with Figures 10–40 and 10–50. The effect persists at least to 2 years.

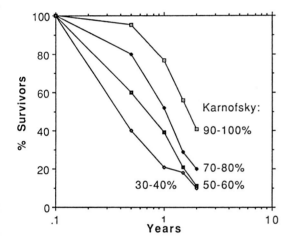

Fig. 10–38. Survival rates of patients with "malignant gliomas" (80% with glioblastoma multiforme and 20% with other gliomas, mostly anaplastic astrocytomas) according to postoperative neurologic status (Karnofsky scale in %; see Table 10–5; data from Shapiro et al.[169]). The effect in most patients rapidly disappears after 1 year, but is still seen in the best patients at 2 years.

Fig. 10–40. Survival rates of patients of different ages with glioblastomas (data from Burger et al.,[77] Cooper et al.,[135] and Nelson et al.[85]); see Figures 10–39 and 10–50. The sizes of the symbols parallel the age groups. The effect in most patients rapidly disappears after 1 year except in the youngest patients. The best curve represents patients under 40 years of age with "malignant gliomas" or astrocytomas of moderate to marked anaplasia, said to be equivalent to Kernohan grades 3 and 4, treated with excision of "as much tumor as possible without undue risk," 6,000 cGy and chemotherapy.[135]

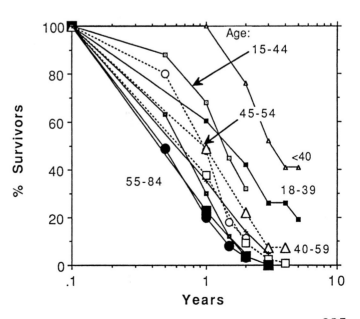

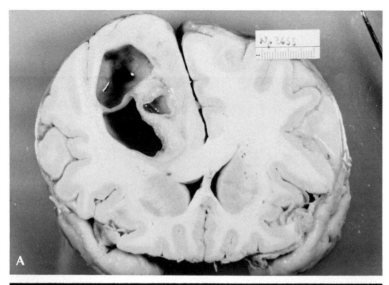

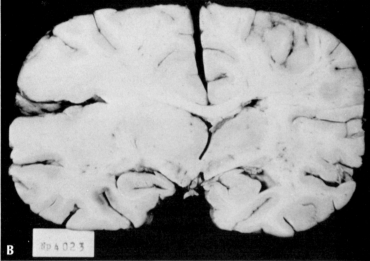

Fig. 10–41. Low-grade astrocytomas of right frontal lobe (A, Np2655) and right cerebral hemisphere (B, Np4023).

sis). Hoshino et al.[151] analyzed "low-grade" astrocytomas, which were said to be histologically equivalent to "grade II" of Kernohan and Sayre[80] but also were described as "moderately anaplastic" astrocytomas, an unfortunate choice of words which will create confusion with other definitions of anaplastic astrocytomas, as described below. Hoshino et al.[151] subdivided these into two groups based on the in vivo incorporation of BrDU of more or less than 1%. The prognoses were appropriately different, the less active ones behaving as would be expected for low-grade astrocytomas (Figs. 10–45 and 10–46), the more active ones behaving like intermediate-grade (anaplastic) astrocytomas, as will be discussed below. No

specific effect of age has been reported but most of the pilocytic astrocytomas (Fig. 10–45) tend to occur in young individuals, under age 59[132] or under age 27 or 29.[140,176]

3. Intermediate-grade astrocytomas are obviously in between glioblastomas and low-grade astrocytomas. They are now most commonly called anaplastic astrocytomas, although there is an unfortunate tendency to believe that this is synonymous with the grade 3 astrocytomas of Kernohan and Sayre.[80] They are not histologically identical since Kernohan and Sayre[80] allowed some necrosis; nor are they prognostically identical, as shown originally by Nelson et al.[86] and more recently by Daumas-Duport et al.[78] in Figure 10–16. Ana-

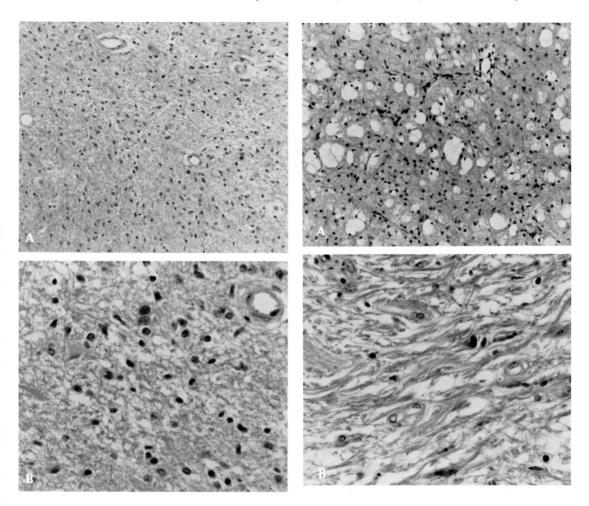

Fig. 10–42. Photomicrographs of low-grade astrocytomas (A, × 200; B, × 500), both Np14018 stained by H&E.

Fig. 10–43. Photomicrographs of low-grade astrocytomas (A, Np13685, microcystic, × 200; B, Np11747, pilocytic, × 500) both stained by H&E.

Fig. 10–44. Survival rates of patients with astrocytomas[78,91,134,138,140,151] of "low-grade." There appear to be 3 patterns: (a) those with LI > 1% who drop off precipitously,[151] (b) a group with practically no failures[78,91,140] (see Fig. 10–45), and (c) an intermediate group with mostly downward curving survival rates (see Fig. 10–46).

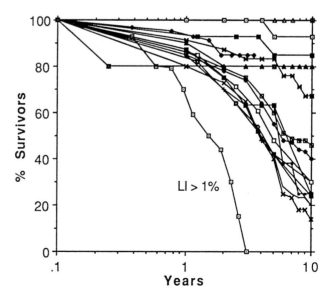

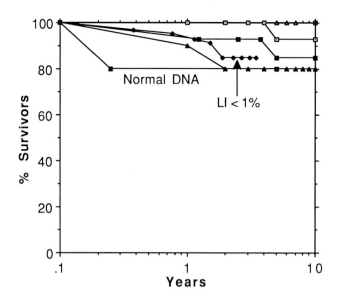

Fig. 10–45. Survival rates of those patients with "low-grade" astrocytomas showing practically no failures (see Fig. 10–44). These include pilocytic astrocytomas[91,140] and cases without any nuclear atypia[78] and may include cases with anaplasia but with little or no mitotic activity (LI < 1%[151] or normal DNA by flow cytometry[134]).

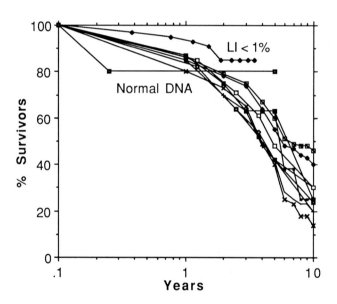

Fig. 10–46. Survival rates of those patients with "low-grade" astrocytomas showing a smoothly curving failure rate (see Fig. 10–44). These include cases considered grades 1 and 2 by the scale of Kernohan and Sayre[80] as reported by others[78,91] or with nuclear atypia only.[78] Those with anaplasia but little or no mitotic activity[134,151] may also belong here (see Fig. 10–45).

plastic astrocytomas have moderate cellular density and nuclear pleomorphism and may have significant mitotic activity and vascular proliferation as in glioblastoma, but the current definition allows no necrosis. Their prognosis is variable (Fig. 10–47). Fulling and Garcia[138] showed that they can be subdivided into two groups based on mitotic activity of more or less than one mitosis per 10 high-power fields with 2- to 3-fold prognostic differences detectable within 2 years and possibly into two other subgroups based on presence or absence of vascular endothelial proliferation with 2-fold differences in prognosis detectable within 5 years (Fig. 10–48). Anaplastic astrocytomas with abnormal DNA by flow cytometry showing evidence of aneuploidy or elevated S or G2-M phases (Coons et al.[134]) have as bad a prognosis as glioblastoma multiforme (Fig. 10–49). The age of the patient also has an effect on the prognosis (Fig. 10–50),[77,85] patients over age 65 with anaplastic astrocytomas dying even more rapidly than comparable patients with glioblastoma multiforme (see Figs.

10–39 and 10–40).[77] The neurologic status of patients with anaplastic astrocytoma is also important (Fig. 10–51).[85]

At least one potentially confusing group of cases can be eliminated from this chapter since "pleomorphic xanthoastrocytomas" occur only in young individuals, those under age 25! These tumors have a much better prognosis than anaplastic astrocytomas occurring in almost comparably young patients.[154–156,161,177] As originally defined by Kepes et al.,[156] they should have no necrosis, so that they could be

confused only with anaplastic astrocytomas; but we have seen some untreated cases with extensive necrosis, so that we suspect that some could also be confused with glioblastomas.

4. Critique: What do we have against the new scheme for classification of astrocytomas presented by Daumas-Duport et al.[78] as "simple and reproducible" and summarized in Table 10–4? Basically, it is too simple and cannot be reproducible without extensive one-on-one instruction! Two of the 4 features (nuclear

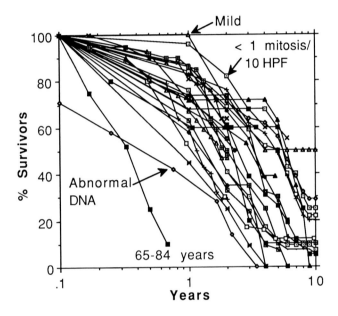

Fig. 10–47. Reported survival rates of patients with anaplastic astrocytomas.[77,78,86,91,134,138,141,145,163,169] Those in patients 65 to 84 years of age[77] or with abnormal DNA by flow cytometry[134] do the worst, those with only "mild" anaplasia[163] or with < 1 mitosis per 10 high power fields[138] do the best; but even after removing these, there is a broad range of survival rates.

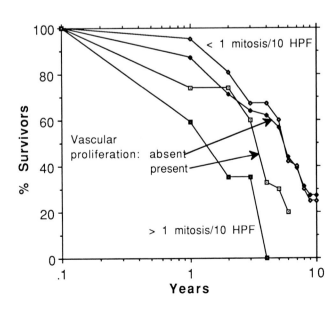

Fig. 10–48. Survival rates of patients with anaplastic astrocytomas (data from Fulling and Garcia[138]) with or without vascular endothelial proliferation (of questionable effect) or containing more or less than 1 mitosis per 10 high power fields (a clear effect).

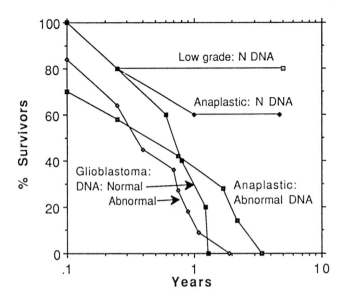

Fig. 10–49. Survival rates of patients with astrocytomas of different grades further subdivided by abnormalities of DNA detected by flow cytometry (data from Coons et al.[134]). Only 4 to 7 patients were in each group.

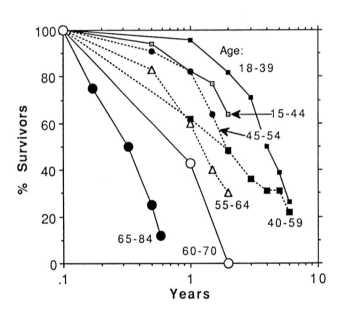

Fig. 10–50. Survival rates of patients of different ages with anaplastic astrocytomas (data from Burger et al.[77] and Nelson et al.[85]); see Figs. 10–39 and 10–40. Three age groups (correlated with sizes of symbols) are apparent with the effect of age persisting for at least 2 years.

atypia and endothelial proliferation) do not occur in all-or-nothing fashion but in a continuum from zero to marked. How can one say that these are present or absent and deserve a corresponding score of 1 or zero? Furthermore, the authors eliminated some of the difficult cases, pleomorphic xanthoastrocytoma and subependymal giant cell astrocytoma, but retained the most difficult, mixed oligoastrocytomas! And most confusing of all, in the next report from the same group (Shaw et al.[91]) they reclassified their new grades 1 and 2 depend-

ing on whether the tumors were pilocytic or gemistocytic or neither. As will become apparent in the discussion of meningiomas below, we are sympathetic to the concept of a scoring system but it should be applicable to all members of the group and it should allow for intermediate scores for those features that do not occur in discrete forms.

From all of the above considerations it should be obvious that we are not completely satisfied with the classification. Astrocytomas are biologically heterogeneous as shown by

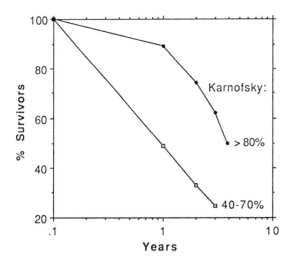

Fig. 10–51. Survival rates of patients with anaplastic astrocytomas with different postoperative Karnofsky scores (data from Nelson et al.[85]).

the significant effect of age and site in the distributions of histologic grades of gliomas and in the durations of their survival. Histologically identical astrocytomas in different locations have different clinical behaviors; e.g., optic nerve or chiasm,[122] cerebellum[65] and spinal cord,[172] and we suspect that astrocytomas in the brainstem or deep or relatively superficial within the cerebral hemispheres should have different prognoses even though we can find no good documentation. Each of these sites, when subdivided by the age of the patient, provides the basis for gliomas with different clinical behaviors; e.g., young patients with optic nerve gliomas[122] or with cerebral astrocytomas (as shown in Figs. 10–39, 10–40, 10–47 and 10–50) have a better prognosis than older patients.

Although predominantly a tumor of children, optic gliomas provide some insight into this problem. There is a broad range of growth rates of optic gliomas (Fig. 10–52). In spite of their histologic homogeneity as low-grade astrocytomas or mixed oligo-astrocytomas, their growth rates not only vary from the most-rapid to the most-slow but also in most cases appear to decelerate (Fig. 10–53). It is not known whether deceleration begins before or after the diagnosis of optic gliomas, but serial MRIs of incidental cases discovered in surveys of families with neurofibromatosis, with which

optic gliomas are frequently associated, should provide the necessary data to prove whether deceleration follows a Gompertz-type curve.[33] At one extreme even infants die within a few months and at the other extreme the last surviving case recurred after 48 years' duration (Fig. 10–54), exactly as predicted by extrapolation of the curve derived from the first 20 years of follow-up.[122] This observation should end the classical argument as to whether optic gliomas are true neoplasms or only hamartomas (congenital malformations that practically do not enlarge) since there is a complete spectrum of growth rates. It is possible, however, that even this observation is a statistical illusion, since Speer et al.[51] have developed a mathematical model that permits long periods of no apparent growth. Even so, especially to be noted in this chapter is the fact that half of the patients over age 50 years with optic gliomas die within 1 year with a glioblastoma and that not all of these glioblastomas are grossly contiguous with the optic glioma that first brought the patient to attention!

As mentioned above, astrocytomas frequently contain small cells without identifiable cytoplasm. The histologic differentiation of oligodendroglia and undifferentiated astrocytes from highly malignant small anaplastic cells is unsatisfactory, to put it mildly. While the existence of "mixed" glial tumors is an accepted fact,[95,96] those with small cells represent especially poorly characterized categories with prognoses varying from relatively benign oligo-astrocytomas to highly malignant small cell glioblastomas. The importance of distinguishing astrocytomas from oligodendrogliomas is shown in Figure 10–37: even the worst of the tumors recognized as oligodendrogliomas has a better prognosis than the best reported for glioblastomas.

In this connection, there is an important asymmetry in the grading introduced by the element of necrosis, which applies only to astrocytomas and separates off those with a bad prognosis (Figs. 10–36 and 10–38 through 10–40 and 10–47 through 10–50) but which does not separate the oligodendrogliomas into different prognostic groups (Figs. 10–26 and 10–27). One is tempted to resolve the issue philosophically by saying that the highest grade of astrocytoma (glioblastoma) includes a high

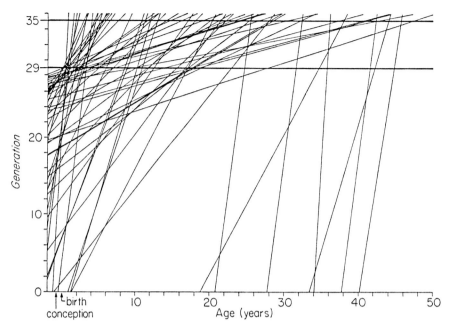

Fig. 10–52. Estimated growth rates of optic gliomas as measured by ages at onset of symptoms and death in 75 patients. For clarity, many overlapping lines are not shown and to save space on the X axis only 3 of the 10 patients over 40 years of age at diagnosis are shown, but all 10 had short courses and correspondingly steep slopes. To construct the graph we assumed that the different sizes of the tumors at the two times (onset of symptoms and death) were approximately the same in every patient. The line joining the two points representing any particular patient can be extrapolated back to the time when the tumor comprised only one cell 20 μ in diameter (that is 29 generations before onset of symptoms) to illustrate growth postulated to have been at a simple exponential rate (doubling at a constant rate). Of the 75 cases, only 23 satisfied this criterion by originating after conception, but at least 42 did not even come close and would require some decelerating growth curve for adequate representation. (From Alvord and Lofton,[122] reprinted by permission of the J. Neurosurg.).

grade of oligodendrogliomas which are so pleomorphic as to be no longer recognizable as oligodendrogliomas. However, this leads immediately to an impasse since the major criterion of necrosis that separates the highest grade of astrocytoma (glioblastoma) from the intermediate grade (anaplastic astrocytoma) does not separate the "good" from the "bad" oligodendrogliomas. It is critically important, therefore, to separate astrocytomas and oligodendrogliomas at the first step in the histologic analysis if the classification of gliomas is to be of any real service in predicting the prognosis of individual patients or in evaluating the results of different treatments of groups of patients.

Gliomas may be regionally heterogeneous in their cellular composition; thus, sampling artifacts can be a significant problem. Several

studies have emphasized that the more striking, classical histologic features of malignancy, such as nuclear atypia (seen in its extreme form in pleomorphic xanthoastrocytomas, as discussed above), are less important than other more subtle substrates of tumor aggressiveness. Multinucleated giant cells are probably end-stage cells, incapable of further growth. The rapidly proliferating, small anaplastic cells are the ones most easily destroyed by irradiation,[170] but only temporarily, since they are the ones that recur and infiltrate.[142,171] Infiltrates of lymphocytes have been variably reported to be correlated with survival, suggesting that immune responses to tumors may[128,136,162] or may not[77] extend survival.

In every diffusely infiltrating glial tumor there is a background population of astrocytes and oligodendroglia normally present in the

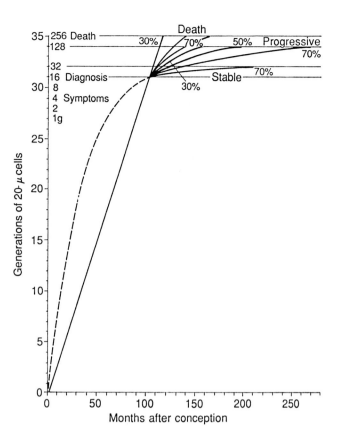

Fig. 10-53. Deceleration of growth rates of optic chiasmal gliomas must occur in order to account for the prolonged survival of most patients after diagnosis. Whether deceleration begins before diagnosis, as suggested by the dashed line, remains to be determined. The multiple lines after diagnosis are for 30%, 50%, and 70% of each of 3 groups of patients: those who remained stable, those who progressed, and those who died.

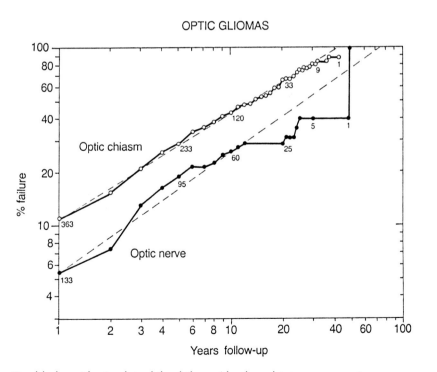

Fig. 10-54. Double-logarithmic plot of the failures (death and tumor progression or recurrence) in 468 patients with optic chiasmal gliomas and in 155 patients with optic nerve gliomas. The numbers indicate the numbers of patients alive at the times indicated. (From Alvord and Lofton,[122] reprinted by permission of the J. Neurosurg.).

243

brain parenchyma, a background which makes it difficult to determine whether the tumor is a low grade glioma, a mixed glioma[95,96] or the edge of a high-grade glioma. Furthermore, the component of reactive gliosis both within and surrounding the main tumor mass can be confused as evidence of astrocytic differentiation of part or all of a neoplasm. We have found the pattern of cell distribution revealed by staining astrocytes for GFAP to be useful: reactive astrocytes may increase in number as well as size but they remain individually separate (Fig. 10–55), not so closely packed together as one would expect of a clone of neoplastic cells (Fig. 10–56). One must be careful

in evaluating the presence of astrocytic fibers, however, since they can be long and extend obliquely through many histologic sections. Thus, the perinuclear cytoplasm, most easily stained by its usual content of GFAP, is the important factor to be recognized, not the more distal fibers, even though they may be quite densely packed.

Since reactive astrocytes are usually plump ("gemästete Glia" in German or gemistocytes in English), their presence can add to the confusion with some astrocytomas that have prominent gemistocytic differentiation and are classified as "gemistocytic astrocytomas." Unfortunately, "gemistocytes" have not been sat-

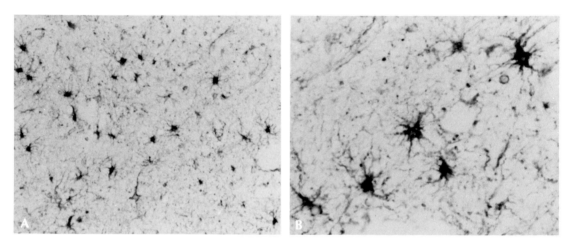

Fig. 10–55. Photomicrographs of sections stained for GFAP illustrating the patterns of cells seen in reactive astrocytic gliosis in an oligodendroglioma (A, × 200; B, × 500; Np15137).

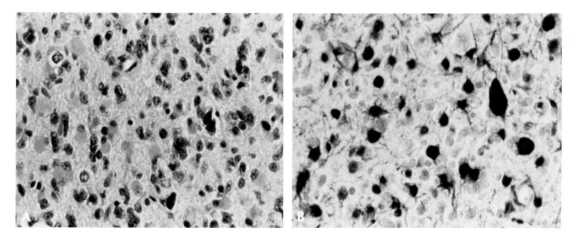

Fig. 10–56. Photomicrographs of an astrocytoma stained by H&E (A) and for GFAP (B), both × 500, Np11603.

isfactorily defined as to just how large they should be or just how they should differ from reactive gliosis, and only one investigator[83] has defined a gemistocytic astrocytoma as one in which "gemistocytes" (otherwise undefined) comprise more than 60% of the population. Shaw et al.[91] noted that low-grade astrocytomas with a significant gemistocytic component behave badly but they provided no actual results. These tumors are probably over-diagnosed when only the edge of a more-rapidly growing glioma is biopsied. Just how much this error contributed to the impression of Shaw et al.[91] that gemistocytic astrocytomas progress more rapidly than expected from their low-grade histologic appearance is difficult to say, but we suspect that it must have played a role in at least some cases since gemistocytic cells have been shown to be end-stage non-proliferating cells.[148]

The maturation of neoplastic and reactive cells can be deduced by comparing autoradiographs of biopsy and autopsy specimens after in vivo labeling with tritiated thymidine, as reported by Hoshino et al.[147] Cells that were dividing rapidly at the time of biopsy will have lost their label after only a few more divisions unless they come to rest in a non-cycling (G_0) phase. Five cell cycles of 2 to 3 days each— about 2 weeks total—should suffice to dilute the label, but a marked variability from case to case was encountered. Two of 5 glioblastomas diluted out the label in 2 to 4 months but the 3 other glioblastomas and the 2 anaplastic astrocytomas retained some labeled neoplastic cells for 3 weeks to 5 months, especially at the growing edge of the tumor. In the one well-differentiated mixed glioma labeled cells remained for 7 years, indicating that either the cells have extremely long cycle times or they enter G_0 and do not return to the cycling pool.

At biopsy many varieties of cells were labeled:[147] astrocytes, oligodendroglia, ependyma, endothelium, lymphocytes, and fibroblasts. Other cells were not labeled: polymorphonuclear leukocytes, macrophages, gemistocytic astrocytes, and peri-necrotic palisading cells. At autopsy most of the neoplastic cells had diluted the label, but other cells were labeled: endothelium, gemistocytic and fibrillary astrocytes, oligodendroglia, microglia, and macrophages. These observations suggest that

gemistocytic astrocytes must derive from non-gemistocytic elements. Multi-nucleated giant cells were sparsely labeled, but all the nuclei were equally labeled, suggesting repeated division of nuclei without cytoplasmic division, not fusion of several cells. Subependymal astrocytes, either normal or neoplastic, were occasionally heavily labeled, indicating a slow rate of proliferation or rapid entry into G_0.

Polymorphonuclear leukocytes and macrophages were not labeled in the biopsies but were observed at autopsy, probably having been labeled in the bone marrow and having migrated subsequently into the tumor. Lymphocytes, by contrast, were labeled in the biopsies but not in the autopsies, probably because they divide rapidly and dilute the label.[147]

The nuclear atypia, reactive gliosis and necrosis following ionizing radiation therapy preclude accurate grading of a treated glioma. This is unfortunate because the question frequently arises, has the tumor evolved into a more malignant form or is it still biologically the same as it was before treatment? Astrocytomas often change in histologic appearance during the natural course of disease, as well as in response to therapy, generally becoming more malignant with the duration as well as with the age of the patient. This pattern suggests that there is a malignant progression of astrocytomas due to increasing genetic instability of the tumor cells.[23,124,125,165–169] Indeed, a better prognosis is correlated with longer duration of symptoms, especially seizures for more than 18 months.[120] Computer models have been developed to permit random spurts in growth,[51] which can easily be imagined as related to step-wise segmental chromosomal changes. Such a progression is now being seen more frequently as advanced diagnostic techniques (CT and MRI) contribute to the earlier diagnosis of all types of brain tumors, as we have mentioned above in relation to oligodendrogliomas.[115,118,119]

Most recently Cavenee[131] has reported evidence that glioblastomas arise in two ways, directly from precursor cells and progressively through intermediate stages of astrocytomas ("grades 2 and 3", presumably of Kernohan's grading). The progression begins with heterozygosity for chromosome 17p, then homozygosity of 17p, followed by hemizygosity for chromosome 10 and ending with production of epithelial cell growth factor receptor (EGFR). Since only about half of glioblastomas (and only about one-fourth of anaplastic astrocytomas) possess EGFR, the other half of glioblastomas are thought to arise directly rather than progressively.

With all of the above factors contributing to confusion in diagnosis, it is remarkable that so many important prognostic variables have already been identified. This is all the more remarkable when one recognizes that the prognosis of any tumor patient obviously depends on the amount and type of tumor left behind in the patient, not what was taken out. Since these two critical factors can usually not be measured with any accuracy, the assumption most generally made is that patients will behave in some statistical fashion related to "average" amounts of "the same type" of tumor left behind as was excised. In most patients with astrocytomas the tumor left behind is usually in the walls of the resection site but in some patients it may be "incubating" at some considerable distance (about 10% of gliomas are grossly multicentric). Is the most malignant cellular component of a glioblastoma multiforme the one that is spreading or is there a more gradual cell-to-cell change, perhaps by transfection by DNA fragments diffusing into the surrounding tissue? Alternatively, is there a multiclonal growth at some stage in the development, most easily visualized as occurring at the beginning in the multicentric cases, but probably near the end of a progressively increasing genetic instability in the grossly solitary ones?

5. Mathematical analysis: Recurrences of gliomas are so common that most of our understanding of the biology of brain tumors is derived from them. Some interesting calculations and approximations can be made relating estimations of growth rates and volumes of tumor remaining to actual durations of survival. Gutin et al.[145] presented the results of treating patients with cerebral anaplastic astrocytomas or glioblastomas by implanting ^{125}I in the walls of the tumor that recurred following surgical excision and x-irradiation. They compared these results with similar patients treated by chemotherapy after surgery and x-

ray therapy. Their results are presented here in Figures 10–57 and 10–58 as mortality rates on a semi-logarithmic scale. Although the "control" and "experimental" groups were collected at different times and, therefore, are not strictly comparable, the results are interesting.

Referring back to Figures 10–3 and 10–4, in which the parallel lines were said to represent groups of patients with tumors differing either

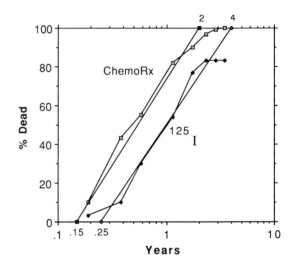

Fig. 10–57. Mortality rates of patients with recurrent glioblastomas following treatment with surgery, x ray, and ^{125}I implantation or with surgery, x-ray, and chemotherapy. Time is after the recurrence, not overall (data from Gutin et al.[145]).

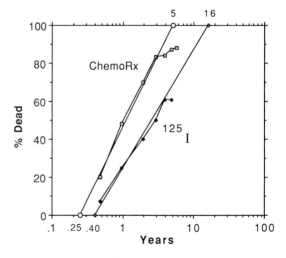

Fig. 10–58. Mortality rates of patients with anaplastic astrocytomas following similar treatments as in Figure 10–57. Time is after the recurrence, not overall (data from Gutin et al.[145]).

by growth rates or by amounts of tumor left behind, one can see that in actuality they represent neither one alone but rather their product, a typical feature underlying Heisenberg's "Uncertainty Principle." Although one cannot define both the growth rate and the amount of tumor left behind in any particular patient, the straight lines representing mortality rates (Figs. 10–57 and 10–58) allow one to calculate the product "time × rate" for a group of patients assuming that the products are evenly distributed through the group. Whatever the range of growth rates and whatever the range of amounts of tumor left behind may be, their products are related such that anaplastic astrocytomas grow about twice (1.6 to 4.0 times) as slowly as comparably treated glioblastomas if one assumes that approximately the same amounts of tumor were left behind in each patient. The actual ratio of growth rates can be defined at arbitrary points, such as the 0%, 50% or 100% mortality rates:

(a) chemotherapy: 0.25/0.15 = 1.7, 1.1/0.54 = 2.0, 5.0/2.0 = 2.5.
(b) ^{125}I: 0.4/0.25 = 1.6, 2.5/1.1 = 2.3, 16/4 = 4.0.

Another conclusion is that ^{125}I destroys about twice as much tumor (measured in number of generations, not grams) as chemotherapy, whether one considers anaplastic astrocytomas or glioblastomas. The actual ratios defined by the 0%, 50% or 100% mortality rates are as follows:

(a) glioblastoma: 0.25/0.15 = 1.7, 1.1/0.54 = 2.0, 4.0/2.0 = 2.0
(b) anaplastic astrocytoma: 0.4/0.25 = 1.6, 2.5/1.1 = 2.3, 16/5 = 3.2.

The improvement in results shown in Figures 10–57 and 10–58 associated with ^{125}I implantation as contrasted with chemotherapy (both following surgery and x-irradiation), similar to the results obtained by extensive surgical excisions,[120,153] can be most easily understood in terms of the amounts of tumor which were probably left behind in the walls of the operative site, as described in Figure 10–6. An almost fatal tumor 5 cm in diameter at the time of operation consists of about 2^{36} cells (64 g, a

large amount, the removal of which a surgeon might well regard as a "total" or "nearly total" removal) but the surrounding 0.5 cm shell consists of about $2^{35.5}$ cells (about 48 g), almost the same amount, which allows less than one more doubling before it is almost fatal again. Of course, the tumor cells in the shell are more diffusely spread through the normal tissue, making their recognition difficult even microscopically. As mentioned previously, if only 6% of the cells in any histologic preparation were neoplastic, only 4 doublings (i.e., to 12%, 24%, 48% and 96%) would be required to bring the tumor up to an equivalent of 100% concentration in this shell and another doubling to return to its original size.

The plateaus shown in Figures 10–57 and 10–58 suggest that some patients may have been cured of their gliomas but further follow-up is obviously necessary since extensive central necrosis of rapidly growing neoplasms can convert exponential growth into much slower linear growth.[40,52,53]

Another example of the probable interaction of cytokinetic factors and amounts of tumor excised is provided by an analysis of the paradoxical results reported by Gaetani et al.[139] and Bookwalter et al.,[127] namely, that patients with glioblastoma died at exactly the same rate regardless of the degree of proliferative activity as measured by the tritiated thymidine labeling index (Fig. 10–59). The nomogram de-

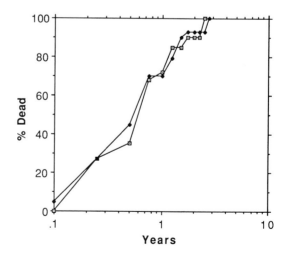

Fig. 10–59. Identical mortality rates reported by Bookwalter et al.[127] for 2 groups of patients with glioblastomas having LI's greater or less than 5%.

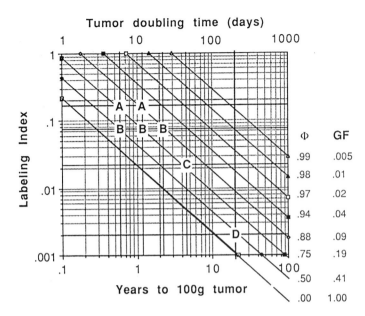

Fig. 10–60. Extremes and medians for LI and survival times reported by Bookwalter et al.[127] and plotted on the nomogram of Figure 10–12 allow estimates of combinations of possible cell loss factors (or growth fractions) and amounts of tumor left behind: 75 to 88% cell loss with 2^0 to $2^{18.25}$ cells (up to 0.3 mg) left behind in the high extreme patient (A), 50 to 88% cell loss with 2^0 to $2^{27.38}$ cells (up to 200 mg) left behind in the median of the high LI group (B), 80% cell loss with $2^{31.94}$ cells (4 g) left behind in the median of the low LI group (C), and 50% cell loss with $2^{35.4}$ cells (44 g) left behind in the low extreme patient (D).

veloped on theoretical considerations (Fig. 10–12) was used as the basis for Figure 10–60, in which are plotted the available data from Bookwalter et al.:[127] extremes of LI (0.2 and 18%), median LI's of the two groups of patients with LI above or below 5% (7.4 and 2.2%, respectively), extremes of survival (0 and 2.5 years), median survival of both groups (0.6 year) and median growth fractions of a few cases in each group (18.9% in 3 cases with low LI, 32% in 5 cases with high LI).

Assuming that each patient or group of patients had only 1 cell left behind so that they all died at the median time (0.6 year) leads to the possible conclusion derived from Figure 10–60 that the group with the high LI's (including the extreme case) must have had at least 50% cell loss (with 80% in the extreme case) but to the impossible conclusion that there was less than zero cell loss for the group with the low LI's. The next easiest possibility to consider is to assume that each had $2^{18.5}$ cells left behind. This at least lets the group with the low LI's fit on the nomogram with zero cell loss, but the extreme lowest must be moved to the right at least to the point of having about 22 g of tumor left behind with zero cell loss. If one assumes "reasonable" degrees of cell loss of the order of 50% to 90%, the estimates of the amounts of tumor left behind would be as follows: 0.3 mg in the case with the highest LI, 200 mg in the median case with LI > 5%, 4 g

in the median case with LI < 5% and 44 g in the case with the lowest LI. Again, as with Heisenberg's "Uncertainty Principle," a product of two factors is involved, this time the LI and the amount of tumor left behind contributing to the range of possible solutions to the problem posed by the original paradox.

Two cases with specific LI's and survival times were also presented by Bookwalter et al.[127] and are illustrated in Figure 10–61. Both would fit with a cell loss factor of 87.5% if only 1 tumor cell had been left behind, but other possibilities include 93.8% cell loss if 0.3 mg of tumor had been left behind, 96.9% cell loss if 200 mg of tumor had been left behind, etc. as the ratio between actual and expected survival times decreases—"expected," that is, on the basis of how great the unmeasured cell loss factor actually was.

The range of cell loss factors estimated in these two cases assumes a growth fraction of 100%, but the determination of actual growth fractions in a few other cases allows another graphic solution to be made (Fig. 10–62). If it is assumed that the cell loss factor (ϕ) was zero, and if the medians of the few cases studied are representative of the medians of their respective groups, the median amounts of tumor left behind can be estimated as $2^{12} = 4,000$ cells and 2^{32} cells (4 g) for the groups with high and low LI's, respectively (using Fig. 10–11 and the ratio of actual and expected sur-

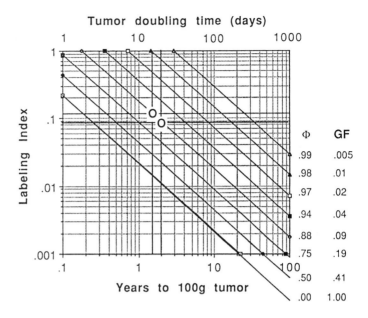

Fig. 10–61. Two cases reported by Bookwalter et al.[127] had specific LI's and survival times which allow estimates of combinations of cell loss factor (or growth fractions) and amount of tumor left behind: 87.5% if 1 cell were left behind, 93.8% if $2^{18.25}$ cells (0.3 mg) were left behind, 96.9% if $2^{27.38}$ cells (200 mg) were left behind, etc.

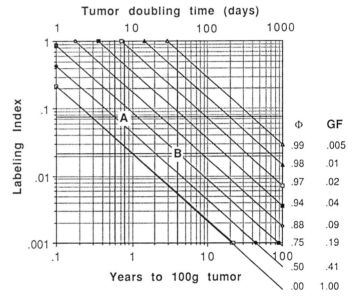

Fig. 10–62. Medians for LI's (all 19 patients in each group) and growth fractions (only 5 of the patients with LI> 5% and only 3 of the patients with LI < 5%) reported by Bookwalter et al.[127] and plotted on the same nomogram allow estimates of amounts of tumor left behind assuming the cell loss factor to be zero and the small samples representative: 2^9 cells (about 500 cells) in the median of the high LI group (A), 2^{31} cells (about 2 g) in the median of the low LI group (B).

vival times defined in Fig. 10–13). Since it is not likely that $\phi = 0$, the expected survival times would be even greater and the ratios correspondingly less; therefore, the amounts of tumor left behind would be even larger.

6. Summary: From all of the above considerations, we believe that 3 *morphologic* tiers of astrocytomas can be defined histologically with reasonable accuracy and reproducibility but by itself such a scheme is not a satisfactory index of prognosis. The prognosis can be better approximated if certain *biologic* features are also considered, such as age, mitotic activity

and DNA abnormalities, as shown in Figure 10–32. Assuming that the amount of tumor left behind is the same in every patient, we can recognize 4 prognostic groups:

The *rapidly recurring astrocytomas* include: (1) practically all glioblastomas as defined by the presence of necrosis[77,86] except those occurring in patients 15 to 44 years of age,[77] (2) "grade 4" astrocytomas of Daumas-Duport et al.,[78] and (3) anaplastic astrocytomas with abnormal DNA[134] or occurring in patients 65 to 84 years of age.[77]

The *intermediate-recurring astrocytomas* include: (1) practically all anaplastic astrocytomas as defined by the absence of necrosis,[77,86] specifically those in patients 45 to 64 years of age[77] and those with one or more mitoses per 10 high-power fields,[138] (2) "grade 3" astrocytomas of Daumas-Duport et al.,[78] (3) glioblastomas occurring in patients 15 to 44 years of age,[77] (4) astrocytomas of grades 1 and 2 of Daumas-Duport et al.[78] with gemistocytic features,[91] and (5) "moderately anaplastic" ("low grade") astrocytomas with BrDU labeling index of 1% or more.[151]

The *slowly recurring astrocytomas* include: (1) astrocytomas of grades 1 and 2 of Daumas-Duport et al.[78] without other characteristics, (2) low-grade astrocytomas with normal DNA,[134] (3) "moderately anaplastic" ("low grade") astrocytomas with BrDU labeling index less than 1%,[151] and (4) anaplastic astrocytomas occurring in patients 15 to 44 years of age,[77] having few or no mitoses[138] or normal DNA.[134]

The very slowly recurring astrocytomas include the pilocytic astrocytomas derived from the astrocytomas of grades 1 and 2 of Daumas-Duport et al.,[78] as also reported by others.[91,132,140,176] In fact, these tumors are almost non-recurring, especially if totally excised, and probably do not respond to x-irradiation.[140,176]

Of course, one must first be certain that the lesion is really neoplastic and not reactive, as in early multiple sclerosis, where we have learned to our embarrassment that the astrocytes can be especially pleomorphic, before one begins to grade it as an astrocytoma. Reference to CT or MR images usually shows the presence of multiple lesions, which prompted the biopsy for presumptive metastatic cancer, but we[181] have seen large single lesions that have required a high index of suspicion (usually prompted by the presence of macrophages, which are unusual in neoplasms) to suggest doing special stains for myelin and axons. Atrophy of the white matter in chronic focal epileptics results in hypercellularity that can also be misinterpreted as a glioma, especially an oligodendroglioma. The asymmetry in classification of astrocytomas and oligodendrogliomas related to the factor of necrosis must also be recognized as such an important factor that this differentiation must also be made before grading even an obvious neoplasm as an astrocytoma; but until we have

specific stains for oligodendroglioma cells, our ability to truly differentiate astrocytomas, oligodendrogliomas and mixed gliomas will remain difficult.

MENINGIOMAS

Meningiomas[10,31,182–213] commonly occur in the elderly. These tumors are usually hemispherical masses attached to the under surface of the dura and are derived from pia, arachnoid and dura (Figs. 10–63 through 10–65). They are generally benign, at least 90% of those that can be completely excised according to Jääskeläinen et al.,[31,197] and thought, therefore, to be slowly growing tumors; but they frequently recur, sometimes incredibly rapidly. One may not be too surprised at recurrence rates of 6 to 12% per year after incomplete removals,[182,205] except perhaps to wonder why the rate is not higher; but how is one to understand the recurrence rates of 1 to 2.5% per year after radically complete excisions, as noted by several recent reports?[31,182,197,205,207] And how is one to understand growth rates (gross volume-doubling times or Td) of a "benign" tumor ranging from 0.3 to 35 months,[10,31] rates remarkably similar to the ranges of those of breast cancers[32] and gliomas (see Figs. 10–25 and 10–29)? Do growth rates correlate with recurrence rates and do histologic appearances of meningiomas correlate with these biologic characteristics?

To begin with the last question, ever since Cushing and Eisenhardt[189] described their "57 varieties" of meningiomas, other investigators have attempted to simplify the scheme. The most popular classification currently includes meningothelial (Fig. 10–66), psammomatous (Fig. 10–67A), transitional, fibroblastic (Fig. 10–67B), angioblastic (Fig. 10–68) and anaplastic or sarcomatous (Fig. 10–69). This classification does not seem to be helpful since about 10% of each of the "benign" types recur, with, of course, an expectedly higher rate for the anaplastic or sarcomatous (Fig. 10–70). Even though these estimates have not been defined actuarily, why should the "benign" ones recur? Why is the recognition of the malignant ones so difficult?[210] Histologic criteria predicting recurrences have been presented by de la Monte et al.,[190] but they studied only

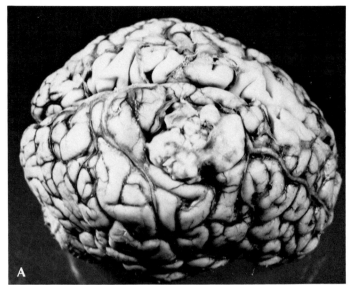

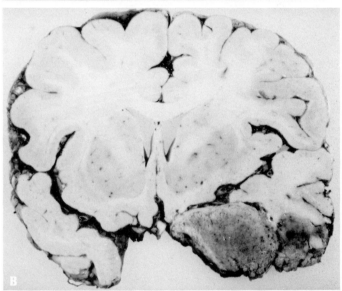

Fig. 10–63. Meningiomas of the right cerebral convexity (A, Np4612) and of the left temporal pole (B, Np12399).

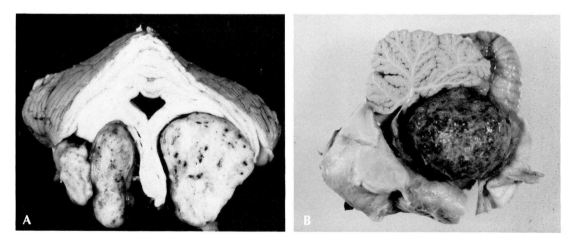

Fig. 10–64. Meningiomas of both cerebello-pontine angles (A, Np3781) and of the posterior foramen magnum extending into the 4th ventricle (B, Np8237).

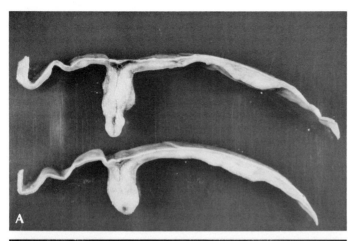

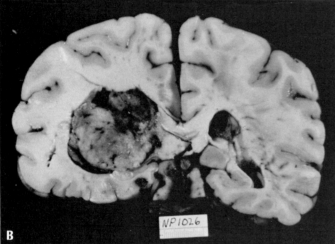

Fig. 10–65. En plaque meningioma of dura and superior sagittal sinus (A, Np8116) and intraventricular meningioma in left trigone (B, Np1026).

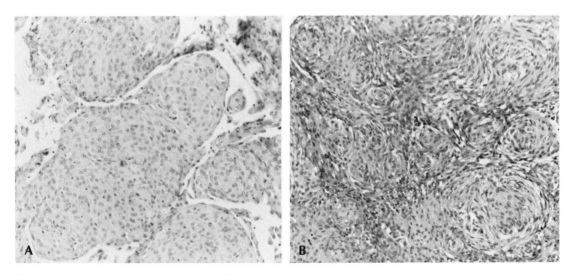

Fig. 10–66.   Photomicrographs of two different fields of a grade 1 meningothelial meningioma (A, H&E, × 200; B, Np11704). Note the better whorl formation in B.

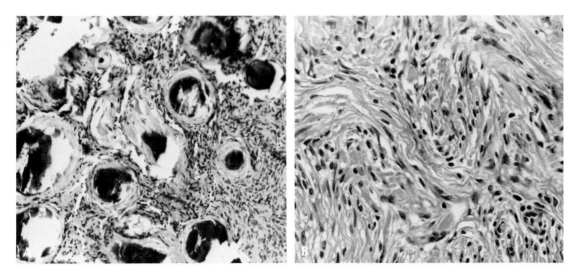

Fig. 10–67. Photomicrographs of grade 1 psammomatous (A, Np15212, × 200) and fibroblastic (B, Np15246 × 500) meningiomas, both stained by H&E.

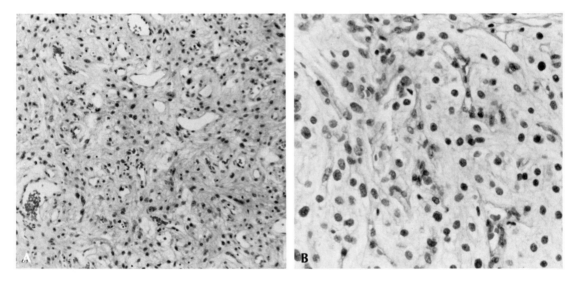

Fig. 10–68. Photomicrographs of angioblastic meningiomas stained by H&E (A, grade 2, Np12314, × 200; B, grade 3, Np14060, × 500).

incompletely removed meningiomas, all of which should have recurred anyway at times at least partly dependent on how much tumor had been left behind, which, needless to say, was not reported. May et al.[204] have used flow cytometric measurements on paraffin-embedded specimens from completely excised tumors, some of which recurred and some did not. Nine of the 15 recurrent cases had >20% for the total of S and G2/M phases, whereas

none of the 18 non-recurrent cases were this high. A new histologic scheme proposed by Haltia in a series of studies by Jääskeläinen et al.[31,197] uses other characteristics in a semi-quantitative way to reach cummulative scores that define grades 1, 2, 3 and 4 (Table 10–6).

The value of Haltia's scheme is clearly seen in the results reported by Jääskeläinen et al.[31,197,198] showing that practically all grade 3 meningiomas recur within 6 years, about half

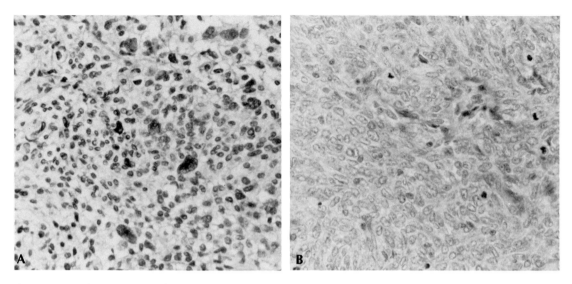

Fig. 10-69. Photomicrographs of an anaplastic focus (grade 3) in the angioblastic meningioma shown in Figure 10-68B (A, × 500) and of a sarcomatous (grade 4) meningioma (B, Np5409, × 500) both stained by H&E.

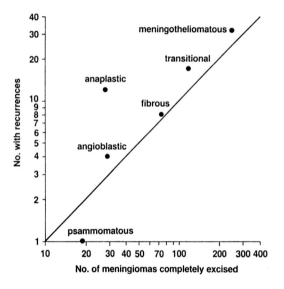

Fig. 10-70. About 10% of "completely excised" meningiomas recur regardless of classical histologic type as shown by the dots being near the diagonal straight line, but about 4 times as many of the anaplastic meningiomas recur (data from M. Kujas in Philippon et al.[207]).

of grade 2 meningiomas recur within 12 years, and 20% of grade 1 meningiomas recur within 24 years (Fig. 10-71). If the 20% were really 25%, we would see a very precise double exponential relationship between recurrence rate

and time, which has a certain esthetic elegance that contributes a useful mnemonic aid! Hemangiopericytomas[199] (Fig. 10-72), which some would include with angioblastic meningiomas, behave like grade 2 to 3 meningiomas, about 50% recurring within 8 to 9 years (Fig. 10-73). As with gliomas (see Fig. 10-32), perhaps a combination of histologic features (Table 10-6) and biologic features[204] will predict recurrences better than either alone but unfortunately May et al.[204] used the wrong (i.e., classical) histologic scheme which does not recognize intermediate grades of malignancy!

Of the several published reports concerning grossly "complete" excisions of meningiomas,[10,31,182,197,205,207,209,210] two have been the

TABLE 10-6. Haltia's Criteria for Histologic Grading of Meningiomas (Jääskeläinen et al.[31])

Histologic features	Potential score
Loss of architecture	0-1-2-3
Increased cellularity	0-1-2-3
Nuclear pleomorphism	0-1-2-3
Mitotic figures	0-1-2-3
Focal necroses	0-1-2-3
Brain infiltration	0------3
Total score for Grade 1:	0-2
2:	3-6
3:	7-11
4:	12-18

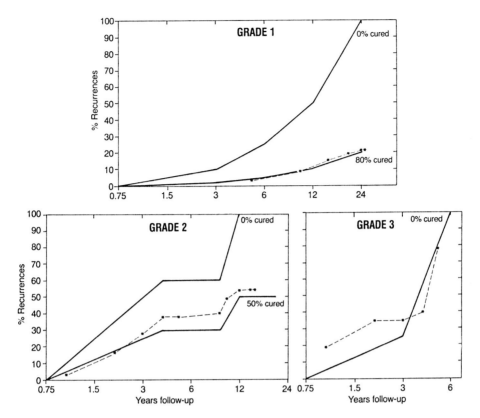

Fig. 10–71. Recurrence rates (dashed lines) of completely excised meningiomas graded by Haltia (data provided by Jääskeläinen) and compared with expected recurrence rates (solid lines) if 0, 50, or 80% cure rates had been obtained.

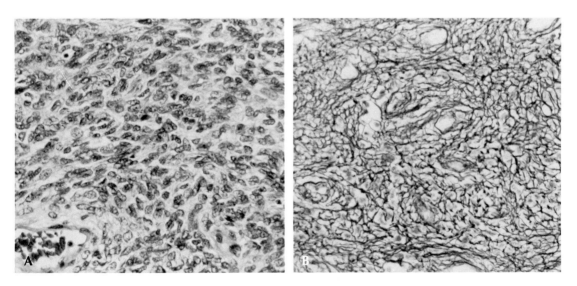

Fig. 10–72. Hemangiopericytoma with abundant reticulin surrounding thin sheets of tumor cells (Np14473, × 500; A, H&E; B, reticulin stain).

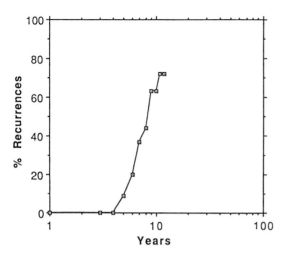

Fig. 10–73. Recurrence rate of completely excised intracranial hemangiopericytomas (data from Jääskeläinen et al.[199]). The curve is intermediate between those for meningiomas of grades 2 and 3 (see Fig. 10–71).

most valuable for estimating growth rates. The first was that of Philippon et al.,[207] who divided their patients with recurrences into 2 groups: those followed for 5 to 10 years (20 cases) and those followed for 10 to 15 years (25 cases). Even though this study incorporates one error that we will comment on below, it is clear that the longer one follows patients, the more recurrences are found (Fig. 10–74). This is not surprising but it does not permit much more analysis. The second was the series of re-

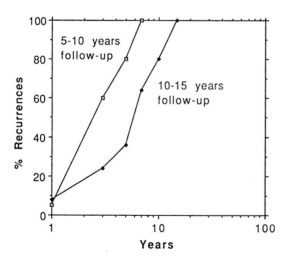

Fig. 10–74. Recurrence rates of completely excised meningiomas followed for 5 to 10 years or for 10 to 15 years (data from Philippon et al.[207]).

ports of Jääskeläinen et al.,[31,197] who have made extensive comparisons of a large number of patients that have been followed over even longer periods of time than those of Philippon et al.[207] Jääskeläinen generously provided the data regarding the actual times of recurrences so that, following the suggestion of Berkson and Gage,[75] we could group patients for exact durations of "risk to follow-up" of 3, 6, 12, and 24 years, an arbitrarily exponential progression. Figure 10–75 shows the results for all the known recurrences following "complete" excision of all histologic grades of meningiomas (98 cases). It should be noted that there is still no overlapping of the curves at 12 and 24 years, suggesting that even 24 years is not a sufficiently long follow-up.

To understand this last suggestion, one may perform an imaginary experiment: suppose that a theoretical tumor is being studied, all of whose recurrences will occur before 15 years of follow-up. If one group of these patients is followed for exactly 5 years, a certain number of recurrences will be observed and can be identified as 100% at 5 years and corresponding percentages calculated for the recurrences at years 1, 2, etc., and plotted (Fig. 10–76). If another group of patients is followed for exactly 10 years, another number of recurrences will be observed, but the total can still be identified as 100% at 10 years follow-up, with corresponding annual percentages of recurrences calculated and plotted. If still other patients are followed for exactly 15 years, still another number of recurrences will be observed and the total identified as 100% at 15 years follow-up, the annual recurrence percentages calculated and plotted. Any group of patients followed for more than 15 years will yield a line that overlaps this 15-year group and will show a plateau at 100% from 15 years on.

What one must be careful not to do—but what is almost always done in medical reports—is to add the recurrences occurring in one group of patients (e.g., those followed up to 5 years) to another group of patients (e.g., those followed up to 10 years) and say that they have been followed for "5 to 10 years" or "up to 10 years" without any correction for possible inadequacy of follow-up of either group. In our theoretical example above, both of the groups with follow-ups only for 5 and

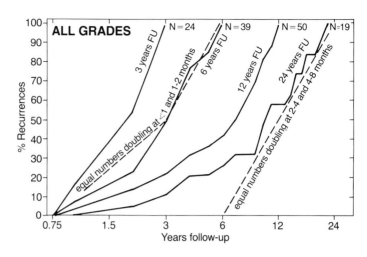

Fig. 10–75. Recurrence rates of completely excised meningiomas (all grades combined) compared with expected results if there were single cells left behind to double every 0.5 to 2 months or every 2 to 8 months (these ranges are twice as broad as the ones shown in Figs. 10–3 and 10–4; thus, the slopes are half as steep).

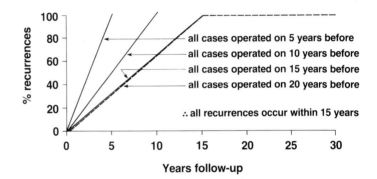

Fig. 10–76. Recurrences of a theoretical tumor "completely removed" in patients followed for exactly 5, 10, 15 or 20 years.

10 years obviously fall short of the 15 years necessary to obtain all the recurrences. Although each group of patients can have rapidly growing tumors, only those with the longer follow-ups can have the slower growing tumors. That is, as Berkson and Gage[75] pointed out, one must define the patients "exposed to the risk for surviving 5 years," 10 years, etc. The common practice of grouping patients as having been followed 0 to 5 years, 5 to 10 years, etc., as in Figure 10–74, has exactly this fallacy of attempting to average disparate patients, disparate because even within apparently similar durations of follow-up, those followed for 5 years have a different risk for surviving 10 years as compared to those actually followed for 10 years.

To return to the real world of meningiomas, we see in Figure 10–75 evidence that even 24 years is not long enough follow-up for all meningiomas. Figure 10–77 shows the same for the benign grade 1 meningiomas that comprise 90% of the total. However, for grades 2 and 3,

all of the recurrences occur within 12 and 6 years, respectively (Figs. 10–78 and 10–79).

But why should any tumor that has been "completely excised" recur? The obvious answer is that some tumor was left behind. But how much and where? Was one cell or more than one cell left behind? What is the growth rate of that cell or of those cells left behind? Just as with Heisenberg's "Uncertainty Principle" mentioned in the Introduction, one cannot define precisely both the amount of tumor that must have been left behind after "complete" excision and the growth rate, although some reasonable limits can be estimated. Figures 10–77, 10–78 and 10–79 show that the growth rates of recurrent meningiomas correlate with the histologic gradings and fit with the hypothesis that recurrent meningiomas develop from masses of tumor left behind that vary from a single cell to 18 to 27 generations of cells (up to about 0.25 to 125 mg, respectively), as shown in Table 10–7 and Figure 10–80. Cures occur in about 80% of grade 1 ("be-

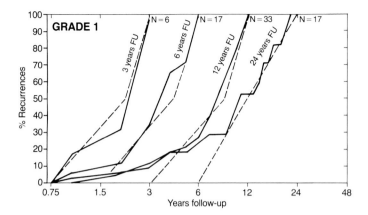

Fig. 10-77. Recurrences of grade 1 meningiomas in patients followed for exactly 3, 6, 12 or 24 years (data provided by Jääskeläinen). The dashed lines represent expected results if equal numbers of patients had 1 cell or 2^{18} cells left behind to double every 4 to 8 months.

nign'') meningiomas and in about 50% of grade 2 ("atypical") meningiomas when not even 1 cell is left behind; but since at least 18 generations of tumor are left behind in grade 3 ("anaplastic") meningiomas, no cures appear possible by surgical excision.

An independent approach is to use Figure 10–12 as a basis for plotting the data for 4 meningiomas studied by Cho et al.[10] From the LI and the Td reported for each case (Fig. 10–81) one can obtain both the cell loss factor (or its approximate inverse, the growth fraction) and the expected time to recurrence. Since there is little evidence of cell loss due to necrosis or

metastasis, the growth fraction is most likely to be the critical factor. Assuming 100 g for the recurrence, only 1 generation larger than the median of 64 g measured by Jääskeläinen et al.,[31,197] one can estimate growth fractions of about 4 to 16% and amounts of tumor left behind of 90 cells to 4 g (Fig. 10–81). Another dozen meningiomas with LI's only were reported by Cho et al.[10] and Fukui et al.[193] and are plotted in Figure 10–82. Even if only 1 cell had been left behind, growth fractions must have been only about 4 to 41%. The cases to the left in Figure 10–82, most of which were known to have been subtotally resected, can

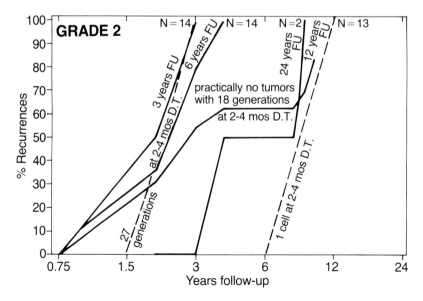

Fig. 10-78. Recurrences of grade 2 meningiomas in patients followed for exactly 3, 6, 12 or 24 years (data provided by Jääskeläinen). The dashed lines represent expected results if 1 cell or 2^{27} cells had been left behind to double every 2 to 4 months. Note that there must have been practically no patients with 2^{18} cells left behind.

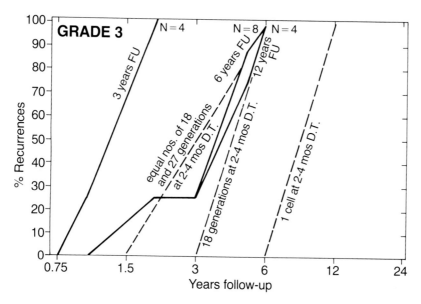

Fig. 10–79. Recurrences of grade 3 meningiomas in patients followed for exactly 3, 6 or 12 years (data provided by Jääskeläinen). The dashed lines represent expected results if 1 cell, 2^{18} or 2^{27} cells had been left behind to double every 2 to 4 months. Note that there could have been no cases with only 1 cell left behind.

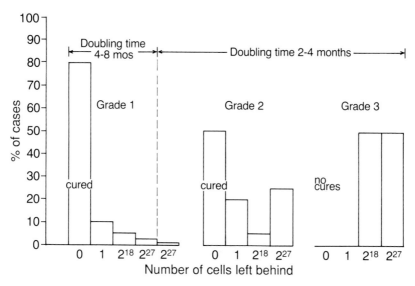

Fig. 10–80. Theoretical distributions of numbers of meningioma cells of various grades left behind following "complete" excision with doubling times of 2 to 4 months or 4 to 8 months, distributions that would fit the results shown in Figures 10–77 through 10–79.

TABLE 10–7. Distribution of Cases with Cured or Recurrent Meningiomas as Functions of Growth Rates and Amounts of Tumor Left Behind*

Growth rate (doubling time)	Number of cells left behind				
	0	1	2^{18}	2^{27}	Total
4–8 months	80%		5%	2%	⎫
2–4 months 0		10%0	01	%	⎬ Grade 1 = 92%
2–4 months	50%	20%	5%	25%	Grade 2 = 6%
2–4 months	0	0	50%	50%	Grade 3 = 2%

*based on data provided by Jääskeläinen.[197]

259

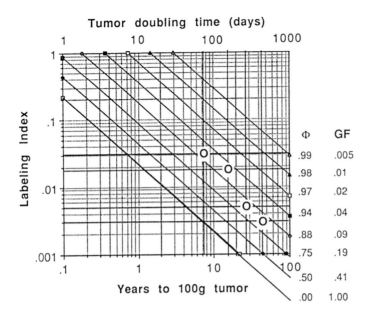

Fig. 10–81. In 4 meningiomas reported by Cho et al.[10] the LI's and Td's were reported as well as the times to recurrences. Either the cell loss factor was 82 to 92% or the growth fraction was about 5 to 16%. On the assumption that the recurrences were about 100 g, the amounts of tumor left behind could be estimated to be about 90 cells, 48 mg, 100 mg and 4 g.

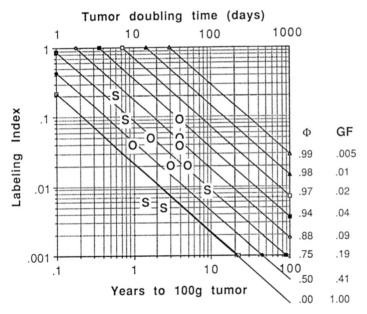

Fig. 10–82. In another dozen meningiomas reported by Cho et al.[10] and Fukui et al.[193] the LI's and times to recurrence allow estimates of the cell loss factor to be 50 to 94% (or the growth fraction to be about 4 to 41%). Those 5 tumors identified with "S" were known to have been subtotally resected and could, therefore, be moved to the right to the average 87.5% cell loss (or 9% growth fraction), allowing estimates of the amounts of tumor left behind to be about 0.2 to 4 mg in 3 cases and about 16 g in 2 cases.

be moved to the right to the oblique line representing the average estimated growth fraction of about 9%, close to the 6.2 to 8.2% measured by Yoshii et al.[63] This change yields estimated amounts of tumor left behind of 0.2 mg to 16 g.

These two different approaches give gratifyingly similar results: between 1 and 2^{27} cells (i.e., up to about 125 mg) usually left behind as grossly invisible at the time of "complete" excision (Figs. 10–80 and 10–81), with only 2 cases estimated to have had what should have

been grossly visible amounts, 4 to 16 g, left behind (Fig. 10–81). These amounts of microscopic invasiveness define the limits of curability by excision. They also define the interval between "complete" excision and recurrence when combined with the growth rates, which by the first estimate appear to range only between 2 and 8 months doubling time (Fig. 10–83) and by actual measurement to 75 to 440 days (or 2.5 to 15 months) according to Cho et al.[10] It is of some interest that the histologic grade appears to define the degree of invasive-

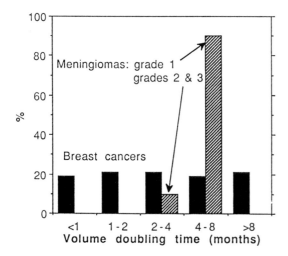

Fig. 10–83. Distribution of doubling times of meningiomas (see Fig. 10–80) and breast cancers (data from Kusama et al.[32]).

ness (i.e., the amount of tumor left behind) more than the growth rate. Also of note is the similarity in cell loss factors (or the approximate inverse, the growth fractions) of benign meningiomas (Figs. 10–81 and 10–82) and of highly malignant glioblastomas (Figs. 10–60 through 10–62).

The problem of recurrences of meningiomas has been known for many decades, most dramatically pointed out by Cushing and Eisenhardt[189] in several specific cases, and has usually been dismissed as merely the result of incomplete excision. Simpson[209] was the first formally to suggest a systematic analysis of these surgical failures. He proposed grading the extent of removal of meningiomas as follows: surgical grades 1 and 2 represent macroscopically complete removal of the tumor with excision (grade 1) or coagulation (grade 2) of the dural attachment, surgical grade 3 macroscopically complete without resection or coagulation of the dural attachment, surgical grade 4 partial removal and surgical grade 5 simple decompression. The series reported by Jääskeläinen et al.[31,197] and used in the present analysis included only surgical grades 1 and 2 but other published series have varied: Adegbite et al.[182] followed Simpson[209] exactly but Mirimanoff et al.[205] not at all, reporting only "total" and "subtotal" resections. Philippon et al.[207] generally grouped surgical grades 1, 2 and 3 together and, indeed, Adegbite et al.[182]

found little or no difference between surgical grades 1, 2 and 3. Borovich et al.[185] have proposed adding a "surgical grade 0" which would represent a wide resection of the dura around the attachment zone of the completely removed meningioma in an attempt to excise the regionally multicentric tumors that Borovich and Doron[184] reported.

Simpson's analysis[209] pointed to the dural attachment as being the site of the cell(s) left behind, since about 30% of his surgical grade 3 removals ultimately recurred, as compared to only about 10% and 15% for surgical grades 1 and 2, respectively. Similar results were reported by Philippon et al.[207] with 8, 10 and 24% recurrences for surgical grades 1, 2 and 3, respectively. Neither Simpson[209] nor Philippon et al.[207] expressed their results as life-table or actuarial analyses so that both sets of results must be regarded with some suspicion. The absence of any recurrences in the surgical grade 3 excisions reported by Adegbite et al.,[182] even better than their results with surgical grades 1 and 2, suggests that the base of the tumor is less important than the leptomeningeal surface; however, there were only 7 cases in their surgical grade 3, so that these results also must be regarded with suspicion.

Study of our meningiomas, especially at autopsy where the microscopic relationships can be seen better (Fig. 10–84), confirms the recent report of Nakasu et al.[206] Invasion of the pia and of the subpial brain tissue is relatively common even in histologically otherwise-benign meningiomas. This observation suggests that the fundus of the tumor extending into the brain may be at least as likely a site as the base of the tumor at the dura for the persistence of the cell(s) remaining.

Another possibility is that these "recurrences" are "second primaries" developing in genetically predisposed individuals with a tendency to lose all or part of chromosome 22.[186,200,208] Just why such a genetic defect should promote another primary at essentially the same site rather than randomly somewhere else is, however, difficult to imagine.

ACOUSTIC NEURILEMMOMAS

The diagnosis of acoustic neurilemmomas (neurinomas or schwannomas)[60,214–216] is usu-

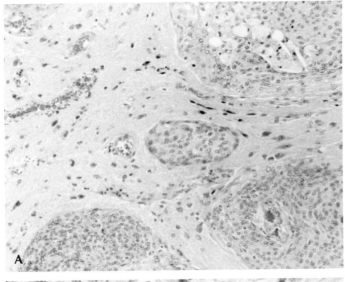

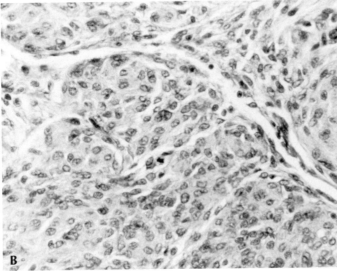

Fig. 10–84. Microscopic invasion of grade 2 meningioma through the pia into the brain (Np9041, H&E; A, × 200; B, × 500). Note the mitosis in B.

ally relatively easy, as Cushing[214] noted as early as 1917: unilateral tinnitus and deafness (and less often vertigo) in a slowly progressive rather than an episodic pattern, the latter being more characteristic of Menière's syndrome with attacks of vertigo and falling. In the elderly, however, who frequently have an insidiously progressive deafness as part of their aging, the recognition of an additional deafness can be difficult. This is to be especially regretted since modern diagnostic techniques permit the discovery of these tumors when they are of the order of 1 cm in diameter, practically entirely within the internal auditory meatus (Fig. 10–85). This is long before they

expand to compress the brainstem and other cranial nerves, such as the trigeminal and facial. Obviously, the smaller the tumor, the easier the surgical removal.

The microscopic appearance is usually typical (Fig. 10–86): interlacing bundles of spindle cells with nuclear palisades (Verocay bodies) comprise Antoni type A elements and masses of vacuolated or foamy cells comprise Antoni type B elements. Reticulin stains demonstrate parallel fibers surrounding each of the spindle cells. By electron microscopy these fibers are basal laminae that characteristically surround each Schwann cell. Occasionally nuclear pleomorphism may be extreme, leading to the di-

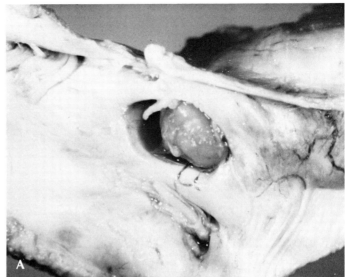

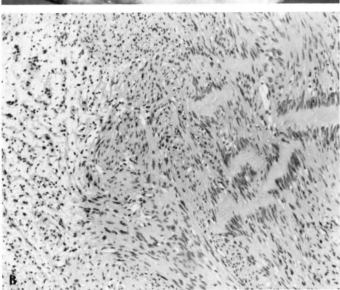

Fig. 10–85. Small (1 cm) acoustic neurilemmoma in right internal auditory meatus, an incidental observation at autopsy (A, Np372). Photomicrograph of another tumor showing Antoni A and B patterns (B, Np15094, H&E, × 200).

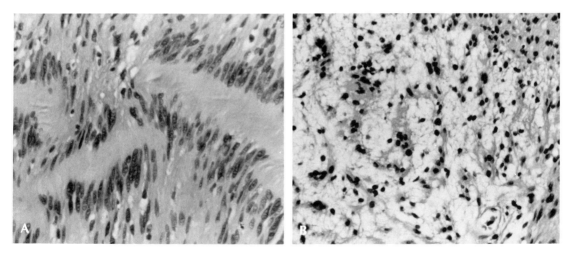

Fig. 10–86. Photomicrographs of the same acoustic neurilemmoma shown in Figure 10–85 B with nuclear palisading characteristic of a Verocay body (A) and with foamy Antoni B cells (B), both H&E × 500.

263

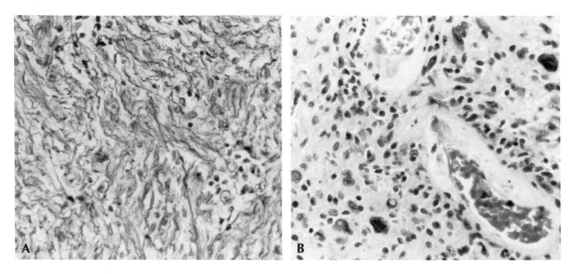

Fig. 10–87. Photomicrographs of another acoustic neurilemmoma (Np8290) showing delicate reticulin fibers (basement membranes by EM) parallel to each bipolar Schwann cell (A, × 500). B illustrates the pleomorphism characteristic of an "ancient" Schwannoma (Np15278, H&E, × 500).

agnosis of an "ancient" schwannoma; although the benign prognosis is thought to be the same, we cannot find good documentation for this opinion (Fig. 10–87).

The growth rates of acoustic neurilemmomas have recently been measured in serial CT scans by Laasonen and Troupp[215] and found to

be extremely slow, as compared not only to breast cancers (Fig. 10–88) but also to meningiomas (see Fig. 10–83), with Td's up to 64 months or more! The most rapid acoustic neurilemmoma required about 4 months to double, implying that the youngest possible patient would have to be at least 10 years old (30 doublings would produce about 1 g of tumor). This implication is confirmed in Figure 10–89,

Growth Rates

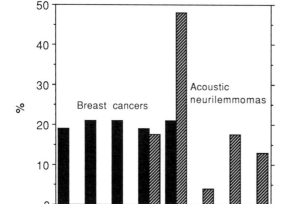

Fig. 10–88. Distribution of doubling times of acoustic neurilemmomas (data from Laasonen and Troupp[215]) as compared to those of breast cancers (data from Kusama et al.[32]).

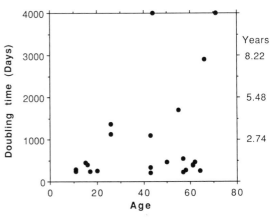

Fig. 10–89. Distribution of doubling times of acoustic neurilemmomas in patients of various ages (data from Laasonen and Troupp[215]). Only older people can have slowly growing tumors, whereas rapidly growing tumors can occur at any age.

which also shows that the elderly can have either rapidly or slowly growing tumors, whereas the young can have only relatively rapidly growing tumors. However, for those patients with a slowly growing tumor a partial resection may be quite all that is needed for an extended life with little or no disability, the only caveat being that one must think in terms of numbers of generations, not mass, left behind (see Fig. 10–7 and Table 10–1). One explanation for the long Tds may derive from the two observations of Yoshii et al.[63] of a growth fraction of only about 4%, equivalent to a cell loss factor of about 94%. Burger et al.[7] found an even smaller growth fraction, 0.2%, using Ki-67 antigen as a marker of all cells except those in G_0. If so few cells are really all that are dividing, no wonder the Tds are so long!

The effectiveness of x-irradiation therapy with $>4,500$ cGy can be seen in those patients whose tumors were incompletely removed, but the difference is convincing only for acoustic neurilemmomas,[60] not for other intracranial neurilemmomas.[216]

From the results presented by Wallner et al.[60] one can make some interesting calculations based on the times to clinical recurrence after "subtotal" (defined as <90%) or "near-total" (defined as 90 to 99%) removals of acoustic neurilemmomas. Since it requires only 1 to 3.2 doublings for a subtotally removed tumor to return to its original size (Fig. 10–7), the recurrences at 0.25 to 10.5 years in half of the non-irradiated patients would indicate doubling times of 3 months to 4.5 years in most, and of 3.5 to 10.5 years in only one patient. Even the slowest of these would be included in the slowest one-third measured by Laasonen and Troupp.[215] For the single recurrence at 2 years following x-irradiation a similar calculation would indicate a doubling time of 0.7 to 2 years, again well within the range of those measured.[215] By contrast, since it requires only 3.3 to 6.6 doublings for a near-totally removed tumor to return to its original size (Fig. 10–7), the single recurrence at 1 year in the x-irradiated group would indicate a doubling time of 56 to 104 days, 2 to 4 times faster than the most rapid one measured by Laasonen and Troupp.[215] Perhaps this patient received only "subtotal" excision!

PITUITARY ADENOMAS

If the etiology and pathogenesis of a disease are poorly understood, as is generally true of neoplasms, the classification and grading become perpetually controversial. New technologies may help to clarify some aspects of the disease but can also add fuel to the controversies. In most disease entities, new techniques produce new results that represent progress in our understanding, which helps in the formulation of an improved diagnosis and treatment.

The evolution of our understanding of the pathology of pituitary adenomas[217–264] follows this pattern almost archetypically and shows the limitations of classical histopathology which has dominated all of medical science for so long and has been regarded as the basis for the definition of so many diseases. Contemporary laboratory techniques, especially microassays of hormones, have developed far beyond the upper limits of classical histopathology, causing many frustrations for surgical pathologists in the 1960s and 1970s. The incorporation of modern immunocytochemical and ultrastructural techniques has allowed the histopathologic diagnoses of pituitary adenomas at last to catch up.

The history of the pathology of pituitary adenomas is intimately related to the history of Neurosurgery, especially with the development of various neurosurgical techniques to reach this formerly "inaccessible" organ. Both the physiology of the gland as well as the histopathology of its tumors were developed by pioneer neurosurgeons, especially Harvey Cushing and his colleagues.

The pituitary gland, known since ancient days, was regarded as a single organ until the epoch-making embryologic study in 1838 by Rathke,[258] who demonstrated that the pituitary gland consisted of two parts, each of different origins: epithelial and neural. Pituitary adenomas arise from the epithelial part, also known as the adenohypophysis, pars distalis, or anterior lobe. Tumors arising from the neurohypophysis, or posterior lobe, are rare, specialized forms of astrocytomas known as infundibulomas; since they show no predilection to involve older patients, they will not be further discussed.

Credit has generally been given to Flesh[227] in 1884 for recognizing two types of cells, chromophil and chromophobe, in the adenohypophysis. However, the histologic recognition of pituitary adenomas has been credited to Benda,[220] who recognized chromophil and chromophobe adenomas in 1900.

It is difficult to tell exactly who discovered the first pituitary adenoma and when it occurred. "Obesity" and "acromegaly" (hypertrophy of the extremities[251]) were known as early as 1886 to be associated with an enlarged pituitary gland.[252,253] The first successful surgical resection of a pituitary adenoma in 1907 is usually credited to Schloffer,[259] who used a transphenoidal approach. The surgical technique was improved in the next few years by Kocher,[243] Kanavel,[142] and von Eiselberg.[261] A still better and less mutilating approach was reported by Hirsch[239] but the sublabial method that Halstead[231] introduced in 1910 became more or less standard for the following 15 years. Harvey Cushing,[221-223] who is regarded as "the father of Neurosurgery," was intensely interested not only in pituitary tumors, but also in the physiology of the pituitary gland. He performed many animal experiments to define the functions of the gland and published extensively, many of these early contributions remaining as classics even today. Cushing[221,222] recognized three types of pathologic conditions of the pars distalis of the hypophysis: hyperpituitarism resulting in acromegaly or gigantism, hypopituitarism causing excessive deposition of fat with persistence of infantile sexual characteristics, and dyspituitarism in which both hyper- and hypopituitarism coexisted in the same patient. These functional disturbances might be due to tumors, hyperplasia, or hypoplasia and surgery was recommended when they were due to tumor.

In 1912 Cushing[222] published his famous monograph, *The Pituitary Body and Its Disorders*, in which he classified diseases of the pituitary gland into the following groups:

Group I. Cases of dyspituitarism with altered glandular activity and signs indicating distortion of neighboring structures

Group II. Cases with symptoms of neighboring structures only

Group III. Cases with glandular symptoms only

Group IV. Cases with distant cerebral lesions with secondary pituitary involvement

Group V. Cases with polyglandular syndromes.

These concepts were developed long before it was discovered that the pituitary gland produces several different kinds of hormones and long before the functions of the hypothalamus were known. In this monograph Cushing reported in great detail his experiences with 47 cases of pituitary tumors, most of which had been operated upon by the transphenoidal route.

Three types of cells were recognized depending upon the types of granules contained in the cytoplasm of the cells: acidophilic, basophilic, or chromophobic. The terminology was based on the belief that one type of granule has an affinity for acid dyes and the other for basic dyes. This belief was shown to be wrong and Bailey and Davidoff[217] proposed calling acidophilic cells *alpha* and basophilic cells *beta*. Chromophobic cells were also known as reserve or chief cells and were variously considered to be cells that had failed to develop granules, had not yet developed granules or had lost their granules. Chromophilic and chromophobic cells were thought to be the same cells at different stages of development, chromophobes being less differentiated. Bailey and Davidoff[217] described the microscopic findings in the surgical specimens from 35 acromegalic patients, reviewed an additional 17 cases reported in the literature and came to the conclusion that the constant pathologic feature was an adenoma composed of alpha cells. There were, however, 2 cases reported in the literature, in which the tumor was not eosinophilic. Bailey and Davidoff[217] attributed the failure in one of them as being due to autolysis related to a delayed autopsy and in the other as probably representing a patient with dyspituitarism with some acromegalic features but not a true acromegalic patient due to hyperpituitarism. The results of 162 operated cases of pituitary adenomas in Cushing's series were reported by Dott and Bailey,[224] who created another type of adenoma, namely a mixed type of adenoma. All of these tumors were grossly recognizable as large adenomas.

In 1932 Cushing[223] described 12 patients who showed what he called a "polyglandular syndrome," now commonly known as "Cushing's syndrome." Six of 8 cases at autopsy showed small pituitary adenomas, 3 of which were definitely basophilic, 2 undifferentiated adenomas and 1 an adenomatous structure in a fibrotic area of the pituitary gland. These tumors were too small to have been a surgical object in those days but were the forerunner of "microadenomas" as we know them today.

Cushing's series was further expanded to 338 cases,[237] including rare adenocarcinomas and the three principal varieties of adenoma (chromophobe, acidophil, and basophil). Chromophobe adenomas were by far the most common and usually produced such inconstant secondary constitutional disturbances due to pituitary insufficiency that the disorder was not likely to be recognized clinically until the tumor became large enough to compress the optic chiasm or nerves. The adenomas associated with acromegaly were composed of acidophilic cells. The basophilic microadenomas causing the polyglandular syndrome rarely attained a large enough size to become the object for surgical removal. Thirty-two cases of mixed acidophil-chromophobe adenomas showed a mixture of signs of hyper- and hypopituitarism, were called "fugitive acromegaly" and were included in the chromophobe group. The 338 cases in Cushing's series[237] represented 17.8% of his total of 2023 brain tumors, the highest incidence in any brain tumor series. By contrast, 292 pituitary adenomas reported from Olivecrona's service constituted only 8.9% of his total brain tumors.[218] Cushing[237] did about 75% of his cases through the transphenoidal route, which was relatively safe and effective in relieving the compression of the optic chiasm immediately. However, complete removal of the tumor was difficult and visualization at the depths of the operative field was poor. Subsequently the surgical approach gradually shifted to the transfrontal route, which became the preferred technique for hypophyseal surgery and remained so until the 1950s even though the transphenoidal approach was continued with

successful results by a few surgeons, such as Dott[224] and Hirsch.[240]

Our knowledge about the morphology and function of the adenohypophysis has expanded immensely following the development of newer cytologic, histophysiologic, cytochemical, and electron microscopic techniques. Through experimental studies on various species of animals and observations on human subjects at least 5 different hormones (7, if gonadotropin is divided into LH and FSH and if corticotropin is divided into ACTH and MSH) are now known to be produced by the pituitary. Different types of cells corresponding to their different functional capacities have been characterized mainly by immunocytochemical (ICC)[265,266] and electron microscopic (EM) studies. Unfortunately, the ordinary light microscopy using combinations of dyes to stain different types of cells fell way behind these new techniques and became extremely complicated and less specific for the identification of cells other than the traditional acidophilic, basophilic and chromophobic cells.

Thus, the number of cell types has increased to 7 or more (including non-secretory cells) from the original 3. Different functional types of adenomas arising from each of these many types of cells were soon discovered but it took quite a few years before it was realized that tumors did not necessarily contain normal-appearing granules.

The first of these new adenomas was recognized in 1954, when Forbes et al.[228] reported a series of 15 young women who had amenorrhea and galactorrhea without evidence of pregnancy or acromegaly. Eight had a pituitary adenoma, a chromophobe adenoma being confirmed by biopsy in three. They[228] proposed that all of these patients had overproduction of prolactin. This report was followed by a wave of reports describing ICC-proven prolactinomas, which soon became the most common pituitary adenoma, accounting for approximately 30% and becoming the "Cinderella" of pituitary adenomas.[244] Much less common thyrotropin-producing chromophobe adenomas[232] and gonadotropin-producing adenomas[260,264] soon filled in most of the blank spaces.

As noted above, the transphenoidal route for hypophysectomy and resection of pituitary tumors was developed in the early 1900s but was gradually replaced by the transfrontal craniotomy as the mortality rate in the latter was lowered to an acceptable level. The transphenoidal technique was revived in the late 1950s[229,232,233] and gradually achieved general popularity. The timing of this revival was almost perfect, especially when aided by newly developed microsurgical techniques including the microscope and the availability of televised intraoperative radiofluoroscopic control. Within a few years this became the technique of choice for surgical resection for small pituitary adenomas.

Furthermore, microimmunoassays of hormones, CT scans and MR images were timely contributions for diagnosing and locating microadenomas. Microadenomas which are too small to produce clinical symptoms or to produce any diagnostic radiologic changes may still be diagnosed by microimmunoassays of serum hormones and can be found selectively under high magnification through an operating microscope and resected.[234]

Most of these new microadenomas contain "chromophobe" cells. Originally considered to be a specific type of cell, the "chromophobe" can now be seen to be any one of the following: an immature cell, an inherently non-hormone-producing cell, an exhausted cell, a cell in a resting stage or a cell actively producing and simultaneously secreting any type of hormone so that no hormonal granules are retained in the cytoplasm. Therefore, a chromophobe adenoma is not always hypofunctional, as the classical macroadenomas were, but can be a tumor with hyperpituitarism, such as the usual prolactinoma is.

The different sizes, shapes, and numbers of granules found in different functional types of cells by EM in the normal pituitary gland of humans and animals were expected to be seen in pituitary adenomas but are not. Small granules are usually seen in the region of Golgi's apparatus and are considered to be immature granules. They fuse and become larger as they move toward the surface to exit from the cells. Since granules in actively secreting cells tend to be smaller than normal, EM cannot be used to diagnose different types of functional adenomas merely by the size and shape of the granules. It is useful in demonstrating synthesizing activity, secretory activity and other fea-

tures, e.g., oncocytes, filamentous aggregates, Crooke's hyaline changes, exocytosis, and autophages.

Light microscopy cannot be dismissed as an old-fashioned and useless technique. It is essential to establish a diagnosis of adenoma and to make a differential diagnosis of other types of tumor, such as craniopharyngioma, glioma, ganglioglioma, choristoma or meningioma, and other pathologic conditions, such as hypophysitis. ICC is excellent only when it is positive. EM is significant only when the specimen can be verified as a tumor.

A new classification of pituitary adenomas has been proposed[244,247] based on the lessons we have learned during the last 2 decades with these newly available techniques. A complete shift from the old 3 types of adenomas to the new classification incorporating ICC and EM has been slow because the new classification requires new laboratory facilities. Only when the new facilities are universally available and new techniques become routine will the complete switch become possible. In the meantime we recognize a variety of classifications depending on the availability of EM and ICC:

A. Classification based on tinctorial characteristics:
   1. chromophobe adenoma
   2. acidophilic adenoma
   3. basophilic adenoma
   4. mixed adenoma
B. Classification by light microscopy with ICC:[265,266]
   1. Lactotrophic adenoma (prolactinoma)
   2. Somatotrophic adenoma (growth hormone-producing adenoma)
   3. Corticotrophic adenoma (ACTH-producing adenoma)
   4. Thyrotrophic adenoma
   5. Gonadotrophic adenoma
   6. Mixed (types to be designated) adenoma
   7. Non-functional adenoma
C. Classification by light microscopy with ICC (as in B) with EM findings appended:
   a. number and size of hormone granules
   b. biological state of tumor cells
   c. presence of other features, e.g., fila-

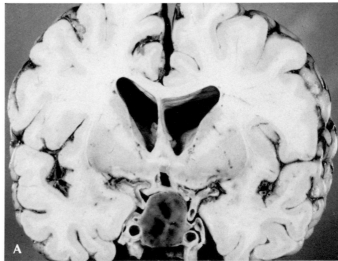

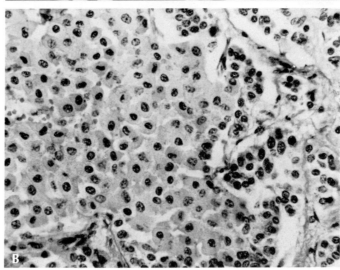

Fig. 10–90. A, Non-functional chromophobe adenoma (oncocytoma) of pituitary with small hemorrhages secondary to needle biopsy. Note slight elevation of optic chiasm causing bitemporal hemianopsia (Np273). B is a photomicrograph of an H&E-stained section of a similar tumor (Np4264, × 500).

mentous aggregates, Crooks' hyaline changes,

d. specific non-functional adenomas, e.g., oncocytoma or null-cell adenoma.

EM is especially important for the diagnosis of non-functional adenomas (Figs. 10–90 and 10–91). Oncocytomas, in which the tumor cells are stuffed with mitochondria, appear as otherwise-unspecifiable chromophobe adenomas when stained by H&E (Fig. 10–90B). They can be occasionally diagnosed without EM when the resolution is good in sections stained by phosphotungstic acid-hematoxylin but we have not found this stain to be sensitive enough for routine screening of tumors. Am-

yloid deposits, calcifications, cyst formations, and old hemorrhages are seen in some adenomas but these changes are not specific for any one type of tumor.

The evolution of the above concepts of pituitary adenomas not only affected the histopathologic classification, but also markedly changed the epidemiologic statistics. It is extremely difficult, if not impossible, to compare relatively large series reported from different medical centers before and after about 1970. Incidental adenomas frequently found in autopsy series pose other problems and different questions and will not be further discussed here. Most series have dealt with surgically resected adenomas. Practically all of the older series dealt with macroadenomas since micro-

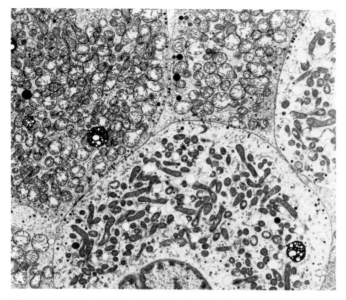

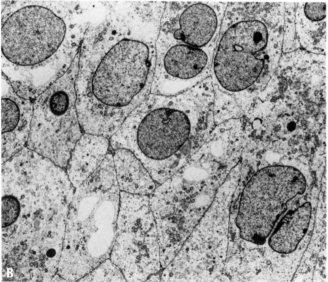

Fig. 10–91. Electronmicrographs of an oncocytoma (A, Np14057, × 6000) and of a null-cell adenoma of the pituitary (B, Np11144, × 4000).

adenomas were not diagnosable or operatively discoverable until the advent of modern techniques. Chromophobe adenomas, almost synonymous with non-functional adenomas in those days, occupied more than 75% of those series prior to the "epidemic" of prolactinomas.[218,226,237,255] Even in some post-1970 publications, non-functional or chromophobe adenomas might still be the major type if older cases were included in the series.[225,229] In these older series the average age of the patients with an adenoma was generally older because of the inclusion of a large number of non-functional chromophobe adenomas with a

peak incidence in the 5th or 6th decade in contrast to the younger average age of chromophilic adenomas.[218,226,237,255]

The newer series reported after the development of microneurosurgery usually include a much higher incidence of hyper-secreting pituitary adenomas, especially prolactinomas, which now comprise 25 to 41% of many large series.[235,250,257,262] As a result, the incidence of non-functional adenomas has decreased to 16.5 to 29%.[246,262] The average age of patients with an adenoma is also lower because prolactinomas tend to affect young women.

The following analyses are based on 319

histologically verified pituitary adenomas from the files of the Neuropathology Laboratory, University of Washington Medical School, from 1960 to the present. No case of an incidental pituitary adenoma found either at autopsy or surgery is included. Pituitary lesions other than adenoma were also excluded. The age of the patients in the following tables represents the age when the histologic diagnosis was made for the first time irrespective of the number of subsequent operations in each patient.

All pathologically verified pituitary adenomas were divided into four groups: lactotrophic, somatotrophic, corticotrophic, and non-functional adenomas (Tables 10–8 and 10–9). Non-functional adenomas were further divided into oncocytoma,[244,248] null-cell adenoma[246] and unspecified (Table 10–10). The diagnoses were made by light histology, ICC and EM as well as by clinical presentation and endocrinologic data but not all of these techniques were available in all cases, especially some of the older cases prior to the 1970s, in which the diagnosis of somatotrophic and corticotrophic adenomas was made by assumption when the clinical and light histologic findings were typical. We have seen no cases of thyrotrophic or gonadotrophic adenomas.

TABLE 10–8. Numbers and Types of Pituitary Adenomas Seen at the University of Washington Medical Center

Type of adenoma	Male	Female	Total
Lactotrophic	18	105	123
Somatotrophic	22	20	42
Corticotrophic	8	28	36
Non-functional	73	45	118
	121	198	319

TABLE 10–10. Age Distribution of Various Types of Non-Functional Pituitary Adenomas

Age	Oncocytoma	Null-cell	Unspecified	Total
20–29	0	3	6	9
30–39	0	7	6	13
40–49	7	4	4	15
50–59	9	10	10	29
60–69	15	10	5	30
70–79	10	2	6	18
> 80	4	0	0	4
Total	45	36	37	118

Table 10–8 shows the four types of adenomas and their sex distribution. Prolactinomas (lactotrophic adenomas) and non-functional adenomas each make up about one-third of the total. The high incidence of prolactinomas and the marked female preponderance for prolactinomas and ACTH-producing adenomas have also been noted by many other investigators.

Table 10–9 shows the age distributions of the four different types of adenomas. Pituitary adenomas, regardless of type, practically do not occur in young children. Lactotrophic adenoma (prolactinoma) is a tumor predominantly seen in young women: 105 females and 18 males, the youngest patient 16 and the oldest 65 years of age. Prolactinoma is uncommon after age 50, only 2 out of 123 cases, both females aged 61 and 65. One patient had a macroadenoma with suprasellar extension and manifested unilateral ptosis clinically. The other patient had a history of psychiatric problems for many years, a large sella and a serum prolactin of 400. The sella was found to be empty but the soft tissue in the wall of the cyst proved to be a prolactinoma by light histology and ICC. Randall et al.[256,257] also found 2 patients who were over 60 years old among their 100 cases of prolactinoma. Both patients were

TABLE 10–9. Age Distribution of Various Types of Pituitary Adenomas

Age	Lactotrophic	Somatotrophic	Corticotrophic	Non-functional	Total
0–9	0	0	0	0	0
10–19	9	2	2	0	13
20–29	63	5	9	9	86
30–39	38	14	12	13	77
40–49	11	6	5	15	37
50–59	0	9	5	29	43
60–69	2	5	2	30	39
70–79	0	0	1	18	19
> 80	0	1	0	4	5
Total	123	42	36	118	319

male and the tumors were large. Male patients are generally older (39 versus 26 years in females) and their tumors larger because the clinical endocrinologic symptoms are less obvious in male patients.[256] Table 10–9 also shows that there is no age predilection among patients with somatotrophic and corticotrophic adenomas, ranging between 10 to 15 and 76 to 82 years. The male:female ratio is about equal in acromegalic patients but there is a significant female preponderance in ACTH-producing adenomas. Non-functional adenomas, which are usually large and cause neurological symptoms by compression, are the adenoma predominantly seen in older adults (Tables 10–10 and 10–11).

Since the diagnosis of oncocytoma and null-cell adenoma requires EM, which was not always used in our cases, the 118 cases of non-functional adenomas were further divided into 3 groups: oncocytoma, null-cell adenoma and unspecified non-functional adenoma (Tables 10–10 and 10–11). It should be pointed out that EM is not absolutely necessary for the diagnosis of oncocytoma. A 1-μ thick section of epon-embedded tissue stained with either toluidine blue or methylene blue usually gives satisfactory resolution to differentiate secretory granules and mitochondria under high magnification light microscopy. Non-functional chromophobe adenomas, which were not further differentiated by special techniques into oncocytoma and null-cell adenoma, are included in the unspecified group. Table 10-10 shows that the patients with an oncocytoma are generally older than those with a null-cell adenoma. There were no cases of oncocytoma under 40 years of age. Oncocytomas were clustered above the fifth decades, whereas the null-cell adenomas were more or less evenly distributed between the third and eighth decades.

TABLE 10–11. Types of Pituitary Adenomas Seen in Persons 60 Years of Age and Older

Lactotrophic adenoma		2
Somatotrophic adenoma		6
Corticotrophic adenoma		3
Non-functional adenomas		52
oncocytoma	29	
null-cell adenoma	12	
unspecified	11	
	Total	63

There were 63 patients over 60 years of age with a pituitary adenoma in our series (Table 10–11). The great majority of these patients had a non-functional adenoma (82.5%). Oncocytoma seems to be the most common adenoma of the older population, whereas prolactinoma is quite uncommon. Somatotrophic and corticotrophic adenomas show no specific age preference.

As for proliferative potential and growth rates relatively little information is available. Landolt et al.[249] have measured the growth fraction of 31 pituitary adenomas by using monoclonal antibody Ki-67. They found a range of only 0.1 to 3.7% and a mean of 1% of cycling cells, with lower values (0.2 to 1.0%) in endocrine-inactive adenomas and higher but overlapping values in endocrine-active tumors. Nagashima et al.[254] reported BrDU labeling indices for pituitary adenomas up to only 1.5% with a median of 0.16%. If these were independent variables, as shown in Figure 10–92, the outrageous conclusion would be that 1000 years would be required to produce 100 g of pituitary adenoma, 800 years to produce a 1-g macroadenoma, and 550 years even for an ultramicroadenoma of only 1 mg. Obviously, the two sets of figures cannot be combined in such a simple fashion. Indeed, from equations (1), (3), and (5) on page 215 and assuming $\lambda Ts = 0.22$, one can calculate the cell cycle duration (Tc) to be 2 days and the tumor doubling time (Td) to be 138 days for the usual pituitary adenoma.

METASTATIC NEOPLASMS

About 10% of all malignant neoplasms metastasize to the brain.[80,267–276] This is approximately the same number as primary intracranial neoplasms. About 30% of the metastases are "solitary." All 3 of these statistics are surprisingly difficult to obtain. Each hospital, each physician has peculiarly personal characteristics serving as magnets attracting or repelling each kind of patient: witness Cushing's high incidence of pituitary adenomas![237] One would think that Veterans Administration hospitals would be a good source of relatively old patients, relatively well cared for both medically and surgically with a relatively high autopsy rate, but practically no women; therefore,

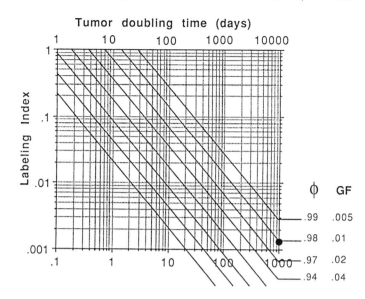

Fig. 10–92. The combination of the median LI[7,254] and the mean GF[249] suggested for pituitary adenomas requires that another log scale be added to Figure 10–12 to accommodate such small fractions. As explained in the text (pages 218 and 272), such a simple combination cannot be made.

practically no cancers of the breast, which happen to be one of the common sources of metastases to the brain. And so on, eliminating one by one practically all of the possible sources of such statistics, after which one begins to wonder why the numbers seemed so important in the first place. After all, when you come right down to it, the statistics do not help much when it is really a question of the individual patient and the individual physician. The answer is usually 0% or 100%, the patient has it or not, whatever *it* may be. Where statistics usually become helpful is in prioritizing the order of the search for the ultimately correct diagnosis. Unfortunately, this prioritizing is being translated into cost-effectiveness, then into cost per se, by which time the search has been delayed so long that the treatment becomes ineffective, too late to be effective, completing the circular reasoning which began by saying that it would not be cost-effective! The lay and medical media are increasingly wringing their hands in despair as over-crowded medical facilities and rising costs of medical diagnosis and care are combining to force limitations on medical delivery—and the elderly, having lived so long and having become accustomed to the older slower ways, will be the first to be restricted and the last to recognize the restriction.

The brain is one of the favorite sites of metastasis for carcinomas of the lung, breast, kidney, gastrointestinal tract, testis, and melanoma (Table 10–12). Although carcinoma of

the prostate practically never metastasizes to the brain or spinal cord itself, the skull and vertebrae are frequently involved, as are pelvic perineural lymphatics; thus, neurologic signs occur frequently with prostatic cancer, the one that notoriously increases in incidence with increasing age.

Metastatic neoplasms to the brain are usually multiple, spherical, and sharply delineated (Figs. 10–93 and 10–94). Some appear diffusely within the leptomeninges—a rule of thumb that we have learned the hard way being that we can grossly miss a layer of cells proven microscopically to be a half-dozen cells thick! Some metastases may be confined to the dura, either subdural or epidural.

Microscopically most metastases are composed of such large cells with such hyperchromatic nuclei that one can usually recognize the

TABLE 10–12.   Distribution of Sources of Metastases to the Brain*

Primary tumor	This % of primary tumors	Metastasize to the brain, accounting for this % of all metastases to the brain
1. Carcinoma of		
Lung	15–30	20–60
Breast	5–15	10–25
Kidney	10–20	5–20
Large intestine	10	5–10
Testis	30	5
2. Melanoma	50–90	5–10
3. Lymphoma	3	5

*data from Earle,[268] Kernohan and Sayre,[80] Störtebecker,[274] and Willis.[275]

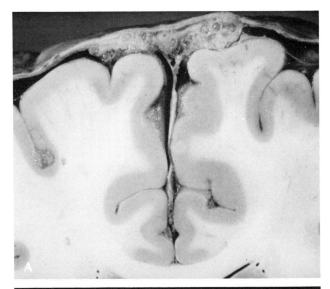

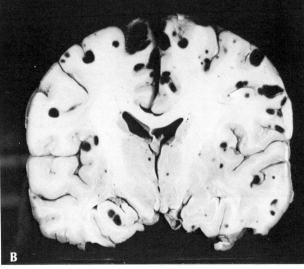

Fig. 10–93. A, Metastatic adenocarcinoma from lung to superior sagittal sinus, subdural space, cerebral cortex, and white matter (Np241). B, Metastatic melanoma to cerebral cortex, cortico-medullary junction, and thalamus (N-57).

metastasis with the naked eye alone—practically only medulloblastomas are so hematoxyphilic, especially compared to the generally eosinophilic CNS tissue in the background. If something special (e.g., melanin, colloid, mucus, or neurosecretory granules) can be recognized, increasingly precisely so with ICC reagents,[265,266] one can guess intelligently as to the site of the primary (see Table 10–12). Otherwise one can really only guess, and the best guess is either metastatic bronchogenic carcinoma or glioblastoma multiforme, each close to half of all the metastatic or primary tumors in the brain.

The brain is so frequently involved by metastatic carcinomas from the lung that one of the advances in treatment of this primary neoplasm has been prophylactic x-irradiation of the whole head. Initially confined to small cell carcinomas, this practice is being extended to include all histologic types of bronchogenic carcinoma since there is relatively little difference in incidence of metastases to the brain from the various types of cancer of the lung.

If one includes bone and dura, the statistics in Table 10–12 change considerably. Carcinoma of the nasopharynx usually invades directly through the base of the skull, producing

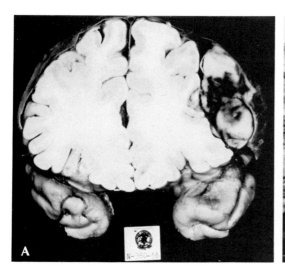
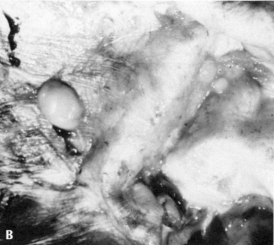

Fig. 10–94.   A, Metastatic myeloma to left subdural space (VA-56-380). B, Metastatic leukemia to under surface of dura (A-64-33).

progressive paralysis of multiple cranial nerves and pain, as in Babe Ruth, whose hoarse farewell in Yankee Stadium still haunts the air of those old enough and fortunate enough to own the recording.

Surgical treatment of solitary metastases to the brain is also being extended to multiple metastases in selected cases, depending on the expected duration of survival related to the extent of neoplasm in the whole patient. Measurements of growth rates of individual metastases should prove beneficial in deciding how much treatment of particular metastases may be of value to the patient.

Metastases to the spinal cord itself are rare but compression of the spinal cord by metastases to the vertebrae or to the epidural space is common. Back pain is the most common presenting symptom and may be present for weeks, following which neurologic symptoms usually progress rapidly: weakness, sensory changes, bowel and bladder paralysis leading to complete paraplegia within hours or a few days. The prognosis depends on the rapidity of diagnosis and treatment since "patients who are not ambulatory before treatment do not regain function after treatment."[271] The metastases can usually be treated by steroids and local x-irradiation but surgical decompression may be necessary if the signs of spinal cord compression do not rapidly reverse.

Malignant lymphomas, formerly most commonly seen as one of the spinal epidural metastases, are now increasingly appearing as primary brain tumors. This is especially so in patients with AIDS (acquired immunodeficiency syndrome due to infection by one of the human-immunodeficiency viruses, HIV)—therefore, not so commonly seen in the elderly! For reasons that are not at all clear, however, primary lymphomas of the brain are increasingly frequent also in HIV-negative individuals. Some of this increase may be attributed to an increased awareness of the possibility of lymphoma involving the CNS and even more to an increased sensitivity and specificity of the diagnostic reagents (monoclonal antibodies to the many epitopes on human T and B cells and macrophages). There is no basic reason that we can think of to explain the increase in numbers of glioma-like masses in contrast to the subdural masses (Fig. 10–94) and leukemia-like leptomeningitis or encephalitis that tended to occur in former decades. Nakhleh et al.[270] note that the immuno-compromised patients are younger (average age 34), the non-immuno-compromised patients older (average age 62) in primary CNS lymphomas, and that each group is 12 to 18 years older than patients with systemic lymphomas and secondary involvement of the CNS. Of their 26 cases, all but 2 were B-cell lymphomas.

DISCUSSION

The elderly can have many diseases other than neoplasms. At least some of these are treatable, a few even curable. One should not leap too quickly to the diagnosis of a primary or metastatic neoplasm, either clinically or microscopically. We know only too well that a single large mass-expanding lesion can be the first detectable lesion of multiple sclerosis,[181] even in a person over 65 years of age. Amyloid angiopathy and other vascular lesions can also mimic neoplasms both clinically and imagewise, as can abscesses, etc. The popular suggestion of withholding treatment and allowing the elderly to die in peace must be tempered by good judgment. It usually takes a tough old bird to live to become elderly. By the same token, we do not advocate not performing an autopsy "because he or she has suffered enough." We have much still to learn. And if we do not see for ourselves, to translate the word *autopsy* into the deed itself and the accompanying investigative research attitude of doing the autopsy properly, who is going to teach the next generation? Will they have to learn everything by themselves as we old duffers make way for them to correct our mistakes, to fill in our areas of ignorance?

As we have pointed out throughout this chapter, major uncertainties persist in our understanding of neoplasms. We know little of their natural histories (causes, times of onset, growth rates, times of invasion and/or metastasis and correlations of histologic types and grades with growth rates, invasiveness/metastasis and prognosis) and not much more of their histories as modified by various therapies.

There have been major advances in our understanding of tumor cell kinetics, especially concerning rates of production but to a much lesser extent, rates of loss of cells. In the Introduction (Figs. 10–1 through 10–14) we have attempted to show the mathematical relationships between S-phase measures and labeling indices (LI), growth fractions (GF), cell loss factors (ϕ), potential doubling times (Tp), actual doubling times (Td) and amounts of tumor left behind. In spite of the variety of factors that can be measured, they all exert their influence through Td. Thus, Td could theoretically be calculated from all of these factors that could be measured at a single point in time. The major question, whether Td is constant, still requires multiple observations over time. While two points determine a line and three points a circle, at least four points in time are needed to define a decelerating Gompertzian curve such as many investigators believe to be generally the case for many cancers[33] and such as we have emphasized must happen with most optic gliomas (Fig. 10–53). Unfortunately, the evidence for deceleration in other human tumors is not convincing and we are not persuaded that deceleration applies to other than a few exceptional types.

The concept of all cells doubling at a constant rate without cell loss (Figs. 10–1 and 10–2) developed by Collins et al.[12] has been criticized for being over-simplified but, even as modified with S-phase measurements, growth fractions and cell loss factors, the mathematical formulation still produces a growth rate that remains a simple exponential. It is surprising how many tumors appear to follow a straight line on semi-logarithmic paper over long periods of time. Regardless of how accurate the model really is, the clinically visible portion of the natural history of human tumors must represent only a small portion of the total history of the tumor (Figs. 10–2, 10–52 and 10–53). How far back one can extrapolate to the origin of a tumor, as Hirakawa et al.[25] did for medulloblastomas, is problematic, but a Gompertzian curve will extrapolate back to a later date than a simple exponential. The problem, of course, is how long the inductive phase may be, how long before the tumor really takes off? Even after surgical therapy, estimates of the amount of tumor left behind and the amount of tumor detectable at autopsy would still be useful pieces of information on which to improve our understanding of the actual behavior of particular neoplasms by defining any necessary modifications of Figure 10–12.

From an entirely different perspective 60 years ago, Heisenberg[24] developed the "Uncertainty Principle" to explain why, at the level of subatomic physics and with discontinuities in time and space, it was impossible to locate electrons accurately.[21] He wrote, of course, in German and since then his "Uncertainty Principle" has been re-worded in a variety of ways. At least two of these expressions can be interpreted as applying directly to some of the important problems in the diagnosis and treatment of cancer: (1) "There is no way that we can know simultaneously the position and the momentum of a moving particle," and (2) The observer influences the observed or " . . . we cannot observe something without changing it."[64]

The first of these expressions has been repeatedly emphasized in this chapter. The discontinuities in space-time of theoretical physics illustrated by Heisenberg[24] are readily discernible not only in the obviously episodic mitotic activity of normal cell growth, but also in other possibly random spurts of cancer growth.[51] Furthermore, the most common type of cancer research includes the making of a histologic diagnosis of cancer, the institution of a treatment and the measurement of the duration of survival. By analogy with Heisenberg's "Uncertainty Principle," as shown in Figure 10-5, a "position" is observed (the histologic appearance) and a "momentum" predicted (the duration of survival or prognosis). Several examples have been presented to illustrate the fallacy of this procedure, including studies of optic gliomas,[122] oligodendrogliomas,[108,115-118] ependymomas,[105] neurilemmomas[215] and meningiomas,[31,197,198] but studies of cancers of the breast[32] and kidney[277] extend these neuropathologic examples into general pathology.

From the study of breast cancer by Kusama et al.[32] one can estimate the times at which metastases must have begun: progressively earlier in each of the progressively more-slowly growing cancers.[36] The recent improvement in treatment of breast cancer by systemic chemotherapy[278] designed to kill the widely disseminated subclinical micrometastases fits well with these calculations.

That still-older data concerning kidney cancers[277] also fit with the concept of simple exponential growth is gratifying. The straight line in Figure 10-95 indicates no metastasis if the primary was at the stage of 33 generations and 100% of cases with metastases if the primary was at 40 generations. One can interpret these observations as follows: if Bell[277] saw no gross metastasis when the renal primary was

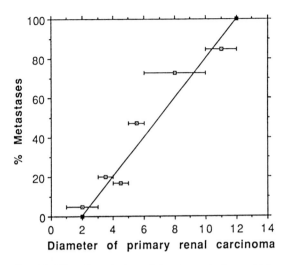

Fig. 10–95. Correlation of the size of primary kidney tumors and the incidence of gross metastases discovered at autopsy (data from Bell[277]). The straight line could be sigmoid without significantly changing the deductions possible.

at a size corresponding to 33 generations, how large a metastasis could he have missed? We need an approximate answer to this question in order to understand how at least one metastasis can become grossly visible in 14% of cases coming to autopsy with the primary only one generation later. Depending on how thin Bell[277] cut the various organs, he could have missed a mass corresponding to 29 generations (1 cm in diameter or 0.5 g) and almost certainly would have missed most masses corresponding to 20 generations (1 cu mm). With the linear increase in percentage of cases with gross metastases up to 100% at a size of the primary corresponding to 40 generations (Fig. 10-95), one can estimate that at the time when the primary was at the size of 33 generations, there were a few cases (14%) with an occult metastasis at 28 generations, ready to become visible with one more doubling; a few more cases (another 14%) with an occult metastasis at 27 generations, ready to become visible with 2 more doublings; etc., until by 40 generations for the primary every case has at least 1 grossly visible metastasis which had required only the last 7 generations to become visible. Thus, the first metastasis in each 14% of cases must have begun about 28 generations before the 33 to 40 generations of the primary which were seen at autopsy, that is, when the primary was at about 5 to 12 generations. Each of these 7 early generations must have contributed metastases in about one-seventh or 14% of the cases. Now, the thinner Bell[277] cut the gross tissues, the smaller the grossly visible metastasis, but the error could hardly be more than 10 generations.

At its "best," a long time ago, the problems inherent in cancer research related to Heisenberg's "Uncertainty Principle" were not so bad since the results of treatment did not seriously affect the natural history of the tumor and data could be collected in a relatively unbiased fashion. For some decades, however, the situation has been changing as the available treatments have been improving; and now, at its "worst," we have a pattern leading to chaos.

Why this relatively sudden development of a marked difference between "best" and "worst"? Not only because of the improvements in treatments but also because modern medicine is introducing new methods leading to earlier and different diagnoses and almost simultaneously changing the criteria for particular diagnoses. Feinstein et al.[279] have called attention to the "Will Rogers' phenomenon" (he is said to have joked that the Okies leaving the dust bowl in Oklahoma and moving to California in the 1930s raised the average intelligence level in both places). Translated to cancer, this means that earlier diagnoses leading to the inclusion of smaller tumors among the cases being treated will necessarily result in a lengthening of the group's survival time regardless of the treatment. Most present day staging schemes of cancers of the breast, kidney, or other organs include as one criterion the size of the primary, usually only larger or smaller than 3 cm in diameter, with no recognition of the fact that this size corresponds to about 34 doublings of an average 10-μ tumor cell and that doubling or halving the diameter represents not only 3 generations but also 8-fold changes in volume. The same improvements in diagnosis will also lead to earlier detection of metastases, so that "stage migration" will contribute to statistical improvement in survival regardless of any improvement in therapy.[279]

In the treatment of cancer we rely essentially on several determinations (the size, distribution, and histologic appearance of the tumor)

at one point in time (the time of diagnosis and the beginning of treatment). Only in rare cases do we have observations at two points in time sufficiently far apart and uninfluenced by treatment to permit calculation of the actual growth rate. Indeed, most treatments are based on the expected growth rate derived from past experiences with the particular histologic appearance of the tumor, including the results of any particular type of treatment for any specific cancer, and are generally expressed in terms of survival times (e.g., 50% or median survival times, 5-year survival percentages, etc.).

The problem, of course, is that the growth rates actually observed in occasional cases or approximated by observations of the complete range of survival times in any series of cases cover a broad range for any particular histologic type. For a most extreme example see Figure 10–52 for optic gliomas! This problem is only compounded when different pathologists attempt to interpret and then apply any published scheme of classification or, even worse, when different pathologists formally change the criteria for making particular diagnoses. The most recent example of this is the claim by Murovic et al.[159] that there are 6% "complete responders" to treatment of glioblastoma and anaplastic astrocytoma. If the pathologist contaminated the series with a significant number of inherently less malignant oligodendrogliomas—the recognition of which cannot be easily excluded by the histologic scheme used—exactly this pattern of pseudo-responders might be expected. This hypothesis is supported by the absence of any oligodendrogliomas in the series of tumors with labeling indices reported by Hoshino et al.[30] from the same institution.

These problems, which can be derived from the first version of Heisenberg's "Uncertainty Principle," are raised exponentially when problems related to the second version also enter; i.e., when the therapist enters additional factors into the formula that specifies the treatment of a particular patient—and even more so when the therapist is also the histologic diagnostician. One of us (ECA) knows first-hand from a study of muscle biopsies[280] how difficult histologic observations can become when clinical information is available before recording

Neoplasms Affecting the Nervous System of the Elderly

the histologic characteristics. The ability of one such clinically-informed observer to challenge the independent observations of 3 other uninformed observers was most remarkable! In such situations it becomes essentially impossible to obtain an unbiased sampling of the population of cancer patients from which randomly selected subsamples can be treated differently and then compared as to survival rates.

Consideration of Heisenberg's "Uncertainty Principle" is most appropriate at this time since we are perturbing the patient population with (1) earlier diagnosis with techniques, such as CT, MRI and cytologic screening, (2) alteration in the patient outcome with multiple varieties of treatment, each personalized without adequate long-term follow-up of other patients, (3) alteration in histologic classification by treatment (e.g., radiation therapy of pineal tumors followed by biopsy at recurrence or biopsy of gliomas followed by chemo- or radiotreatment and later debulking), and (4) continuous modification of the histologic classification of tumors by new techniques (e.g., diagnostic monoclonal antibodies, flow cytometry, and various molecular probes).

It is the essence of the Heisenberg "Uncertainty Principle" to be observing a patient's neoplasm from two different and rapidly changing perspectives: (1) refining the pathologic classification with new measuring techniques, and (2) modifying the patient population with new techniques for earlier diagnosis and a variety of treatment modalities. We do not see these two perspectives as independent phenomena, rather each modifies our perception of the mutual goals of better therapy and better outcome. Perhaps a common language based on tumor kinetic theory with clinical and pathologic inputs may better correlate with these common goals and foster better communication concerning the nature of the disease process. Such a "language" is attempted in Figure 10–12, where labeling index (LI), gross doubling time (Td), cell loss factor (ϕ), growth fraction (GF) and time to recurrence based on amount of tumor left behind are collected in one nomogram illustrating their interactions. It is remarkable how many pairs of products there are in the mathematical analysis of the biology of cancer, any one of

which would resemble the product "time times rate = distance" characteristic of Heisenberg's "Uncertainty Principle."

SUMMARY

As illustrated in Figure 10–96, many more factors must be considered in the staging of cancer patients than just the histology of the tumor: its growth rate and degree of invasiveness, the clinical status of the patient, and the amount of tumor left behind being minimal criteria. Although admittedly an over-simplification, the concept of "simple" exponential growth and the staging of tumors in terms of the total amount of tumor equated to approximately numbers of doublings has much to recommend its routine use, even if one begins by measuring only volumes rather than diameters as a reference standard. This over-simplified model can be modified relatively easily to accommodate newer cytokinetic factors, such as mitotic and proliferative activities, S-phase measurements, labeling indices (LI), cell loss factor (ϕ) and growth fraction (GF) as well as potential (Tp) and actual (Td) doubling

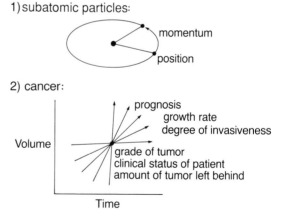

1) subatomic particles:

momentum

position

2) cancer:

Volume

prognosis
growth rate
degree of invasiveness

grade of tumor
clinical status of patient
amount of tumor left behind

Time

Fig. 10–96. Heisenberg's "Uncertainty Principle" and an expanded concept of how current techniques still fall short of predicting the prognosis of cancer patients. The most important variables cannot be measured (degree of invasiveness and amount of tumor left behind), the growth rate is rarely measured and the clinical status of the patient on admission is uncommonly considered in publications concerning the follow-up of groups of patients.

times (Fig. 10–12). The importance of following patients with repeated observations over time, including the final observation at autopsy, must be emphasized if we are to come to quantitative grips with either benign or malignant neoplasms.

ACKNOWLEDGMENTS

Dr. Todd Richards helped in the preparation of the many graphs concerning prognosis. Drs. Steven Lofton and George Swan provided helpful comments concerning factors affecting growth rates. Dr. William Kelly performed practically all of the operations on the patients with pituitary tumors and Dr. George Ojemann on those with epilepsy. To each of these and many others, including many residents who have studied with us, we are most grateful for the many surgical and autopsy specimens provided us during the past several decades. We are especially grateful to Drs. Juha Jääskeläinen and Matti Haltia, who generously provided their data concerning recurrences of meningiomas.

REFERENCES

1. Alvord, E.C., Jr.: Why do gliomas not metastasize? Arch. Neurol., 33:73, 1976.
2. Alvord, E.C., Jr.: Hypothesis: Growth rates of epidermoid tumors. Ann. Neurol., 2:367, 1977.
3. Barlogie, B., et al.: Flow cytometry in clinical cancer research. Cancer Res., 43:3982, 1983.
4. Barnard, N.J., Hall, P.A., Lemoine, N.R., et al.: Proliferative index in breast carcinoma determined in situ by Ki67 immunostaining and its relationship to clinical and pathological variables. J. Path., 152:287, 1987.
5. Begg, A.C., McNally, N.J., Shrieve, D.C., et al.: A method to measure the duraction of DNA synthesis and the potential doubling time from a single sample. Cytometry, 6:620, 1985.
6. Bonnin, J.M., and Rubinstein, L.J.: Astroblastomas: A pathological study of 23 tumors, with a postoperative follow-up in 13 patients. Neurosurgery, 25:6, 1989.
7. Burger, P.C., Shibata, T., and Kleihues, P.: The use of the monoclonal antibody Ki-67 in the identification of proliferating cells: Application to surgical neuropathology. Amer. J. Surg. Path., 10:611, 1986.
8. Cardiff, R.D.: Cellular and molecular aspects of neoplastic progression in the mammary gland. Eur. J. Cancer Clin. Oncol., 24:15, 1988.
9. Charpin, C., et al.: Multiparametric evaluation (SAMBA) of growth fraction (monoclonal Ki67) in breast carcinoma tissue sections. Cancer Res., 48:4368, 1988.
10. Cho, K.G., et al.: Prediction of tumor doubling time in recurrent meningiomas. Cell kinetics studies with bromodeoxyuridine labeling. J. Neurosurg., 65:790, 1986.
11. Clark, G.M., et al.: Prediction of relapse or survival in patients with node-negative breast cancer by DNA flow cytometry. New Engl. J. Med., 320:627, 1989.
12. Collins, V.P., Loeffler, R.K., and Tivey, H.: Observations on growth rates of human tumors. Am. J. Roentgenol. Radium Ther. Nucl. Med., 76:988, 1956.
13. Concannon, J.C., Kramer, S., and Berry, R.: The extent of intracranial gliomata at autopsy and its relation to techniques used in radiation therapy of brain tumors. Am. J. Roentgenol. Radium Ther. Nucl. Med., 84:99, 1960.
14. Danova, M., et al.: Ploidy and proliferative activity of human brain tumors. Oncology, 44:102, 1987.
15. Danova, M., et al.: Cell kinetics of human brain tumors: In vivo study with bromodeoxyuridine and flow cytometry. Eur. J. Cancer Clin. Oncol., 24:873, 1988.
16. Darzynkiewicz, Z.: Cytochemical probes of cycling and quiescent cells applicable to flow cytometry. In: Techniques in Cell Cycle Analysis. (Eds.) J.E. Gray and Z. Darzynkiewicz. Clifton, N.J., Humana Press., Inc., 1986, pp. 255–290.
17. Falini, B., et al.: Evolutionary conservation in various mammalian species of the human proliferation-associated epitope recognized by the Ki-67 monoclonal antibody. J. Histochem. Cytochem., 37:1471, 1989.
18. Gerdes, J.: An immunohistological method of estimating cell growth fractions in rapid histopathological diagnosis during surgery. Int. J. Cancer, 35:169, 1985.
19. Gerdes, J., et al.: Cell cycle analysis of a cell proliferation-associated human nuclear antigen defined by the monoclonal antibody Ki-67. J. Immunol., 133:1710, 1984.
20. Gray, J.W.: Quantitative cytokinetics: Cellular response to cell cycle specific agents. Intl. Ency. Pharm. Therap., 121:44, 1984.
21. Hawking, S.W.: A Brief History of Time. From the Big Bang to Black Holes. Toronto, Bantam Books, 1988, pp. 53–61, 187.
22. Hedley, D.W., Rugg, C.A., and Gelber, R.D.: Association of DNA index and S-phase fraction with prognosis of nodes positive early breast cancer. Cancer Res., 47:4729, 1987.
23. Heim, S., and Mitelman, F.: Numerical chromosome aberrations in human neoplasia. Cancer Genet. Cytogenet., 22:99, 1986.
24. Heisenberg, W.: Über den anschaulichen Inhalt der quantentheoretischen Kinematik und Mechanik. Zts. Physik, 43:172, 1927.
25. Hirakawa, K., Suzuki, K., Ueda, S., et al.: Fetal origin of the medulloblastoma: Evidence from growth analysis of two cases. Acta Neuropathol. (Berlin), 70:277, 1986.
26. Hoshino, T., and Wilson, C.B.: Review of basic concepts of cell kinetics as applied to brain tumors. J. Neurosurg., 42:123, 1975.
27. Hoshino, T., and Wilson, C.B.: Cell kinetic analyses of human malignant brain tumors (gliomas). Cancer, 44:956, 1979.
28. Hoshino, T., Wilson, C.B., Rosenblum, M.L., et al.: Chemotherapeutic implications of growth fraction and cell cycle time in glioblastomas. J. Neurosurg., 43:127, 1975.
29. Hoshino, T., et al.: In situ cell kinetics studies on

human neuroectodermal tumors with bromodeoxy-uridine labeling. J. Neurosurg., *64*:453, 1986.

30. Hoshino, T., et al.: S-Phase fraction of human brain tumors *in situ* measured by uptake of bromodeoxy-uridine. Int. J. Cancer, *38*:369, 1986.

31. Jääskeläinen, J., et al.: The growth rate of intracranial meningiomas and its relation to histology. An analysis of 43 patients. Surg. Neurol., *24*:165, 1985.

32. Kusama, S., et al.: The gross rates of growth of human mammary carcinoma. Cancer, *30*:594, 1972.

33. Laird, A.K.: Dynamics of tumour growth: Comparison of growth rates and extrapolation of growth curve to one cell. Br. J. Cancer, *19*:278, 1965.

34. Lellé, R.J., Heidenreich, W., Stauch, G., et al.: The correlation of growth fractions with histologic grading and lymph node status in human mammary carcinoma. Cancer, *59*:83, 1987.

35. Lellé, R.J., et al.: Determination of growth fractions in benign breast disease (BBD) with monoclonal antibody Ki-67. J. Cancer Res. Clin. Oncol., *113*:73, 1987.

36. Lemire, R.J., Loeser, J.D., Leech, R.W., et al.: *Normal and Abnormal Development of the Human Nervous System.* Hagerstown, Harper & Row, 1975, pp. 344–350.

37. Malaise, E.P., Chavaudra, N., Charbit, A., et al.: Relationship between the growth rate of human metastases, survival and pathological type. Europ. J. Cancer, *10*:451, 1974.

38. Malaise, E.P., Chavaudra, N., and Tubiana, M.: The relationship between growth rate, labelling index and histological type of human solid tumours. Europ. J. Cancer, *9*:305, 1973.

39. Mandybur, T.I., Sawaya, R., and Ormsby, I.: The morphology and biologic behavior of human glioblastoma growing in nude mice. Cancer, *58*:1061, 1986.

40. Mayneord, W.V.: On a law of growth of Jensen's rat sarcoma. Amer. J. Cancer, *16*:841, 1932.

41. McDivitt, R.W., et al.: A proposed classification of breast cancer based on kinetic information derived from a comparison of risk factors in 168 primary operable breast cancers. Cancer, *57*:269, 1986.

42. McGurrin, J.F., et al.: Assessment of tumor cell kinetics by immunohistochemistry in carcinoma of breast. Cancer, *59*:1744, 1987.

43. Mendelsohn, M.L.: Autoradiographic analysis of cell proliferation in spontaneous breast cancer of C3H mouse. III. The growth fraction. J. Nat. Cancer Inst., *28*:1015, 1962.

44. Meyer, J.S.: Growth and cell kinetic measurements in human tumors. Path. Ann., *16*:53, 1981.

45. Meyer, J.S.: Cell kinetics of breast and breast tumors. In: *Cancer of the Breast.* 3rd Ed. (Eds.) W.L. Donegan, and J.S. Spratt, Philadelphia, W.B. Saunders Co., 1988, pp. 250–269.

46. Meyer, J.S., Prey, M.U., Babcock, D.S., et al.: Breast carcinoma cell kinetics, morphology, stage and host characteristics. A thymidine labeling study. Lab. Invest., *54*:41, 1986.

47. Rabinovitch, P.S.: Regulation of human fibroblast growth rate by both noncycling cell fraction and transition probability is shown by growth in 5-bro-modeoxyuridine followed by Hoechst 33258 flow cytometry. Proc. Natl. Acad. Sci. USA, *80*:2951, 1983.

48. Riccardi, A., et al.: Cell kinetics in human malignancies studied with *in vivo* administration of bromodeoxyuridine and flow cytometry. Cancer Res., *48*:6238, 1988.

49. Silvestrini, R., Sanfilippo, O., and Tedesco, G.: Kinetics of human mammary carcinomas and their correlation with the cancer and host characteristics. Cancer, *34*:1252, 1974.

50. Spaar, F.W., et al.: Flow-cytophotometry of nuclear DNA in biopsies of 45 human gliomas and after primary culture in vitro. Clin. Neuropath., *5*:157, 1986.

51. Speer, J.F., et al.: A stochastic numerical model of breast cancer growth that simulates clinical data. Cancer Res., *44*:4124, 1984.

52. Spratt, J.S., and Spratt, J.A.: Growth rates. In: *Cancer of the Breast.* 2nd Ed. (Eds.) W.L. Donegan and J.S. Spratt, Philadelphia, W.B. Saunders Co., 1979, pp. 197–220.

53. Spratt, J.S., and Spratt, J.A.: Growth rates. In: *Cancer of the Breast.* 3rd Ed. (Eds.) W.L. Donegan and J.S. Spratt, Philadelphia, W.B. Saunders Co., 1988, pp. 270–302.

54. Steel, G.G.: Cell loss from experimental tumours. Cell Tissue Kinet., *1*:193, 1968.

55. Steel, G.G.: *Growth Kinetics of Tumours. Cell Population Kinetics in Relation to the Growth and Treatment of Cancer.* Oxford, Clarendon Press, 1977.

56. Swan, G.W.: Tumor growth models and cancer chemotherapy. In: *Cancer Modeling.* (Eds.) J.R. Thompson and B.W. Brown. New York, Marcel Dekker, Inc., 1987.

57. Tubiana, M.: Tumor cell proliferation kinetics and tumor growth rate. Acta Oncol., *28*:113, 1989.

58. Tubiana, M., et al.: The long-term prognostic significance of the thymidine labelling index in breast cancer. Int. J. Cancer, *33*:441, 1984.

59. von Fournier, D., et al.: Growth rate of 147 mammary carcinomas. Cancer, *45*:2198, 1980.

60. Wallner, K.E., et al.: Efficacy of irradiation for incompletely excised acoustic neurilemmomas. J. Neurosurg., *67*:857, 1987.

61. Wilson, G.D., et al.: Measurement of cell kinetics in human tumours *in vivo* using bromodeoxyuridine incorporation and flow cytometry. Br. J. Cancer, *58*:423, 1988.

62. Yanagisawa, M., Dolbeare, F., Todoroki, T., et al.: Cell cycle analysis using numerical simulation of bivariate DNA/bromodeoxyuridine distributions. Cytometry, *6*:550, 1985.

63. Yoshii, Y., et al.: Estimation of growth fraction with bromodeoxyurdine in human central nervous system tumors. J. Neurosurg., *65*:659, 1986.

64. Zukav, G.: *The Dancing Wu Li Masters, An Overview of the New Physics.* Toronto, Bantam Books, 1979, pp. 27, 112.

65. Austin, E.J., and Alvord, E.C., Jr.: Recurrences of cerebellar astrocytomas: A violation of Collins' Law. J. Neurosurg., *68*:41, 1988.

66. Cushing, H.: Experiences with the cerebellar astrocytomas. A critical review of seventy-six cases. Surg. Gynecol. Obstet., *52*:129, 1931.

67. Elvidge, A., Penfield, W., and Cone, W.: The gliomas of the central nervous system. Res. Publ. Ass. Nerv. Ment. Dis., *16*:107, 1935.

68. Gol, A., and McKissock, W.: The cerebellar astrocytomas. A report on 98 verified cases. J. Neurosurg., *16*:287, 1959.

69. Kepes, J.J., et al.: Cerebellar astrocytomas in elderly patients with very long preoperative histories: Report of three cases. Neurosurg., *25*:258, 1989.

70. Kitaoka, K., Tashiro, K., Abe, H., et al.: A clinical survey of cerebellar astrocytoma—Comparison be-

tween childhood and adult cases. No Shinkei Geka, 8:55, 1980.

71. Mabon, R.F., et al.: Astrocytomas of the cerebellum. Arch. Neurol. Psychiat., 64:74, 1950.

72. Ringertz, N., and Nordenstam, H.: Cerebellar astrocytoma. J. Neuropath. Exp. Neurol., 10:343, 1951.

73. Zülch, K.-J.: Über das "sog." Kleinhirnastrocytom. Virchows Arch. path. Anat., 307:222, 1940.

74. Bailey, P., and Cushing, H.: *A Classification of the Tumors of the Glioma Group on a Histogenetic Basis with a Correlated Study of Prognosis.* Philadelphia, J.B. Lippincott Co., 1926 (reprinted, New York, Argosy-Antiquarian Ltd., 1971).

75. Berkson, J., and Gage, R.P.: Calculation of survival rates for cancer. Proc. Staff Meet. Mayo Clin., 25:270, 1950.

76. Burger, P.C., and Vogel, F.S.: *Surgical Pathology of the Nervous System and Its Coverings.* 2nd Ed., New York, John Wiley and Sons, 1982, pp. 223–458.

77. Burger, P.C., et al.: Glioblastoma and anaplastic astrocytoma: Pathologic criteria and prognostic implications. Cancer, 56:1106, 1985.

78. Daumas-Duport, C., Scheithauer, B., O'Fallon, J., et al.: Grading of astrocytomas: A simple and reproducible method. Cancer, 62:2152, 1988.

79. Greenfield, J.G.: The pathological examination of forty intracranial neoplasms. Brain, 42:29, 1915.

80. Kernohan, J.W., and Sayre, G.P.: Section X—Fascicles 35 and 37. *Tumors of the Central Nervous System.* Washington, D.C., Armed Forces Institute of Pathology, 1952.

81. Kernohan, J.W., et al.: A simplified classification of the gliomas. Proc. Staff Meet. Mayo Clin., 24:71, 1949.

82. Levin, V.A., et al.: Phase II study of combined carmustine, 5-fluorouracil, hydroxyurea, and 6-mercaptopurine (BFHM) for the treatment of malignant gliomas. Cancer Treat. Rep., 70:1271, 1986.

83. Levin, V.A., et al.: Phase I-II study of eflornithine and mitoguazone combined in the treatment of recurrent primary brain tumors. Cancer Treat. Rep., 71:459, 1987.

84. McComb, R.D., and Burger, P.C.: Pathologic analysis of primary brain tumors. Neurol. Clin., 3:711, 1985.

85. Nelson, D.F., et al.: Survival and prognosis of patients with astrocytoma with atypical or anaplastic features. J. Neuro-Oncol., 3:99, 1985.

86. Nelson, J.S., et al.: Necrosis as a prognostic criterion in malignant supratentorial, astrocytic gliomas. Cancer, 52:550, 1983.

87. Ringertz, N.: Grading of gliomas. Acta Path. Microbiol. Scand., 27:51, 1950.

88. Rubinstein, L.J.: *Tumors of the Central Nervous System. AFIP Atlas of Tumor Pathology,* Series 2, Fascicle 6. Washington, D.C., Armed Forces Institute of Pathology, 1972, pp. 32–34.

89. Russell, D.S., and Rubinstein, L.J.: *Pathology of Tumours of the Nervous System.* 5th Ed. Baltimore, Williams & Wilkins, 1989.

90. Scherer, H.J.: Cerebral astrocytomas and their derivatives. Amer. J. Cancer, 40:159, 1940.

91. Shaw, E.G., et al.: Radiation therapy in the management of low-grade supratentorial astrocytomas. J. Neurosurg., 70:853, 1989.

92. Tooth, H.H.: Some observations on the growth and survival-period of intracranial tumours, based on the records of 500 cases, with special reference to the pathology of gliomata. Brain, 35:61, 1912.

93. Zülch, K.J.: *Histological Typing of Tumours of the Central Nervous System.* Geneva, World Health Organization, 1979.

94. Zülch, K.J.: *Brain Tumors. Their Biology and Pathology.* 3rd Ed., Berlin, Springer-Verlag, 1986.

95. Hart, M.N., Petito, C.K., and Earle, K.M.: Mixed gliomas. Cancer, 33:134, 1974.

96. Herpers, M.J.H.M., and Budka, H.: Glial fibrillary acidic protein (GFAP) in oligodendroglial tumors: Gliofibrillary oligodendroglioma and transitional oligoastrocytoma as subtypes of oligodendroglioma. Acta Neuropath. (Wien), 64:265, 1984.

97. Scheithauer, B.W.: Neuropathology of pineal region tumors. Clin. Neurosurg., 32:351, 1984.

98. Alvord, E.C., Jr.: Head circumference, brain weight, and tumor burden. J. Child Neurol., 1:240, 1986.

99. Centeno, R.S., et al.: Supratentorial ependymomas: Neuroimaging and clinicopathological correlation. J. Neurosurg., 64:209, 1986.

100. Chin, H.W., Maruyama, Y., Markesbery, W., et al.: Intracranial ependymoma: Results of radiotherapy at the University of Kentucky. Cancer, 49:2276, 1982.

101. Garrett, P.G., and Simpson, W.J.K.: Ependymomas: Results of radiation treatment. Int. J. Rad. Oncol. Biol. Phys., 9:1121, 1983.

102. Marks, J.E., and Adler, S.J.: A comparative study of ependymomas by site of origin. Int. J. Rad. Oncol. Biol. Phys., 8:37, 1982.

103. Pierre-Kahn, A., et al.: Intracranial ependymomas in childhood: Survival and functional results of 47 cases. Child's Brain, 10:145, 1983.

104. Salazar, O.M., et al.: Improved survival in cases of intracranial ependymoma after radiation therapy. Late report and recommendations. J. Neurosurg., 59:652, 1983.

105. Shuman, R.M., Alvord, E.C., Jr., and Leech, R.W.: The biology of childhood ependymomas. Arch. Neurol., 32:731, 1975.

106. West, C.R., Bruce, D.A., and Duffner, P.K.: Ependymomas: Factors in clinical and diagnostic staging. Cancer, 56:1812, 1985.

107. Bullard, D.E., et al.: Oligodendroglioma. An analysis of the value of radiation therapy. Cancer, 60:2179, 1987.

108. Burger, P.C., et al.: Clinicopathologic correlations in the oligodendroglioma. Cancer, 59:1345, 1987.

109. Cairncross, J.G., and Macdonald, D.R.: Successful chemotherapy for recurrent malignant oligodendroglioma. Ann. Neurol., 23:360, 1988.

110. Choi, B.H.: Myelin-forming oligodendrocytes of developing mouse spinal cord: Immunocytochemical and ultrastructural studies. J. Neuropath. Exp. Neurol., 45:513, 1986.

111. Choi, B.H., and Kim, R.C.: Expression of glial fibrillary acidic protein by immature oligodendroglia and its implications. J. Neuroimmunol., 8:215, 1985.

112. De Reuck, J., et al.: Cytophotometric DNA determination in human oligodendroglial tumours. Histopath. 4:225, 1980.

113. Helseth, A., and Mørk, S.J.: Neoplasms of the central nervous system in Norway. III. Epidemiological characteristics of intracranial gliomas according to histology. APMIS, 97:547, 1989.

114. Kondziolka, D., et al.: Significance of hemorrhage into brain tumors: Clinicopathological study. J. Neurosurg., 67:852, 1987.

115. Lindegaard, K.-F., et al.: Statistical analysis of clinicopathological features, radiotherapy, and survival in 170 cases of oligodendroglioma. J. Neurosurg., 67:224, 1987.

116. Ludwig, C.L., et al.: A clinicopathological study of 323 patients with oligodendrogliomas. Ann Neurol., 19:15, 1986.

117. Mørk, S.J., et al.: Oligodendroglioma: Incidence and biological behavior in a defined population. J. Neurosurg., 63:881, 1985.

118. Mørk, S.J., et al.: Oligodendroglioma: Histologic evaluation and prognosis. J. Neuropath. Exp. Neurol., 45:65, 1986.

119. Wallner, K.E., et al.: Treatment of oligodendrogliomas with or without postoperative irradiation. J. Neurosurg., 68:684, 1988.

120. Winger, M.J., Macdonald, D.R., and Cairncross, J.G.: Supratentorial anaplastic gliomas in adults. The prognostic importance of extent of resection and prior low-grade glioma. J. Neurosurg., 71:487, 1989.

121. Karnofsky, D.A., Abelmann, W.H., Craver, L.F., et al.: The use of the nitrogen mustards in the palliative treatment of carcinoma with particular reference to bronchogenic carcinoma. Cancer, 1:634, 1948.

122. Alvord, E.C., Jr., and Lofton, S.: Gliomas of the optic nerve or chiasm: Outcome by patients' age, tumor site, and treatment. J. Neurosurg., 68:85, 1988.

123. Bell, E., Jr., and Karnosh, L.J.: Cerebral hemispherectomy. Report of a case ten years after operation. J. Neurosurg., 6:285, 1949.

124. Bigner, S.H., Bjerkvig, R., and Laerum, O.D.: DNA content and chromosomal composition of malignant human gliomas. Neurol. Clin., 3:769, 1985.

125. Bigner, S.H., et al.: Chromosomal evolution in malignant human gliomas starts with specific and usually numerical deviations. Cancer Genet. Cytogenet., 22:121, 1986.

126. Black, K.L., et al.: Use of thallium-201 SPECT to quantitate malignancy grade of gliomas. J. Neurosurg., 71:342, 1989.

127. Bookwalter, J.W., III, et al.: Brain-tumor cell kinetics correlated with survival. J. Neurosurg., 65:795, 1986.

128. Brooks, W.H., et al.: Relationship of lymphocyte invasion and survival of brain tumor patients. Ann. Neurol., 4:219, 1978.

129. Burger, P.C., and Green, S.B.: Patient age, histologic features, and length of survival in patients with glioblastoma multiforme. Cancer, 59:1617, 1987.

130. Burger, P.C., et al.: Topographic anatomy and CT correlations in the untreated glioblastoma multiforme. J. Neurosurg., 68:698, 1988.

131. Cavenee, W.K.: Molecular genetics of brain tumor progression. Amer. Assoc. Neuropath., June 18, 1989.

132. Clark, G.B., Henry, J.M., and McKeever, P.E.: Cerebral pilocytic astrocytoma. Cancer, 56:1128, 1985.

133. Cohadon, F., et al.: Histologic and non-histologic factors correlated with survival time in supratentorial astrocytic tumors. J. Neuro-Oncol., 3:105, 1985.

134. Coons, S.W., Davis, J.R., and Way, D.L.: Correlation of DNA content and histology in prognosis of astrocytomas. Amer. J. Clin. Path., 90:289, 1988.

135. Cooper, J.S., Borok, T.L., Ransohoff, J., and Carella, R.J.: Malignant glioma. Results of combined modality therapy. JAMA, 248:62, 1982.

136. Di Lorenzo, N., Palma, L., and Nicole, S.: Lymphocytic infiltration in long-survival glioblastomas: Possible host's resistance. Acta Neurochir., 39:27, 1977.

137. Fitzgibbons, P.L., et al.: Flow cytometric DNA and nuclear antigen content in astrocytic neoplasms. Amer. J. Clin. Pathol., 89:640, 1988.

138. Fulling, K.H., and Garcia, D.M.: Anaplastic astrocytoma of the adult cerebrum: Prognostic value of histologic features. Cancer, 55:928, 1985.

139. Gaetani, P., et al.: Cell kinetics aspect of human malignant neuroepithelial tumors: A follow-up study. Tumori, 74:145, 1988.

140. Garcia, D.M., and Fulling, K.H.: Juvenile pilocytic astrocytomas of the cerebrum in adults. A distinctive neoplasm with favorable prognosis. J. Neurosurg., 63:382, 1985.

141. Garcia, D.M., Fulling, K.H., and Marks, J.E.: The value of radiation therapy in addition to surgery for astrocytomas of the adult cerebrum. Cancer, 55:919, 1985.

142. Giangaspero, F., and Burger, P.C.: Correlations between cytologic composition and biologic behavior in the glioblastoma multiforme: A postmortem study of 50 cases. Cancer, 52:2320, 1983.

143. Giangaspero, F., Chieco, P., Lisignoli, G., et al.: Comparison of cytologic composition with microfluorometric DNA analysis of the glioblastoma multiforme and anaplastic astrocytoma. Cancer, 60:59, 1987.

144. Green, S.B., et al.: Comparisons of carmustine, procarbazine, and high-dose methylprednisolone as additions to surgery and radiotherapy for the treatment of malignant glioma. Cancer Treat. Rep., 67:121, 1983.

145. Gutin, P.H., et al.: Recurrent malignant gliomas: Survival following interstitial brachytherapy with high-activity iodine-125 sources. J. Neurosurg., 67:864, 1987.

146. Hoshino, T.: A commentary on the biology and growth kinetics of low-grade and high-grade gliomas. J. Neurosurg., 61:895, 1984.

147. Hoshino, T., Townsend, J.J., Muraoka, I., and Wilson, C.B.: An autoradiographic study of human gliomas: Growth kinetics of anaplastic astrocytoma and glioblastoma multiforme. Brain, 103:967, 1980.

148. Hoshino, T., Wilson, C.B., and Ellis, W.G.: Gemistocytic astrocytes in gliomas: An autoradiographic study. J. Neuropath. Exp. Neurol., 34:263, 1975.

149. Hoshino, T., et al.: The distribution of nuclear DNA from human brain-tumor cells. Flow cytometric studies. J. Neurosurg., 49:13, 1978.

150. Hoshino, T., et al.: Cell kinetic studies of in situ human brain tumors with bromodeoxyuridine. Cytometry, 6:627, 1985.

151. Hoshino, T., et al.: Prognostic implications of the proliferative potential of low-grade astrocytomas. J. Neurosurg., 69:839, 1988.

152. Hoshino, T., et al.: Prognostic implications of the bromodeoxyuridine labeling index of human gliomas. J. Neurosurg., 71:335, 1989.

153. Jelsma, R., and Bucy, P.C.: Glioblastoma multiforme. Its treatment and some factors affecting survival. Arch. Neurol., 20:161, 1969.

154. Kepes, J.J., and Rubinstein, L.J.: Malignant gliomas with heavily lipidized (foamy) tumor cells. A report of three cases with immunoperoxidase study. Cancer, 47:2451, 1981.

155. Kepes, J.J., Kepes, M., and Slowik, F.: Fibrous xanthomas and xanthosarcomas of the meninges and the brain. Acta Neuropathol. (Wien), 23:187, 1973.

156. Kepes, J.J., Rubinstein, L.J., and Eng, L.F.: Pleomorphic xanthoastrocytoma: A distinctive meningocerebral glioma of young subjects with relatively favorable prognosis. A study of 12 cases. Cancer, 44:1835, 1979.

157. Laramore, G.E., et al.: Randomized neutron dose searching study for malignant gliomas of the brain:

Results of an RTOG study. Int. J. Rad. Oncol. Biol. Phys. *14*:1093, 1988.

158. Levy, L.F., and Elvidge, A.R.: Astrocytoma of the brain and spinal cord: A review of 176 cases, 1940–1949. J. Neurosurg., *13*:413, 1956.

159. Murovic, J., et al.: Computerized tomography in the prognosis of malignant gliomas. J. Neurosurg., *65*:799, 1986.

160. Nagashima, T., DeArmond, S.J., Murovic, J., et al.: Immunocytochemical demonstration of S-phase cells by antibromodeoxyuridine monoclonal antibody in human brain tumor tissues. Acta Neuropathol. (Berlin), *67*:155, 1985.

161. Pasquier, B., et al.: Le xanthoastrocytome du sujet jeune. Revue de la littérature à propos de deux observations d'évolution discordante. Ann. Pathol., *5*:29, 1985.

162. Ridley, A., and Cavanagh, J.B.: Lymphocytic infiltration in gliomas: Evidence of possible host resistance. Brain, *94*:117, 1971.

163. Schiffer, D., et al.: Prognostic value of histologic factors in adult cerebral astrocytoma. Cancer, *61*:1386, 1988.

164. Schold, C.S., et al.: Chemotherapy for malignant gliomas? Ann. Neurol., *25*:88, 1989.

165. Shapiro, J.R., and Shapiro, W.R.: Clonal tumor cell heterogeneity. Prog. Exp. Tumor Res., *27*:49, 1984.

166. Shapiro, J.R., and Shapiro, W.R.: The subpopulations and isolated cell types of freshly resected high grade gliomas: Their influence on the tumor's evolution *in vivo* and behavior and therapy *in vitro*. Cancer Metas. Rev., *4*:107, 1985.

167. Shapiro, J.R., Yung, W.-K.A., and Shapiro, W.R.: Isolation, karyotype and clonal growth of heterogeneous subpopulations of human malignant gliomas. Cancer Res., *41*:2349, 1981.

168. Shapiro, W.R.: Therapy of adult malignant brain tumors: What have the clinical trials taught us? Sem. Oncol., *13*:38, 1986.

169. Shapiro, W.R., et al.: Randomized trial of three chemotherapy regimens and two radiotherapy regimens in postoperative treatment of malignant glioma: Brain Tumor Cooperative Group trial 8001. J. Neurosurg., *71*:1, 1989.

170. Shaw, C.M., et al.: Fast neutron irradiation of glioblastoma multiforme. J. Neurosurg., *49*:1, 1978.

171. Sieben, G., et al.: The influence of AZQ on the DNA distribution of human cerebral tumours in short-term culture. Eur. J. Cancer, *21*:217, 1985.

172. Slooff, J.L., Kernohan, J.W., and MacCarty, C.S.: *Primary Intramedullary Tumors of the Spinal Cord and Filum Terminale.* Philadelphia, W.B. Saunders Co., 1964.

173. Stage, W.S., and Stein, J.J.: Treatment of malignant astrocytomas. Amer. J. Roetgen. Rad. Ther. Nucl. Med., *120*:7, 1974.

174. Walker, M.D., et al.: Evaluation of BCNU and/or radiotherapy in the treatment of anaplastic gliomas: A cooperative clinical trial. J. Neurosurg., *49*:333, 1978.

175. Walker, M.D., et al.: Randomized comparisons of radiotherapy and nitrosoureas for the treatment of malignant glioma after surgery. N. Engl. J. Med., *303*:1323, 1980.

176. Wallner, K.E., et al.: Treatment results of juvenile pilocytic astrocytoma. J. Neurosurg., *69*:171, 1988.

177. Whittle, I.R., et al.: Pleomorphic xanthoastrocytoma. Report of four cases. J. Neurosurg., *70*:463, 1989.

178. Wood, J.R., Green, S.B., and Shapiro, W.R.: The prognostic importance of tumor size in malignant gliomas: A computed tomographic scan study by the Brain Tumor Cooperative Group. J. Clin. Oncol., *6*:338, 1988.

179. Yamashita, T., and Kuwabara, T.: Estimation of rate of growth of malignant brain tumors by computed tomography scanning. Surg. Neurol., *20*:464, 1983.

180. Zaprianov, Z., and Christov, K.: Histological grading, DNA content, cell proliferation and survival of patients with astroglial tumors. Cytometry, *9*:380, 1988.

181. Garbern, J., Spence, A.M., and Alvord, E.C., Jr.: Balo's concentric demyelination diagnosed premortem. Neurology, *36*:1610, 1986.

182. Adegbite, A.B., Khan, M.I., Paine, K.W.E., et al.: The recurrence of intracranial meningiomas after surgical treatment. J. Neurosurg., *58*:51, 1983.

183. Böker, D.-K., Meurer, H., and Gullotta, F.: Recurring intracranial meningiomas: Evaluation of some factors predisposing for tumor recurrence. J. Neurosurg. Sci., *29*:11, 1985.

184. Borovich, B., and Doron, Y.: Recurrence of intracranial meningiomas: The role played by regional multicentricity. J. Neurosurg., *64*:58, 1986.

185. Borovich, B., et al.: Recurrence of intracranial meningiomas: The role played by regional multicentricity. Part 2: Clinical and radiological aspects. J. Neurosurg., *65*:168, 1986.

186. Boylan, S.E., and McCunniff, A.J.: Recurrent meningioma. Cancer, *61*:1447, 1988.

187. Chan, R.C., and Thompson, G.B.: Morbidity, mortality, and quality of life following surgery for intracranial meningiomas: A retrospective study in 257 cases. J. Neurosurg., *60*:52, 1984.

188. Christensen, D., Laursen, H., and Klinken, L.: Prediction of recurrence in meningiomas after surgical treatment: A quantitative approach. Acta Neuropathol. (Berlin), *61*:130, 1983.

189. Cushing, H., and Eisenhardt, L.: *Meningiomas, Their Classification, Regional Behavior, Life History, and Surgical End Results.* Springfield, Charles C Thomas, 1938.

190. de la Monte, S.M., Flickinger, J., and Linggood, R.M.: Histopathologic features predicting recurrence of meningiomas following subtotal resection. Amer. J. Surg. Path., *10*:836, 1986.

191. Forbes, A.R., and Goldberg, I.D.: Radiation therapy in the treatment of meningioma: The Joint Center for Radiation Therapy experience 1970 to 1982. J. Clin. Oncol., *2*:1139, 1984.

192. Frederiksen, P., Reske-Nielsen, E., and Bichel, P.: DNA content of meningiomas. Acta Neuropathol. (Berlin), *46*:65, 1979.

193. Fukui, M., et al.: Proliferative activity of meningiomas as evaluated by bromodeoxyuridine uptake examination. Acta Neurochir. (Wein), *81*:135, 1986.

194. Globus, J.H.: The meningiomas: Their origin, divergence in structure and relationship to contiguous tissues in the light of the phylogenesis and ontogenesis of the meninges; with a suggestion of a simplified classification of meningeal neoplasms. Res. Publ. Assoc. Res. Nerv. Ment. Dis., *16*:210, 1937.

195. Hoshino, T., et al.: Proliferative potential of human meningiomas of the brain. A cell kinetics study with bromodeoxyuridine. Cancer, *58*:1466, 1986.

196. Inoue, H., et al: Clinical pathology of malignant meningiomas. Acta Neurochir., *73*:179, 1984.

197. Jääskeläinen, J.: Seemingly complete removal of histologically benign intracranial meningioma: Late re-

currence rate and factors predicting recurrence in 657 patients. A multivariate analysis. Surg. Neurol., 26:461, 1986.

198. Jääskeläinen, J., Haltia, M., and Servo, A.: Atypical and anaplastic meningiomas: Radiology, surgery, radiotherapy, and outcome. Surg. Neurol., 25:233, 1986.

199. Jääskeläinen, J., et al.: Intracranial hemangiopericytoma: Radiology, surgery, radiotherapy, and outcome in 21 patients. Surg. Neurol., 23:227, 1985.

200. Katsuyama, J., et al.: Chromosome abnormalities in meningiomas. Cancer Genet. Cytogenet., 22:63, 1986.

201. King, D.L., Chang, C.H., and Pool, J.L.: Radiotherapy in the management of meningiomas. Acta Radiol. Ther. Phys. Biol., 5:26, 1966.

202. Kupersmith, M.J., Warren, F.A., Newell, J., et al.: Irradiation of meningiomas of the intracranial anterior visual pathway. Ann. Neurol., 21:131, 1987.

203. MacCarty, C.S., and Taylor, W.F.: Intracranial meningiomas: Experiences at the Mayo Clinic. Neurol. Med. Chir. (Tokyo), 19:569, 1979.

204. May, P.L., et al.: The prediction of recurrence in meningiomas. A flow cytometric study of paraffin-embedded archival material. J. Neurosurg., 71:347, 1989.

205. Mirimanoff, R.O., et al.: Meningioma: Analysis of recurrence and progression following neurosurgical resection. J. Neurosurg., 62:18, 1985.

206. Nakasu, S., et al.: Interface between the meningioma and the brain. Surg. Neurol., 32:206, 1989.

207. Philippon, J., et al.: Les méningiomes récidivants. The recurrence of meningiomas. Neurochirurgie, 32 (Suppl. 1):1, 1986.

208. Seizinger, B.R., et al.: Molecular genetic approach to human meningioma: Loss of genes on chromosome 22. Proc. Natl. Acad. Sci. USA, 84:5419, 1987.

209. Simpson, D.: The recurrence of intracranial meningiomas after surgical treatment. J. Neurol. Neurosurg. Psychiat., 20:22, 1957.

210. Thomas, H.G., Dolman, C.L., and Berry, K.: Malignant meningioma: Clinical and pathological features. J. Neurosurg., 55:929, 1981.

211. Wara, W.M., et al.: Radiation therapy of meningiomas. Am. J. Roentgen. Radium Ther. Nucl. Med., 123:453, 1975.

212. Yamashita, J., et al.: Recurrence of intracranial meningiomas, with special reference to radiotherapy. Surg. Neurol., 14:33, 1980.

213. Zülch, K.J., and Mennel, H.D.: The question of malignancy in meningiomas. Acta Neurochir., 31:275, 1975.

214. Cushing, H.: Tumors of the Nervus Acusticus and the Syndrome of the Cerebellopontile Angle. New York, Hafner Publ. Co., 1963 (orig. ed., 1917).

215. Laasonen, E.M., and Troupp, H.: Volume growth rate of acoustic neurinomas. Neurorad., 28:203, 1986.

216. Wallner, K.E., Pitts, L.H., Davis, R.L., et al.: Radiation therapy for the treatment of non-eighth nerve intracranial neurilemmoma. Int. J. Rad. Oncol. Biol. Phys., 14:287, 1988.

217. Bailey, P., and Davidoff, L.M.: Concerning the microscopic structure of the hypophysis cerebri in acromegaly. Amer. J. Path., 1:185, 1925.

218. Bakay, L.: The results of 300 pituitary adenoma operations (Prof. Herbert Olivecorna's series). J. Neurosurg., 7:240, 1950.

219. Banna, M.: Terminology, embryology and anatomy. Major Problems Neurology, 6:1, 1976.

220. Benda, C.: Beitrage zur normalen and pathologischen Histologie der menschlichen Hypophysis Cerebri. Arch. Anat. Physiol. 214:373, 1900.

221. Cushing, H.: The hypophysis cerebri: Clinical states of hyperpituitarism and of hypopituitarism. JAMA, 53:249, 1909.

222. Cushing, H.: The Pituitary Body and Its Disorders: Clinical States Produced by Disorders of the Hypophysis Cerebri. Philadelphia, J.B. Lippincott Co., 1912.

223. Cushing, H.: The basophilic adenomas of the pituitary body and their clinical manifestations (pituitary basophilism). Bull. Johns Hopkins Hosp., 50:137, 1932.

224. Dott, N.M., and Bailey, P.: Hypophysial adenomata. Br. J. Surg., 13:314, 1925.

225. Earle, K.M., and Dillard, S.H.: Pathology of adenomas of the pituitary gland. In: Diagnosis and Treatment of Pituitary Tumors. (Eds.) P.O. Kohler and G.T. Ross. New York, American Elsevier Publ. Co., 1973, pp. 3–16.

226. Elkington, S.G., and McKissock, W.: Pituitary adenoma: Results of combined surgical and radiotherapeutic treatment of 260 patients. Br. Med. J., 1:263, 1967.

227. Flesch, M. (1884). Tageblat der 57 Naturforscher Versämmlung (Magd). Quoted by M. Banna.[219]

228. Forbes, A.P., Henneman, P.H., Griswold, G.C., et al.: Syndrome characterized by galactorrhea, amenorrhea and low urinary FSH: Comparison with acromegaly and normal lactation. J. Clin. Endocrin. Metabol., 14:265, 1954.

229. Guiot, G.: Transsphenoidal approach in surgical treatment of pituitary adenomas: General principles and indications in non-functioning adenomas. In: Diagnosis and Treatment of Pituitary Tumors. (Eds.) P.O. Kohler and G.T. Ross. Amsterdam, Excerpta Medica, International Congress Series No. 303, 1973, pp. 159–178.

230. Guiot, G., Rougerie, J., and Hertzog, E.: L'utilisation de l'amplificateur de brillance en neurochirurgie. Sem. Hop. Paris, 12:689, 1958.

231. Halstead, A.E.: Remarks on the operative treatment of tumors of hypophysis. Trans. Amer. Surg. Assoc., 27:75, 1910.

232. Hamilton, C.R., Jr., Adams, L.C., and Maloof, F.: Hyperthyroidism due to thyrotropin-producing pituitary chromophobe adenoma. N. Engl. J. Med., 283:1077, 1970.

233. Hardy, J.: Transsphenoidal microsurgery of the normal and pathological pituitary. Clin. Neurosurg., 16:185, 1969.

234. Hardy, J.: Transsphenoidal surgery of hypersecreting pituitary tumors. In: Diagnosis and Treatment of Pituitary Tumors. (Eds.) P.O. Kohler and G.T. Ross. New York, American Elsevier, 1973, pp. 179–194.

235. Hardy, J., and Vezina, J.L.: Transsphenoidal neurosurgery of intracranial neoplasms. Adv. Neurol., 15:216, 1976.

236. Hardy, J., and Wigser, S.: Transsphenoidal surgery of pituitary fossa tumors with televised radiofluoroscopic control. J. Neurosurg., 23:612, 1965.

237. Henderson, W.R.: The pituitary adenomata, a follow-up study of the surgical results in 338 cases (Dr. Harvey Cushing's series). Br. J. Surg., 26:809, 1939.

238. Heuer, G.J.: The surgical approach and the treatment

of tumors and other lesions about the optic chiasm. Surg. Gyn. Obstet., 53:489, 1931.

239. Hirsch, O.: Endonasal methods of removal of hypophyseal tumors with report of two successful cases. JAMA, 55:772, 1910.

240. Hirsch, O.: Pituitary tumors. A borderland between cranial and trans-sphenoidal surgery. N. Engl. J. Med., 254:937, 1955.

241. Horrax, G.: Historical Sketches of Neurosurgery. Springfield, Charles C Thomas, 1952.

242. Kanavel, A.B.: Removal of tumors of the pituitary body by an infranasal route. JAMA, 53:1704, 1909.

243. Kocher, T.: Ein Fall von Hypophysis-Tumor mit operative Heilung. Dtsch. Zts. Chir., 100:13, 1909.

244. Kovacs, K., and Horvath, E.: Pituitary "chromophobe" adenoma composed of oncocytes. Arch. Path., 95:235, 1973.

245. Kovacs, K., and Horvath, E.: Tumors of the Pituitary Gland. Atlas of Tumor Pathology, Second series, Fascicle 21. AFIP, Washington, DC, 1986.

246. Kovacs, K., et al.: Null cell adenoma of the human pituitary. Virchows Arch. path. Anat., 387:165, 1980.

247. Landolt, A.M.: Ultrastructure of human sella tumors. Correlations of clinical findings and morphology. Acta Neurochir. (Supplement), 22:1, 1975.

248. Landolt, A.M., and Oswald, U.W.: Histology and ultrastructure of an oncocytic adenoma of the human pituitary. Cancer, 31:1099, 1973.

249. Landolt, A.M., Shibata, T., and Kleihues, P.: Growth rate of human pituitary adenomas. J. Neurosurg., 67:803, 1987.

250. Laws, E.R., Jr.: Pituitary adenomas. In: Current Therapy in Neurologic Diseases 1985–1986. (Ed.) R.T. Johnson. St. Louis, CV Mosby Co., 1985, pp. 220–225.

251. Marie, P.: Sur deux cas d'acromegalie: Hypertrophie singulière non-congenitale des extrémités supérieures, inférieures et céphaliques. Rev. Med., 6:297, 1886.

252. Marie, P., and Marinesco, G.: Sur l'anatomie pathologique de l'acromegalie. Arch. Med. Exper. Anat. Path., 3:539, 1891.

253. Minkowski, O.: Ueber einen Fall von Akromegalie. Berl. klin. Wchnschr., 24:371, 1887.

254. Nagashima, T., et al.: The proliferative potential of human pituitary tumors in situ. J. Neurosurg., 64:588, 1986.

255. Poppen, J.L.: Changing concepts in the treatment of pituitary adenomas: The Charles A. Elseberg lecture. Bull. New York Acad. Med., 39:21, 1963.

256. Randall, R.V., et al.: Transsphenoidal microsurgical treatment of prolactin-producing pituitary adenomas, results in 100 patients. Proc. Staff Meet. Mayo Clin., 58:108, 1983.

257. Randall, R.V., et al.: Pituitary adenomas associated with hyperprolactinemia: A clinical and immunohistological study of 97 patients operated transsphenoidally. Proc. Staff Meet. Mayo Clin., 60:753, 1985.

258. Rathke, H.: Ueber die Entstehung der Glandula Pituitaria. Muellers Arch. Anat. Physiol. Wissensch. Med., 5:482, 1838.

259. Schloffer, H.: Erfolgreiche Operation eines Hypophysentumors auf nasalen Wege. Wien. klin. Wochenschr. 20:621, 1907.

260. Snyder, P.J., and Sterling, F.H.: Hypersecretion of

LH and FSH by a pituitary adenoma. J. Clin. Endocrin. Metab., 42:544, 1976.

261. von Eiselberg, A.F.: My experience about operation upon the hypophysis. Trans. Amer. Surg. Assoc., 28:55, 1910.

262. Wilson, C.B.: A decade of pituitary microsurgery. The Herbert Olivecrona Lecture. J. Neurosurg., 61:814, 1984.

263. Wilson, C.B., and Dempsey, L.C.: Transsphenoidal microsurgical removal of 250 pituitary adenomas. J. Neurosurg., 48:13, 1978.

264. Woolf, P.D., and Schenk, E.A.: An FSH-producing pituitary tumor in a patient with hypogonadism. J. Clin. Endocrinol. Metab., 38:561, 1974.

265. DeLellis, R.A. (ed.): Advances in Immunohistochemistry. New York, Raven Press, 1988.

266. Wick, M.R., and Siegal, G.P. (eds.): Monoclonal Antibodies in Diagnostic Immunohistochemistry. New York, Marcel Dekker, Inc., 1988.

267. Eapen, L., et al.: Brain metastases with an unknown primary: A clinical perspective. J. Neuro-Oncol., 6:31, 1988.

268. Earle, K.M.: Metastatic and primary intracranial tumors of the adult male. J. Neuropath. Exp. Neurol., 13:448, 1954.

269. Le Chevalier, T., et al.: Early metastatic cancer of unknown primary origin at presentation. A clinical study of 302 consecutive autopsied patients. Arch. Intern. Med., 148:2035, 1988.

270. Nakhleh, R.E., Manivel, J.C., Hurd, D., et al.: Central nervous system lymphomas. Immunohistochemical and clinicopathologic study of 26 autopsy cases. Arch. Pathol. Lab. Med., 113:1050, 1989.

271. Patchell, R.A., and Posner, J.B.: Neurologic complications of systemic cancer. Neurol. Clin., 3:729, 1985.

272. Sheline, G.E., and Brady, L.W.: Radiation therapy for brain metastases. J. Neuro-Oncol., 4:219, 1987.

273. Slatkin, N.E., and Posner, J.B.: Management of spinal epidural metastases. Clin. Neurosurg., 3:698, 1982.

274. Störtebecker, T.P.: Metastatic tumors of the brain from a neurosurgical point of view. A follow-up study of 158 cases. J. Neurosurg., 11:84, 1954.

275. Willis, R.A.: Pathology of Tumors. 2nd Ed. London, Butterworth, 1953.

276. Young, H.F., and Becker, D.P.: Indications for resection of intracranial metastasis. Surg. Rounds, 8(Mch.):42, 1985.

277. Bell, E.T.: Renal Diseases. 2nd Ed. Philadelphia, Lea & Febiger, 1950, pp 435–437.

278. Early Breast Cancer Trialists' Collaborative Group: Effects of adjuvant tamoxifen and of cytotoxic therapy on mortality in early breast cancer. An overview of 61 randomized trials among 28,896 women. N. Engl. J. Med., 319:1681, 1988.

279. Feinstein, A.R., Sosin, D.M., and Wells, C.K.: The Will Rogers phenomenon: Stage migration and new diagnostic techniques as a source of misleading statistics for survival in cancer. N. Engl. J. Med., 312:1604, 1985.

280. Greenfield, J.G., Shy, G.M., Alvord, E.C., Jr., et al.: An Atlas of Muscle Pathology in Neuromuscular Diseases. Edinburgh, E.&S. Livingstone, Ltd., 1957.

11

Immunologic Diseases

J. BRUCE SMITH and
MICHAEL E. SHY

That aging is "usual and successful"[1] may in part be related to preservation of immune function and to a selective advantage conferred by having certain specific human leukocyte antigen (HLA), haplotypes, or individual HLA antigens.[2-4] The genes of the major histocompatibility complex (MHC) encode the cell surface HLA antigens through which immune cell interactions occur[5,6] and may define individuals at risk for the development of various diseases.[7-9] Aging is often accompanied by measurable and sometimes striking impairments of immune functions.[10-14] Thus the increased incidence of certain diseases in the aging population[15-19] may be related to both HLA genes and antigens and to attrition of immunologic functions.

In this chapter we will present a brief overview of the immune response, discuss changes in the immune system that have been noted to occur with age, review immune/nervous system interactions and conditions of the elderly in which immunologic impairments may be directly involved.

OVERVIEW OF THE IMMUNE RESPONSE

An immune response results from the interactions of lymphocytes and macrophages when these cells are activated in the various lymphoid tissues (bone marrow, spleen, lymph nodes, thymus, gut-associated lymphoid tissue) that form a functional organ by virtue of being interconnected by a network of lymphatic vessels. The organization of these tissues is such that entrapped immunogens (antigens) are in the proximity of cells that are able to effect an immune response. For example, when an immunogen in sufficient dosage arrives in a lymph node, it is ingested by macrophages and is partially degraded by lysosomal enzymes which is a process known as "antigen processing." Antigenic components are then redistributed on the cell surface where they are available for recognition by T lymphocytes.[20] Activation of T helper (Th) lymphocytes and their clonal expansion is prerequisite to the induction of all aspects of an immune response with the exception of a restricted number of T cell independent responses by B lymphocytes[21] and the activation of some memory B cells[22] which are responsible for secondary or recall antibody responses. Once an immune response is initiated, a series of events occur that result in amplification of the response by cytokines (see below), activation of cytotoxic T lymphocytes (Tc) if appropriate, antibody synthesis and secretion by B lymphocytes, and eventual down regulation of the response by T suppressor (Ts) cells or antiidiotypic antibodies (see below).

Antigen presenting cells: Antigen presenting cells (APC) are classically thought of as cells of the monocyte-macrophage series and arise, like all cells of the immune and hematopoetic systems, from stem cells resident in the bone marrow (Fig. 11–1). These cells enter the cir-

culation as monocytes and migrate to various lymphoid and other tissues where they can be identified as cells that are positive for expression of surface HLA class II determinants (HLA-DR, -DP, -DQ). These cells are part of the reticuloendothelial system (RES) and can be found in the skin (Langerhan's cells, dendritic cells), liver (Kupffer's cells), brain (microglial cells), lung (alveolar macrophages) and are present as dendritic cells in the spleen, lymph nodes, and thymus. In the thymus these cells may play an important role in the deletion of auto-reactive T cell clones as T cells undergo maturation to functional lymphocytes.

As part of the RES, macrophages perform two primary functions. They are scavenger cells which ingest foreign particulate matter as a first step in its elimination from the organism, and they "process" antigens for presentation to lymphocytes as noted above. Macrophages that scavenge are generally low in expression of surface class II molecules, while APC tend to express class II antigens more ex-

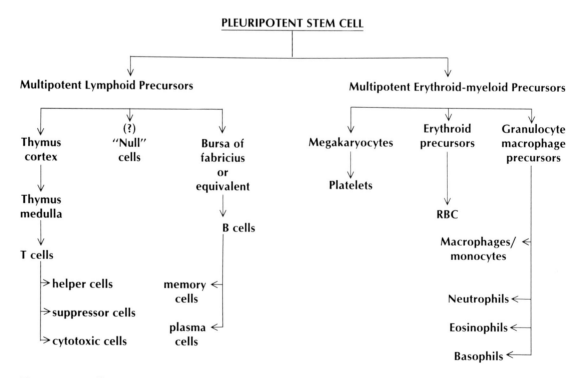

Fig. 11–1. Differentiation of lymphoid and myeloid cells from pleuripotent cells in bone marrow. (Modified from Clark and Kamen, 1987.)

uberantly.[23] Macrophage surface markers include HLA antigens of both class I and class II types, and it is now known that processed antigens attach to class II molecules on the cell surface via specific interactions between amino acid sequences held in common by antigens and the histocompatibility determinants.[24,25] Macrophages also have receptors for the Fc (crystalizable fragment) portion of antibody molecules and the third component of complement (C3). While a number of cell types can be induced to express HLA class II determinants by exposure to various cytokines (see below), constitutive expression of these molecules is generally restricted to cells with antigen presenting capability. A list of cells with class II expression and their potential for antigen presentation is given in Table 11–1.

T CELLS

T lymphocytes, which account for about 70% of peripheral blood lymphocytes (PBL), arise from precursors in the marrow and mature in the thymus (Fig. 11–1). They can be identified by various functional attributes[26,27] which include their participation in delayed-type hypersensitivity (DTH) reactions, help for the development of Tc and B cell responses, mediation of graft vs. host disease, allograft rejection, and suppression of various immune responses. In addition, there are more general functional markers for T cells which include naturally occurring substances (lectins) that trigger T cell proliferation of a polyclonal nature when they bind to T cell surfaces. The best known of these mitogens are phytohemagglutinin (PHA) which causes proliferation of most T cells, and concanavalin-A (Con-A)

TABLE 11–1. Cells with Constitutive Antigen Presenting Capacity

Cell type	Location	Class II antigen exp.
Macrophages	Spleen, Lymph Nodes, Marrow	+
Monocytes	Peripheral Blood	+
Microglial Cells	Brain	+
Dendritic Cells	Skin, Spleen, Lymph Node, Thymus	+
Langerhans Cells	Skin	+
Kupffer Cells	Liver	+
Alveolar Macrophages	Lung	+

TABLE 11–2. Human T Cell Markers: Distribution and Functional Correlations

Cell distribution and/or functional activities	
Cortical Thymocytes, T Cell Leukemias, Thymic Langerhans Cells	CD1
All T Cells, Thymocytes, Srbc Receptor	CD2
All T Cells, Thymocytes, Transduces Mitogenic Signals	CD3
T Helper Cells, Mature Thymocytes, Interacts with HLA Class II	CD4
T Cytotoxic/Suppressor Cells, Some NK Cells, Mature Thymocytes, Interacts with HLA Class I	CD8
Activated T Cells, IL-2 Receptor, Tac	CD25

CD = Cluster designation after World Health Organization recommendations, 1984.

T = Nomenclature used by commercial producers Ortho and Coulter.

Leu = Nomenclature employed by Becton-Dickinson.

which tends to stimulate proliferation of suppressor cells.[28]

The best known cell surface marker for T cells in general is the receptor for Sheep red blood cells (Srbc).[29] Rosette formation with Srbc is commonly used to enumerate T cells and is routinely used in the laboratory to separate T cells from non-T cells in gradient centrifugation techniques. Moretta et al.[30] first described separation of human T cells into functionally distinct populations. T cells bearing Fc receptors for IgM provided help for B cell responses, while those with Fc receptors for IgG suppressed B cell activity. A variety of cell surface alloantigens also serve to distinguish T cells and T cell subsets.[31] Recently the development of monoclonal antibody technology has resulted in the generation of a number of reagents that identify cell surface antigens acquired by functionally different subsets of T cells during their maturation in the thymus.[32] A list of these markers and the correlating T cell functions are given in Table 11–2. The Srbc receptor is identified by the monoclonal antibody (MAB) known as T11, while another pan-T cell marker is the MAB that reacts with the antigen known as T3.[33,34] Th cells generally bear the marker T4 (also known as leu 3) and Ts and Tc are identified by the presence of T8 (also known as leu 2). Since a given subset of T cells may be identified by antibodies to different epitopes (or antigenic determinants) on the same marker molecule, T cell markers that define subsets have been assigned cluster designations (CD). Thus Th are known as CD4 positive cells and Ts and Tc are known as CD8 positive cells.[35] CD4 cells make up about 60 to 70% of the circulating T cells and the majority of the remainder are CD8 positive making the ratio of T helper to T suppressor or cytotoxic cells between 1.5 and 2 to 1. CD4 cells can now be divided into two functionally distinct subpopulations which bear markers known as 4B4 and 2H4 and these identify classical Th and those that function as inducers of suppressor cells.[36]

In addition to the above cell surface markers, resting (unactivated) T cells express HLA class I but not class II surface determinants. Activated T cells, whether through mitogen stimulation or during an antigen-specific response do express class II antigens. This is probably the result of induction of these molecules by interferon and other soluble mediators produced during an immune response.[37,38] T cells that are participating in an immune response also develop receptors for the growth factor interleukin-2 (IL-2), which is discussed below. The receptor for IL-2 (CD25) can be identified by a monoclonal antibody known as anti-Tac.[39]

T Cell Recognition of Antigens. Antigens are recognized by T cells after they are processed by macrophages and redistributed on the cell surface bound to class I and class II molecules. Th (CD4) cells respond to antigen when they recognize it in the context of (or bound to) class II MHC determinants,[40] and Tc (CD8) cells recognize and respond to antigen in combination with class I molecules.[41] It is not entirely clear how Ts respond to antigens but it is probably in the context of class II cell surface determinants. T helper and cytotoxic cells interact with antigen on APC via a specific receptor[6] that is biologically functional only when it contacts antigen and MHC determinants simultaneously. The T cell receptor for antigen has only recently been described and is an area of current intense investigation. The T cell receptor is a two chain structure that is functionally composed of the T3 (CD3) molecular complex and an antigen-binding portion (Ti). It is also functionally associated with either the CD4 molecule in the case of Th, or the CD8 molecule in the case of Tc. The CD4 structure is thought to transmit mitogenic signals to the cell interior since certain of the

monoclonal antibodies to this determinant are mitogenic for T cells. The antigen-binding portion of the complex is made up of two chains (alpha and beta) which are invariant (idiotypic) from clone-to-clone. Ti has antigen specificity that is genetically conferred in a manner similar to the generation of specific antigen binding sites on antibody molecules. At the gene level variable (V), diversity (D), and joining (J) genes rearrange to create a functional antigen binding receptor on the cell surface in much the same way that antibodies of various specificities are formed by B cells.[42,43]

In Figure 11–2 the basic structures of some of the cell surface molecules that act as antigen receptors are shown in diagrammatic fashion. All of these immunologically relevant structures are similar in basic configuration and all are encoded by what is now known as the immunoglobulin gene superfamily. These include the immunoglobulins, T cell receptors, and MHC class I and II molecules.[43]

B CELLS

B lymphocytes make up from 1 to 15% of peripheral blood lymphocytes. B cells are the precursors of plasma cells which are end-stage cells that secrete the immunoglobulins comprising the gamma globulins of serum. B cells, like T cells, arise from a common stem cell (Fig. 11–1). In mammals this occurs in the marrow, and in birds it occurs in a specialized gut-associated organ, the Bursa of Fabricius. B cells differentiate in these organs prior to migrating to the various lymphoid tissues, where they are likely to encounter antigens.[44] Mature B cells are characterized by the presence of cell surface immunoglobulin of the IgM and IgD types. Differentiation of a B cell begins with the rearrangement of its V, D, and J genes to generate the gene for the *mu* heavy (H) chain (IgM).[43] Once this rearrangement is successful, the mu chain is synthesized in the cytoplasm and the cell is known as a "pre-B" cell. With subsequent V and J gene rearrangement, light (L) chain monomeric IgM is produced in the cytoplasm and it is then inserted into the cell membrane. At this point the immature B cell bears a functional receptor for antigen in the form of surface IgM, but it does not achieve

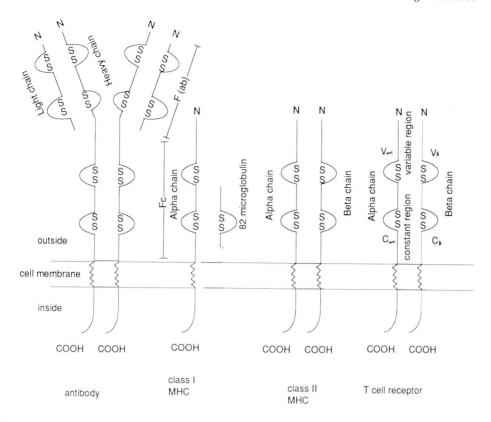

Fig. 11–2. Diagrammatic representation of several immunologically important cell surface molecules.

the ability to actually respond to antigen until surface IgD is present as well.[44,45] The functional significance of this series of events is not entirely clear but it may have to do with the deletion of IgM only bearing B cell clones that produce antibodies having self-specificity.[46] Mature B cells are characterized by the presence of both surface IgM (sIgM) and sIgD and it is these determinants that allow proliferation of B cells when the appropriate antigen is encountered. Once stimulated by antigen, B cells undergo further differentiation and maturation into either antibody-secreting plasma cells or memory cells with surface Ig of the same antigen specificity as the original B cell.[22] With T cell help, B cells can switch from IgM to IgG or IgA producing cells but the antibodies produced by a given clone of B cells always exhibit the same antigen binding specificity regardless of the Ig isotype produced.

In addition to the presence of sIg, B cells also bear several other markers that help differentiate them from other lymphocytes (Table 11–3). These include Fc and C3 receptors,[47] receptors for the Epstein-Barr virus (C3d), and histocompatibility antigens of both class I and class II types. Under certain experimental conditions B cells can be shown to function as antigen presenting cells.[48]

B cell functional tests are readily accomplished in mice and both specific antibody and

TABLE 11–3. Human B Cell Markers and Functions

Cell distribution/function	Marker
Pre B Cells	cytoplas. IgM heavy chain (mu) HLA Class I and II
Immature B Cell	surface IgM HLA Class I and II
Mature B Cell	
○ Resting B cells proliferate in response to antigen	surface IgM and IgD FcR:binds Ig Fc C3R:binds activated C3 C3dR:binds Epstein-Barr virus
○ Differentiate to plasma cell	HLA-Class I and II
○ Memory B cells	Above, but with sIgG or IgA

polyclonal antibody responses can be measured in vitro and in vivo. Murine B cells also respond with proliferation when exposed to mitogens such as bacterial endotoxins and anti-Ig antibodies.[49] Human tonsillar B cells will also respond to mitogens[50] and will proliferate and synthesize antibody when cultured in the presence of Staphlococcus protein-A plus interleukin-2.[51] Peripheral blood B cells can be stimulated to synthesize antibody in a polyclonal fashion by culture in the presence of anti-CD3 activated T helper cells.[52]

Null-cells: Lymphocytes that bear neither T nor B cell markers have classically been referred to as the "null-cell" subset or as "third population" cells. The differentiation pathway for Null-cells is not well understood but they probably represent a branch of the T cell lineage (Fig. 11–1). Null-cells make up about 5% of the peripheral blood lymphocytes and morphologically can be identified as large granular lymphocytes (LGL). LGL have Fc receptors for IgG but lack C3 receptors.[53,54] The null-cell set contains most of the lymphocytes having natural killer (NK) capability and that function as effector cells in antibody dependent cellular cytotoxicity (ADCC). NK cells have the ability to lyse, without prior sensitization, certain RNA virus-infected tumor cells and a limited number of cell lines maintained in vitro.[55] ADCC cells kill "antibody sensitized" target cells when they bind via Fc receptors to target cells that have antibody bound to their surfaces.[56,57] Both of these cell types have been postulated to play a role in immunosurveillance against the occurrence of malignant cells.

IMMUNOGLOBULINS

The products of B lymphocytes and plasma cells circulate in the plasma and are known collectively as immunoglobulins or gamma globulins. They are glycoproteins which can be divided into five classes (or isotypes) based on electrophoretic, physical, chemical and functional properties (Table 11–4). The gamma globulins are present in adult serum in a concentration of about 1500 mg/dl. IgG accounts for about 1100 mg/dl of this, while IgM and IgA have concentrations in the range of 100 and 200 mg/dl respectively. IgD and IgE are present in serum only in trace amounts. All antibody molecules have the same basic structural unit.[58,59] This consists of two light (L) and two heavy (H) polypeptide chains which are linked by disulfide bonds (Fig. 11–2). The light chains are about 200 amino acids long and have a molecular weight of about 23,000. Light chains are of either kappa or lambda types and can be identified by structural or antigenic differences. A given antibody molecule contains either two lambda or two kappa L chains but never one of each. In humans kappa chains occur in about 60% of antibody molecules. Heavy chains are 2-to-3 times the size of light chains and contain roughly 400 amino acids. The five types of heavy chains, mu, delta, gamma, alpha, and epsilon, can be identified by structural differences that occur at their carboxy termini and these are what characterize antibody molecules as IgM, IgD, IgG, IgA, or IgE. Heavy chain classes can be divided into subclasses based on the occurrence of highly related amino acid sequences. Thus, IgG, IgM, and IgA have 4, 2, and 2 subclasses respectively.

Every H and L chain has two regions.[59,60] The variable (V) regions occur at the amino (N) terminal portion of the chains and exhibit wide variation in amino acid sequences. Both heavy and light chain V regions (VH and VL) also contain hypervariable regions which are in-

TABLE 11–4.   Characteristics of Immunoglobulins in Human Serum

Property	IgG₁	IgG₂	IgG₃	IgG₄	IgA	IgM	IgD	IgE
Mol. wt. ($\times 10^{-3}$)	146	146	170	146	160	950	184	188
½ life in serum (wks)	3	3	1	3	1	1.5	.5	.5
Approx. serum conc. (mg/dl)	900	300	100	50	200	125	3	.1
C' fixation	+ +	+	+ + +	−	−	+ + +	−	−
Activates alternate C' pathway	−	−	−	−	+	−	−	−
Placental transfer	+	−	+	−	−	−	−	−
Binds to FcR (on monocytes)	+	−	+	−	−	−	−	−
Binds to mast cells	−	−	−	−	−	−	−	+

volved in creating the antigen binding site of the antibody molecule. The constant (C) regions of H and L chains are invariant in amino acid sequence from molecule to molecule in a given class. In addition, each Ig chain can be divided into domains on the basis of the globular structure conferred by intrachain disulfide bonds. H chains have four or five domains, one in the variable region and three or four in the constant regions. Gamma, alpha, and delta chains have four domains (one variable and three constant), while mu and epsilon chains have five domains (one variable and four constant).

Antibody molecules can be fragmented by enzyme treatment.[61] The Fab (antibody) fragment contains a whole light chain plus the variable and first constant domains of the H chain. The Fab fragment contains the antigen binding site of an antibody molecule. The Fc (crystalizable) fragment contains the carboxy terminal portion of the heavy chains. This portion of the molecule binds complement and confers other biologic activities such as placental transfer and Fc receptor binding.[62]

As noted above IgG is the major Ig of human serum. It is a monomer with two identical H and two identical L chains and has a molecular weight of 150,000. It is the only Ig that can cross the placenta and has an important immunoprotective role in the developing fetus and in the neonate during the first few months after birth. IgG has a half life of 3 weeks in the serum and is the major antibody produced in secondary or memory responses. As shown in Table 11–4, IgG can be divided into 4 subclasses that exhibit distinct biologic and functional activities. All subclasses except IgG4 can bind complement. IgG is also important with regard to phagocytosis as IgG1 and IgG3 bind to the Fc receptors of macrophages and neutrophils and provide a mechanism whereby antibody-coated (opsonized) microorganisms can be bound and ingested.

Serum IgA is also usually in the form of a monomer although dimers, trimers, and tetramers occur.[58] When it is polymeric, the dimers are joined at their carboxy terminal portions by a glycopeptide known as the J chain. IgA does not activate complement by the classical pathway but can activate the alternate (properdin) pathway which bypasses the requirements for C1, C4, and C2 and which can be triggered by microbial cell surfaces, complex polysaccharides, and endotoxins.[63] Secretory IgA is a special form of the antibody found in saliva, tears, breast milk, and in gastrointestinal and other secretions.[64] It is a divalent form of IgA which has in addition to the J chain a secretory component. The latter is a single polypeptide chain with a molecular weight of about 70,000 which is produced by epithelial cells and which acts as a receptor for IgA produced by plasma cells and B lymphocytes in submucosal areas. Secretory component allows IgA to be transported through mucosal tissues into secretions without loss of antibody activity. IgA forms a major line of defense against organisms that would otherwise invade the body through mucosal surfaces.

IgM occurs in serum as a pentamer with the monomeric units linked by J chains. It is the predominant antibody in primary immune responses and is the most efficient of all Ig molecules with regard to binding complement. In the serum it has a half-life of about 5 days. Because of a hydrophobic component of the H chain, monomeric IgM is incorporated into the membranes of B lymphocytes where it acts as the antigen receptor for these cells.

IgD is present in only trace amounts in serum. Its biologic functions are not known and its half-life is only 2 or 3 days. It occurs on the surface of B lymphocytes and is probably involved in B cell activation.[65]

IgE is also present in only trace amounts in serum. It is a monomer with a molecular weight of about 190,000. IgE has a half-life in the serum of 2 to 3 days. IgE does not fix complement but it does bind to mast cells, basophils, and skin by FcR specific for IgE on these cells. Mast cell bound IgE that binds antigen results in release of a variety of vasoactive peptides and other substances from these cells and is associated with immediate hypersensitivity reactions. It is also associated with immunity to various parasitic infections.

ANTIBODY DIVERSITY

Antibodies vary not only by class, but they also bear several other markers. Allotypes are genetic variations in antibody proteins that are inherited in a Mendelian fashion.[66] Allotypic markers are found on heavy chains and light chains in the constant regions and can be identified by specific antisera. Allotypic markers on gamma chains are designated Gm, while those on alpha chains are termed Am. The allotypic markers of kappa chains are designated *Km* or *Inv*. Antigenic determinants that are unique to certain antibodies are known as idiotypes.[67] They may be associated with only one antibody clone in which case they are referred to as private idiotypes, or they may be shared among several clones and are then known as public idiotypes. Anti-idiotypic antibodies sometimes react with the antigen binding portions of antibody molecules and such antibodies have proven extremely useful in studies to elucidate the fine specificity of humoral immune responses and the nature of antibody binding sites for antigen.

Antigen binding diversity is generated by rearranging a limited number of genes that specify construction of useful antibodies[42,43] and to some extent by somatic mutation.[68] The genes that encode H chains are found on chromosome 14, while the genes that specify the amino acid sequences of kappa and light chains are found on chromosomes 2 and 22 respectively. As stated above, the amino acid sequences of constant regions are relatively fixed and do not show much variation from molecule to molecule, while the amino acid sequences of the variable regions are quite distinct and vary greatly. Analysis of the immunoglobulin genes has shown that in germ line (egg and sperm) DNA, there are constant region genes that specify the five different isotypes and subclasses of constant regions of the heavy chains, four J (joining) genes along with a number of D (diversity) and V region genes. For light chains, there are similar V genes, several J genes, and constant region genes for kappa and lambda. These genes (or exxons) are separated by introns which are segments of DNA not translated into peptides. When a B-cell is maturing to an antibody producing cell, the H chain genes are rearranged by a series of enzymatic events in which the introns are excised causing appropriate V, D, and J region genes to abut each other after which they are spliced together. RNA transcripts are made from these rearranged genes and form a whole constant region gene. These RNA transcripts are then connected to form the entire heavy chain transcript and this is subsequently translated into the polypeptide chain. Light chains are formed in a similar manner. Heavy and light chains are then assembled into the antibody molecule in the endoplasmic reticulum of the cell. By utilizing various combinations of V, D, and J genes and heavy chain genes, an enormous diversity of antibody specificities can be generated from a relatively conservative number of genes. In addition, post-translational modification and somatic cell mutations account for some alterations in binding specificity and affinity of the final product. The heavy chain genes are arranged in the following sequence: mu, delta, gamma, alpha, and epsilon. Class switching, for example from IgM to IgG, involves bringing the same VDJ gene segment to the constant region gene for the gamma chain to be used and eliminating the delta chain constant region gene in between. Once switched, a B cell cannot return to the synthesis of an earlier class of antibody. In general both copies of genes inherited from either parent are expressed. However, in the case of antibodies, allelic exclusion prevents co-dominant expression. The mechanism for this is not well understood but it appears that once a productive (functional) rearrangement has occurred on one allele, the other is fixed in its embryonic (germline) configuration. As a result, non-productive rearrangements are avoided and the problem of the heavy chains of a given antibody molecule associating with different light chains is avoided. Thus allelic exclusion ensures that antibody molecules will have the same light chains with the same specificity and that they will be functionally divalent with regard to antigen binding.

CYTOKINES

Once a specific immune response is initiated it can be amplified by the action of a variety of soluble factors produced by the cells participating in an immune response.[37,38,69] The best known of these factors are interleukin-1 (IL-1) and interleukin-2 (IL-2). IL-1 is a hormone-like polypeptide with a molecular weight of approximately 17,000 and is produced primarily by cells of the monocyte/macrophage series.

TABLE 11–5. Functions of Interleukin-1

EFFECTS ON LEUKOCYTE TARGETS
  Induces IL-2 receptors on T cells
  Enhances production of various T cell factors IL-2,
    CSF, BCGF, IFN, chemotactic factors
  _____ Promotes proliferation of T cells
  Enhances helper T cell activity
  Enhances suppressor T cell activity
  Inc. B cell expression of surface immunoglobulin
  Inc. antibody secretion by B cells
  Causes B cell proliferation
EFFECTS ON NON-LEUKOCYTE TARGETS
  Fever induction (endogenous pyrogen)
  Stimulates production of acute phase proteins
  Inc. synthesis of prostaglandins
  Stimulates bone resorption
  Stimulates cartilage breakdown
  Stimulates proliferation of various cell types
  Promotes slow-wave sleep
  Causes anorexia/cachexia
  Causes alterations in levels of divalent cations (dec.
    iron, zinc: inc. copper)
  Stimulates pituitary adrenal axis (Inc. ACTH and Glu-
    cocorticoids)
  Stimulates release of insulin and glucagon
  Inc. skeletal muscle proteolysis
  Inc. amino acid oxidation

Under certain experimental conditions it can also be produced by a number of different cell types most of which are able to participate in an immune response as antigen presenting cells. IL-1 has a wide range of biologic activities and has effects on both lymphocyte and non-lymphocyte targets as shown in Table 11–5. Prominent among these biologic activities are fever induction (IL-1 was originally re-

ferred to as endogenous pyrogen) and its function as a co-factor for hematopoetic growth factors. IL-1 can be inhibited by hydrocortisone, prostaglandin E-2, lipoxygenase pathway inhibitors, age, immunosuppressive drugs, UV irradiation, and suppressor T cells. Immunoregulatory pathways in which IL-1 is involved are depicted in Fig. 11–3.

IL-2 is a product of T cells which was originally known as T cell growth factor (TCGF).[70] It is a glycoprotein with a molecular weight of about 15,000. IL-2 supports growth (proliferation) of T cells, enhances NK cell activity, augments generation of cytotoxic T cells, and enhances production of other cytokines. It also enhances B cell differentiation and antibody synthesis. IL-2 binds to T cells by a specific receptor (IL-2R, Tac)[39] which is induced by IL-1.[71] As an immune response increases, the affinity of the IL-2R increases and proliferation of T cells is enhanced. After the peak of an immune response the number and affinity of IL-2R decreases and this decrease in IL-2R parallels the waning of the immune response. IL-2 has recently been shown to induce cytotoxic cells of uncertain lineage that have anti-tumor activity. These lymphokine-activated killer cells (LAK cells) have been used successfully to treat some patients with certain types of malignancies, most notably melanoma and renal carcinoma.[72] Other interleukins include IL-4 and IL-5. IL-4 is a growth factor for activated

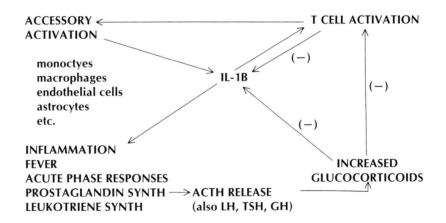

(−) = down-regulating effects

Fig. 11–3. IL-1 regulatory pathways.

B cells and is also known as B cell stimulating factor-1 (BCSF-1).[73] IL-4 also increases cytotoxic activity of T cells and is a growth factor for mast cells. IL-5, or T cell replacing factor, induces expression of IL-2 receptors on B cells and synergizes with IL-2 in inducing Ig production by B cells.

The colony stimulating factors are a heterogeneous group of cytokines which are responsible for stimulating outgrowth of specific cell lineages from pluripotent stem cells in the marrow.[74] IL-3 supports growth of a variety of cell lineages in the marrow including erythrocyte precursors, megakaryocytes. granulocytes, macrophages, mast cells, and eosinophils. GM-CSF stimulates growth of eosinophil, macrophage, and neutrophil colonies, while G-CSF and M-CSF stimulate outgrowth of granulocyte and macrophage colonies respectively. The genes for all of these factors have been cloned and it is hoped that they will find clinical usefulness in enhancing recovery of patients after bone marrow transplantation.

Interferons (alpha, beta, and gamma) are also actively involved in enhancing and modulating immune responses.[38] Immune interferon (interferon gamma) is a product of activated T cells and a potent adjuvant for immune responses. It enhances immune responses by functioning as a macrophage activating factor and by increasing expression of HLA class II determinants on antigen presenting cells. The latter results in enhanced T helper cell interaction with these cells. It also induces HLA class II expression on endothelial cells, fibroblasts, and epithelial cells,[75] thus making it theoretically possible for these cells to actively participate in an immune response. Immune interferon also enhances expression of class I determinants and can thus augment cytotoxic T cell responses. Gamma IFN enhances NK cell activity and it is currently undergoing clinical trials as an anti-cancer agent. In addition to the above mentioned immune enhancing effects, it has recently been shown that gamma IFN can act as a co-factor in the induction of IL-1 production by vascular endothelial cells.[76] While it has immune potentiating activities, gamma IFN has also been shown to have anti-proliferative activities in several in vitro and in vivo systems. Alpha interferon is produced by T and B cells and macrophages. Beta interferon is produced primarily by fibroblasts and epithelial cells.[77] Both promote anti-viral activity and can act as differentiation factors for numerous cell types.

Regulation of the immune responses: Control of the types and magnitude of immune responses can occur at several levels. Genes of the major histocompatibility complex have been shown to be responsible for the magnitude of immune responses to certain well defined synthetic antigens and immune responses to some antigens in humans.[8,78,79] For example, hyperresponses to ragweed antigen and to collagen, and low responses to tetanus toxoid and some streptococcal antigens are associated with certain of the HLA antigens. Genes of the MHC, as noted above, place other regulatory constraints on immune responses through the mechanism of MHC restriction (of Th responses in association with class II molecules and Tc responses in association with Class I determinants). Regulation of antibody production also occurs at the gene level in the form of class switching. In addition, serum antibody levels have been shown to be regulated by feedback mechanisms.[80] In the clinical situation, gamma globulin depletion after plasmapheresis procedures is often followed by overproduction of Ig and this can have serious consequences in patients with pathology related to auto-antibody production.[81] Since idiotypic determinants are unique and often involve the antigen binding sites of antibody molecules, they can be recognized as foreign. Anti-idiotypic antibodies have been shown to down regulate antibody formation through their effects on Th and B cells. This is the basis of the idiotype-anti-idiotype network theory of immune regulation proposed by Jerne.[82] Experimental evidence for anti-idiotypic antibody regulation of immune responses has been reported in several systems.[83,84] Regulation of the immune response also is mediated by Ts which can effect Th cells, Tc cells and B cells either through direct contact or by the production of soluble factors.[28,85,86] T suppressor cells can occur naturally,[87-89] can be induced by exposure to autologous class II MHC determinants in the absence of nominal antigen,[90] by specific antigens,[91,92] and as part of feedback circuits.[93–95]

One of the most important aspects of immunoregulation is the development and maintenance of self tolerance.[96–98] All individuals have the capacity for making antibodies, and perhaps cell-mediated responses, to self antigens. A breakdown in the mechanisms that control these responses can lead to autoimmune diseases that range in nature from specific autoantibody responses like those that occur in myasthenia gravis, thyroiditis, juvenile diabetes, and other organ-specific disorders, to organ non-specific diseases such as SLE and other pathologic conditions of connective tissue. Tolerance to self antigens (and environmental antigens as well) is most easily induced during embryonic or neonatal stages of life and in adult animals that have been immunocompromised with x-irradiation or immunosuppressive drug treatment. Tolerance is also more easily induced by antigens that are not readily degradable and which have a large polymeric structure. Both T cells and B cells are susceptible to tolerance induction. T cell tolerance is probably initiated in the thymus either by deletion of clones of autoreactive cells,[46] or by down regulation of autoreactive clones by suppressor cells.[99] The clonal deletion theory holds that immature T cells or B cells having self-specificity are destroyed when their high affinity receptors for self molecules are occupied. Evidence for this is not strong but includes studies showing that developing B cells that bear only surface IgM become unresponsive to that antigen after exposure to it, while B cells that bear both surface IgM and IgD make immune responses to the same antigen. Likewise, mice injected neonatally with T cell dependent antigens became tolerant to those antigens but their spleen or lymph node cells could be used to transfer to irradiated recipient mice all immune responses except those to which they were tolerant. Early studies on tolerance[96] also established that tolerance was antigen dose dependent in that low doses of antigen induced tolerance by affecting T helper cells, whereas high doses of immunogen caused tolerance by affecting B cells— probably by extensively cross-linking antibody (receptor) molecules on the cell surface making them immobile and unable to transmit positive signals to the cell interior.

ALTERATIONS IN IMMUNE RESPONSES RELATED TO AGING

General considerations: A recent book[100] and several reviews[11,13,18,101] present in excellent detail the multiple and complex immune deficiencies that occur in conjunction with the aging process in mammals. As is noted in these reviews, virtually all aspects of the immune response undergo some alteration with age. Some of these are due to intrinsic problems with aging cells; others may result from the environments in which aging cells reside. We will review here the effects of some non-immunologic factors that appear to have direct bearing on immune attrition with age along with non-specific and specific changes that occur in T and B cell functions. Studies accomplished in both humans and in laboratory animals will be reviewed as many experimental approaches that have been instrumental in our understanding of the aging process are possible only in laboratory animals. A variety of non-immunologic biologic factors actively influence the function of the immune system and may be related to changes in immune responses noted to occur with age. Certain age related immune defects occur earlier in females than they do in males. Examples of these include attrition of mitogenic responses of T cells[102] and the increase in incidence of autoantibodies.[103] Nutrition also may play a role and there is evidence that poor dietary habits in the elderly could contribute to immune dysfunction. Poor nutrition is associated with a reduction in size of the thymus[104] and T cell deficiency and dysfunction have both been observed in protein-calorie malnutrition and zinc deficiency.[105] Conversely, increased longevity in experimental animals can be induced by dietary restrictions[106] and studies on calorie restricted mice have shown preservation of T and B cell functions in old age.[107,108] In unmanipulated aging mice a decrease in the number of precursor cells for T cell responses has previously been noted,[109] but preservation of precursors for immunologically reactive lymphoctes occurs in diet-restricted mice with increased lifespans.[110]

MHC GENES

As previously noted, the genes in the MHC are important in determining disease susceptibility or resistance, the magnitude of many immune responses, and they encode the cell surface molecules (HLA antigens) that are the recognition structures employed in immune cell interactions. The genes of the MHC would therefore be expected to have some effect on longevity. In mice, longevity can be associated with vigorous responses of T cells to mitogens[7] and with genes in or linked to the MHC.[12] Direct evidence for a role of the MHC in survival is not available in humans, however, circumstantial evidence suggests that certain MHC genes do influence longevity. Takata et al.[4] have shown a low frequency of HLA DRw9 and a high frequency of DR1 in Okinawan subjects over age 90. Hodge and Walford[111] also reported a high frequency of individuals homozygous for HLA B4 and B6 in nonagenerians. In that regard it is interesting that there is an age related decrease in individuals with HLA A1,B8 among females but not males.[10,112] This may be due to the association of autoimmune diseases (which predominate in females) with these HLA types and the negative influence of autoimmune disease on survival. Interestingly, the "autoimmune" phenotype is now known to be A1,B8,DR3 and it has been shown that healthy DR3 positive individuals do not generate suppressor cells with the same vigor as non-DR3 individuals.[113]

THYMUS AND STEM CELL

Involution of the thymus begins in humans at puberty and this can be related to several aspects of immune deficiency. Production of thymic hormones begins to decline as early as the third decade of life and reaches its nadir in the 60 to 70 year age group.[114,115] Treatment of mice with exogenous thymic hormones increases their lifespan compared to control animals.[116] Since thymic hormones influence differentiation of T cells in the thymus, alterations in the maturation of T lymphocytes in the involuting thymus would be predicted. While the number of lymphocytes in peripheral blood remains relatively constant during aging,[117-119] the percentage of lymphocytes in the peripheral blood that form rosettes with Sheep red blood cells (T cells) undergoes some attrition with age.[115] Alterations in T cell subsets have also been noted. A general increase in CD4 positive (helper) lymphocytes and a concomitant decrease in CD8 positive (suppressor/cytotoxic) cells has been reported.[120] Others[121,122] have not found CD4 cells to be increased, however, they did find that CD8 cells were decreased. Hallgren et al.[122] made the interesting observation that the absolute number of T3 cells were decreased in elderly females but not males and that a significant increase in the early T cell marker, T10, occurred in the aging population of both males and females. This observation is consistent with the idea that a defect in T cell maturation occurs with precursor cells passing through the thymus without undergoing differentiation to mature subpopulations. It is also consistent with the observation from the same laboratory that LDH isoenzyme patterns in lymphocytes obtained from elderly individuals exhibit a pattern associated with less differentiated cells.[123]

The quality of the stem cells passing through the thymus and the environment in which they finally reside may also play an important role regarding their function in the aging organism. Astle and Harrison[124] have reported findings consistent with the hypothesis that bone marrow cells from aged mice, when transplanted into an aged environment, produce suppressor cells and/or factors but not when they reside in a young environment. Gorczynski and Chang[125] have also examined the cytotoxic T cell responses at the clonal level after transplantation of marrow from young or old donors into young or old immunocompromised recipients. They found not only an intrinsic defect in Tc precursors in aged marrow but a defect in the repertoire of cytotoxic T cells in an aged environment. Thus, old marrow into old recipients failed to recognize as wide a variety of allospecificities within a given MHC haplotype as young unmanipulated mice or as T cells that resulted after a young-young marrow-recipient combination. The mechanism for this finding is not known but could be accounted for by suppressor factors or cells or problems with antigen presentation in aging mice.

T CELLS AND CYTOKINES

Makinodan and Peterson[126] first demonstrated deficiency of T cell dependent antibody responses to Sheep rbc in aging mice and since then numerous studies have provided details on a variety of other T cell responses that change relative to age. Age-related Th responses in the ability of carrier-primed T cells to initiate antibody responses to a hapten were noted by Krosgrud and Perkins[127] and Callard and Basten[128] who found similar losses with age in thymus dependent responses. Delayed-type hypersensitivity (DTH) reactions which are mediated by T lymphocytes and measured by skin test reactivity to recall antigens such as monilla, histoplasmin, and PPD have been shown to decline with age.[129-131] Also, cutaneous DTH to antigens such as dinitrochlorobenzine is defective in elderly individuals.[129] Mitogen-induced proliferation of T cells from human peripheral blood is deficient in elderly humans[132,133] and mitogen-induced T cell colony formation by human peripheral blood lymphocytes in agar are also reduced in elderly persons compared to young controls.[134] The ability of T cells to respond to allogeneic stimulation in mixed lymphocyte cultures is depressed in aging mice[135] and in humans.[131,133]

Uptake of tritiated thymidine (3HTdR) which is incorporated into newly synthesized DNA is generally taken as a measure of cell proliferation. However, decreased uptake does not solely reflect decreased proliferation and the attrition with age of T cell uptake of 3HTdR after stimulation by specific antigen, allogeneic cells, or mitogens could have several explanations. Mechanisms for which there is experimental evidence include decrease in the number of cells able to make a particular response, damage to responding cells by radiation from the isotopes used to measure DNA synthesis, and failure to respond to or produce growth factors such as IL-2. Decrease in the number of T cells able to make particular responses has been demonstrated in humans and in experimental animals. Inkeles et al.[118] and Antel et al.[136] used limiting dilution analysis to show that the number of lymphocytes able to respond with increased DNA synthesis after mitogen stimulation was decreased in elderly compared to young donors. Similar studies in aging mice have demonstrated decreased precursor frequency for T cells involved in cytotoxic T cell,[137] and in both antigen-specific and non-specific helper T cell responses.[109]

Radiation damage to proliferating cells in vitro was noted by Pollack et al.[138] and subsequently it has been demonstrated that lymphocytes from elderly humans exhibit increased sensitivity to this sort of damage.[139] Studies in mice[140] and in humans[132,138] have not demonstrated alterations in cell cycle kinetics related to age. However, further studies on this phenomenon[138] indicated that while PHA stimulated lymphocytes from both young and old donors entered the first S to M phases (increased DNA synthesis to mitosis) of the cell cycle with comparable rates, T cells from old donors were less likely to re-enter G1 (pre-DNA synthesis) for another round of cell division.

Age related changes in responses to and production of cytokines has recently been reviewed in some detail[141] and Zatz and Goldstein[142] have also reviewed alterations in production of thymic hormones that accompany the waning immune response. The decrease in thymic hormones seen with age precedes the functional impairments that occur[114,143,144] and injection of mice with thymosin preparations has been shown to restore certain T helper cell functions in aging mice[145] and humans.[146] Thymosin fraction 5 (TH-5) has been shown to increase IL-2 production by lymphocytes from mice[141,147] and humans.[148] Other studies also indicate that decreased production of IL-2 is at least in part responsible for age related immune deficiencies in mice[136,149,150,151] and humans.[152] Administration of IL-2 to mice has recently also been shown to restore cytotoxic T cell responses in aging mice.[144]

Immune cell dysfunction found in elderly individuals has also been examined at the level of other intracellular mediators. Alterations in the levels of cyclic adenosine 3',5'-monophosphate (cAMP) and cyclic guanosine 3'5'-monophosphate (cGMP) have been hypothesized to play roles in the activation of lymphocytes by mitogens. Parker[153] proposed that cAMP exerted a positive effect on mitogenesis. Hadden et al.[154] suggested a negative effect for cAMP but a positive one for cGMP. Resting cell levels of cAMP have been shown to be markedly reduced, while cGMP were elevated by a factor of 10 in elderly compared to young donors.[155] Others, however, have not demonstrated similar changes in humans.[156] Gutowski et al.[157] have also found that cytoplasmic proteins involved in the triggering of DNA synthesis are normal in lymphocytes from aged individuals.

The ability of aging T cells to transduce proliferation signals from the cell surface to the nucleus via activation of protein kinase-C has recently been examined. Miller[158] has shown that this second messenger system is normal in aging T cells in that substances such as phorbol myristate acetate (PMA) plus calcium ionophore can stimulate proliferation similar to that found in young mice. This would suggest a problem with signaling across the membrane in view of the known impairment of proliferation after stimulating cells with mitogens. Further studies indicated that the influx of Ca^{++} after mitogen stimulation was lower in aged compared to young mice[159] suggesting an intramembrane or receptor problem.

HUMORAL IMMUNITY

Many of the defects noted in antibody synthesis in older individuals can be ascribed to T helper cell defects since most antibody responses require T cell help. Thus changes in antibody levels in serum can reflect problems at the level of either T or B cells. Although there is a tendency for IgG and IgA levels to increase and IgM levels to fall with advancing age,[160] there is not a significant change in total gamma globulin in the serum. Individual antibodies do, however, show significant changes with age. The IgM isoantibodies to blood group antigens, which occur independently of T cell help, show a progressive decline with age[161] as do antibody responses to salmonella flagellin.[130] As is the case for T lymphocytes, the total number of B cells in human peripheral blood changes little or not at all with advancing age.[133,162] Studies in aging mice have shown that at the single cell level, the ability of bone marrow to generate B cells as well as the ability of B cells to secrete specific antibody is comparable to that of young

mice.[163] These same workers found that B cell precursors for similar responses in old compared to young mice were markedly diminished when examined in the spleen[163,164] due to the presence of anti-idiotypic antibodies and their down regulating effect on B cells. Szewczuk and Wade[84] have also examined auto-anti-idiotypic antibody regulation of B cell responses in the spleen and in mucosal immunity. They studied the responses of young and aging mice to immunization with trinitrophenyl-bovine gamma globulin (TNP-BGG) as a hapten-carrier complex and found that aging mice of certain strains developed decreased antibody forming cell responses to TNP and that these were not augmentable by culture in the presence of the hapten. The mechanism for this appears to be the presence of anti-idiotypic autoantibodies that inhibit the response.

One of the most striking aspects of immunodysregulation accompanying aging is the occurrence of monoclonal gammopathies.[165,166] "Benign" monoclonal immunoglobulin peaks demonstrable by serum protein electrophoresis and immuno-electrophoretic techniques are rarely found in individuals under 50 years of age but are found with increasing frequency in later years: 10% in individuals over 75 and perhaps 20% of those over 90. Although monoclonal gammopathies are common, the incidence of multiple myeloma with malignant immunoglobulin production in these age groups is only about 0.02%. The relative frequency of immunoglobulin isotypes involved in monoclonal gammopathies are about 50% IgG, 20% IgA, and 10% IgM with IgD and IgE accounting for only 1% or less. Kyle and Garton[167] reviewed the records of 430 patients with IgM monoclonal gammopathies: 56% of individuals had "benign" monoclonal gammopathy, 17% had Waldenstrom's macroglobulinemia, 7% had lymphoma, 5% had chronic lymphocytic leukemia, 1% had primary amyloidosis, and 5% had other lymphoproliferative diseases. In that study, which drew on serum collected over a 22-year period, about 20% of patients initially diagnosed with "benign" gammopathy eventually developed lymphoma. Explanations for the increased frequency of monoclonal gammopathies seen with aging include a gradual breakdown in control mechanisms governing antibody production. Decreased production of anti-idiotype antibodies, decreased activity of suppressor cells, or increased activity of T helper cells could play roles. These same problems with immunoregulation could also be responsible for the increase in incidence of autoantibodies with age. In particular, rheumatoid factors, antinuclear antibodies, antithyroid and antilymphocyte autoantibodies have been demonstrated.[131,168-170]

Because disturbances in regulation of the immune response are common to both autoimmune disease and aging, it has been suggested that some autoimmune diseases may represent a premature aging phenomenon.[171] One way of measuring immunoregulation in vitro is by assessing the proliferative reaction of T lymphocytes when they are cultured with autologous non-T lymphoid cells. This reaction, the autologous mixed lymphocyte reaction (AMLR), is present in all healthy individuals but deficient in patients with autoimmune and lymphoproliferative diseases[172] and in aging.[173] The responder cells in the AMLR are in the subset of helper T cells known as suppressor-inducer cells and experiments have shown that suppressor cells can be recovered from AMLR cultures.[90] Studies in mice also indicate that this reaction represents an aspect of immunoregulation[174] and that it becomes deficient with age.[175] When examined in the autoimmune mouse strain, NZB, the AMLR has been shown to become deficient due to several overlapping mechanisms.[176] Young NZB mice have a normal AMLR when compared to age matched non-autoimmune control strains. A decline in the AMLR precedes the development of overt autoimmune disease in these animals and initially the decrease is due to decreased IL-2 production. Later the decrease is due to that plus the occurrence of suppressor T cells that bear class II histocompatibility surface antigens and finally, as has been noted for other immune responses with aging, there supervenes an absolute decrease in the number of precursor cells able to make an AMLR response.

Not only do immune responses change with age, but the antigenicity of tissues and proteins

change as well. The latter may in part be responsible for the increase with age of antibody responses that exhibit more cross-reactivity[177] and these in turn probably cause the increase in anti-idiotype antibodies that has also been noted with age.[84,178] Tissue antigens include the scenescent cell antigen, an ubiquitous glycoprotein that occurs on aging cell surfaces and which may serve as a target of an immune response for deleting aging cells including cells in the central nervous system.[179]

NEUROIMMUNOLOGY

It has long been known that the immune system and the nervous system are much alike. Both have a memory function, both respond either positively or negatively to autocrine and endocrine types of signals, and both can send signals to diverse cell types. While the brain and the immune system are anatomically separated by the blood brain barrier and the brain does not have a lymphatic drainage system, cells of the brain and immune system share certain surface antigens. The best known of these is the Thy1 antigen which is a marker for all murine T cells and which is also found on cells in the CNS.[180] There are a large number of potential antigens in neural tissue that could act as antigens for an immune response. Glycolipids such as galactosylceramide, various gangliosides and glycosphingolipids are found in high concentration in neural tissue and antibody responses to these have been found in patients after cerebral trauma[181] and in patients with SLE and multiple sclerosis (MS).[181,182] Antibodies to phospholipids (PL), mainly cardiolipin, have also been described in lupus patients with CNS involvement.[183-185] Anticardiolipin antibodies have also been described in patients with Guillain-Barré syndrome[186] and, again, in SLE with neurologic complications such as optic neuritis,[187] and chorea.[188] It is not clear at this time whether these antibodies arise as part of the pathogenesis of these conditions or if they arise secondary to tissue injury. Cell-mediated responses to gangliosides have been reported to occur in MS[189-191] and cell mediated injury to neural tissue in autoimmune CNS disease fits with the current evidence for the pathogenesis of similar diseases in experimental animal models.[192,193]

It seems likely that certain cells in the CNS can actively participate in an immune response. Incubation of rat,[194] mouse,[195] and human fetal[196] astrocytes with immune interferon results in expression of HLA class II surface molecules. Similar results have been obtained with cultured human glioma cells. These cells express low levels of HLA-DR spontaneously[197] and this can be enhanced by culture in the presence of immune interferon.[198] Interferon-beta, which has been shown to oppose some of the effects of immune interferon on macrophages[199,200] has recently been shown to also down regulate expression of induced class II antigen expression on cultured human glioblastoma cells.[201] These sets of circumstances have potential clinical importance. Studies in mice have shown that treatment of mice with experimental allergic encephalomyelitis (EAE) with antibodies to class II antigens interrupts the progression of that disease.[202] For similar reasons, interferon-beta has recently been employed in clinical trials in the treatment of glioblastoma[203,204] and in patients with multiple sclerosis[205] as that disease is also associated with increased HLA class I and HLA class II antigen expression of various cell types in the brain.[206,207] In order for an effective immune response to occur, amplification of specific T cell/antigen presenting cell interaction is required and this is generally accomplished through the actions of cytokines. Glial cell lines have been shown to produce IL-1.[208] More recently, work from the same laboratory indicates that astrocytes secrete more IL-1 on a per cell basis than peripheral monocytes.[209] Thus, certain glial cells can act as antigen presenting cells for T cells that might transgress the blood-brain barrier.

Cytokines also play an important role in normal physiologic responses in the brain. As depicted in Figure 11-3, IL-1 produced locally by astrocytes can mediate a variety of effects including induction of slow-wave sleep, fever, decreased perception of pain, and anorexia.[37,69,210,211] Increased synthesis of leukotrienes and prostaglandins is probably responsible for many of the effects of IL-1. Although IL-1 does not cross the blood brain barrier, injection of IL-1 into the brains of mice results in

production of acute phase reactants by the liver.[212] Increased synthesis of prostaglandins and leukotrines by IL-1 results in release of ACTH and other hormones as shown also in Figure 11-3. The resultant surge in glucocorticoid synthesis has a negative regulatory influence on T cell activation and IL-1 production causing dampening of immune responses. Recent studies suggest that IL-1 is an intrinsic modulator of brain function[213] and can directly affect target cells in the anterior pituitary.[214] Thus a primary role for this cytokine in neurohormonal regulation is implied.

Other cytokines also have effects on the CNS. Tumor necrosis factor (TNF) is a polypeptide cytokine also known as cachectin which lyses a variety of tumor cells in vitro and which has numerous overlapping functions with IL-1[215] including induction of slow-wave sleep.[216] Recently, Robbins et al.[217] have shown that rat astrocytes cultured in the presence of calcium ionophore produce a TNF-like substance that is cytotoxic for oligodendrocytes. Fontana et al.[218] have demonstrated a factor produced by mitogen stimulated spleen cells that stimulates glial cell proliferation and this factor (GSF) may have a role in recovery of inflammatory lesions in the CNS. Likewise nerve growth factor (NGF), which is also produced by mitogen activated lymphocytes, can maintain healthy and functional neurons in culture.[219] Factors that inhibit biologic effects of IL-2 have also been shown to be produced by glioblastoma cells[209] and this may represent an important mechanism of escape of tumor cells from immune attack.

SPECIFIC NEUROLOGIC DISORDERS

Some neuroimmunologic disorders are clearly associated with aging as in neurologic complications of monoclonal gammopathies. In other disorders such as multiple sclerosis or myasthenia gravis, the situation is more complicated with bimodal peaks of disease involving younger and older populations. In this section we will examine the various neurologic disorders that fall into these two groupings beginning with those in which the association with an aging immune system is the most unequivocal.

NEUROLOGIC DISORDERS ASSOCIATED WITH PLASMA CELL DYSCRASIA

As mentioned previously the frequency of plasma cell dyscrasia (PCD) increases with age. The monoclonal antibodies, or "M proteins," may invade bone or tissue as a neoplastic process. If the M proteins are IgG or IgA, these cases are termed multiple myeloma; in the case of IgM paraproteins the diagnosis is Waldenstrom's macroglobulinemia. In approximately one half of individuals with paraproteinemia, however, there is no invasion of tissue and in these patients the monoclonal gammopathy is of uncertain significance.[220] All these forms of PCD may be associated with neurologic sequelae, particularly in the peripheral nervous system (PNS). Approximately 10% of myeloma patients have an associated peripheral neuropathy including 50% of cases in which the myeloma is of the "osteosclerotic" variety.[221,222] In Waldenstrom's the frequency of neuropathy is as high as 25%.[221] In some cases such as neuropathies, radiculopathies, or mononeuritis multiplex, clinical presentations may be caused by direct invasion of roots or nerves by plasma cells.[222] However, in many cases no evidence of invasion is detectable. Many of these neuropathies may be caused by M proteins binding immunologically to specific PNS epitopes with resultant damage to the peripheral nerve. The most extensively studied example is with patients with IgM M proteins which immunologically bind carbohydrate determinants shared by the myelin associated glycoprotein (MAG)[223] and several other glycoproteins[224] and glycolipids[225] of peripheral nerve. These patients usually have distal sensory loss which evolves into a chronic slowly progressing demyelinating sensorimotor neuropathy.[226] On sural nerve biopsy IgM is detected on affected nerve by fluorescence immunohistochemistry[227,228] [Fig. 11–4]. The M proteins seem likely to cause the neuropathy since in some patients the neuropathy responds to plasma exchange or immunosuppressive therapy.[223,229–233] Moreover, serum from patients, but not controls, has been shown to induce demyelination when injected into cat nerve.[234]

IgG M proteins are likely to induce neurop-

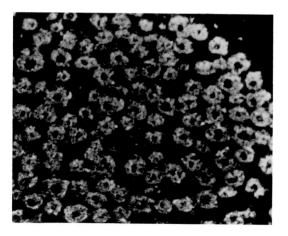

Fig. 11–4. Binding of human monoclonal antibodies to myelin associated glycoprotein (MAG) in tissue sections of normal human peripheral nerve demonstrated by immunofluorescence histochemistry. The bound IgM was made visible by fluorescein-conjugated goat antihuman IgM. Reprinted with permission from Nobile-Orazio et al.

athy in patients with the osteosclerotic form of myeloma. Osteosclerotic patients constitute only 3% of total myeloma cases but 50% of patients with the osteosclerotic form have an associated neuropathy.[235] Some of these patients have the so-called "POEMS" syndrome (Polyneuropathy, Organomegaly, Endocrinopathy, Myeloma, Skin changes) also known as the Crowe Fukase syndrome.[236–238] When the myeloma is treated by radiation or chemotherapy, the neuropathy frequently improves. Recently, IgG binding to pituitary tissue by Western blot and immunohistochemistry has been demonstrated in a patient with POEMS syndrome. As no binding was detected in other affected organs such as nerve, skin, or muscle, the authors felt the pituitary may be a primary target for the antibodies.[239] Conceivably, lesions in the hypophysis could induce secondary endocrinopathy and skin changes. However, it is unclear how antibodies binding to pituitary tissue could induce a neuropathy and the explanation for at least the neurologic component of this disorder remains unknown.

In addition to neuropathy, PCD has been implicated in some cases of motor neuron disease (MND). A higher frequency of MND patients have PCD than the general population.[240] This is particularly the case with IgM M proteins and the lower motor neuron form of MND known as progressive spinal muscular atrophy (PSMA). Several of these patients have IgM M proteins which bind specifically to the galactose (β1-3) N-acetylgalactosamine moiety shared by gangliosides GM§1 and GD§ 1§b.[240-242] It is not known for certain that the M proteins induce the MND but patients have been described who improved with therapy directed towards lowering the M protein concentration.[221] In addition, using anti-GM-1 antibodies, patients without PCD have been detected in MND[243] and in multifocal motor neuropathies[244,245] and these individuals have also improved with immunotherapy.

COLLAGEN VASCULAR DISEASE

Several of the collagen vascular disorders are more frequent in older people.

TEMPORAL ARTERITIS

Temporal (giant cell) arteritis characteristically occurs in patients over the age of 60. In this disorder visual loss may occur as a result of ischemia of the optic nerve and/or retina. The visual loss is usually accompanied or preceded by vague systemic complaints such as myalgias, malaise, and fever. Typically, the patient has a high erythrocyte sedimentation rate (ESR) and tender, pulseless arteries of the scalp. The arteries most frequently involved are the temporal, posterior auricular, or cervical.[246] The arteritis is documented by biopsy of the affected artery. It should be emphasized that biopsies may miss the lesion due to the multifocal nature of the disorder.

A related disease, polymyalgia rheumatica, also occurs in older patients. Polymyalgia rheumatica patients have myalgias, malaise, and fever but without the eye findings and scalp artery changes of temporal arteritis. However, up to 40% of patients with temporal arteritis also have polymyalgia rheumatica.[247] The peak incidence for both sexes is between 70 and 79 years.[248] Disability is more related to pain and stiffness than weakness. When the muscle disease is active the ESR is nearly always elevated to greater than 40 mm/h.[248] It may be that polymyalgia rheumatica and temporal arteritis are different manifestations of

the same disease. Both of these syndromes respond well to corticosteroid therapy.[249] However, polymyalgia rheumatica without temporal arteritis frequently requires much lower doses for treatment (10 to 20 mg of prednisone per day). The pathogenesis of both disorders is unclear but is thought to involve an autoimmune inflammatory arteritis of the vessels in question. Despite the frequent mylagias there are no characteristic pathologic findings in muscle.[248]

POLYMYOSITIS/DERMATOMYOSITIS

Polymyositis (PM) and dermatomyositis (DM) most likely encompass a group of autoimmune disorders involving muscle and, in the case of DM, skin. Particularly for DM, there are two age peaks; one during childhood and the other in the fifth or sixth decade.[250] It is likely that the adult form of disease is a different disorder as it has a different pathologic expression and is associated with many abnormalities not found in the pediatric form of DM. In adult forms, black patients are more likely to be affected than whites and in all ages there is a female predominance.[250] Typically PM-DM begins insidiously with slowly progressive weakness of proximal muscles of the limb girdle, shoulder, and neck flexors. The course may be over weeks, months, or even years. Atypical weakness may be present localized to one limb or a single group of muscles such as the quadriceps.[251,252] Pain is present in approximately $\frac{1}{3}$ of cases. In dermatomyositis, weakness is accompanied by characteristic skin changes. These skin changes, which may not all be present in the same patient consist of heliotrope discoloration and edema of the eyelids, a raised scaly erythematous rash on the face, shoulders, and upper trunk as well as on the extensor surfaces of the limbs. This rash is particularly frequent over the knuckles, wrists, elbows, and knees.[253] The diagnosis of PM is based on the clinical picture as well as results from serum levels of muscle enzymes, the EMG, and from muscle biopsy. The most important muscle enzyme is the creatine kinase (CK) which is released from damaged muscle and is elevated in most but not all cases. The ESR is elevated in fewer than half of the cases and does not correlate well with the clinical status of the patient.[250] EMG in most cases gives a myopathic picture of small, low amplitude, fragmented narrow motor units and recruitment patterns which fill earlier than expected. However, the EMG may also be normal, particularly in chronic cases. In patients with active PM and DM there is likely to be evidence of acute changes on EMG as illustrated by fibrillation potentials and positive waves.[254] Muscle biopsy is the most important diagnostic procedure and reveals differences between PM and DM as well as distinguishing between the adult and juvenile forms of PM. In both PM and DM there is usually evidence of necrosis as well as regeneration of muscle fibers. Necrosis is illustrated early on by obliteration of the striations of muscle fiber. Later, the muscle fiber becomes swollen and invaded both by macrophages and lymphocytes and sarcoplasmic components exhibit various stages of degeneration.[250] Regeneration is also seen with muscle fibers exhibiting basophilic cytoplasm on hematoxylin and eosin staining along with large, peripherally or centrally placed nuclei with prominent nucleoli. In addition to changes of necrosis and regeneration, muscle biopsies in PM-DM frequently contain foci of inflammatory cells [Fig. 11–5]. Lymphocytes, plasma cells, and histiocytes are frequent in the perimysium and endomysium. In PM but not DM T lymphocytes and occasional macrophages surround and invade normal appearing muscle fibers.[250] Arahata and Engle[255] have shown that T8 + cytotoxic T cells are the predominant cells in PM infiltrates but not in those of DM. DM of children differs from that of the adult by the presence of perifascicular atrophy in which muscle fibers at the periphery of the muscle fascicle atrophy out of proportion to those in the center. Childhood DM also differs from the adult form by the presence of areas of ischemia as well as endothelial hyperplasia of intramuscular blood vessels.

The adult forms of PM-DM are associated with other autoimmune disorders such as the collagen vascular diseases. These include scleroderma, systemic lupus erythematosis, and rheumatoid arthritis. Though there is debate with PM,[256] there is an increased incidence of malignancy associated with DM. This

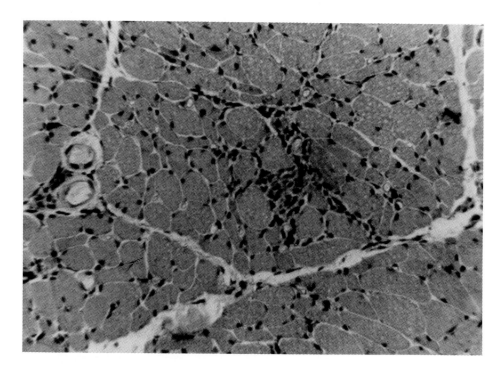

Fig. 11–5. Acute polymyositis demonstrating perivascular infiltrate, phagocytosis of degenerating muscle fiber and early evidence of regeneration. (Courtesy of T. Heiman-Patterson, M.D., Philadelphia, PA.)

may suggest changes in the immune system associated with age or in some cases DM may represent a paraneoplastic syndrome.

PERIARTERITIS NODOSA

The peak incidence of periarteritis nodosa is in the fifth and sixth decades. Angiography reveals characteristic arterial beading [Fig. 11–6]. The disorder is rare but clinically detectable neuropathy may be the dominating feature and is present in almost two thirds of cases at some stage of the disease.[257] Other organ involvement with pericarditis, renal failure, abdominal pain, hypertension, and fever usually, but not always, precede the neuropathy. The neuropathy usually presents as a mononeuritis multiplex with branches of the radial, median, and sciatic nerves being particularly susceptible.[258] Eventually the disorder evolves into a symmetrical, sensorimotor, predominantly distal axonal polyneuropathy. The pathogenesis of the neuropathy is probably ischemic and arteriolar occlusion is probably secondary to inflammatory fibrinoid necrosis.[259]

PARANEOPLASTIC SYNDROMES

It is becoming increasingly evident that many of the remote effects of carcinoma, the paraneoplastic syndromes, may be mediated by products of the immune system. Thus, IL-1 and TNF, as well as other cytokines, may cause the fever, anemia, cachexia, and malaise associated with malignancy and antibodies may mediate more specific forms of paraneoplastic syndromes. These syndromes tend to increase with age as they follow the incidence of the tumors with which they are typically associated. Three syndromes that are probably antibody mediated syndromes are peripheral neuropathies, cerebellar degeneration, and the Lambert Eaton syndrome.

PERIPHERAL NEUROPATHY

Various forms of neuropathy have been associated with malignancy. Some, such as those associated with plasma cell dyscrasia, have already been discussed. Acute sensorimotor neuropathy resembling the Guillain-Barre syn-

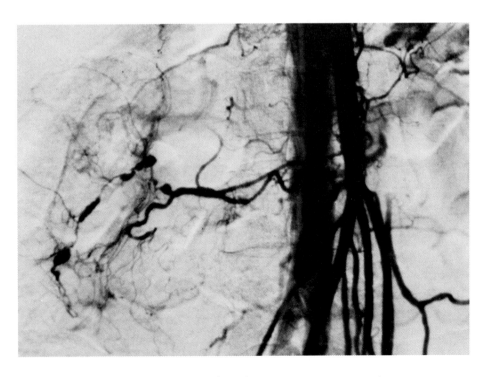

Fig. 11–6. Beading of renal artery in periarteritis nodosa.

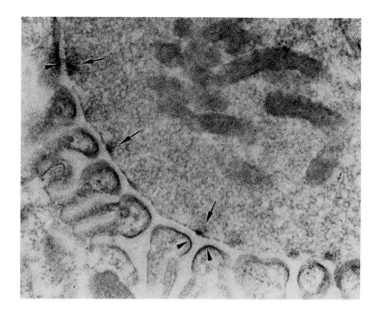

Fig. 11-7. Localization with immunoperoxidase of human IgG in mice treated with IgG from patient with Lambert-Eaton syndrome. Immunoreactive zones identified by arrow. (Reprinted with permissions from Fukuoka et al. Ann. Neurol., 22:200, 1987.)

drome have been said to be more frequent in patients with Hodgkin's disease.[260,261] Subacute to chronic relapsing and progressive sensorimotor neuropathies are associated with malignancy.[262] These are typically axonal in form though some may be demyelinating. The pathogenesis in most has not, at least yet, been demonstrated to be immunologic. One paraneoplastic neuropathy that appears to be clearly immunologic is the pure sensory neuropathy that is frequently associated with carcinoma of the breast or small cell carcinoma of the lung. Autoantibodies have been detected in some of these patients and these may cause the neuropathy by cross reacting with tumor antigens.[263]

CEREBELLAR DEGENERATION

Antibody mediated disease of the cerebellum is a well-recognized paraneoplastic syndrome.[264] IgG antibodies have been detected which bind to Purkinje cells in the cerebellum, particularly in cases of ovarian carcinoma. Clinically these cases rarely occur prior to the age of 30[265] and may precede or follow detection of the tumor. Symptoms of cerebellar dysfunction can come on acutely over a period of days or chronically over a period of months. Over 50% of patients have nystagmus and the cerebellar deficit may be severe enough to incapacitate the patient. Pathologically, there is

a predominant loss of Purkinje cells and, to a lesser extent, cells in the granular layer of the cerebellum.[256] Occasional reports cite improvement of the cerebellar deficits with treatment of the tumor but overall the clinical course is likely to be poor in this disorder.

LAMBERT EATON SYNDROME

The Lambert Eaton syndrome (LES) is an autoimmune disorder involving the neuromuscular junction. In approximately one half of the cases it is associated with a tumor; particularly small cell carcinoma of the lung.[266] In these cases it is likely that IgG binds to and damages presynaptic voltage gated calcium channels (VGCC) on the presynaptic terminal of the neuromuscular junction[267] [Fig. 11-7]. Therefore, there is a reduction in the number of quanta of acetylcholine (ACh) released from the presynaptic terminal. It may be that there is shared antigenicity between the VGCC of the tumor and that of the presynaptic terminal of the NMJ. Clinically, the LES may present similarly to another disorder of the neuromuscular junction, myasthenia gravis (MG). Both disorders typically present with weakness and fatigability.[266] Unlike MG, however, autonomic features are frequently present in LES. These include dry mouth, sexual impotence, and difficulties with sphincter muscle control. Since detection of IgG reacting with the VGCC is not generally available to the clinician, the diagnosis of LES is usually made by nerve conduction studies. A single stimulation of a peripheral nerve generates a smaller than normal compound muscle action potential (CMAP) because of the reduced number of ACh quanta released. Because of a process termed facilitation, more quanta are released following a brief period of tetanic contraction and a subsequent stimulus generates a CMAP that is more than 100% increased in amplitude. This increase is characteristic of presynaptic disorders involving the neuromuscular junction and thus is characteristic of the LES. In addition to the presence of IgG on the presynaptic terminals, other evidence supports an autoimmune pathogenesis for the LES. Plasmapheresis improves the reduction in the initial CMAP amplitude[268] and may be associated with clinical improvement. Also, LES IgG injected into mice induces many of the physiologic changes of the disease.[269] The role of the neoplasms in those cases associated with tumors is unclear. The neurologic disorder may precede evidence of tumor by up to 4 years.[266] It may be that there are shared antigens on the tumor and the presynaptic terminal. Particularly in the non-carcinomatous form of the disease, there is an association with other autoimmune disorders and a significant increase in the frequency of HLA B8.[270] Particularly because of the association with carcinoma, this syndrome tends not to strike a younger population but is more frequent in older patients who are more susceptible to lung cancer.

MULTIPLE SCLEROSIS

Although MS is usually thought of as a disease affecting young people, particularly women, there is a second population peak affected after the age of 40 with many cases beginning after 60 years of age. Clinically the older group typically has a progressive spastic para- or quadriparesis without the relapsing-remitting course of younger patients. There are no histopathologic features which clearly distinguish MS occurring in young people from those with the onset over 40 years of age. In both cases there are multiple foci of partial to complete destruction of CNS but not PNS myelin with sparing of the axon cylinders. Both

younger and older patients have neuroglial scarring and acutely exhibit perivascular infiltration of mononuclear cells and lymphocytes. In more chronic lesions there are fewer cellular infiltrates and more acellular fibroglial tissue.

The evidence that MS is an autoimmune disease will only be summarized here. The reader is invited to look elsewhere for a more extensive discussion [See Chap. 13]. MS patients do not appear to have a generalized disturbance of their immune system. There are no immunologic abnormalities which are thought to be specific for MS. However, MS patients have a decrease in avid T cell rosette formation and a reduction in concanavalin A (con A) induced suppressor activity.[271] There is general acceptance of a reduction in T-suppressor cells, as defined by the T8 (CD8) monoclonal antibody, in acute exacerbations of MS. Eighty to 90% of patients with definite MS have multiple clones of IgG in their CSF (oligoclonal bands). The antigenic specificity of these bands remains unknown. An immunologic model of MS, experimental allergic encephalitis (EAE), can be induced by injecting CNS homogenates and immunologic adjuvants such as complete Freund's adjuvant into rats.[272,273]

As noted above, patients who contract MS over the age of 40 tend to have a steadily progressive course of spastic paraparesis as opposed to the typical relapsing-remitting course of younger patients. It has been thought that the differing clinical course is related to changes occurring in the immune system in MS.[274]

MYASTHENIA GRAVIS

Myasthenia gravis is a disorder in which autoantibodies induce weakness in patients through binding to the postsynaptic membrane of the neuromuscular junction.[275] MG may be present at any age but the incidence in women peaks in the third decade, while that in men peaks in the sixth to seventh decade of life. Twenty eight is the mean age of onset for women, while that for men is 42.[275] The overall male to female ratio is 6:4. There is an increased incidence of HLA-A1, B8, and DR3 in patients under the age of 40 while patients over 40 are more likely to exhibit the A3, B7, DR2 haplotype.[275] Older patients with MG are more likely to have an associated thymoma or thymus involution, while younger patients are more likely to have thymic hyperplasia.[268]

Pathologically there is damage to the postsynaptic portion of the nicotinamide neuromuscular junction in MG[276] and this is probably antibody mediated. In addition, considering the favorable response of many patients to thymectomy, there are abnormalities of the thymus gland which are likely to be related to the disease. Approximately 10% of patients, particularly the older group, have actual thymomas, while about 80% of remaining patients demonstrate hyperplasia of lymphoid follicles in the medulla of the thymus. Abnormalities in the thymus may reflect the autoimmune nature of the disease. During development of the immune system T lymphocytes are processed in the thymus where they mature into functioning T cells,[277] and aberrations in thymus function may result in problems with tolerance or nonresponsiveness to self-antigens.

Clinically, MG is characterized by weakness in skeletal muscles which may be more severe following exercise. In about 60% of patients weakness first involves the eye muscles and these are involved ultimately in approximately 90% of cases. The diagnosis is typically made by history and examination as well as results from three tests. The first is the edrophonium (Tensilon) test in which up to 10 mg of the anticholinesterase agent, edrophonium, is injected intravenously into the patient. This prevents acetylcholine from being degraded in the neuromuscular junction and allows ACh to act for a longer period of time on a damaged postsynaptic receptor [See below]. In many but not all cases this is translated clinically into dramatic increases of strength in previously weak muscles. In repetitive stimulation a nerve, typically the median nerve, is stimulated supramaximally at a frequency of 3 HZ and recording electrodes are placed over a muscle innervated by the nerve, in this case, the abductor pollicis brevis (APB). Normally there should be less than a 10% decrement between the amplitudes of the first and fifth compound muscle action potential [CMAP] evoked by the stimulus. Because of the damaged postsynaptic receptor in the NMJ it is more difficult for the quanta of ACh to generate an action po-

tential and the decrement may become greater than 10% in a myasthenic patient and greater than 20% if the patient is made to exercise prior to the test. The most specific test for MG is the presence in the serum of antibodies to the Acetylcholine receptor (AchR) which will be discussed below.

The evidence for an autoimmune basis for MG is substantial. Nearly 90% of myasthenic patients have anti-AchR antibodies when tested by a radioimmunoassay measuring antibodies to human muscle AchR.[278] When immunoglobulin fractions from these patients are passively transferred into mice they develop the characteristic features of MG.[279] In humans approximately 1 in 8 babies of myasthenic mothers develop "neonatal MG" which is a transient form of the disease induced by maternal IgG which has crossed the placenta.[280] Electron microscopic studies have demonstrated IgG and complement at the postsynaptic membranes of the NMJ.[281] Plasmapheresis, to reduce the concentration of anti-AchR antibodies, as well as immunosuppressive therapy are mainstays of treatment. MG is frequently associated with other autoimmune diseases. These include Hashimoto's thyroiditis, systemic lupus erythematosus, and rheumatoid arthritis.[282] Furthermore, an immunologic animal model for MG exists. Experimental autoimmune myasthenia gravis (EAMG) is induced when purified ACh receptor is injected along with Freund's adjuvant.[283] The resulting syndrome mimics many of the clinical and pathologic findings in MG.

The disorders listed above are the main neuroimmunologic disorders which increase in frequency with the age of the patient. As pointed out in the earlier portion of the chapter, the immune system is quite complicated and while abnormalities secondary to immune dysfunction occur in all age groups, attrition of certain immune responses and increased autoantibody production appear to be directly involved in the pathogenesis of certain nervous system diseases that also exhibit increased prevalence in the aging population.

REFERENCES

1. Rowe, J.W., and Kahn, R.L.: Human ageing: Usual and successful. Science, 237:143, 1987.

2. Watson, A.L., and Yunis, E.J.: Immunogenetics and Longevity. Prog. Clin. Biol. Res., *133*:77, 1983.

3. Kafetz, K.: The main histocompatibility complex and ageing in mice and men. Age Ageing, *13*:291, 1984.

4. Takata, H., et al.: Influence of major histocompatibility complex region genes on human longevity among Okinawan-Japanese centenarians and nonagenarians. Lancet, *2*:824, 1987.

5. Katz, D.H., and Benacerraf, B.: The regulatory influence of activated T cells on B cell responses to antigen. Adv. Immunol., *15*:1, 1972.

6. Haskins, K., Kappler, J., and Marrack, P.: The major histocompatibility complex-restricted antigen receptor on T cells. Ann. Rev. Immunol., *2*:51, 1984.

7. Meredith, P.J., and Walford, R.L.: Autoimmunity, histocompatibility and ageing. Mech. Ageing Dev., *9*:61, 1979.

8. McDevitt, H.O.: Regulation of the immune response by the major histocompatibility system. N. Engl. J. Med., *303*:1514, 1980.

9. Moller, G.: HLA and disease susceptibility. Immunol. Rev., *70*:1, 1983.

10. Makinodan, T., and Kay, M.M.B.: Age influence on the immune system. Adv. Immunol., *29*:287, 1980.

11. Kay, M.M., and Makinodan, T.: Relationship between ageing and the immune system. Prog. Allergy, *29*:134, 1981.

12. Walford, R.L., et al.: Immunological and biochemical studies of Down's syndrome as a model of accelerated ageing. In: *Immunological Aspects of Ageing.* (Eds.) D. Segre, and L. Smith. New York, Marcel Dekker, 1981.

13. Weksler, M.E.: Senescence of the immune system. Med. Clin. N. Am., *67*:263, 1983.

14. Makinodan, T., and Hirayama, R.: Age-related changes in immunologic and hormonal activities. IARC. Sci. Publ., *58*:55, 1985.

15. Felser, J.M., and Raff, M.J.: Infectious diseases and ageing: Immunologic perspectives. J. Am. Geriatr. Sci., *31*:802, 1983.

16. Proust, J., Rosenzweig, P., Debouzy, C., et al.: Lymphopenia induced by acute bacterial infections in the elderly: a sign of age-related immune dysfunction of major prognostic significance. Gerontology, *31*:178, 1985.

17. Lipschitz, D.A., et al.: Cancer in the elderly: basic science and clinical aspects. Ann. Intern. Med., *102*:218, 1985.

18. Busby, J., and Caranasos, G.L.: Immune function, autoimmunity and selective immunoprophylaxis in the aged. Med. Clin. N. Am., *69*:465, 1985.

19. Schmucker, D. L., and Daniels, C.K.: Ageing, gastrointestinal infections and mucosal immunity. J. Am. Geriatr. Soc., *34*:377, 1986.

20. Grey, H.M., and Chesnut, R.: Antigen processing and presentation to T cells. Immunol. Today, *6*:101, 1985.

21. Mosier, D.E., and Johnson, B.M.: Ontogeny of mouse lymphocyte function. I. Development of the ability to produce antibody is modulated by T lymphocytes. J. Exp. Med., *141*:216, 1975.

22. Miller, J.F.A.P.: Immunological memory. Contemp. Top. Immunobiol., *2*:151, 1973.

23. Unanue, E.R., and Allen, P.M.: The basis for the immunoregulatory role of macrophages and other accessory cells. Science, *236*:551, 1987.

24. Buus, S., et al.: The relation between major histocompatibility complex (MHC) restriction and the capacity of Ia to bind immunogenic peptides. Science, *235*:1353, 1987.

25. Guillet, J.G., et al.: Interaction of peptide hormones and class II major histocompatibility complex antigens. Nature, *324*:260, 1987.

26. Raff, M.C.: T and B lymphocytes and immune response. Nature, *242*:19, 1973.

27. Gershon, R.K., Cohen, P., Hencin, R., et al.: Suppressor T cells. J. Immunol., *108*:586, 1972.

28. Rich, R.R., and Pierce, C.W.: Biological expressions of lymphocyte activation. I. Effects of phytomitogens on antibody synthesis in vitro. J. Exp. Med., *137*:205, 1973.

29. Jondal, M.: Surface markers on human B and T lymphocytes. IV. Distribution of surface markers on resting and blasttransformed lymphocytes. Scand. J. Immunol., *3*:739, 1974.

30. Moretta, L., et al.: Functional analysis of two human T cell subpopulations: Help and suppression of B-cell responses by T cell bearing receptors for IgM or IgG. J. Exp. Med., *146*:184, 1977.

31. Boyse, E.A., and Cantor, H.: Surface characteristics of T-lymphocyte subpopulations. Hospital Practice, *12*:81, 1977.

32. Reinherz, E.L., and Schlossman, S.F.: Current concepts in immunology. Regulation of the immune response-inducer and suppressor T-lymphocyte subsets in human beings. N. Engl. J. Med., *303*:370, 1980.

33. Reinherz, E.L., et al.: Antigen recognition by human T lymphocytes is linked to surface expression of the T3 molecular complex. Cell, *30*:735, 1982.

34. Clevers, H., et al.: The T cell receptor/CD3 complex: A dynamic protein ensemble. Ann. Rev. Immunol., *6*:629, 1988.

35. Shaw, S.: Characterization of human leukocyte differentiation antigens. Immunol. Today, *8*:1, 1987.

36. Takeuchi, T., Schlossman, S.F., and Morimoto, C.: The T4 molecule differentially regulating the activation of subpopulations of T4+ cells. J. Immunol., *139*:665, 1987.

37. Oppenheim, J.J., et al.: Lymphokines: Their role in lymphocyte responses. Properties of interleukin-1. Fed. Proc., *41*:257, 1982.

38. Dinarello, C.A., and Mier, J.W.: Current concepts: Lymphokines. N. Engl. J. Med., *137*:940, 1987.

39. Robb, R.J., Greene, W.C., and Rusk, C.M.: Low and high affinity cellular receptors for IL-2: Implications for the level of Tac antigen. J. Exp. Med., *160*:1126, 1984.

40. Singer, A., Hathcock, K.S., and Hodes, R.J.: Cellular and genetic control of antibody responses. V. Helper T cell recognition of H-2 determinants on accessory cells but not B cells. J. Exp. Med., *149*:1208, 1979.

41. Zinkernagl, R.M., and Doherty, P.C.: Immunological surveillance against altered self components by sensitized T lymphocytes in lymphocytic choriomeningitis. Nature, *251*:547, 1974.

42. Mak, T.W., et al.: Genes encoding the gamma- chains of the human T cell antigen receptor. Prog. Immunol., *6*:176, 1986.

43. Hunkapiller, T., and Hood, L.: Diversification of immunoglobulins and T cell receptors. Prog. Immunol. *6*:106, 1986.

44. Cooper, M.D.: B cell development in birds and mammals. Prog. Immunol., *6*:18, 1986.

45. Vitetta, E.S., and Uhr, J.: Immunoglobulin receptors revisited. A model for the differentiation of bone

marrow-derived lymphocytes is described. Science, *189*:964, 1975.

46. Burnet, F.M.: Clonal selection and after. In: *Theoretical Immunology.* (Eds.) G.I. Bell, A.S. Perelson, and G.H. Pimley, Jr. New York, Marcel Dekker, 1978.

47. Parrish, C.R., and Hayward, J.A.: The lymphocyte surface: I. Relation between Fc receptors, C'3 receptors and surface immunoglobulin. Proc. Roy. Soc. Land., *187*:47, 1974.

48. Chesnut, R.W., and Grey, H.M.: Studies on the capacity of B cells to serve as antigen presenting cells. J. Immunol., *126*:1075, 1981.

49. Doenhoff, M.J., et al.: Lymphocyte activation: VI. A reevaluation of factors affecting the selectivity of polyclonal mitogens for mouse T and B cells. Clin. Exp. Immunol., *17*:475, 1974.

50. Greaves, M., Janossy, G., and Doenhoff, M.: Selective triggering of human T and B lymphocytes in vitro by polyclonal mitogens. J. Exp. Med., *140*:1, 1974.

51. Jelinek, D.F., Splauski, J.B., and Lipsky, P.E.: The roles of interleukin-2 and interferon in human B cell activation, growth and differentiation. Eur. J. Immunol., *16*:925, 1986.

52. Hirohata, S., Jelinek, D.F., and Lipsky, P.E.: T cell dependent activation of B cell proliferation and differentiation by immunobilized monoclonal antibodies to CD3. J. Immunol., *140*:3726, 1988.

53. Sakselo, E., Timonen, T., Ranki, A., et al.: Morphological and functional characterization of isolated effector cells responsible to human natural killer activity to fetal fibroblasts and to cultured cell line targets. Immunol. Rev., *44*:71, 1979.

54. Tedder, T.F., Fearon, D.T., Gartland, G.L., et al.: Expression of C3b receptors on human B cells and myelomonocytic cells but not natural killer cells. J. Immunol., *130*:1668, 1983.

55. Santoli, D., and Koprowski, H.: Mechanism of activation of human natural killer cells against tumor and virus infected cells. Immunol. Rev., *44*:125, 1979.

56. Perlmann, P., Perlmann, H., and Wigzell, H.: Lymphocyte mediated cytotoxicity in vitro. Induction and inhibition by humoral antibody and nature of effector cells. Transplant Review, *13*:91, 1972.

57. Sugamura, K., and Smith, J.B.: Reversible blocking of antibody-dependent cell-mediated cytotoxicity. Cell. Immunol., *30*:353, 1977.

58. Natvig, J.B., and Kunkel, H.G.: Human immunoglobulins, classes, subclasses, genetic variante, and idiotypes. Adv. Immunol., *16*:1, 1973.

59. Kabat, E.A.: Antibody complimentarity and antibody structure. J. Immunol., *141*:525, 1988.

60. Weigert, M., and Riblet, R.: Genetic control of antibody variable region. Cold Spring Harbor. Symp. Quant. Biol., *41*:837, 1976.

61. Zappacosta, S., Nisonoff, A., and Mandy, W.J.: Mechanism of cleavage of rabbit IgG in vitro stage by soluble papean and reducing agent. J. Immunol., *100*:1268, 1968.

62. Davies, D.R., and Metzger, H.: Structural basis of antibody function. Ann. Rev. Immunol., *87*, 1983.

63. Ruddy, S.: Complement. In: *Manual of Clinical Laboratory Immunology,* 3rd ed., (Eds.) N.R. Rose, H. Friedman, and J.L. Fahey. Am. Soc. Microbiol., *175*:3, 1986.

64. Lamm, M.E.: Cellular aspects of immunoglobulin A. Adv. Immunol., *22*:223, 1976.

65. Zan-Bar, I., Strober, S., and Vitetta, E.S.: The relationship between surface immunoglobulin isotype and immune function of murine B lymphocytes. IV. Role of IgD-bearing cells in the propagation of immunologic memory. J. Immunol., *123*:925, 1979.

66. Herzenberg, L.A., McDevitt, H.O., and Herzenberg, L.A.: Genetics of antibodies. Ann. Rev. Genet., *2*:209, 1968.

67. Kuettner, M.G., Wang, A.L., and Nisonoff, A.: Quantitative investigators of idiotypic antibodies. VI. Idiotypic specificity as a potential genetic marker for the valuable regions of mouse immunoglobulin polypeptide chains. J. Exp. Med., *135*:579, 1972.

68. Cumano, A., et al.: Mutation and selection of antibodies. Prog. Immunol., *6*:130, 1986.

69. Oppenheim, J.J., et al.: The role of cytokines in promoting accessory cell function. Prog. Immunol., *5*:285, 1983.

70. Ruscetti, F.W., and Gallo, R.C.: Human T-lymphocyte growth factor: Regulation of growth and function of T lymphocytes. Blood, *57*:379, 1981.

71. Kaye, J., et al.: Growth of a cloned helper T cell line induced by a monoclonal antibody specific for the antigen receptor: Interleukin-1 is required for the expression of receptors for interleukin-2. J. Immunol., *133*:1339, 1984.

72. Grimm, E.A., Mazumder, A., Zhang, H.Z., et al.: Lymphokine activated killer cell phenomenon: lysis of natural killer resistant fresh solid teemer cells by interleukin-2 activated autologous human peripheral blood lymphocytes. J. Exp. Med., *155*:1823, 1982.

73. Paul, W.E., and O'Hara, J.: B-cell stimulatory factor-1/interleukin-4. Ann. Rev. Immunol., *5*:429, 1987.

74. Clark, S.C., and Kamen, R.: The human hematopoetic colony stimulating factors. Science, *236*:1229, 1987.

75. Halloran, P.F., Wadgymar, A., and Autenreid, P.: The regulation of expression of major histocompatibility complex products. Transplantation, *41*:413, 1986.

76. Miossec, P., and Ziff, M.: Immune interferon enhances the production of interleukin-1 by human endothelial cells stimulated with lipopolysaccharide. J. Immunol., *137*:2848, 1986.

77. Stiehm, E.R., et al.: Interferon: Immunobiology and clinical significance. Ann. Intern. Med., *96*:80, 1982.

78. Dausset, J., Degos, L., and Hors, J.: The association of the HLA antigens with diseases. Clin. Immunol. Immunopathol., *3*:127, 1974.

79. McDevitt, H.O.: The HLA system and its relation to disease. Hospital Practice, *20*:57, 1985.

80. Bystryn, J.C., Graf, M.W., and Uhr, J.W.: Regulation of antibody formation by serum antibody. II. Removal of specific antibody by means of exchange transfusion. J. Exp. Med., *132*:1279, 1970.

81. Schlansky, R., DeHoratius, R.J., Pinius, T., et al.: Plasmapheresis in systemic lupus erythematosus: A cautionary note. Arth. Rheum., *24*:49, 1981.

82. Jerne, N.K.: The immune system. Sci. Am., *229(1)*: 1973.

83. Rowley, D.A., et al.: Suppression by autologous complementary idiotypes: the priority of the first response. J. Exp. Med., *144*:946, 1976.

84. Szewczuk, M.R., and Wade, A.W.: Age-related strain differences in the development of auto-anti-idiotypic antibody regulation in the splenic and mucosal-associated lymphoid systems. Gerontology, *31*:251, 1985.

85. Dorf, M.E., and Benacerraf, B.: Suppressor cells and immunoregulation. Ann. Rev. Immunol., 2:127, 1984.

86. Wolos, J.A., Spagnoli, B., and Smith, J.B.: Suppression of a polyclonal B-cell response by supernatants from murine autologous mixed lymphocyte reaction. Cell Immunol., 96:61, 1985.

87. Mosier, D.E., Mathieson, B.J., and Campbell, D.: Ly phenotype and mechanism of action of mouse neonatal suppressor T cells. J. Exp. Med., 146:59, 1977.

88. Calkins, C.E., and Stutman, O.: Changes in suppressor mechanisms during post-natal development in mice. J. Exp. Med., 141:1376, 1978.

89. Smith, J.B., and Eaton, G.J.: Suppressor cells in spleens from "nude" mice: Their effect on the mitogenic response of B lymphocytes. J. Immunol., 117:319, 1976.

90. Smith, J.B., and Knowlton, K.P.: Activation of suppressor T cells in human autologous mixed lymphocyte culture. J. Immunol., 123:419, 1979.

91. Tada, T., Tanguelin, M., and Takemori, T.: Properties of primed suppressor T cells and their products. Transplant. Rev., 26:107, 1975.

92. Feldman, M., and Kontiainen, S.: Suppressor cell induction in vitro. II. Cellular requirements of suppressor cell induction. Eur. J. Immunol., 6:302, 1976.

93. Calkins, C.E., et al.: Cell interaction in the suppression of in vitro antibody responses. J. Exp. Med., 143:1421, 1976.

94. Green, D.R., et al.: Immunoregulatory circuits which modulate responsiveness to suppressor cell signals: characterization of an effector cell in the controsuppressor circuit. Eur. J. Immunol., 11:973, 1981.

95. Hausman, P.B., Sherr, D.H., and Dorf, M.E.: An in vitro system for the requirement for B cells in their induction. J. Immunol., 134:1388, 1985.

96. Weigle, W.O.: Immunological unresponsiveness. Adv. Immunol., 16:61, 1973.

97. Nossel, G.J.V.: Cellular mechanisms of immunological tolerance. Ann. Rev. Immunol., 1:33, 1983.

98. Roitt, I.M., and Cooke, A.: Idiotypes and autoimmunity. Progress Immunol., 6:512, 1986.

99. Miller, R.C., and Calkins, C.E.: Development of self-tolerance in normal mice: Appearance of suppressor cells that maintain adult self-tolerance follows the neonatal antibody response. J. Immunol., 141:2206, 1988.

100. Goidl, E.A.: Ageing and the Immune Response: Cellular and Humoral Aspects. New York, Marcel Dekker, 1987.

101. Makinodan, T., Lubinski, J., and Fong, T.C.: Cellular, biochemical, and molecular basis of T cell senescence. Arch. Pathol. Lab. Med., 111:910, 1987.

102. Mascart-Lemone, F., Delepresse, G., Servais, G., et al.: Characterization of immunoregulatory T lymphocytes during ageing by monoclonal antibodies. Clin. Exp. Immunol., 48:148, 1982.

103. Whittinghams, S., et al.: Diabetes mellitus autoimmunity and ageing. Lancet, 1:763, 1971.

104. Kendall, M.D.: Have we understood the importance of the thymus in man. Experientia, 40:1181, 1984.

105. Thompson, J.S., Robbins, J., and Cooper, J.K.: Nutrition and immune function in the geriatric population. Clin. Geriatr. Med., 3:309, 1987.

106. Ross, M.H.: Nutrition and longevity in experimental animals. Nutr. Ageing, p. 43, 1976.

107. Walford, R.L., et al.: Long-term dietary restriction and immune function in mice: response to sheep red blood cells and to mitogenic agents. Mech. Age. Dev., 2:447, 1974.

108. Weindruch, R., Gottesman, S.R.S., and Walford, R.L.: Modification of age-related immune decline in mice dietary restricted from or after midadulthood. Proc. Natl. Acad. Sci. (USA), 79:898, 1982.

109. Miller, R.A.: Age-associated decline in precursor frequency for different T cell mediated reactions with preservation of helper or cytotoxic effect per precursor cell. J. Immunol., 132:63, 1984.

110. Miller, R.A., and Harrison, D.E.: Delayed reduction in T cell precursor frequencies accompanies diet-induced lifespan extension. J. Immunol., 134:1426, 1985.

111. Hodge, S., and Walford, R.L.: HLA distribution in aged normals. In: Report of the Eighth International Workshop on Histocompatibility Testing. (Ed.) P.I. Teraski. Los Angeles, UCLA tissue typing laboratory, 1980.

112. Greenberg, L.J., and Yunis, E.J.: Histocompatibility determinants, immune responsiveness and ageing in man. Fed. Proc., 37:1258, 1978.

113. Ambinder, J.M., et al.: Special characteristics of cellular immune function in normal individuals of the HLA-DR3 type. Clin. Immunol. Immunopathol. 23:269, 1982.

114. Lewis, V.M., et al.: Age, thymic involution, and circulating thymic hormone activity. J. Clin. Endocr. Metab., 47:145, 1978.

115. Singh, V., and Singh, A.K.: Age related changes in human thymus. Clin. Exp. Immunol., 37:507, 1979.

116. Hiramoto, R.N., Ghanta, V.K., and Soong, S.J.: Effect of thymic hormones on immunity and life-span. In Ageing and the Immune Response. Edited E.A. Goidl. New York, Marcel Dekker, 1987.

117. Diaz-Johnson, E., Williams, Jr., R.C., and Strickland, R.G.: Age-related changes in T and B cells. Lancet, 1:660, 1974.

118. Inkeles, B., et al.: Immunological studies of ageing. III. Cytokineric basis for the impaired response of lymphocytes from aged humans to plant lectins, J. Exp. Med., 145:1176, 1977.

119. Kay, M.M.B.: Role of physiological autoantibody in the removal of senescent human red cells. J. Supramol. Struct., 9:555, 1978.

120. Moody, C.E., et al.: Lymphocyte transformation induced by autologous cells. XI. The effect of age on the autologous mixed lymphocyte reaction. Immunol., 44:431, 1981.

121. Nagel, J.E., Chrest, F.J., and Adler, W.H.: Enumeration of T lymphocyte subsets by monoclonal antibodies in young and aged humans. J. Immunol., 127:2086, 1981.

122. Hallgren, H.M., Jackola, D.R., and O'Leary, J.J.: Unusual pattern of surface marker expression on peripheral lymphocytes from aged humans suggestive of a population of less differentiated cells. J. Immunol., 131:191, 1983.

123. O'Leary, J.J., et al.: Evidence for a less differentiated subpopulation of lymphocytes in advanced age. Mech. Ageing. Dev., 21:109, 1983.

124. Astle, C.M., and Harrison, D.E.: Effects of marrow donor and recipient age on immune responses. J. Immunol., 132:673, 1984.

125. Gorczyniski, R.M., and Chang, M.P.: Significant expansion of the CLp repetoire taking place in the periphery, beyond the early appearing specificities present in the thymus: Defect in the peripheral en-

vironment of aged mice that results in altered expansion of the thymic CTLp repertoire. In addition, there is an intrinsic difference in bone marrow precursor cells of CTLp in aged mice that is revealed only in an aged environment. J. Immunol., 133:2382, 1984.

126. Makinodan, T., and Peterson, W.J.: Relative antibody forming capacity of spleen cells as a function of age. Proc. Natl. Acad. Sci. (USA), 48:234, 1962.

127. Krogsrud, R.L., and Perkins, E.H.: Age-related changes in T cell function. J. Immunol., 118:1607, 1977.

128. Callard, R.E., Basten, A., and Waters, L.K.: Immune function in aged mice. II. B-cell function. Cell. Immunol., 31:26, 1977.

129. Waldorf, D.S., Wilkens, R.R., and Decker, J.L.: Impaired delayed hypersensitivity in an ageing population. Association with antinuclear reactivity and rheumatoid factor. JAMA, 203:831, 1968.

130. Roberts-Thomson, I.C., Youngchaiyud, U., Whittingham, S., et al.: Ageing, immune response and mortality. Lancet 2:368, 1974.

131. Goodwin, J.S., Searles, R.P., and Tung, K.S.K.: Immunological responses of a healthy elderly population. Clin. Exp. Immunol., 48:403, 1982.

132. Hefton, et al.: Immunological studies of ageing. V. Impaired proliferation of PHA response human lymphocytes in culture. J. Immunol., 125:1007, 1980.

133. Weksler, W.E., and Hutteroth, J.H.: Impaired lymphocyte function in aged humans. J. Clin. Invest., 53:99, 1974.

134. Kay, M.M.: Age effects on a colony-forming human peripheral blood T and B cell. Gerontology, 31:278, 1985.

135. Gershon, H., Merhav, S., and Abraham, C.: T-cell division and ageing. Mech. Ageing. Dev., 9:27, 1979.

136. Antel, J.P., et al.: Reduced T lymphocyte cell reactivity as a function of human ageing. Cell. Immunol., 54:184, 1980.

137. Miller, R.A., and Stutman, O.: Decline in ageing of mice, of the anti-TNP cytotoxic response attributable to loss of Lyt-2, IL-2 producing helper cell function. Eur. J. Immunol., 11:751, 1981.

138. Pollack, A., Bagwell, C.B., and Irvin, III, G.L.: Radiation from H-TdR perturbs the cell cycle progression of stimulated lymphoctyes. Science, 203:1025, 1979.

139. Staiano-Coico, L., et al.: Increased sensitivity of lymphocytes from people over 65 to cell cycle arrest and chromosomal damage. Science, 219:1335.

140. Abraham, C., Tal, Y., and Gershon, H.: Reduced in vitro response to concavalin A and lipopolysaccharide in senescent mice: a function of reduced number of responding cells. Eur. J. Immunol., 7:301, 1977.

141. de Weck, A.L., et al.: Lymphocyte proliferation, lymphokine production, and lymphocyte receptors in ageing and various clinical conditions. Springer Semin. Immunopathol., 7:273, 1984.

142. Zatz, M.M., and Goldstein, A.L.: Thymosins, lymphokines and the immunology of ageing. Gerontology, 31:263, 1985.

143. Bach, J.F., Bach, M.A., and Blanot, D.: Thymic serum factor. Bull. Inst. Pasteur. 76:325, 1978.

144. McClure, J.E., Lameris, N., Wara, D.W., et al.: Immunochemical studies on thymosin: radioimmunoassay of thymosid. J. Immunol., 128:368, 1982.

145. Thoman, M.L., and Weigle, W.O.: Reconstitution of in vivo cell-mediated lympholysis 10 responses in aged mice with interleukin-2. J. Immunol., 134:949, 1985.

146. Ershler, W.B., Moore, A.L., and Spcomsli, M.A.: Influenza and ageing: age related changes and the effects of thymosin on the antibody response to influenza vaccine. J. Clin. Immunol., 4:453, 1984.

147. Ghanta, et. al.: Alloreactivity I. Effects of age and thymic hormone treatment on cell mediated immunity in C57 BL6 mice. Mech. Ageing. Dev. 22:309, 1983.

148. Zatz, M.M., et al.: Thymosin increases production of T-cell growth factor by normal human peripheral blood lymphocytes. Proc. Nat. Acad. Sci. (USA), 81:2882, 1984.

149. Chang, M.P., Makinodan, T., Peterson, W.J., et al.: Role of T cells and adherent cells in age-related decline in murine interleukin-2 production. J. Immunol., 129:2426, 1982.

150. Thoman, M.L., and Weigle, W.O.: Cell-mediated immunity in aged mice: an underlying lesion in IL-2 synthesis. J. Immunol., 128:2358, 1982.

151. Thoman, M.L.: Role of interleukin-2 in the age-related impairment of immune function. J. Am. Geriatr. Soc., 33:781, 1985.

152. Sohnle, P.G., Larson, S.E., Colling-Lech, C., et al.: Failure of lymphokine-producing lymphocytes from aged humans to undergo activation by recall antigens. J. Immunol., 124:2169, 1980.

153. Parker, C.W.: cAMP and lectin-induced mitogenesis in lymphocytes—possible implications for neoplastic cell growth. Advances in Cyclic Nucleotide Research, 9:647, 1979.

154. Hadden, J.W., Hadden, E.M., Haddox, M.K., et al.: Guanosine 3′, 5′-cyclic monophosphate: a possible intracellular mediator of mitogenic influence in lymphocytes. Proc. Natl. Acad. Sci., 69:3024, 1972.

155. Tam, C.F., and Walford, R.L.: Alterations in cyclic nucleotides and cyclase-specific activities in T lymphocytes of ageing normal humans and patients with Down's syndrome. J. Immunol., 125:1665, 1980.

156. Mark, A.U., and Weksler, M.D.: Immunologic studies of ageing VIII: no change in cyclic nucleotide concentration in T lymphocytes from old humans despite their depressed proliferation response. J. Immunol., 129:2323, 1982.

157. Gutowski, J.K., Innes, J., Weksler, M.E., et al.: Induction of DNA synthesis in isolated nuclei by cytoplasmic factors. II. normal generation of cytoplasmic stimulatory factors by lymphocytes from aged humans with depressed proliferative responses. J. Immunol., 132:559, 1984.

158. Miller, R.A.: Immunodeficiency of ageing: Restorative effects of phorbol ester combined with calcium ionophore. J. Immunol., 137:805, 1986.

159. Miller, R.A., Jacobson, B., Weil, G., et al.: Diminished calcium influx in lectin-stimulated T cells from old mice. J. Cell. Phy., 132:337, 1987.

160. Hallgren, H.M., Buckley, C.E., Gilbertsen, V.A., et al.: Lymphocyte phytohemagglutinin responsiveness immunoglobulins and autoantibodies ageing humans. J. Immunol., 111:1101, 1973.

161. Somers, H., and Kuhns, W.: Blood group antibodies in old age. Proc. Soc. Exp. Biol. Med., 141,1104, 1975.

162. Becker, M.J., et al.: Cell-mediated cytotoxicity in humans: age-related decline as measured by xenogeneic assay. Clin. Immunol. Immunopathol., 14:204, 1979.

163. Zahary, D., and Klinman, N.R.: Antigen responsiveness of the mature and generative B cell population of aged mice. J. Exp. Med., 157:1300, 1983.

164. Zahary, D., and Klinman, N.R.: The effects of ageing on murine B cell responsiveness. In: *Ageing and the Immune Response*. Ed. E.A. Goidl. New York, Marcel Dekker, 1987.

165. Axelsson, U., Bachman, R., and Hallen, J.: Frequency of pathological proteins (M-components) on 6995 sera from an adult population. Acta. Med. Scand., *179*:235, 1966.

166. Crawford Eye, M.R., and Cohen, H.J.: Evaluation of monoclonal gammaopathies in the "well" elderly. Am. J. Med., *82*:39, 1987.

167. Kyle, R.A., and Garton, J.P.: The spectrum of IgM monoclonal gammopathy in 430 cases. Mayo. Clin. proc., *62*:719, 1987.

168. Cammarata, R.J., Rodman, G.P., and Fennell, R.H.: Serum antigammaglobulin and antinuclear factors in the aged. JAMA, *199*:456, 1967.

169. McKay, I.R.: Ageing and immunological functions in man. Gerontology, *18*:285, 1972.

170. Koopman, W.J., and Schrohenloher, R.E.: In vitro synthesis of IgM RF by lymphocytes from healthy adults. J. Immunol., *125*:934, 1988.

171. Good, R.A., and Yunis, E.: Association of autoimmunity immunodeficiency and ageing in man, rabbits and mice. Fed. Proc., *33*:2040, 1974.

172. Smith, J.B., and Talal, N.: Significance of self-recognition and Interleukin-2 for immunoregulation, autoimmunity and cancer. Scand. J. Immunol., *16*:269, 1982.

173. Fernandez, L.A., and MacSween, J.M.: Decreased autologous mixed lymphocyte reaction with ageing. Mech. Age. Dev., *12*:245, 1980.

174. Smith, J.B., Wolos, J.A., and Bocchieri, M.H.: Mechanisms of help and suppression in the AMLR: Studies in normal and NZB mice. Behring. Inst. Mitteil., *72*:37, 1983.

175. Hom, J.T., and Talal, N.: Decreased syngeneic mixed lymphocyte response in autoimmune susceptible mice. Scand. J. Immunol., *15*:195, 1982.

176. Bocchieri, M.H., and Smith, J.B.: Detection of autologous mixed lymphocyte reaction responding cells and their precursor frequency in NZB mice. Cell. Immunol., *74*:345, 1982.

177. Johnson, R.C., and Wang, A.C.: DNA repair, antibody diversity, and ageing. Gerontology, *31*:203, 1985.

178. Szewczuk, M.R., and Campbell, R.J.: Loss of immune competence with age may be due to auto-anti-idiotypic antibody regulation. Nature (Land). *286*:164, 1980.

179. Kay, M.M.B., Bosman, G., Notter, M., et al.: Life and death of neurons: The role of senescent cell antigen. Ann. N.Y. Acad. Sci., *521*:155, 1988.

180. Reif, A.E., and Allen, J.M.V.: The AKR thymic antigen and its distribution in leukemias and nervous tissues. J. Exp. Med., *120*:413, 1964.

181. Endo, T., et al.: Antibodies to glycosphingolipids in patients with multiple sclerosis. Ann. N.Y. Acad. Sci., *436*:213, 1984.

182. Endo, T., et al.: Antibodies to glycosphingolipids in patients with multiple sclerosis and SLE. J. Immunol., *132*:1793, 1984.

183. Asherson, R.A., et al.: Recurrent stroke and multi-infarct dementia in systemic lupus erythematosus: association with antiphospholipid antibodies. Ann. Rheum. Dis., *46*:605, 1987.

184. Harris, E.N., et al.: Cerebral infarction in systemic lupus: association with anticardiolipin antibodies. Clin. Exp. Rheum., *2*:47, 1984.

185. Harris, E.N., et al.: Lupoid sclerosis: a possible pathogenetic role for antiphospholipid antibodies. Ann. Rheum. Dis., *44*:281, 1985.

186. Harris, E.N.: Antiphospholipid antibodies in acute Guillain-Barre syndrome. Lancet, *2*:1361, 1983.

187. Oppenheimer, S., and Hoffbrand, B.I.: Optic neuritis and myelopathy in systemic lupus erythematosus. Can. J. Neurol. Sci., *13*:129, 1986.

188. Asherson, R.A., et al.: Chorea in systemic lupus and lupus-like disease. Association with antiphospholipid antibodies. Arth. Rheum., *29*:S95, 1986.

189. Offner, H., and Konat, G.: Stimulation of active E-rosette forming lymphocytes from multiple sclerosis patients by gangliosides and cerebrosides. J. Neurol. Sci., *46*:101, 1980.

190. Offner, H., Konat, G., and Sela, B.: Multi-sialo brain gangliosides are powerful stimulators of active E-rosetting lymphocytes from multiple sclerosis patients. J. Neurol. Sci., *52*:279, 1981.

191. Lyas, A.A., and Davidson, A.N.: Cellular hypersensitivity to gangliosides and myelin basic protein in multiple sclerosis. J. Neurol. Sci., *59*:85, 1983.

192. Linthicum, D.S., and Frelinger, J.A.: Acute autoimmune encephalonigelifis in mice. J. Exp. Med., *155*:31, 1982.

193. Doherty, P., and Simpson, E.: Murine models of multiple sclerosis. Nature, *299*:106, 1982.

194. Fierz, W., et al.: Astrocytes as antigen-presenting cells. I. Induction of Ia antigen expression on astrocytes by T cells via immune interferon and its effect on antigen presentation. J. Immunol., *134*:3785, 1985.

195. Wong, G.H.W., et al.: Inducible expression of H-2 and Ia antigens on brain cells. Nature, *310*:688, 1984.

196. Pelver, M. Carrel, S. Mach, J.P., et al.: Cultured human fetal astrocytes can be induced by gamma interferon to express HLA-DR. J. Neuroimmunol., *14*:123, 1987.

197. Carrel, S, deTribolet, A., and Gross, N.: Expression of HLA-DR and common acute lymphoblastic leukemia antigens on glioma cells. Eur. J. Immunol., *12*:354, 1982.

198. Piguet, V., et al.: Heterogeneity of the induction of HLA-DR expression by human immune interferon on glioma cell lines and their clones. J. Natl. Cancer Inst. *76*:223, 1986.

199. Ling, P.D., Warren, M.K., and Vogel, S.N.: Antaginistic effect of interferon beta on interferon gamma induced expression of Ia antigen in murine macrophages. J. Immunol., *135*:1857, 1985.

200. Inaba, K., et al.: Contrasting effect of alpha/beta and gamma interferon on expression of macrophage Ia antigens. J. Exp. Med., *163*:1030, 1986.

201. Joseph, J., Knobler, R.L., D'Imperio, C., et al.: Down-regulation of interferon g-induced class II expression on human glioma cells by recombinant interferon-B effects of dosage treatment schedule. J. Neuroimmunol, *20*:39, 1988.

202. Siram, S., and Steinman, L.: Anti-IA antibody suppresses active encephalomyelitis: Treatment model for diseases linked to IR genes. J. Exp. Med., *158*:1362, 1983.

203. Nagai, M., Arai, T., Kohno, S., et al.: Local application of interferon to malignant brain tumors. Tex. Rep. Biol. Med., *41*:693, 1981.

204. Duff, T.A., et al.: Phase II trial of interferon beta for treatment of recurrent glioblastoma multiforme. J. Neurosurg., *64*:408, 1986.

205. Greenstein, J.I., et al.: A phase I clinical trial of

human recombinant beta interferon in relapsing-remitting multiple sclerosis. J. Neuroimmunol., 7:121, 1987.

206. Traugott, U., Reinherz, E.L., and Raine, C.S.: Multiple sclerosis-distribution of T cells, T cell subsets and Ia-positive macrophages in lesions of different ages. J. Neuroimmunol., 4:201, 1983.

207. Hauser, S.L., et al.: Immunohistochemical staining of human brain with monoclonal antibodies that identify lymphocytes, monocytes, and the Ia antigen. J. Neuroimmunol., 5:197, 1983.

208. Fontana, A., et al.: Production of prostaglandin E and interleukin 1-like factors by cultures of astrocytes and C-6 glioma cells. J. Immunol., 129:2413, 1982.

209. Fontana, A., et al.: Glioblastoma cells release interleukin 1 and factors inhibiting interleukin 2 mediated effects. J. Immunol., 132:1837, 1984.

210. Kruegar, J.M., et al.: Sleep promoting effects of endogenous pyrogen (Interleukin 1). Am. J. Physiol., 246:994, 1984.

211. Dinarello, C.A., et al.: The influence of lipoxygenase inhibitors on the in vitro production of human leukocytic pyrogen and lymphocyte activating factor (interleukin 1). Int. J. Immunopharmacol., 6:43, 1984.

212. Turchik, J.B., and Bornstein, D.L.: Role of the central nervous system in acute phase responses to leukocytic pyrogen. Infect. Immun., 30:439, 1980.

213. Breder, C.D., Dinarello, C.A., and Saper, C.B.: Interleukin-1 immunoreactive innovation of the human hypothalmus. Science, 240:321, 1988.

214. Bernton, E.W., et al.: Release of multiple hormones by a direct action of interleukin 1 on pituitary cells. Science, 238:519, 1987.

215. Le, J., and Vilcek, J.: Tumor necrosis factor and interleukin-1: cytokines with multiple overlapping biological activities. Lab. Invest., 56:234, 1987.

216. Soham, S., et al.: Recombinant tumor necrosis factor and interleukin-1 enhance slow wave sleep. Am. J. Physiol., 253:R142, 1987.

217. Robbins, D.S., et al.: Production of cytotoxic factor for oligiodendrosytes by stimulated ostrocytes. J. Immunol., 139:2593, 1987.

218. Fontana, A., et al.: Glia cell stimulating factor (GSF): a new lymphokine. Part 1. Cellular sources and partial purification of murine GSF, role of cytoskeleton and protein synthesis in its production. J Neuroimmunol., 2:71, 1982.

219. Gozes, Y., Muskowitz, M.A., Strom, T.B., et al.: Conditioned media from activated lymphocytes maintain sympathetic neurons in culture. Div. Brain Res., 6:97, 1983.

220. Saleun, J.P., Vicariot, M., Deroff, P., et al.: Monoclonal gammapathies in the adult population of Finistere France. J. Clin. Pathol., 35:63, 1982.

221. Latov, N.: Waldenstrom's macroglobulinemia and nonmalignant IgM monoclonal gammapathies. In: Polyneuropathies Associated with Plasma Cell Dyscrasia. (Eds.) J.J. Kell, R.A. Kyle, and N. Latov. Boston, Martinus Nijhoff Publishing, 1987.

222. Kelly, Jr., J.J.: Epidemiology of polyneuropathies associated with plasma cell dyscrasias. In: Polyneuropathies Associated with Plasma Cell Dyscrasias, (Eds.) J.J. Kelly, R.A. Kyle Jr., and N. Latov. Boston, Martinus Nijhoff Publishers, 1987.

223. Latov, N., et al.: Plasma cell dyscrasia and peripheral neuropathy: Identification of the myelin antigens that react with the human paraproteins. Proc. Natl. Acad. Sci. (USA), 78:7139, 1981.

224. Nobile-Orazio, E., et al.: Specificity of mouse and human monoclonal antibodies to myelin associated glycoprotein. Neurology, 34:1336, 1984.

225. Ilyas, A.A., et al.: Igm in a human neuropathy related to paraproteinemia binds to a carbohydrate determinant in the mylein associated glycoprotein and to a ganglioside. Proc. Natl. Acad. Sci. (USA), 81:1225, 1984.

226. Hafler, D.A., et al.: Monoclonal gammapathy and neuropathy: myelin associated glycoprotein reactivity and clinical characteristics. Neurology, 36:75, 1986.

227. Takatsu, M., et al.: Immunofluorescence study of patients with neuropathy and IgM M proteins. Ann. Neurol., 18:173, 1985.

228. Mendell, J.R., et al.: Polyneuropathy and IgM monoclonal gammapathy: studies on the pathogenetic role of antimyelin associated glycoprotein antibody. Ann. Neurol., 17:243, 1985.

229. Krieger, C., and Melmed, K.: A cure of amyotrophic lateral sclerosis and paraproteinemia. Neurology, 32:896, 1982.

230. Steck, A.J., et al.: Demyelinating neuropathy and monoclonal IgM antibody to myelin associated glycoprotein. Neurology, 33:19, 1983.

231. Steffanson, K., et al.: Neuropathy accompanying IgM plasma cell dyscrasia. Acta. Neuropath. (Berl) 59:255, 1983.

232. Nemni, R.G., et al.: Polyneuropathy in nonmalignant IgM plasma cell dyscrasia: a morphological study. Ann. Neurol., 14:43, 1983.

233. Sherman, W.H., et al.: Monoclonal IgM,k antibody precipitating with chondroitin sulfate C from patients with axonal polyneuropathy and epidermolysis. Neurology (NY) 33:192, 1984.

234. Hays, A.P., Latov, N., Takatsu, M., et al.: Experimental dymyelination of nerve induced by serum of patients with neuropathy and an anti MAG IsgMM protein. Ann. Neurol., (In press) 1989.

235. Kyle, R.A.: Osteosclerotic myeloma. In: Polyneuropathies Associated with Plasma Cell Dyscrasias. (Eds.) J.J. Kelly, R.A. Kyle, and N.Latov. Boston, Martinus Nijhoff Publishers, 1987.

236. Bardwick, P.A., et al.: Plasma cell dyscrasia with polyneuropathy, organomegaly, endocrinopathy, M protein and skin changes the POEMS syndrome: report on two cases and a review of the literature. Medicine, 59:311, 1980.

237. Nakonishi, T., et al.: The Crow Fukase syndrome: a study of 102 cases in Japan. Neurol., 34:712, 1984.

238. Meier, C., et al.: Polyneuropathy in Waldenstrom's macroglobulinemia: reduction of endoneurial IgM deposits after treatment with chlorambucil and plasmapheresis. Acta Neuropathol. (Berl), 64:297, 1984.

239. Reulecke, M., Dumas, M., and Meier, C.: Specific antibody activity against neuroendocrine tissue in a case of POEMS syndrome with IgG gammapathy. Neurology, 38:614, 1988.

240. Shy, M.E., et al.: Motor neuron disease and plasma cell dyscrasia. Neurology, 36:1429, 1986.

241. Freddo, L., et al.: Gangliosides GM1 and GD1b are antigens for IgM M proteins in a patient with motor neuron disease. Neurology, 36:454, 1986.

242. Nardelli, E., et al.: Neuropathy and monoclonal IgM M protein with antibody activity against gangliosides. J. Neuroimmunol., 16:132, 1987.

243. Shy, M.E., et al.: Antibodies to GM1 and GD1b in patients with motor neuron disease without plasma cell dyscrasia. Ann. Neurol., 25:511, 1989.

244. Pestronk, A., et al.: A treatable chronic multifocal polyneuropathy associated with antibodies to a defined neural antigen. Ann. Neurol., 22:119A, 1987.

245. Pestronk, A., et al.: Multifocal motor neuropathy: Clinical features of patients with anti GM1 ganglioside antibodies. Neurol., 38:(1), 251, 1988.

246. Goodman, B.W.: Temporal arteritis. Am. J. Med., 77:839, 1979.

247. Chuang, T.Y., Hunder, G.G., Ilstrup, D.M., et al.: Polymyalgia rheumatica. A 10 year epidemiologic and clinical study. Ann. Intern. Med., 97:672, 1982.

248. Banker, B.Q.: Other inflammatory myopathies. In: Myology. (Eds.) A.G. Engel, and B.Q. Banker. New York, McGraw-Hill, 1986.

249. Lisak, R.P.: Neurologic manifestations of collagen vascular disease. In: Diseases of the Nervous System: Clinical Neurobiology. (Eds.) A.K. Asbury, G.M. Mckhann, and W.I. McDonald. Philadelphia, W.B. Saunders Co., 1986.

250. Banker, B.Q., Engel, A.G.: The polymyositis and dermatomyositis syndromes. In: Myology. (Eds.) A.G. Engel and B.Q. Banker. New York, McGraw-Hill, 1986.

251. Mastaglia, F.L., and Ojeda, V.J.: Inflammatory Myopathies: Part One. Ann. Neurol., 17:215, 1985.

252. Mastaglia, F.L., and Ojeda, V.J.: Inflammatory Myopathies: Part Two. Ann. Neurol., 17:317, 1985.

253. Morgan Hughes, J.A.: Diseases of striated muscle. In: Diseases of the Nervous System: Clinical Neurobiology. (Eds.) A.K. Asbury, G.M. McKhann, and W.I McDonald. Philadelphia, W.B. Saunders Co., 1986.

254. Kimura, J.: Electrodiagnosis in Diseases of the Nerve and Muscle: Principles and Practice. Philadelphia, F.A. Davis Co., 1983.

255. Arahata, K., and Engel, A.G.: Monoclonal antibody analysis of mononuclear cells in myopathies. V: Identification and quantitation of T8+ suppressor cells. Ann. Neurol., 23:493, 1988.

256. Henson, R.A.: Neurologic manifestations of paraneoplastic disorders. In: Diseases of the Nervous System: Clinical Neurobiology. (Eds.) A.K. Asbury, G.M. McKhann, and W.I. McDonald. Philadelphia, W.B. Saunders Co., 1986.

257. Kernohan, J.W., and Woltman, H.W.: Periarteritis nodosa: a clinico pathologic study with special reference to the nervous system. Arch. Neurol., 139:655, 1983.

258. Schaumberg, H.H., Spencer, P.S., Thomas, P.K., (eds.): Disorders of Peripheral Nerve. Philadelphia, F.A. Davis Co., 1983.

259. Eames, R.A., and Lange, L.S.: Clinical and pathological study of ischemic neuropathy. J. Neurol., Neurosurg, Psychiatry, 30:215, 1967.

260. Lisak, R.P., et al.: Guillain Barre syndrome and Hodgkin's disease, three cases with immunological studies. Ann. Neurol., 1:72, 1977.

261. Henson, R.A., and Urich, H.: Cancer and the Nervous System. Oxford, Blackwell Scientific Publications, 1982.

262. Asbury, A.K.: Disorders of peripheral nerve. In: Diseases of the Nervous System: Clinical Neurobiology. (Eds.) A.K. Asbury, G.M. McKhann, and W.I. McDonald. Philadelphia, W.B. Saunders Co., 1986.

263. Anderson, N.E., et al.: Autoantibodies in paraneoplastic syndromes associated with small cell carcinoma. Neurology, 38:1391, 1988.

264. Cunningham, F., Grais, F., Anderson, N., et al.: Partial characterization of the Purkinje cell antigens in paraneoplastic cerebellar degeneration. Neurology, 36:1163, 1986.

265. Thomas, C., Zengerling, W., and Noetzzel, H.: Neurologische Formen. Paraneoplastichen Syndromes, Stuttgart, F.K. Schattauer, 1972.

266. Drachman, D.B.: Pathophysiology of the neuromuscular junction. In: Diseases of the Nervous System: Clinical Neurobiology. (Eds.) A.K. Asbury, G.M. McKhann, and W.I. McDonald. Philadelphia, W.B. Saunders Co., 1986.

267. Kim, Y.I., and Neher, E.: IgG from patients with Lambert Eaton syndrome blocks voltage dependent calcium channels. Science, 239:405, 1988.

268. Newsom Davis, J.: Diseases of the neuromuscular junction. In: Diseases of the Nervous System. (Eds.) A.K. Asbury, G.M. McKhann, and W.I. McDonald. Philadelphia, W.B. Saunders Co., 1986.

269. Lang, B., et al.: Autoimmune etiology for myasthenic (Eaton Lambert) syndrome. Lancet, 2:224, 1981.

270. Willcox, M., et al.: Increased frequency of IgG heavy chain marker Glm (2) and of HLA B8 in Lambert Eaton myasthenic syndrome with and without associated lung carcinoma. Hum. Immunol., 14:29, 1985.

271. Arnason, B.G.W., Antel, J.P., and Reder, A.T.: Immunoregulation in multiple sclerosis. Ann. New York Acad. Sci., 436:133, 1984.

272. Raine, C.S., and Traugott, U.: Experimental autoimmune demyelination, chronic relapsing models and their therapeutic implications for multiple sclerosis. Ann New York Acad. Sci., 426:33, 1984.

273. Lublin, F.D., Mauer, P.H., Berry, R.G., et al.: Delayed relapsing experimental allergic encephalomyelitis in mice. J. Immunol., 126(3):819, 1981.

274. Noseworthy, J., et al.: Multiple sclerosis under the age of 50. Neurology, 33:1537, 1983.

275. Engel, A.G.: Acquired autoimmune myasthenia gravis. In: Myology. (Eds.) A.G. Engel, and B.Q. Banker. New York, McGraw-Hill, 1986.

276. Fambrough, D., Brachman, D.B., and Satyamurti, S.: Neuromuscular junction in myasthenia gravis. Decreased acetylcholine receptors. Science, 182:293, 1973.

277. Roitt, I., Brosteff, J., and Male, D.: Cells involved in the immune response. In: Immunology. (Eds.) I. Roitt, J. Brosteff, and D. Male. St. Louis, C.V. Mosby Co., 1985.

278. Lindstrom, J.M., et al.: Antibody to acetylcholine receptor in myasthenia gravis. Prevalence, clinical correlates and diagnostic value. Neurology, 26:1054, 1976.

279. Toyka, K.V., et al.: Myasthenia gravis; study of humoral immune mechanisms by passive transfer to mice. N. Engl. J. Med., 296:125, 1977.

280. Lefvert, A.K., and Osterman, P.O.: Newborn infants to myasthenic mothers: A clinical study and an investigation of acetyl choline receptor antibodies in 17 children. Neurology, 33:133, 1983.

281. Engel, A.G. Morphologic and immunopathologic findings in myasthenia gravis and in congenital myasthenic syndromes. J. Neurol., Neurosurg., Psychiat., 43:577, 1980.

282. Simpson, J.A.: Myasthenia gravis: a new hypothesis. Scot. Med. J., 5:419, 1960.

283. Patrick, J., and Lindstrom, J.M.: Autoimmune response to acetylcholine receptor. Science, 180:871, 1973.

12

Demyelinating Disorders of the Aged Brain

ROBERT L. KNOBLER

Among the many changes that occur with the normal process of aging are changes within the nervous system. These changes are those which are widely recognized to contribute to a measurable slowing of reaction time. Despite the accumulation of wisdom with age and experiences over the passage of time, it is now widely recognized that there is an irreversible and progressive decline in neuronal cell numbers in different regions of the central nervous system and peripheral ganglia, as well as loss of arborization of the neuronal dendritic tree. There is also slowing of the conduction of nerve impulses and an increase in synaptic delay.

The present chapter will focus on diseases of the aging myelinated fiber pathways of the white matter of the central nervous system, demyelinating diseases more commonly seen with aging. Although it is well recognized that diseases which affect the myelinated fibers of the central nervous system are more common in younger individuals, it is clear that both clinical and pathologic evidence documents

the presence of demyelination as the underlying lesion in a variety of conditions which present in adulthood. As a result of this emphasis, the more common demyelinating diseases in younger individuals, such as multiple sclerosis and the dysmyelinating syndromes, will only be briefly discussed.

Rather than reflecting the universal occurrence of neuronal cell dropout with aging and secondary loss of myelinated fiber pathways as the principal source of these changes, the focus in this chapter is on those pathologic processes that increase the specific involvement of the white matter with age. Despite this emphasis, it will be recognized that some of the processes that lead to clinical disease of the white matter in the older or aging individual may have actually started earlier in their lifetime without becoming symptomatic until later in life. There are at least three concepts to keep in mind to help explain this phenomenon [Table 12–1].

The first concept is related to the "safety factor" inherent in the normal functioning of the

TABLE 12-1.   Reasons for the Late Appearance of Symptoms and Signs

Lesion size overcomes redundancy within individual myelinated central nervous system pathways (safety factor).
Time course of lesion onset is slowly progressive.
Lesion size overcomes redundancy of multiple nervous system pathways mediating integrated functions.

nervous system. In this context, the "safety factor" is not referred to in its axon physiology sense,[1] which regards axonal properties important in nerve conduction, but instead, the reserve built into the organization of each neural pathway. This reserve is in large part due to redundancy in the number of fibers and connections mediating the neural function of the particular pathway. The degree of redundancy is variable for different pathways and in different individuals. Because there are more functioning fibers than the minimum required to mediate the principal neural activity of a given pathway, a percentage of the pathway can be rendered nonfunctional before recognizable neurologic symptoms or signs become apparent.

In this way, a person could theoretically remain clinically asymptomatic until perhaps 80% of a particular pathway became pathologically altered. At this time symptoms would then occur. The symptoms would be progressively worse depending on how much more than 80% loss was present. Related issues for "myelinated fibers" are that there may be fluctuations in function of the remaining fibers depending upon their state of myelination (for example, thinly remyelinated fibers may decompensate in function more readily with increasing body temperature,[2] as after physical activity, in febrile states or high ambient temperatures) or other metabolic conditions which may alter the functioning of the remaining neurons supplying the affected pathway.

The second concept is related to the time course of symptom development. A slowly progressive process may take a long time to involve enough fibers to lead to the appearance of neurologic symptoms. In this way, much of a lifetime may go by before the patient becomes symptomatic. There are genetically determined factors that may play a role in influencing the developmental expression of gene products. In this way damage occurs "developmentally", at a timepoint when the required but defective gene product is needed. Alternatively, damage may occur because of the slow accumulation of toxic products as a result of a genetically defective product necessary for its clearance. In contrast, a rapidly expanding mass, a hemorrhage or even the edema associated with an inflammatory cell infiltrate may produce devastating functional deficits rapidly because of the way in which these processes may disrupt the normal cytoarchitecture of the myelinated fibers. This in part accounts for the recognized clinical effectiveness of steroid hormone therapies when they are therapeutically administered to treat the edema associated with brain tumors and inflammatory demyelinating conditions.

The third concept is related to the normal role of the myelinated fiber [Table 12-2A], and how it is modified from its normal function by demyelinating diseases [Table 12-2B]. Regardless of the neural pathway in question, the myelinated fiber serves three functions. These are to promote speed of impulse transmission, to enhance capacity for repetitive impulse transmission over a given time period, and for conservation of the energy of nerve impulse transmission.[3] The integration of these nerve impulses into patterns which we recognize as behavior (through such physiologic events as spatial and temporal summation) is contingent upon the ability for myelinated nerve fibers to repetitively discharge within a defined frame-

TABLE 12-2A.   Functions of the Myelin Sheath

Rapid nerve impulse conduction (saltatory conduction).
Facilitate repetitive impulse conduction.
Conserve energy required for nerve impulse conduction.

TABLE 12-2B.   Myelin Physiology— Considerations in Axon Function

Saltatory conduction—nodes of Ranvier.
 Relationship between axon diameter, internode length and speed of the nerve impulse.
 The energy requirement of conducting a nerve impulse.
 Temperature dependence of impulse conduction.
Sodium/Potassium channel distribution.
 Sodium channels at the node of Ranvier.
 Potassium channels at the paranodal region.
Conduction block—potassium channel redistribution, extending to the node.

work of time. When myelinated nerve fibers are lost or compromised functionally, these patterns become disrupted, and the normally orchestrated ebb and flow of neural impulses is reduced to a meaningless cacophony of neuroelectric noise. Because multiple systems may contribute to the execution of a behavior, there is a "plasticity" by which one of the remaining intact systems may continue to maintain the behavior while some function of the affected pathway remains intact. When this plasticity becomes overtaxed by virtue of a greater loss of the affected pathway, symptoms may then become apparent.

In this context, it is not simply the nerve impulse that is lost, but it is also the higher order processing of integrated nerve impulses that becomes affected. Such a loss is only recognizable as neurologic symptoms or signs when the lesion size in the specific anatomic pathways affected exceeds the "safety factor," or reserve of the integrated neurologic function being evaluated. Alternatively, because myelin loss affects the speed and repetitiveness of nerve impulse transmission, such loss may be manifested as a disruption of the "timing" of arrival of neural impulses. Since there are accumulative effects, culminating in a "go" or "no go" firing signal of a target cell, which are based upon the timing of the arrival of input nerve impulses at this target cell, alterations of the timing of signal transmission can completely disrupt normal neural transmission.

In the present chapter, I will review some of the principles of normal development and maintenance of the cells and structures of the white matter, and then indicate a variety of pathologic processes that have been documented to affect these structures, with specific emphasis to the aged population.

MYELIN DEVELOPMENT AND MAINTENANCE

The white matter is named for its glistening white appearance on fresh cut sections of whole brain. Its white appearance is contrasted to the gray of the collections of nerve cell bodies that comprises the cortices of the cerebral and cerebellar hemispheres, as well as the deep collections of nerve cell bodies (nuclei) of the basal ganglia, the brainstem nuclei

and the gray matter of the spinal cord. The term myelin is derived from the Greek root for marrow, a descriptive term originally applied because of the appearance of the marrow-like appearance of the most externally located white matter fiber pathways of the spinal cord within the spinal column.

MYELIN FORMING CELLS

Oligodendrocytes are the myelin forming and maintaining cells of the central nervous system. Their name was originally derived from their appearance in light microscopic preparations, as a cell (cyte) with few (oligo) branches (dendro). Subsequent studies have estimated that a single oligodendrocyte has between 5 and 50 connections to central myelin sheaths established during development,[4] but despite this, the original name has remained. The oligodendrocyte is histologically defined by its connection to the myelin sheath, although antibodies to oligodendrocyte specific molecules have allowed immunocytochemical definition in recent years and characterization of the stages of development of this cell type.[5] The myelin sheath, a concentric arrangement of thick major dense lines and thinner intraperiod lines, is derived from modified cell membranes of the oligodendrocyte.[4] The major dense line morphologically represents the outermost portions (external surface) of the oligodendrocyte membranes, while the intraperiod line represents the apposition of the innermost (cytoplasmic surfaces) of the oligodendrocyte membranes.[6]

Each myelin sheath segment formed by a myelin forming cell is referred to as an internode, because it is bounded on either end by a node of Ranvier. Each node occurs between segments of the myelin sheath aligned along the length of a single nerve fiber at which the nerve impulse is propagated. This arrangement allows the nerve impulse to travel down the length of the nerve fiber by saltatory (to jump) conduction [Table 12–2B]. There is a specific and directly proportional arrangement between the diameter of the nerve fiber and both the thickness of the myelin sheath and the length of the internode.[7,8] In this way, larger diameter nerve fibers have thicker sheaths and longer internodes. This facilitates most rapid impulse conduction along the largest fibers. In remyelination, it is unlikely that either the same thickness or length of the original internode will be reproduced, although the remyelinated segment greatly improves function when compared to the demyelinated segment.[3,6,9,10]

A related issue is the redistribution of sodium and potassium channels at the node of Ranvier. Normally, a highly simplistic view is that the nodal area is rich in conduction facilitating sodium channels, while the paranodal region is rich in conduction blocking potassium channels. During demyelination, there is believed to be spread of the potassium channel rich paranodal area over the normally sodium channel bearing area.[3,11] This redistribution is thought to resolve coincidently with the return of conduction along the length of the nerve fiber, leaving a more normal distribution of sodium channels at the nodal-like structure present.

The multiple sheaths formed by a single oligodendrocyte are ususally intermingled with those sheaths made by nearby oligodendrocytes. In this way, loss of a single oligodendrocyte may affect more than a single pathway alone. Adjacent compacted central myelin sheaths usually abut upon one another, without an intervening basal lamina or much visible oligodendrocyte cytoplasm. The only location in which oligodendrocyte cytoplasm is regularly observed in association with the compact myelin sheath is at the paranodal region, the site adjacent to the node of Ranvier.[4] Interestingly, this is frequently found to be a site at which stripping away of myelin by macrophages occurs in a variety of pathologic states.

In the immature central nervous system oligodendrocyte cytoplasm retained within the lamellae of the myelin sheath (the cleft of Schmidt-Lantermann), and connections between the oligodendrocyte and the mature myelin sheath may be observed. However, under pathologic circumstances, clefts of Schmidt-Lantermann and connections between the oligodendrocyte and the myelin sheaths may be observed even within the mature nervous system. The latter is considered direct evidence that oligodendrocytes can re-

myelinate central axons that have been demyelinated.[12]

In some instances, however, it is the myelin forming cell of the peripheral nervous system, the Schwann cell,[13] that remyelinates central axons. This occurs primarily in the vicinity of root entry and exit zones. The Schwann cell, in contrast to the oligodendrocyte, forms only one internode of mature myelin, and is surrounded by a basal lamina. These morphologic features allow this cell type to be identified in sections of central nervous sytem tissue they have invaded.[4]

MYELINOGENIC CYCLES

Myelination of central nervous system pathways does not occur at the same time for each pathway.[14] In fact, myelination continues into the late teens and early twenties for some of the pathways in the cerebral hemispheres. In contrast, those pathways of the vestibulospinal system and corticospinal tracts, pathways stimulated by, as well as essential for the earliest coordinated movements, are among the first to become myelinated. It is the myelination of these spinal cord pathways that correlates with the ability to refine motor movements to the point of initiating patterns of walking movements in late infancy.[15] Of note, myelin is formed earlier and more abundantly in females than males. This correlates with an earlier capacity of females for finer motor skills as compared to males, and has been attributed to hormonal effects such as exposure to estrogens.[16,17] There is a slightly larger diameter to the nerves of females,[18] which considering the observations of Duncan and Murray[7,8] on the proportional increase in myelination with increased axonal diameter may have a bearing on increased myelination in females as well. However, the reasons for these anatomic and physiologic differences between the sexes remain poorly understood at the present time.

Developmental Changes. Tissue culture parallels between myelin markers being expressed and developmental changes in the intact animal have been well documented.[5] Of particular relevance are the studies that show a dependence on the correct milieu to provide a permissive environment for the development of these cells. An intact thyroid axis during myelinogenesis is one such requirement for normal myelination.[19] A permissive role for insulin and insulin-like growth factor (IGF) during myelinogenesis and remyelination has also been shown.[20] In contrast, there is the suggestion that the lymphokine interleukin-2 (IL-2), a product of stimulated helper lymphocytes, may restrict the proliferation of oligodendrocyte progenitor cells in a defined-medium system in tissue culture.[21] The in vivo implication of this observation would be limited remyelination in the presence of IL-2, such as in the presence of helper lymphocyte infiltration, and the possibility that this molecule may also function in negative regulation of the proliferation of oligodendroctye precursors during normal development. Tissue culture data in a serum containing medium (a far more variable milieu than defined medium) have been presented suggesting that IL-2 may stimulate proliferation of oligodendrocyte progenitor cells,[22] so that further work on the specific role, if any, of IL-2 in this system is needed. Finally, there is the suggestion that antibodies directed against spinal cord antigens may have a stimulatory effect on the proliferation of oligodendrocyte precursor cells.[23] A possible explanation would be increased expression of a specific determinant on oligodendrocyte progenitor cells at this stage of development to which this antibody binds and then stimulates proliferation or differentiation (myelin formation) of these cells.

The significance in developmental changes lies both in their dependency on exogenous substances in a permissive role as well as the re-emergence in expression of molecules present initially only during development. The implications of in vitro studies to date suggest that successful remyelination will require the correct milieu.[20,21] The expression of marker molecules previously present only during earlier stages of development suggests a role as receptors for specific molecules required for progenitor proliferation. Re-expression of such markers may render these precursor cells more vulnerable, in that these markers may serve as receptors for viruses or targets for immune-mediated attack. This will likely prove to be a fertile area for future investigation.

MYELIN CHEMISTRY

Molecular Organization of Myelin Membrane. Myelin was one of the first substances studied ultrastructurally, because of its ready availability and unusual but highly recognizable structure. It soon became apparent that myelin was an extension of the cell membrane of the myelin-forming cell that spiraled around the ensheathed nerve fiber.[24] The recognition of the fluid mosaic nature of cell membranes,[25] and that varied proteins existed in different membranes as structural elements and receptors, led to a greater understanding of how myelin could be of different chemical composition than the oligodendrocyte or Schwann cell membrane, although originating as an extension of their membranes and cytoplasm. Furthermore, in contrast to the chemical composition of the cell membrane of most other cells of the body, myelin is approximately 70% lipid and 30% protein, and contains several unqiue lipid and protein molecules in the central [Table 12-3A], and peripheral nervous systems [Table 12-3B]. The unique nature of this composition provides a means for differentiating myelin from other cell membranes biochemically and immunologically, and a means for better understanding both the pathogenesis of immune-mediated myelin disorders, and the genetic basis of inherited disorders of myelin composition [dysmyelination syndromes, Tables 12-4A and 12-4B]. Ironically, although myelin basic protein has been identified as the principal antigen toward which the immune system can be

TABLE 12-3A. Myelin Composition: Major CNS Components*

CNS Structural Proteins
  Proteolipid protein (PLP)
  Myelin basic protein (MBP): 18.5K, 14K, 17K, and
    21.5K forms
  Myelin associated glycoprotein (MAG)
CNS enzymatic protein
  Wolfgram protein: 2',3'-cyclic nucleotide 3'-
    phosphohydrolase (CNP)
  Carbonic anhydrase (CA)
Lipids
  Galactocerebroside
  Sulfatide
  Cholesterol
  Phospholipid

*Partial listing of central myelin components, with only the major constituents represented.

TABLE 12–3B.   Myelin Composition: Major PNS Components*

PNS Structural Proteins
  P_0 Protein: Major PNS structural protein, a glycoprotein
  P_1 Protein: Analogous to CNS 18.5K MBP
  P_r Protein: Analogous to CNS 14K MBP
  P_2 Protein: Unique PNS protein
  Myelin associated glycoprotein (MAG): Similar to CNS MAG
PNS enzymatic protein
  Wolfgram protein: 2′,3′-cyclic nucleotide 3′-phosphohydrolase (CNP)
  Carbonic anhydrase (CA)
Lipids
  Galactocerebroside
  Sulfatide
  Cholesterol
  Phospholipid

*Partial listing of peripheral myelin components, with only the major constituents represented.

TABLE 12–4A.   Dysmyelinating Diseases (Hereditary Metabolic Diseases)

Adrenoleukodystrophies
Alexander's Disease (Dysmyelinogenic Leukodystrophy)
Canavan's Disease (Spongy Degeneration of the White Matter)
Hereditary Leukodystrophy of Adult-Onset
Krabbe's Disease (Globoid-cell Leukodystrophy)
Metachromatic Leukodystrophy (MLD)—Sulfatide Lipidosis
Pelizaeus-Merzbacher Disease (Sudanophilic Leukodystrophy)

TABLE 12–4B.   The Adrenoleukodystrophies (ALD)*—Adrenal Disease and Demyelination

Neonatal Form—Peroxisomal deficiency disorders.
  Neonatal ALD—Autosomal recessive.
  Dysmorphic features, hypotonia, seizures, psychomotor retardation.
Childhood Form—An X-linked ALD, most common and most severe.
  Attention deficit disorder, strabismus, seizures.
Adolescent Form—An X-linked ALD.
  Resembles childhood form except for later age of onset.
Adult Cerebral Form—An X-linked ALD.
  Schizophrenia-like psychosis, dementia, or cerebral deficit.
Adrenomyeloneuropathy (AMN)—An X-linked ALD, spastic paraparesis.
  With adrenal insufficiency disease.
  Without adrenal disease.
  ALD Heterozygous Women—minimal adrenal disease and mild AMN.
Addison's Disease Only—VLCFA storage in the absence of neurologic findings.

*Adapted from Hugo Moser. ALDs represent storage of very long chain fatty acids (VLCFA).

directed in experimental encephalomyelitis (EAE), it has been shown to be located internally, at the level of the cytoplasmic surfaces that fuse to form the major dense lines of the central myelin sheath. In contrast, proteolipid protein has been demonstrated to be located within the more hydrophobic, lipid-rich bilayer of the myelin membrane.

Molecular Genetics and Clinical Disorders of Myelin Metabolism.   In recent years, the genes for proteolipid protein and myelin basic protein have come to be identified and sequenced. Because of defects in the genes for these specific myelin components, the myelin sheath does not undergo its normal sequence of biochemical and morphologic development. The resulting defective development of the myelin sheath leads to clinical symptoms, and is identified as dysmyelination [Tables 12–4A and 12–4B].

There are mutant mouse models which have clinical syndromes virtually identical to human dysmyelinating diseases. For example, Pelizaeus-Merzbacher disease (sudanophilic leukodystrophy) is an X-linked human dysmyelinating disorder, which occurs exclusively in males. It is characterized by progressive deterioration in function in early childhood, which could include dementia, optic atrophy, tremor, progressive ataxia and spasticity. Children could survive for variable periods of time, with death usually the result of intercurrent infection. There is a related mouse model of an inherited disorder of proteolipid protein. This disease in the mouse is known as the Jimpy mutant. They are both X-linked recessively inherited disorders. Although a human counterpart has not yet been identified, another mutant that has been described in the mouse is due to a defect in the myelin basic protein gene, the Shiverer mutant. The Twitcher mutant reflects a defect in galactosylceramide beta-galactosidase, which gives rise to a clinical and pathologic picture identical to human Krabbe's disease, or globoid cell leukodystrophy. The availability of these and other dysmyelinating mutations in mice allows the study of both the molecular mechanisms of myelinogenesis as well as the development of approaches for the prevention or treatment of such disorders.

Nutritional and Endocrine Influences on Myelin Metabolism. Recognition of the need for nutritional cofactors and a specific hormonal milieu in the normal development and maintenance of the integrity of the myelin sheath has increased through the understanding of the underlying biochemistry and molecular biology of myelinogenesis. In this context, at least two specific examples come to mind. These are copper, as an essential element for normal myelination,[26] and normal levels of thyroid hormone,[19] particularly during myelination.

Immunogenicity. Immune mediated diseases leading to loss of myelin have been studied experimentally since the discovery of neurologic reactions to the injection of rabies vaccines consisting of a series of injections of infected dessicated rabbit spinal cord. More formal studies of this phenomenon were undertaken by Rivers, who injected whole spinal cord emulsion.[27,28] Subsequently, it was learned that myelin basic protein,[29] proteolipid protein[30] and galactocerebroside[31] could serve as the substrate for immune mediated reactivity. While cellular reactivity appears to be the principal response against the two proteins, humoral immunity plays the more important role in reactivity directed against galactocerebroside. It is now recognized that there are several myelin components which are potentially immunogenic [Table 12–5].

The concept of molecular mimicry is important in this context.[32] This reflects the possibility in which either the primary amino acid sequence, the secondary structural configuration of a molecule present in myelin, or both, are also found in a component of a pathogen. During an immune response to the pathogen, an immune response to the host antigen is also generated. In this fashion, a normal host immune response may give rise to autoimmune disease. Clinical examples of this phenomenon include autoimmune hemolytic anemia secondary to drugs, Chaga's disease, rheumatic fever, and Sydenham's chorea among others, at the present time. This group of diseases will likely be increased in years to come as greater understanding of the shared sequences in nature and human biology occurs.

A potentially related issue is associated with the established turnover of myelin components. In this context, establishment of a persistent infection of an oligodendrocyte with a non-lytic virus infection could theoretically influence the production of myelin components and thus their ability to serve as targets for "autoimmune disease," or to play a role in spontaneous demyelination. As with molecular mimicry, this possibility awaits further documentation. However, transgenic mice containing genetic elements of the JC virus will undergo spontaneous demyelination.[33] In contrast, other mice persistently infected with the mouse coronavirus MHV-A59 or MHV-4, undergo remyelination.[34,35]

DEMYELINATING DISEASES

The loss of an intact myelin sheath is known as demyelination. When this occurs following the loss of an axon, so that both the axon and its surrounding myelin sheath degenerate, the process is referred to as secondary demyelination. An example of this would be the loss of myelin which occurs during Wallerian degeneration. In contrast, when the loss of the myelin sheath occurs but the axon is left intact, the process is known as primary demyelination. The focus of this chapter will be on the primary demyelinating diseases affecting the central nervous system. These have vascular, infectious, traumatic, inflammatory/immune, toxic/metabolic, iatrogenic, neoplastic and developmental/congenital causes [Table 12-6]. Demyelinating diseases are also to be differentiated from the dysmyelinating diseases [Tables 12–4A and 12–4B], which reflect impairment in the development of the myelin sheath. These in turn have primarily a genetic basis, and reflect abnormalities of either myelin proteins or enzymes important in the synthesis or turnover of the myelin sheath. Although the mechanisms of these diseases are

TABLE 12–5. Immunogenic CNS Myelin Components*

Galactocerebroside
Myelin Associated Glycoprotein
Myelin Basic Protein
Proteolipid Protein

*Partial listing of central myelin components, with major immunoreactive constituents represented.

TABLE 12–6. Major Causes of Primary Demyelinating Diseases (VITAMIN D Mnemonic)

Vascular
Infectious
Traumatic
Autoimmune
Metabolic/Toxic
Iatrogenic
Neoplastic
Developmental/Congenital

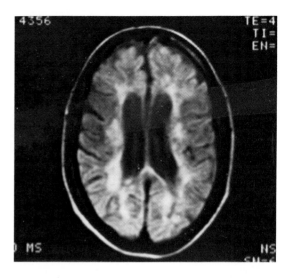

different, the symptoms will overlap somewhat because they reflect the loss of the myelin sheath, and the resulting functional limitations of the demyelinated axon [Table 12–2B].

VASCULAR

Perhaps the most common lesion of the white matter currently recognized in the elderly is that which occurs in a periventricular distribution. It is found in asymptomatic individuals, as well as those with multi-infarct dementia (MID) and senile dementia of the Alzheimer's type (SDAT), and other disorders.[36–40] Clinical correlation to relate the significance of these periventricular lesions to a specific finding is lacking at the present time, although the suspicion is that cognitive functioning is most likely to be affected. This is based on recent correlative studies in younger patients with white matter lesions in this location and cognitive losses due to multiple sclerosis (MS),[41,42] or findings in older patients with similarly placed lesions and either MID or SDAT.

The true incidence and prevalence of this white matter finding is not known at the present time. However, since the introduction of magnetic resonance imaging (MRI), periventricular white matter lesions have been more commonly found and frequently described as periventricular hyperintensity (PVH) [Fig. 12–1]. Although PVH may be found in a number of clinical syndromes, as well as in neurologically "normal" individuals, it is neither a specific finding for any one disease entity, nor is it always associated with gross pathologic changes in the periventricular white matter when examining fresh brain tissue at the time of autopsy. It is perhaps for the latter reason that the periventricular white matter had not

Fig. 12–1. A magnetic resonance image (MRI) which demonstrates periventricular hyperintensity (PVH) in a patient with a history of hypertension. This finding is nonspecific, and must be interpreted in the context of the overall clinical picture. However, a history of hypertension accompanied by intermittent mental confusion and focal neurologic deficits would not be inconsistent with this MRI finding called leuko-araiosis.

routinely been evaluated by careful histopathologic examination. Therefore, the frequency and degree of histopathologic abnormalities remains only partially characterized at present.

Histopathologic and clinical correlation with the MRI finding of PVH in asymptomatic patients and those with MID and SDAT, have shown several specific vascular changes in the periventricular white matter (See Fig. 3–8). These vascular changes, although resulting in primary demyelination, differ from other causes of primary demyelination, such as occurs in MS or progressive multifocal leukoencephalopathy (PML). Pallor of the periventricular white matter is noted when myelin stains of whole brain sections are prepared. However, subcortical U-fibers typically are spared, although lesions may extend into the surrounding white matter of the centrum semiovale. In the most severe cases ventricular dilatation may be found as a result of loss of the periventricular white matter.

Sparing of the subcortical U-fibers presumably reflects a rich vascular supply. These nerve pathways connect adjacent cortical gyri, and derive their blood supply from the same vessels that nourish the cerebral cortex. In contrast, the periventricular and surrounding white matter is supplied by the terminal extensions of long-penetrating vessels. These behave as watershed vessels, which are less well perfused during hypotension. Oligodendrocytes are particuarly vulnerable to hypoxia. Therefore, it is not surprising to find demyelination with relative sparing of axons associated with this mechanism. Hypertension and associated arteriolosclerosis complicate matters by further reducing the effective vessel lumen diameter. This restricts the vascular supply even more during a hypotensive episode, and increases the severity of the lesion. It is not yet clear what degree of tissue destruction in this location is necessary before clinical symptoms will become apparent. However, based upon this hypothetical vascular mechanism as described, it should be noted that these periventricular lesions may coexist with other pathologic processes in the brain, and any source of anoxia or ischemia can yield such lesions.[43] Therefore, although PVH may be found in SDAT, it likely reflects a separate pathologic mechanism in those patients.

Microscopically, there usually is a loss of myelin and oligodendroglia with relative sparing of axons. Astrocytosis is frequently present. There is often arteriolar fibrohyaline thickening and sclerosis, which may greatly narrow the vessel lumen. The perivascular space becomes dilated. The constellation of dilated perivascular space, arteriolosclerosis and vascular ectasia has been referred to as "etat crible."

A generic term to describe the appearance of the white matter has been suggested.[44] It is leuko-araiosis (L-A), which refers to the decreased density of the white matter radiographically, initially recognized on computerized tomographs (CT) of the brain, and then extended with MRI studies. A differential diagnosis of L-A is provided in Table 12–7. As can be seen from review of this table, there are many possible causes of grossly similar appearing white matter changes.

INFECTIOUS

When considering an infectious etiology for demyelinating diseases, it should be recog-

TABLE 12–7.   Differential Diagnosis of Leuko-Araiosis

Vascular
  Amyloid Angiopathy—Hemorrhagic
  Granulomatous Angiitis
  Hypotension (Watershed Stroke)
  MID (Multi-Infarct Dementia)
  Subarachnoid Hemorrhage
Infectious
  AIDS (Acquired Immunodeficiency Syndrome)
    AIDS Encephalopathy
    Progressive Leukoencephalopathy of AIDS
  HTLV-1 Infection
  Lyme Disease
  PML (Progressive Multifocal Leukoencephalopathy)
  Progressive Rubella Panencephalitis
  Subacute Sclerosing Panencephalitis
  Vasculitis (Meningitis)
Trauma
  Cerebral Edema
    Acute Compression
  Barbotage of CSF
Autoimmune Diseases
  Acute Hemorrhagic Leukoencephalopathy
  Bechet's Syndrome
  Chronic Inflammatory Demyelinating Neuropathy (CIDP)
  MS (Multiple Sclerosis)
    Postinfectious Encephalomyelitis
  Sjogren's Syndrome
  SLE (Systemic Lupus Erythematosus)
  Vogt-Koyanaga-Hirada Syndrome
Metabolic-Toxic
  Alcohol
    Central Pontine Myelinolysis
    Marchiafava-Bignami Disease: Corpus Callosum, Anterior Commissure
  Dysmyelinating Syndromes [See Tables 12–4A and 12–4B]
  Heavy Metal Exposure—Arsenic, Lead, Mercury
  Hepatic/Renal Failure
  Hypoglycemia
  Hypoxia (Carbon Monoxide Poisoning, Cyanide)
  Metabolic Dysfunction
  Vitamin Deficiencies
    Subacute Combined Degeneration (Vitamin B_{12} Deficiency)
    Vitamin B_1 Deficiency
    Vitamin B_6 Deficiency
    Vitamin E Deficiency
  Organic Solvent Exposure
  Organophosphate Exposure
Iatrogenic
  Cyclosporin
  Methotrexate
  Radiation Leukoencephalopathy
  Rapid Correction of Electrolyte Imbalance
Neoplastic
  Cerebral Edema Secondary to Tumor
  Lymphoma
  Remote Effect of Malignant Disease
Developmental-Congenital
  Arnold-Chiari Malformation
  Basilar Impression
  Hydrocephalus
  Periventricular Leukomalacia of Prematurity

nized that the more common of these are the result of an opportunistic infection in which the patient was immunocompromised. However, there are less frequent diseases such as subacute sclerosing panencephalitis[45-47] caused by infection with measles virus, or progressive rubella panencephalitis[48,49] caused by infection with the rubella virus, which occur without any specific underlying disease causing immunosuppression, other than perhaps the immunosuppressive state (von Pirquet's phenomenon) caused by the infection with the virus.[50] These are more common in younger individuals. Nevertheless, there are two specific infectious diseases which are of great importance at the present time as causes of demyelinating disease in older individuals. These are progressive multifocal leukoencephalopathy (PML), and AIDS encephalopathy.

PML has long been recognized as a neurologic complication of infectious etiology which may occur in the context of malignant disease, particularly chronic lymphocytic leukemia and Hodgkin's disease.[51] In recent years, PML has also been recognized to occur with increased frequency as a complicating secondary infection of the central nervous system in AIDS.[52-54] There is a separate central nervous system demyelinating component in AIDS, which is due to infiltration of the central nervous system with HIV-1 infected macrophages.[55] In addition, there have been cases of multifocal varicella-zoster viral leukoencephalitis,[56] which have occurred at different time periods after shingles, and cytomegalovirus-induced demyelination[57] in patients with AIDS. These should be considered separately [Table 12–8].

PML is most commonly caused by the JC virus, which is a polyomavirus named after the

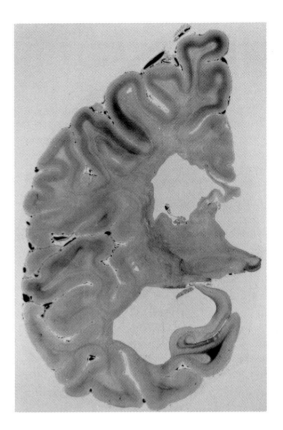

Fig. 12–2. This gross section of the cerebral white matter shows the extensive loss of myelin which can be found in progressive multifocal leukoencephalopathy (PML). It is not uncommon for confluence of several smaller lesions to occur. This may lead to compensatory enlargement of the cerebral ventricles. Loyez (myelin) stain.

TABLE 12–8.   Infectious Causes of Primary Demyelination

AIDS (Acquired Immunodeficiency Syndrome)
  AIDS Encephalopathy
    Cytomegalovirus-induced Demyelination
    Progressive Leukoencephalopathy of AIDS
Herpes Zoster Encephalomyelitis
PML (Progressive Multifocal Leukoencephalopathy)
Progressive Rubella Panencephalitis
Subacute Sclerosing Panencephalitis
Tropical Spastic Paraparesis (HTLV-1 Infection)
Vasculitis (Meningitis)

initials of the first patient from whom this virus was isolated.[58] The JC virus has an additional unusual property of being able to induce brain tumors in several species of animals into which it is injected intracerebrally. It is a common human virus.[59] In man PML is considered an opportunistic infection and is characterized by an insidious course that is ultimately fatal. The disease is thought to be due to reactivation of a latent infection with the JC virus during immunosuppression, although this is not proven. Some cases of PML caused by the SV40 virus have been reported as well.[60]

Pathologically there is the loss of myelin [Fig. 12–2], with the relative preservation of axons. Typically, oligodendrocytes, which support the replication of the virus, contain enlarged nuclei with viral inclusion bodies in the form of a crystalline array. There is demonstration of JC viral antigens within these cells, and demonstration of the JC virus genome within these cells by in situ hybridization.[61] A second interesting feature is the appearance of enlarged, bizarre, giant astrocytes, which is not thought to represent a direct effect of virus replication in these cells. There is often relatively little in the way of an inflammatory reaction in this infection, although phagocytic macrophages are regularly noted engulfing myelin breakdown products, and on occasion perivascular cuffs have been observed. Of note, there may infrequently be the presence of malignant tumors of glial origin,[62] or additional opportunistic infections.

It is interesting to speculate on whether the evolving immunocompromised state in PML patients is solely a function of the underlying disease, such as chronic lymphocytic leukemia (CLL) or Hodgkin's disease, or whether it represents direct effects of the JC virus on the brain or immune organs, or indirect effects on immune organs mediated through infection of the brain. Work in my laboratory, with mouse hepatitis virus type-4 (MHV-4), suggests that virus infection of the nervous system may lead to compromise of immune function.[63] This intriguing hypothesis is under further study at the present time, but raises the interesting possibility that an insidious central nervous system infection could contribute to the state of immunosuppression, and a more permissive state for virus replication. Such a mechanism, evolving over time, would be an additional way in which the onset of symptoms may greatly lag behind the onset of the disease process.

In contrast to PML, the demyelination of HIV encephalopathy does not have evidence for infection of the oligodendrocyte with HIV or any other pathogen in the specimens studied to date. There are no oligodendrocyte inclusions, and there is no oligodendrocyte hypertrophy. Astrocytes do not form the same type of bizarre cell as in PML, but instead form multinucleated giant cells, with the nuclei arranged along the periphery of these giant cells. Generally, the demyelinating lesions observed in the cerebral hemispheres are small and scattered about, rarely coalescing to form enlarged areas of demyelination as so often occurs in

PML. There may be a foamy appearance to the tissue microscopically, because of the huge numbers of vacuolated macrophages phagocytosing myelin debris. A vacuolated myelopathy has been described in which the lesions are confined to the spinal cord.[64]

On occasion, the lesions of HIV encephalopathy may be large and resemble PML in their clinical features and by MRI criteria.[65,66] However, in some patients these huge white matter lesions were confined to the posterior fossa, a relatively infrequent site for involvement in PML. Subsequent hybridization analysis with nucleic acid probes to the papovavirus JC, herpes simplex I, herpes zoster, cytomegalovirus, hepatitis B, HIV-1 and HTLV-1 demonstrated infection with HIV-1 alone.[67]

In other studies of HIV encephalopathy, the virus has been demonstrated to be localized to within infiltrating macrophages,[68,69] with the implication that the virus in the brain may be a variant virus.[70] This macrophage route of entry into the brain has been described as analogous to "Trojan horses" carrying the virus into the central nervous system, as in other retrovirus infections of the central nervous system with other members of the lentiviruses.[71]

The mechanisms of demyelination produced by cytomegalovirus and herpes zoster remain to be elucidated. It should be noted that cytomegalovirus has been identified as a virus associated with demyelinating disease in AIDS,[57] where other pathogens, including HIV-1, may be playing a significant, albeit as yet poorly understood role, as well. Infection with varicella zoster virus has been described as a multifocal leukoencephalitis[56] in cancer patients with a prior history of shingles. Eosinophilic Cowdry Type A intranuclear inclusions have been observed in neurons, astrocytes, and oligodendrocytes. Cortical or subcortical hemorrhages may occur, since the lesions have a greater prevalence at the gray-white junction. More tissue swelling, likely reflecting the occurrence of hemorrhages, may be present in this condition than in PML, which it otherwise may closely resemble.

HTLV-1 has recently gained recognition because it may give rise to a cutaneous form of lymphoma,[72] adult T-cell leukemia,[73,74] or to a demyelinating disease resembling multiple sclerosis,[75,76] which is also known as tropical spastic paraparesis (TSP) and HTLV-1 associated myelopathy (HAM). Familial cases of HTLV-1 associated myelopathy have been reported, suggesting the possibility of genetic regulation of susceptibility to infection with this virus.[77] Because of its resemblance to MS, efforts have recently been undertaken to isolate this virus from the tissue of individuals with multiple sclerosis,[78,79] but these data remain controversial at the present time.[76]

Vasculitis may result as a complication of meningitis. This should be mentioned because it may in turn lead to white matter ischemia and demyelination.

TRAUMA

The principal way in which a traumatic lesion can subsequently contribute to white matter demyelination, other than by direct destruction and Wallerian degeneration, is through edema [Table 12-9]. Cerebral edema may also result from primary or metastatic tumors invading the central nervous system. Acute tissue compression from a traumatic lesion, and barbotage of CSF as when medications are injected intrathecally, are other mechanisms in which trauma can lead to demyelination. Myelinated fibers are extremely sensitive to pressure effects, and subsequently breakdown. The fibers with the largest diameter myelin sheaths are the most sensitive.

AUTOIMMUNE

Autoimmune mechanisms of white matter disease most often are manifested as multiple sclerosis (MS), although systemic lupus erythematosus (SLE), Sjögren's syndrome, Behçet's syndrome and postinfectious encephalomyelitis should also be considered [Table 12-10]. In addition, there are additional clinical syndromes. These may include transverse myelitis, a disorder of unknown etiology and chronic inflammatory demyelinating neuropa-

TABLE 12-9. Traumatic Causes of Primary Demyelination

Acute Compression
Barbotage of CSF
Cerebral Edema

TABLE 12-10. Autoimmune Causes of Primary Demyelination

Acute Hemorrhagic Leukoencephalopathy
Bechet's Syndrome
Chronic Inflammatory Demyelinating Polyneuropathy
  (CIDP)
MS (Multiple Sclerosis)
  Postinfectious Encephalomyelitis
SLE (Systemic Lupus Erythematosus)
Sjogren's Syndrome
Vogt-Koyanaga-Hirada Syndrome

thy (CIDP). In CIDP, although the principal lesion affects peripheral nerves, there may be involvement of the central nervous system as well.[80]

Multiple sclerosis (MS) is the most common demyelinating disease of the central nervous system. It most often becomes clinically apparent in young adults, although it may go undiagnosed for many years. In recent years, because of the increased use of MRI examinations, the presence of white matter lesions consistent with the diagnosis of MS may be found in a relatively asymptomatic individual at any age. Demyelination of the cerebral white matter in MS is readily detected pathologically [Fig. 12-3], and by MRI [Fig. 12-4]. MS should always be considered in the differential diagnosis of a progressive neurologic disorder first apparent in the elderly when other more common causes of dysfunction have been excluded.

MS affects women more often than men by almost a 2 to 1 ratio. It is believed to be an immune mediated disease triggered by exposure to an environmental agent, such as a virus, in a genetically predisposed individual. The neuropathology of multiple sclerosis has been reviewed by many investigators, however, the findings of Prineas[81] deserve special mention. He emphasizes the immunopathogenic mechanisms in play, describing the characteristic perivascular distribution of cells, with infiltration into the surrounding tissue. Prineas hypothesizes that this lesion morphology resembles the organization within lymphoid follicular structures. In addition, he has described coated vesicles in association with the macrophages involved in the active stripping of myelin from the axon. This finding is believed to be unique in "immune-mediated" demyelination.[82-84]

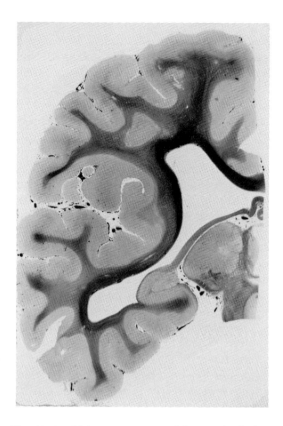

phates, cyanide, heavy metals such as arsenic, lead and mercury [Table 12–11], are directly toxic on the oligodendrocyte, and thus interfere with the integrity of the myelin sheath. Awareness of this sensitivity, and exposure to such agents should be sought in the evaluation of patients with unexplained neurologic symptoms involving the white matter of the brain.

Open heart surgery and cardiopulmonary compromise from any cause could lead to a relative hypoxic state, which although not severe enough to compromise neuronal cell function, may impair oligodendrocyte metabolism to a sufficient degree to affect the structural integrity of the white matter.

There are inborn errors of metabolism which lead to dysmyelinating syndromes in which myelin synthesis is incomplete.[85] Some forms may be present in infancy and childhood, while other forms, even with the same enzymatic defect, are not present until adulthood. The reasons for these discrepancies are not clear at the present time. However, the occurrence of multiple forms or alleles of the genes

Fig. 12–3. This gross section of the cerebral white matter shows the extensive loss of myelin which can be found in multiple sclerosis (MS). It is common to find multiple lesions of variable age and size in MS. There may be compensatory enlargement of the cerebral ventricles in MS as a result of extensive destruction and loss of the white matter. On occasion, concentric rings of demyelination and remyelination are found (Balo's concentric sclerosis). Loyez (myelin) stain.

METABOLIC/TOXIC

Because of the high level of metabolic activity within the oligodendrocyte at all stages of development, and the involvement of multiple gene products in the ordered sequence of events characterizing the development and maintenance of the myelin sheath, there are many ways in which disorders of metabolism, exposure to toxic agents or inborn errors of metabolic pathways can lead to either disruption of normal myelination or failure of maintenance of the oligodendrocyte-myelin unit.

Hypoxia/anoxia, carbon monoxide poisoning, exposure to organic solvents, organophos-

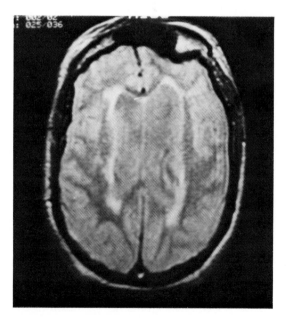

Fig. 12–4. A MRI which demonstrates periventricular hyperintensity in a patient with multiple sclerosis (MS). Although this pattern is nonspecific and must be interpreted in the context of the overall clinical picture, this MRI finding is consistent with the history of MS, relapses and remissions of focal neurologic deficits.

TABLE 12–11. Metabolic/Toxic Causes of Primary Demyelination

Alcohol
    Central Pontine Myelinolysis
    Marchiafava-Bignami Disease: Corpus Callosum, Anterior Commissure
Dysmyelinating Syndromes [See Tables 12–4A and 12–4B]
Heavy Metal Exposure—Arsenic, Lead, Mercury
Metabolic Dysfunction
    Hepatic/Renal Failure
    Hypoglycemia
    Hypoxia (Carbon Monoxide Poisoning, Cyanide)
    Vitamin Deficiencies
        Subacute Combined Degeneration (Vitamin B_{12} Deficiency)
    Vitamin B_1 Deficiency
    Vitamin B_6 Deficiency
    Vitamin E Deficiency
Organic Solvent Exposure
Organophosphate Exposure
Phenylketonuria (PKU)
Refsum's Disease (Phytanic Acid Storage Disease)

which code for the enzymes affected provides a possible explanation.

For example, metachromatic leukodystrophy (sulfatide lipidosis) may be present in an infantile, childhood, or adult onset form. The major defect in this disease is in the enzyme arylsulfatase A, although a variant involving multiple arylsulfatase enzymes exists as well. As a result of the enzyme defect, the synthesis of sulfatide, a lipid component of the myelin sheath in both the central and peripheral nervous system, is impaired. Myelin formation is therefore affected in both central and peripheral nerves, and symptoms of involvement of these tissues, as well as other sulfatide containing organs, provide important clues to this diagnosis. There have been at least four clinical patterns described. These include the late infantile, juvenile, and adult variants, as well as the variant due to multiple sulfatase deficiency. The adult variant differs from the others in being more gradual in onset and having a presentation more of intellectual decline initially than of spasticity and peripheral neuropathy as is found with the other forms of metachromatic leukodystrophy. The name metachromatic leukodystrophy (MLD) has been applied to this disorder because of the change in color or metachromatic pattern obtained when staining these affected structures with a stain such as toluidine blue.

Other inherited forms of leukodystrophy

occur exclusively in adulthood, such as adult-onset hereditary leukodystrophy. This condition has only recently been described,[86] but had been previously misdiagnosed as a familial form of multiple sclerosis. This category also includes the inherited leukodystrophies with adrenal involvement,[85] the adrenoleukodystrophies [Table 12–4B].

Alcohol is an important cause of neurologic disease. Alcohol can lead to demyelination by direct toxic effects or by associated problems with malnutrition. Marchiafava-Bignami disease involves specific demyelination of the corpus callosum and anterior commissure.[87] It was first described in older Italian men who drank red wines, but has not been confined to this group. The etiology and pathogenesis of this rare disorder remains poorly understood. The condition exists as mostly a neuropathologic curiosity to this day. Central pontine myelinolysis (CPM),[88,89] in contrast, remains of current interest. This condition is more frequent, and has both been diagnosed in living patients and in recent years provided with a prospective etiopathogenesis. Experimental work has pointed toward the rapid correction of electrolyte imbalance, particularly through the use of hypertonic saline solutions for the correction of hyponatremia,[90,91] as a possible mechanism of disease.[92] Of interest in this regard is the association of alcohol with the syndrome of inappropriate antidiuretic hormone secretion (SIADH), as a precipitant of the hyponatremic state.

Vitamin deficiencies are common effects of malnutrition, and may also be the result of deficiencies of cofactors necessary for their function. It is well recognized that deficiency of vitamin B_{12} can lead to subacute combined degeneration of the spinal cord, in which demyelination of the dorsal columns and the pathways of the dorsolateral columns of the spinal cord is found. This shows its greatest predilection for the thoracic cord initially, but other tracts and levels of the spinal cord can become involved as the disease progresses. There are also effects on the optic nerves and cerebral hemispheres in the central nervous system (CNS), along with involvement of the peripheral nerves. CNS symptoms can also result from deficiencies of vitamins B_1, B_6 and E.[93] It is important to recognize these vitamin deficiencies as early as possible, since they can be corrected with vitamin supplementation early on, but become irreversible later. Of further interest, with a relative deficiency of vitamin B_1 (thiamine), delivery of glucose without this vitamin as a supplement can precipitate Wernicke's syndrome because of the requirement for B_1 as a cofactor in the metabolism of glucose in the brain. For this reason, it is common practice to administer thiamine along with glucose intravenously in anyone presenting clinically in an unconscious state and suspected of being deficient in this vitamin.

In summary, any source of metabolic dysfunction, such as hepatic or renal failure, hypoglycemia, hypoxia, carbon monoxide poisoning, a cause of hypoxia, will interfere with the metabolic integrity of the oligodendrocyte-myelin unit and can lead to primary demyelination.

IATROGENIC

Amongst the iatrogenic causes of demyelinating disease are radiation therapy[94,95] and chemotherapy [Table 12–12]. Of the latter, methotrexate is the most notable chemotherapeutic agent in the development of demyelinating disease.[96,97] Both the dosage and the diluent composition should be considered in the cause of this problem in which toxic effects on the oligodendrocyte lead to demyelination. Other medical therapies associated with demyelination in the central nervous system include Cyclosporin.[98] Another potentially toxic compound is nitrous oxide, used by dentists for anesthesia, which is believed to act by interfering with the vitamin B_{12} pathway.[99] In this regard, gastrectomy and the resulting loss of the cofactor needed for vitamin B_{12} absorption may also play a role in predisposing to demyelinating disease.

Opportunistic infections as causes of demyelination may be secondary to iatrogenically

induced immunosuppression secondary to the use of prednisone and cyclophosphamide, in the treatment of diseases such as chronic lymphocytic leukemia or rheumatoid arthritis. Opportunistic malignancies like primary lymphoma of the central nervous system may also occur. Either of these infectious or malignant opportunistic conditions may be focal or multicentric in their distribution.

There is overlap with other causes of primary demyelination in the iatrogenically induced demyelinating disease category. For example, any form of surgery resulting in either hypoxia, hypotension or severe hypoglycemia may contribute to a multifocal pattern of white matter disease. Rapid correction of hyponatremia has been implicated as a significant factor in the development of central pontine myelinolysis (CPM).[92]

NEOPLASTIC

Primary lymphoma of the central nervous system, as well as the edema associated with both primary and metastatic tumors affecting the white matter of the central nervous system, will be considered in this category [Table 12-13]. Cerebral edema secondary to a primary or metastatic tumor, lymphoma, or remote effect of malignant disease should be considered.[100,101]

DEVELOPMENTAL/CONGENITAL

Table 12-14 lists several of the developmental/congenital conditions in which demyelination may play a significant role. Pressure on white matter pathways is common to all of

TABLE 12–13. Neoplastic Causes of Demyelination

Cerebral Edema Secondary to a Primary or Metastatic Tumor
Lymphoma
Remote Effect of Malignant Disease

TABLE 12–12.   Iatrogenic Causes of Demyelination

Cyclosporin
Methotrexate
Nitrous Oxide
Radiation Leukoencephalopathy
Rapid Correction of Electrolyte Imbalance

TABLE 12–14.   Developmental/Congenital Causes of Demyelination

Arnold-Chiari Malformation
Basilar Impression
Hydrocephalus
Periventricular Leukomalacia of Prematurity

these disorders. The pressure is either due to direct compression because of the physical arrangement of the tissues at the craniovertebral junction or periventricularly, or alternatively, due to pressure from blood in the extracellular space. Pressure appears to adversely affect larger diameter nerve fibers exclusively.[102] Although most data have been obtained from studies of the peripheral nervous system, the information applies to the central nervous system as well. These include Arnold-Chiari malformation, basilar impression, hydrocephalus, and the periventricular leukomalacia of prematurity due to periventricular hemorrhage.

SUMMARY AND CONCLUSIONS

The purpose of the present chapter is to provide an overview of the ways in which the integrity of the myelinated fiber pathways of the central nervous system could become compromised by changes associated with aging. Because the myelin forming cell, the oligodendrocyte, is active metabolically throughout life, it is vulnerable to a variety of both metabolic and structural assaults on its integrity throughout the course of the lifetime of the individual. Virtually every medical aspect of an individual's well being will have some impact on the integrity of the myelin-oligodendrocyte unit.

In this way the integrity of the cardiovascular system, the exposure and responses to acute and persistent viral infections, the degree of exposure to trauma, the predisposition and manifestations of autoimmune reactivity, the metabolic integrity of the renal/hepatic axes and their ability to handle toxic exposures, the exposure to various forms of medical intervention, the possibility of underlying malignant disease, or the possibility of developmental/congential or degenerative disease affects the integrity of the oligodendrocyte-myelin unit, and so creates the possibility for demyelinating disease.

As can best be seen from the description of leuko-araiosis in particular, principally a dramatic radiographic observation, there is room remaining for better clinicopathologic correlations between the final pathologic findings and the premorbid diagnosis. Hopefully, the present chapter will stimulate such analyses.

ACKNOWLEDGMENT

The preparation of this chapter was made possible in part through work supported by research grants from the USPHS, NS22145, the National Multiple Sclerosis Society, RG1722, and the Swim Foundation.

REFERENCES

1. Stampfli, R.: Overview of studies on the physiology of conduction in myelinated nerve fibers. In: *Demyelinating Diseases: Basic and Clinical Electrophysiology.* (Eds.) S.G. Waxman, and J.M. Ritchie. Adv. Neurol. *31*:11, 1981.
2. Rasminsky, M.: The effects of temperature on conduction in demyelinated single nerve fibers. Arch. Neurol., *28*:287, 1973.
3. Waxman, S.G.: Membranes, myelin, and the pathophysiology of multiple sclerosis. N. Engl. J. Med., *303*:1529, 1982.
4. Peters, A., Palay, S., and Webster, H.D.: *The Fine Structure of the Nervous System: The Neurons and Supporting Cells.* Philadelphia, W.B. Saunders Co., 1976.
5. Raff, M.C.: Glial cell diversification in the rat optic nerve. Science, 243:1450, 1989.
6. Bunge, R.P.: Glial cells and the central myelin sheath. Physiol. Rev.,*48*:197, 1968.
7. Duncan, D.: A relation between axon diameter and myelination determined by measurement of myelinated spinal root fibers. J. Comp. Neurol., *60*:437, 1934.
8. Murray, J.A., and Blakemore, W.F.: The relationship between internodal length and fibre diameter in the spinal cord of the cat. J. Neurol. Sci., *45*:29, 1980.
9. Kocsis, J.D., and Waxman, S.G.: Demyelination: causes and mechanisms of clinical abnormality and functional recovery. In: *Demyelinating Diseases.* Revised Series 3. (Ed) J.C. Koetsier. *Handbook of Clinical Neurology.* Series edited by P.J. Vinken, G.W. Bruyn, and H.L. Klawans. Amsterdam, Elsevier Science Publishers, *47*, 29, 1985.
10. Prineas, J.W., and Connell, F.: Remyelination in multiple sclerosis. Ann. Neurol., *5*:22, 1979.
11. Ritchie, J.M.: Pathophysiology of conduction in demyelinated fibers. In: *Myelin.* 2nd Ed., (Ed) P. Morell, New York, Plenum Press, 1984, p. 337.
12. Bunge, M.B., Bunge, R.P., and Ris, H.: Ultrastructural study of remyelination in an experimental lesion in adult cat spinal cord. J. Biophys. Biochem. Cytol., *10*:67, 1961.
13. Dal Canto, M.C., and Lipton, H.L.: Schwann cell remyelination and recurrent demyelination in the central nervous system of mice infected with attenuated Theiler's virus. Am. J. Pathol., *98*:101, 1980.
14. Yakovlev, P.I., and Lecours, A.: The myelinogenetic cycles of regional maturation of the brain. In: *Regional Development of the Brain in Early Life.* (Ed) A. Minkowski. Oxford, Blackwell, 1967, p. 3.
15. Langworthy, O.R.: Development of behavior patterns and myelinization of tracts in the nervous system. Arch. Neurol. Psych., *28*:1365, 1932.
16. Heim, L.M., and Timiras, P.S.: Gonad-brain relationship: Precocious brain maturation after estradiol in rats. Endocrinology, *72*:598, 1963.
17. Curry, J.J., and Heim, L.M.: Brain myelination after neonatal administration of oestradiol. Nature, *209*:915, 1966.

18. Ide, K.: On the size of the largest nerve fibers in the median and sciatic nerves of the albino rat according to sex. J. Comp. Neurol., *50*:137, 1930.

19. Hamburgh, M.: An analysis of the action of thryoid hormone on development based on in vivo and in vitro studies. Gen. Comp. Endocrinol., *10*:198, 1968.

20. Mozell, R.L., and McMorris, F.A.: Insulin-like growth factor-1 stimulates regeneration of oligodendrocytes in vitro. In: *Advances in Neuroimmunology.* (Ed) C.S. Raine. Ann. New York Acad. Sciences, *540*:430, 1988.

21. Knobler, R.L., et al.: Interleukin-2 blocks oligodendrocyte progenitor proliferation. In: *Advances in Neuroimmunology.* (Ed) C.S. Raine. Ann. New York Acad. Sci., *540*:324, 1988.

22. Benveniste, E.N., and Merrill, J.E.: Stimulation of oligodendroglial proliferation and maturation by interleukin-2. Nature, *321*:610, 1986.

23. Rodriguez, M., and Lennon, V.A.: Immunoglobulins promote remyelination in the central nervous system. Ann. Neurol., *27*:12, 1990.

24. Geren, B.B.: The formation from the Schwann cell surface of myelin in the peripheral nerves of chick embryos. Exp. Cell Res., *7*:558, 1954.

25. Singer, S.J., and Nicholson, G.: The fluid mosaic model of the structure of cell membranes. Science, *175*:720, 1972.

26. DiPaolo, R.V., Kanfer, J.N., and Newberne, P.M.: Copper deficiency and the central nervous system: Myelination in the rat-Morphological and biochemical studies. J. Neuropathol. Exp. Neurol., *33*:226, 1974.

27. Rivers, T.M., Sprunt, D.H., and Berry, G.P.: Observations on attempts to produce acute disseminated encephalomyelitis in monkeys. J. Exp. Med., *58*:39, 1933.

28. Rivers, T.M., and Schwentker, F.F.: Encephalomyelitis accompanied by myelin destruction experimentally produced in monkeys. J. Exp. Med., *61*:689, 1935.

29. Alvord, E.C.: Disseminated encephalomyelitis: Its variations in form and their relationships to other diseases of the nervous system. In: *Demyelinating Diseases.* Revised Series 3. (ED) J.C. Koetsier. *Handbook of Clinical Neurology.* Series (ed.) P.J. Vinken, G.W. Bruyn, and H.L. Klawans. Amsterdam, Elsevier Science Publishers, *47*, 467, 1985.

30. Cambi, F., Lees, M.B., Williams, R.M., et al.: Chronic experimental allergic encephalomyelitis produced by bovine proteolipid apoprotein. Ann. Neurol., *13*:303, 1983.

31. Dubois-Dalcq, M., Neidieck, B., and Buyse, M.: Action of anti-cerebroside sera on myelinated nervous tissue cultures. Pathol. Eur., *5*:331, 1970.

32. Fujinami, R.S.: Virus-induced autoimmunity through molecular mimicry. In: *Advances in Neuroimmunology.* (Ed) C.S. Raine. Ann. New York Acad. Sciences, *540*:210, 1988.

33. Small, J.A., et al.: The early region of human papovirus JC induces dysmyelination in transgenic mice. Cell, *46*:13, 1986.

34. Knobler, R.L., Lampert, P.W., and Oldstone, M.B.A.: Virus persistence and recurrent demyelination produced by a temperature-sensitive mutant of MHV-4. Nature, *298*:279, 1982.

35. Kristensson, K., et al.: Increased levels of myelin basic protein transcripts gene in virus-induced demyelination. Nature, *322*:544, 1986.

36. Huang, K., Wu, L., and Luo, Y.: Binswanger's disease: Progressive subcortical encephalopathy or multi-infarct dementia? Can. J. Neurol. Sci., *12*:88, 1985.

37. Aharon-Peretz, J., Cummings, J.L., and Hill, M.A.: Vascular dementia and dementia of the Alzheimer's type: Cognition, ventricular size, and leuko-araiosis. Arch. Neurol, *45*:719, 1988.

38. Benhaiem-Sigaux, N., et al.: Expanding cerebellar lacunes due to dilatation of the perivascular space associated with Binswanger's subcortical arteriosclerotic encephalopathy. Stroke, *18*:1087, 1987.

39. Bogousslavsky, J., Regli, F., and Uske, A.: Leukoencephalopathy in patients with ischemic stroke. Stroke, *18*:896, 1987.

40. McQuinn, B.A., and O'Leary, D.H.: White matter lucencies on computed tomography, subacute arteriosclerotic encephalopathy (Binswanger's disease), and blood pressure. Stroke, *18*:900, 1987.

41. Peyser, J.M., Rao, S.M., LaRocca, N.G., et al.: Guidelines for neuropsychological research in multiple sclerosis. Arch. Neurol., *47*:94, 1990.

42. Minden, S.L. and Schiffer, R.B.: Affective disorders in multiple sclerosis. Review and recommendations for clinical research. Arch. Neurol., *47*:98, 1990.

43. Brucher, J.M.: Leukoencephalopathies in anoxic-ischemic processes. In: *Demyelinating Diseases.* Revised Series 3. (Ed) J.C. Koetsier. *Handbook of Clinical Neurology.* Series edited by P.J. Vinken, G.W. Bruyn, and H.L. Klawans. Amsterdam, Elsevier Science Publishers, *47*, 525, 1985.

44. Hachinski, V.C., Potter, P., and Mersky, H.: Leukoaraiosis. Arch. Neurol., *44*:21, 1987.

45. Cape, C.A., et al.: Adult onset of subacute sclerosing panencephalitis. Arch. Neurol., *28*:124, 1973.

46. Dawson, J.R.: Cellular inclusions in cerebral lesions of lethargic encephalitis. Am. J. Pathol., *9*:7, 1934.

47. Gilden, D.H., Rorke, L.B., and Taraka, R.: Acute SSPE. Arch. Neurol., *32*:644, 1975.

48. Townsend, J.J., Wolinsky, J.S., and Baringer, J.R.: The neuropathology of progressive rubella panencephalitis of late onset. Brain, *99*:81, 1976.

49. Wolinsky, J.S., Berg, B.O., and Maitland, C.J.: Progressive rubella panencephalitis. Arch. Neurol., *33*:722, 1976.

50. McChesney, M.B., and Oldstone, M.B.A.: Viruses perturb lymphocyte functions. Ann. Rev. Immunol., *5*:279, 1987.

51. Walker, D.L.: Progressive multifocal leukoencephalopathy. In: *Demyelinating Diseases.* Revised Series 3. (Ed) J.C. Koetsier. *Handbook of Clinical Neurology.* Series edited by P.J. Vinken, G.W. Bruyn, and H.L. Klawans. Amsterdam, Elsevier Science Publishers, *47*, 503, 1985.

52. Berger, J.R., Kaskovitz, B., Post, M.J., et al.: Progressive multifocal leukoencephalopathy associated with human immunodeficiency virus infection: A review of the literature with a report of sixteen cases. Ann. Intern. Med., *107*:78, 1987.

53. Blum, L.W., Chambers, R.A., Schwartzman, R.J., et al.: Progressive multifocal leukoencephalopathy in acquired immunodeficiency syndrome. Arch. Neurol., *42*:137, 1985.

54. Miller, J.R., et al.: Progressive multifocal leukoencephalopathy in a male homosexual with T-cell immune deficiency. N. Engl. J. Med., *307*:1436, 1982.

55. Price, R.W., and Brew, B.: Infection of the central nervous system by human immunodeficiency virus:

Role of the immune system in pathogenesis. In: *Advances in Neuroimmunology*. (Ed) C.S. Raine. Ann. New York Acad. Sci., *540*:162, 1988.

56. Horten, B., Rice, R.W., and Jimenez, D.: Multifocal varicella-zoster virus leukoencephalitis temporally remote from herpes zoster. Ann. Neurol, *9*:251, 1981.

57. Moskowitz, L.B., Gregorios, J.B., Hensley, G.T., et al.: Cytomegalovirus: Induced demyelination associated with acquired immune deficiency syndrome. Arch. Pathol. Lab. Med., *108*:873, 1984.

58. Padgett, B.L., et al.: Cultivation of papova-like virus from human brain with progressive multifocal leukoencephalopathy. Lancet, *1*:1257, 1971.

59. Brooks, B.R., and Walker, D.L.: Progressive multifocal leukoencephalopathy. Neurol. Clin., *2*:299, 1984.

60. Weiner, L.P., et al.: Isolation of virus related to SV40 from patients with progressive multifocal leukoencephalopathy. N. Engl. J. Med., *286*:385, 1972.

61. Aksamit, A.J., et al.: Diagnosis of progressive multifocal leukoencephalopathy by brain biopsy with biotin labeled DNA: DNA in situ hybridization. J. Neuropathol. Exp. Neurol, *46*:556, 1987.

62. Sima, A.A., Finkelstein, S.D., and McLachlan, D.R.: Multiple malignant astrocytomas in a patient with spontaneous progressive multifocal leukoencephalopathy. Ann. Neurol, *14*:183, 1983.

63. Knobler, R.L., et al.: Immune effects of intracerebral infection with mouse hepatitis virus. In: *Advances in Neuroimmunology*. (Ed) C.S. Raine. Ann. New York Acad. Sci., *540*:642, 1988.

64. Petito, C.K., et al.: Vacuolar myelopathy pathologically resembling subacute combined degeneration in patients with acquired immunodeficiency syndrome (AIDS). N. Engl. J. Med., *312*:874, 1985.

65. Kleihues, P., et al.: Progressive diffuse leukoencephalopathy in patients with acquired immune deficiency syndrome (AIDS). Acta Neuropathol. (Berl.), *68*:333, 1985.

66. Jones, H.R.J., et al.: Acute fulminating fatal leukoencephalopathy as the only manifestation of human immunodeficiency virus infection. Ann. Neurol., *23*:519, 1988.

67. Knobler, R.L., et al.: Progressive leukoencephalopathy in the posterior fossa of patients with AIDS. Neurol., *36*:206, 1986.

68. Koenig, S., et al.: Detection of AIDS virus in macrophages in brain tissue from AIDS patients with encephalopathy. Science, *233*:1089, 1986.

69. Meyenhofer, M.F., Epstein, L.G., Cho, E.-S., et al.: Ultrastructural morphology and intracellular production of human immunodeficiency virus (HIV) in brain. J. Neuropathol. Exp. Neurol, *46*:474, 1987.

70. Koyanogi, Y., et al.: Dual infection of the central nervous system by AIDS viruses with distinct cellular tropisms. Science, *236*:819, 1987.

71. Haase, A.T.: Pathogenesis of lentivirus infections. Nature, *322*:130, 1986.

72. Poiesz, B.J., et al.: Detection and isolation of type C retrovirus particles from fresh and cultured lymphocytes of a patient with cutaneous T-cell lymphoma. Proc. Natl. Acad. Sci. (USA), *77*:7415, 1980.

73. Robert-Guroff, M., et al.: Natural antibodies to human retrovirus HTLV in a cluster of Japanese patients with adult T-cell leukemia. Science, *215*:975, 1982.

74. Broder, S.: Pathogenic human retroviruses. N. Engl. J. Med., *318*:243, 1988.

75. Koprowski, H., et al.: Multiple sclerosis and human T cell lymphotropic retroviruses. Nature, *318*:154, 1985.

76. Grimaldi, L.M.E., et al.: HTLV-1 associated myelopathy: Oligoclonal immunoglobulin G bands contain anti-HTLV-1 p24 antibody. Ann. Neurol., *24*:727, 1988.

77. Miyai, I., et al.: Familial cases of HTLV-1-associated myelopathy. Ann. Neurol, *22*:601, 1987.

78. Koprowski, H., and DeFreitas, E.: HTLV-1 and chronic nervous diseases: Present status and a look into the future. Ann. Neurol., *23 (Suppl)*:S166, 1988.

79. Reddy, E.P., et al.: Amplification and molecular cloning of HTLV-1 sequences from DNA of multiple sclerosis patients. Science, *243*:529, 1989.

80. Pakalnis, A., et al.: Evoked potentials in chronic inflammatory demyelinating polyneuropathy. Arch. Neurol., *45*:1014, 1988.

81. Prineas, J.W.: The neuropathology of multiple sclerosis. In: *Demyelinating Diseases*. Revised Series 3. (Ed) J.C. Koetsier. *Handbook of Clinical Neurology*. Series edited by P.J. Vinken, G.W. Bruyn, and H.L. Klawans. Amsterdam, Elsevier Science Publishers, *47*, 213, 1985.

82. Kuriowa, Y.: Concentric sclerosis. In: *Demyelinating Diseases*. Revised Series 3. (Ed) J.C. Koetsier. *Handbook of Clinical Neurology*. Series edited by P.J. Vinken, G.W. Bruyn, and H.L. Klawans. Amsterdam, Elsevier Science Publishers, *47*, 409, 1985.

83. Kurtzke, J.F.: Epidemiology of multiple sclerosis. In: *Demyelinating Diseases*. Revised Series 3. (Ed) J.C. Koetsier. *Handbook of Clinical Neurology*. Series edited by P.J. Vinken, G.W. Bruyn, and H.L. Klawans. Amsterdam, Elsevier Science Publishers, *47*, 259, 1985.

84. Lampert, P.W.: Autoimmune and virus-induced demyelinating diseases. Am. J. Pathol., *91*:175, 1978.

85. Moser, H.: Leukoencephalopathies caused by metabolic disorders. In: *Demyelinating Diseases*. Revised Series 3. (Ed) J.C. Koetsier. *Handbook of Clinical Neurology*. Series edited by P.J. Vinken, G.W. Bruyn, and H.L. Klawans. Amsterdam, Elsevier Science Publishers, *47*, 583, 1985.

86. Eldridge, R., et al.: Hereditary adult-onset leukodystrophy simulating chronic progressive multiple sclerosis. N. Engl. J. Med., *311*:948, 1984.

87. Merritt, H.H., and Weisman, A.D.: Primary degeneration of the corpus callosum (Marchiafava-Bignami's disease). J. Neuropathol. Exp. Neurol., *4*:155, 1945.

88. Adams, R.D., Victor, M., and Mancall, E.L.: Central pontine myelinolysis. Arch. Neurol. Psychiatry, *81*:184, 1959.

89. Leslie, K.O., Robertson, A.S., and Norenberg, M.D.: Central pontine myelinolysis: An osmotic gradient pathogenesis. J. Neuropathol. Exp. Neurol., *39*:370, 1980.

90. Kleinschmidt-DeMasters, B.K., and Norenberg, M.D.: Rapid correction of hyponatremia causes demyelination: Relation to central pontine myelinolysis. Science, *211*:1068, 1981.

91. Ayus, J.C., Krothapalli, R.K., and Arieff, A.I.: Correction of hyponatremia and its relation to brain damage. N. Engl. J. Med., *318*:1336, 1988.

92. Norenberg, M.D., Leslie, K.O., and Robertson, A.S.: Association between rise in serum sodium and central pontine myelinolysis. Ann. Neurol., *11*:128, 1982.

93. Krendel, D.A., Gilchrist, J.M., Johnson, A.O., et al.: Isolated deficiency of vitamin E with progressive neurologic deterioration. Neurology, 37:538, 1987.
94. Lampert, P.W., and Davis, R.L.: Delayed effects of radiation on the human nervous system. Neurology, 14:912, 1964.
95. Malamud, N., Boldrey, E.B., Welch, W.K., et al.: Necrosis of brain and spinal cord following X-ray therapy. J. Neurosurg., 11:353, 1954.
96. Ojeda, V.J.: Necrotising leukoencephalopathy associated with intrathecal/intraventricular methotrexate therapy. Med. J. Aust., 2:289, 1982.
97. Shapiro, W.R., Chernik, N.L., and Posner, J.B.: Necrotizing encephalopathy following intraventricular instillation of methotrexate. Arch. Neurol., 28:96, 1973.

98. DeGroen, P.C., et al.: Central nervous system toxicity after liver transplantation: The role of cyclosporine and cholesterol. N. Engl. J. Med., 317:861, 1987.
99. Hakim, A.M., Cooper, B.A., Rosenblatt, D.S., et al.: Local cerebral glucose utilization in two models of B12 deficiency. J. Neurochem., 40:1155, 1987.
100. Mancall, E. L., and Rosales, R.K.: Necrotising myelopathy associated with visceral carcinoma. Brain, 87:639, 1964.
101. Ojeda, V.J.: Necrotizing myelopathy associated with malignancy. A clinicopathologic study of two cases and literature review. Cancer, 53:1115, 1984.
102. Strain Jr., R.E., and Olson, W.E.: Selective damage of large diameter peripheral nerve fibers by compression: An application of Laplace's law. Exp. Neurol., 47:68, 1975.

13

Genetic Geriatric Neuropathology

SERGE DUCKETT,
SAMUEL H. MARKIND,
TIMOTHY BLOCK and
RUDOLPH E. TANZI

In 1988 the Office of Human Genome Research was created in the National Institute of Health (NIH). Headed by James D. Watson, the Nobel prize winner for DNA research, its purpose is to map and sequence the human genome. The NIH was joined by the Department of Energy in this enterprise. International cooperation, particularly by European countries and Japan, has led to the formation of the Human Genome Organization (HUGO).[1]

The objective of this vast enterprise is to have a source book containing a complete map and sequence of the 3 billion base pairs of the human genome which correspond to an estimated 50,000 to 100,000 genes. At present about 1500 genes have been mapped to specific chromosomal regions including 600 which have been cloned and sequenced.[2]

There are many imperative reasons for this work. In terms of medicine, the knowledge of the total human genome will permit the genetic diagnosis, the creation of specific diagnostic tests for one human being, and the de-

velopment of methods to interrupt or supplement gene activity.

It is estimated that the mapping and sequencing of the total human genome will take 10 to 15 years at a cost of about $200 million a year. The benefits of this work are already in progress, as new information is announced and acted upon.

Genetic anomalies for a small number of adult onset neurologic syndromes have been identified by examination of the DNA in human chromosomes. The detection of the concerned gene may be achieved by beginning with a classic genetic linkage study to define the abnormal chromosme followed by the isolation of the diseased gene with molecular genetic techniques.[3]

The purpose of this chapter is to review recent information concerning genetically determined neurologic diseases which afflict older men and women. Such diseases may manifest initially in humans 60 years of age and older or may be seen by a physician long after the first symptoms. The family history and clinical presentation of a patient usually identifies the disease in question. However, such identification may be difficult because of the variety of clinical manifestations in members of the family, the inability of the patient to verbalize, and the absence of information.

METHODS OF DETECTION

DIGESTION OF CHROMOSOMAL DNA BY RESTRICTION ENDONUCLEASES

Restriction endonucleases are enzymes, usually isolated from bacteria, that cleave (make double stranded cuts in) double stranded DNA at specific nucleotide seqeunces.[4] For example, EcoR1, isolated from a strain of E. Coli, will cleave a stretch of DNA wherever the sequence 5'GAATTC-3' occurs.[4] If the sequence GAATTC occurs only once within a linear piece of chromosomal DNA, the DNA will be cleaved into two discrete fragments, called restriction fragments. In fact, the human genome (all 46 chromosomes) contains more than 100,000 GAATTC sites and would therefore be cleaved into that many restriction fragments. The key advantage of restriction enzymes is that they always cut at the same sites, as dictated by the DNA sequence [Fig. 13–1].

SEPARATION OF RESTRICTION FRAGMENTS[4]

DNA to be examined is isolated, usually from the peripheral blood of those to be tested, digested with specific restriction enzymes and resolved by electrophoresis through agarose gels [Fig. 13–1].

SOUTHERN BLOTTING AND DNA-DNA HYBRIDIZATION

Following electrophoresis, the restriction fragments, contained in the gel, are transferred to nitrocellulose filters by a blotting technique described by E.M. Southern.[5] The nitrocellulose paper will contain a replica of what was present in the gel and can be used for further experimental manipulations [Fig. 13–1]. For example, the DNA present in the nitrocellulose

paper is hybridized with a radioactively labeled "probe". The probe will typically be a bacterial plasmid or phage into which the human gene of interest has been molecularly cloned. The radioactive probe only "sticks" to the paper where restriction fragments bearing the gene of interest have migrated and allows for visualization of those restriction fragments following autoradiography [Fig. 13–1].

DISCUSSION

Notable among the late onset heritable neurologic diseases are Huntington's chorea, familial Alzheimer's disease, the spinal cerebellar ataxias, choreoacanthocytosis and type I familial amyloidotic polyneuropathy (FAP) [Table 13–1]. The mutations leading to each of these disorders have been associated with defects on specific chromosomes. A brief summary of late onset neurologic diseases associated with heritable defects is provided in Table 13–1.

Although the genes which are responsible for the defects in Table 13–1 have been mapped to their respective chromosomes, except in FAP, the gene products (structural proteins or enzymes) for which they code are not known. Nevertheless, it still may be possible to predict if the offspring has inherited the defective trait or if he/she will be a silent carrier as in the case of disorders with recessive phenotypes. This is possible by making the diagnosis at the molecular level. DNA from the affected individual is examined for the presence of mutations or polymorphisms that are either the cause of the lesion or are in neighboring chromosomal regions often inherited along with the defective allele. The probability of receiving the defective allele can therefore be related to the appearance of characteristic DNA sequences that can result in restriction fragment length polymorphisms (RFLP). RFLPs result when different nucleotides are present within the same chromosomal locus from different people. That is, RFLPs are due to the occurrence of a different restriction endonuclease cleavage site occurring at the same chromosomal site in different people.[6,7] Approximately one base in every 500 nucleotides of chromosomal DNA varies between any two individual

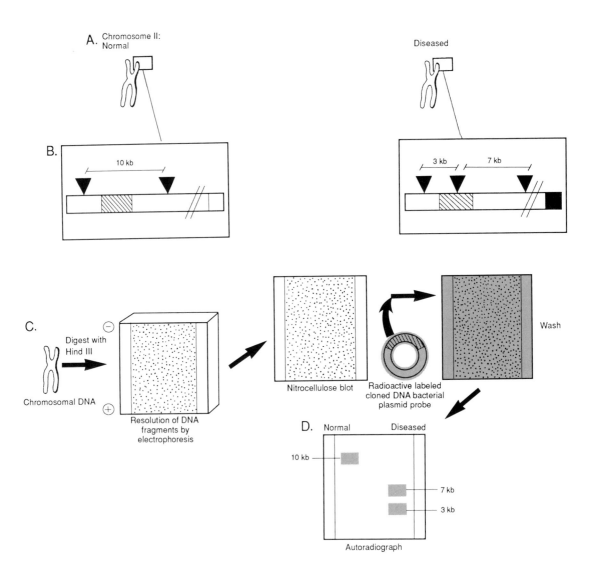

Fig. 13–1. Detection of a hypothetical RFLP. The same chromosomes from two different sources are shown in (A). Expansions of the region of interest are shown in (B) with the "normal" gene presented as a white box at the end of the map, and the diseased allele as a black box at the end of the map. Triangles indicate Hind III sites. Note that the chromosome containing the diseased allele has an additional Hind III site, some distance from the actual diseased gene. Chromosomal DNA from (A) is digested with Hind III endonuclease enzyme and DNA fragments are resolved by electrophoresis (C). The resolved DNA fragments are transferred to nitrocellulose paper. The nitrocellulose paper is incubated with radioactive labeled cloned DNA bacterial probe. DNA cloned into a bacterial plasmid is homologous to the region flanking the additional Hind III site shown as the cross-hatched box in (B) and serves as the radioactive labeled plasmid probe in (C). The nitrocellulose paper is incubated with radioactive labeled probe, washed free of unbound probe and an autoradiograph is made as in (D). Since an additional Hind III site is coinherited with the diseased allele, digestion of chromosomes containing the diseased gene will yield fragments of 7kb and 3kb detected by the probe instead of a single 10kb fragment observed in digests of normal chromosomes.

TABLE 13–1.   Late Onset Neurologic Diseases Associated with a Genetic Linkage and Specific RFLP

	Chromosome #	Reference
Amyloidotic Polyneuropathy	4	8
Huntington's Disease	4	13, 14
Familial Alzheimer's Disease	21	7
Acute Intermittent Porphyria	11	15
Von Recklinghausen Neurofibromatosis NF1	17	16, 17
Bilateral Acoustic Neurofibromatosis NF2	22	18
Manic-Depressive Illness	11	19
Spinocerebellar Ataxia	6	20
Anderson Fabry Disease	X	11
Adrenoleukodystrophy	X	21
Charcot-Marie-Tooth Disease	X	11

chromosomes, chosen at random.[6] Therefore, the human genome is dotted with differences from one person to another. Most of these changes are "neutral" in that they occur outside of structural genes or they do not result in any phenotypic effect. They often, however, result in deletion of common restriction sites or in the creation of new ones. It is these differences that result in RFLPs. If these changes are located near a gene of interest, as defined by the site's co-inheritance with a particular phenotype, they can serve as landmarks along the chromosome and can be used to distinguish one person's chromosomes from another.

Genetically, polymorphisms may be defined as "heritable differences in which the proportion of the population receiving the most common allele does not exceed 99%".[6] Typically, as in the case of type 1 FAP, polymorphisms are revealed by aberrations in the product of this diseased locus, i.e. protein electrophoretic mobility or antigenic variation. Of course, these are directly the result of differences between the DNA sequence from normal and diseased loci. RFLP analysis makes it possible to observe the inheritance pattern probability of syndromes for which no gene product is known. This is done by studying the co-inheritance of polymorphisms of DNA located near or within the affected structural gene.

A hypothetical example of an RFLP analysis to identify the precise location and function of an unknown structural gene responsible for an inherited disease is presented in Figure 13–1. In this hypothetical case, studies reveal that the affected gene is located somewhere on the short arm of chromosome 11 [Fig. 13–1A].

Chromosome 11 has been divided into fragments by restriction endonucleases and has been molecularly cloned in bacteria. An anonymous probe from the chromosome 11 library has been found to hybridize to DNA sequences near the structural gene for this disease, as shown in Figure 13–1C. Individuals receiving the diseased gene frequently contain a polymorphism located within the region of DNA recognized by this probe. The polymorphism resulted in creation of a Hind III site not seen in most of the population, but frequently seen in individuals with the disease [Fig. 13–1B]. Digestion of the individual's chromosomal DNA with Hind III and probing with this anonymous probe can then be used to look for novel restriction fragments which are characteristic of the disease, even though the probe may be recognizing sequences that are millions of base pairs distant from the structural gene responsible for the disease.

Analysis of the enzymatically digested chromosomal DNA from normal and affected individuals is also presented schematically in the figure to show a typical RFLP study. Hundreds of thousands of restriction fragments are generated with a range of molecular weights. These fragments are resolved by electrophoresis, which separates them on the basis of their molecular weight with the larger fragments remaining towards the origin and the smaller migrating towards the bottom [Fig. 13–1C]. The restriction fragment(s) containing the gene of interest will not be visible at this point, since the separation has been on the basis of molecular weight only, and its identity may be obscured by the comigration of thousands of

Chromosome 4:

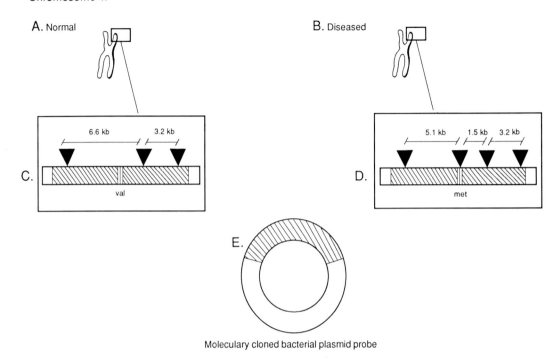

Fig. 13–2. The transthyretin (TTR) gene located on chromosome 4 (2-A) is indicated on the DNA strand as a hatched areas: 2-B. The triangles indicate NsiI sites. The mutant gene (left to A) has an additional NsiI site. The positions of the amino acid valine (val), normal TTR and its substitute methionine (met) (variant TTR in type 1 FAP) are indicated on the DNA strands in the normal and diseased genes in Figure 13–2-B. Figure 13–2-C illustrates the point that a TTR gene has been molecularly cloned and is contained on a bacterial plasmid (hatched box in circle) and serves as a "probe".

other fragments from other parts of the chromosomes. To achieve additional sensitivity for detection, the fragments are transferred to a sheet of nitrocellulose paper by a method referred to as the Southern Blotting Transfer, in recognition of E.M. Southern,[5] who first described the technique [Fig. 13–1C]. The nitrocellulose paper will contain a replica of the gel and can be used for a variety of chemical treatments, including DNA-DNA hybridization. The chromosomal DNA fragments, immobilized on the nitrocellulose paper, are hybridized to a specific "probe" which is homologous to the gene of interest. Only the region of interest is decorated with radioactivity since it binds (hybridizes) to the specific probe. [Fig. 13–1D].

Type 1 FAP provides a good example of RFLP analysis for a disorder in which the structural gene implicated in pathology of disease has been proposed. FAP has been associated with defects within the transthyretin protein, formerly called prealbumin.[8] Figure 13–2 shows that the transthyretin gene is located on chromosome 4 and normally contains three restriction endonuclease NsiI sites. NsiI will make a double stranded cut at every 5' ATGCAT-3" sequence.[4] Therefore, the normal transthyretin gene, as presented here contains three 5'ATGCAT-3 sequences separated by 6.6 and 3.2 kbs. Figure 13–2 also shows that in some type 1 FAP patients, a mutation has occurred that results in a valine to methionine substitution in the protein product. Since the DNA sequence codon that specifies that valine is different from that specifying methionine, an additional NsiI site has also been created in the affected gene.

Digestion of diseased and normal chromosomal DNA with NsiI will result in different sized restriction endonuclease fragments. That is, the transthyretin gene from diseased chromosomal DNA will be contained on different NsiI restriction fragments than is found in a digest of "normal" DNA.

The chromosomal DNA fragments, immobilized on the nitrocellulose paper, are hybridized to a specific probe which is homologous to the gene of interest. In the example shown, the probe is a radioactive copy of the transthyretin gene and will react and bind to any complementary DNA sequences on the nitrocellulose paper. Unbound probe is washed away and only the fragments containing transthyretin sequences outlined in Figure 13–2 are decorated and can be visualized after autoradiography with x-ray film. Here it can been seen that the probe hybridizes 6.6 and 3.2 kb fragments from NsiI digested DNA from a healthy donor. Significantly, a mutation in the transthyretin gene on one chromosome will result in a 5.1 and 1.5 kb fragments, as well as the 6.1 and 3/2 kb fragments contributed by the normal chromosome. The presence of the aberrant restriction fragment is therefore diagnostic for the possession of a diseased genotype since it is part of a specific gene. [See Fig. 13–1 for details about the DNA detection technique.]

The closer the restriction site creating the RFLP is to the structural gene causing the disorder, the more helpful its occurrence will be in predicting inheritance of the defective gene. In the case of FAP, the RFLP was derived from a mutation within the affected genes. In the previous hypothetical case, the RFLP was located some distance from the affected gene, but could still be informative since it was frequently "co-inherited" with the diseased gene. The degree of linkage between two markers is often expressed as a statistical value called the lod score. The lod score is derived from the ratios of likelihoods, to the base of ten, of linkage using pedigree data.[6] For example, a lod score for the linkage of two given markers of 3 indicates that the likelihood of linkage over non-linkage is 1000 to 1. For example, Jackson et al.[9] have reported that the HLA locus and susceptibility to inherited spinocerebellar ataxias are linked on human chromosome number six. After analyzing segregation patterns in 19 members of a kindred, a lod score of 3.15 (at a recombination frequency of 12%) was calculated, suggesting that linkage is favored over

chance by more than 1400 to 1. Studies involving larger sample numbers must be done, however, and it should be noted that some studies dispute a close HLA-dominant hereditary ataxia linkage.[10]

The following conditions must usually be met for DNA diagnosis to be successful. DNA diagnosis is usually done from a blood specimen contributed by the individual along with family members. Diagnosis by RFLP analysis usually requires that the parents be heterozygous and the RFLP must be closely linked to the disease causing locus to minimize the possibility that recombinations between the affected and marker genes have not occurred as this would result in a false-positive. RFLP analysis has indeed served to map various late onset neurologic disorders to specific human chromosomes. However, tests which predict the likelihood of inheriting a diseased locus are available for Huntington's disease, Duchenne's muscular dystrophy, adult onset polycystic kidney disease, and hemophilia B.[11] Since DNA diagnosis requires the isolation of DNA from blood from family members as well as the affected individual, the cooperation of family members is also important.

RFLP analysis is an example of a new technology which offers support to the conventional methods of genetic disease diagnosis, such as recording family history and examination for karyotypic or protein isozyme anomalies (where possible). This kind of DNA diagnosis promises sensitivity and unambiguity and the determination of the presence of defective genetic loci in DNA samples which can be stored and remain stable for long periods of time.[12]

NEUROFIBROMATOSIS

Neurofibromatosis (NF) is a common, inherited disease with an estimated incidence of 1 in 3,000 births.[22] A high rate of spontaneous mutation is associated with this disease. NF presents in a wide variety of ways and exhibits features of both neoplasia and maldevelopment. The cutaneous manifestations of the disease were described as early as 1768 (by Akenside). However, it was Frederick von Recklinghausen, a German pathologist, who first correctly identified the neural origin of the

TABLE 13–2.　Features of NF Categories*

Category	Description	Heritable	CLS	nf	LN	CNS	Other
NF-I	Von Recklinghausen	†	D	D	†	V/F	†
NF-II	Acoustic	†	D	D:F	0	A†	?
NF-III	Mixed	†	D	D:F	?	V/M	?
NF-IV	Variant	†/0	D/?‡	?	?	?	?
NF-V	Segmental	0	L	L	0	?	0
NF-VI	CLS	†/?§	D	0	0	0	?
NF-VII	Late onset	†/?‖	0	D	0	?	?
NF-NOS	Not otherwise specified	?	?	?	?	?	?

*LN, Lisch nodules; nf, neurofibromas; CLS, café-au-lait spots; CNS, central nervous system neural crest-derived tumors; other, phenotypic features considered to be typical or characteristic of NF-I † = present; 0 = absent; ? = possible or uncertain. D, diffuse or widespread distribution; V, variable; F, few; M, multiple; L, limited distribution; A, bilateral acoustic neuromas.

†Infrequently other tumors, especially meningiomas, may be present.

‡Presumably some forms may lack café-au-lait spots.

§Heritability is currently a criterion for assignment to this category, but presumably this restriction is temporary.

‖While no familial cases are known, heritability is not logically excluded.

Reproduced from: Riccardi, V.M.: Neurofibromatosis: Clinical Heterogeneity. *Current Problems in Cancer*, VII(2):3, 1982. Published bimonthly by Year Book Medical Publishers, Inc. Chicago, Il.

neurofibroma and so is credited with the first correct description of the disease that bears his name.

CLASSIFICATION

Clinical attempts to classify neurofibromatosis are quite difficult due to the enormous phenotypic variability with which the disease manifests itself. In their 1986 monograph, Riccardi and Eichner stressed NF's great variety of expression and divided the disease into seven clinical subtypes[23] [Table 13–2]. There is general agreement that a separation exists between central and peripheral forms of the disease; indeed, these are certainly two distinct diseases. The peripheral form—classic von Recklinghausen's disease (NF-1)—is characterized by cutaneous neurofibromas, cafe-au-lait spots (CLS), and pigmented iris hamartomas (Lisch nodules). The hallmark of the central form (NF-2) is a multiplicity of cranial and spinal neoplasms. Bilateral acoustic neuromas are a frequent, but not invariable, component of the central form.[24]

LOCALIZATION

Restriction fragment linked polymorphisms (RFLP) have defined DNA sites near the pericentromeric region of chromosome 17 as being close to the NF-1 locus.[16] For example, two probes, D175133 and pHHO2, recognize

markers that are predicted to be within less than 0.1% recombination units (less than 100 genes) of the actual affected locus in NF-1 and some investigators wonder if this probe recognizes the NF-1 locus itself.[25,26] However, since the location of a functional gene within the pericentromeric region is unprecedented and this is a region saturated with repetitive DNA, investigators wish to accumulate more data before recommending a clinically useful NF-1 diagnostic test. Nevertheless, optimism is high that molecular analysis will eventually provide certainty and objectivity to the diagnosis of NF-1.

Genetic linkage studies locating the defective gene responsible for NF-2 on chromosome 22 are now supported by RFLP analysis. Recently, Rouleau et al. have reported that an RFLP, identified by probe D22S1, occurs in the immediate vicinity of the NF-2 locus.[18] Predictive diagnostic testing is not yet available although it is hoped that, as more closely linked markers are discovered, early detection of tumors and definitive diagnosis will be possible.

CLINICAL MANIFESTATIONS

As the list of clinical manifestations of NF is encyclopedic, we shall limit our attention here to its effects on the nervous system. Tumors are the principal clinical feature of NF in the peripheral nervous system. Neurofibromas can arise anywhere along peripheral nerves, including cranial and autonomic nerves. Clinical symptoms may include weakness, pain or paresthesia, itching, and autonomic dysfunction, in addition to dermatologic complications.[23] Puberty and pregnancy can lead to an increase in the number and size of neurofibromas.[27] Schwannomas can occur widely throughout the peripheral nervous system but are more likely to arise proximally on major nerves or their origins.[23] Interestingly, patients with neurofibromatosis are at an increased risk for malignant peripheral nerve tumors when compared to patients without the disorder.[28]

The list of NF's effects upon the central nervous system is more varied. Several types of CNS tumors are associated with NF.[29] These include acoustic neuromas (which typically present in adulthood and are often bilateral), meningiomas, optic gliomas (which typically occur in children), as well as various other glial tumors such as astrocytomas, medulloblastomas, and ependymomas. Quite a few developmental malformations of the CNS are observed in patients with NF. The lateral thoracic meningocele is a lesion which is fairly specific to NF: 85% of reported cases are afflicted with NF.[29] Other malformative CNS lesions include syringomyelia and hydromyelia, hamartomas of the brain and spinal cord, as well as gray matter heterotopias and cortical architectural anomalies. Among the clinical conditions associated with NF, seizures and mental retardation are more common in NF patients than in the normal population.[29] Cerebrovascular abnormalities are a rare but recognized complication of NF. There is disagreement whether these lesions are primarily due to direct involvement of abnormal neurectodermal tissue or to a primary dysplasia of the arterial wall.[30] Occlusive/stenotic disease, cerebral aneurysm and vertebral arteriovenous fistulas have been described.[30–32] Of note, most cases of occlusive/stenotic disease have been noted in children,[30] and they are frequently associated with Moya-Moya disease.[31,32]

While NF is typically diagnosed in early adulthood or before, the disease certainly expresses itself within the geriatric population. Riccardi, drawing from his large clinical experience, observes that the expression of NF-1 in the seventh decade and beyond is characterized by an apparently slower rate of neurofibroma development and growth, and a fading or loss of cafe-au-lait spots.[33]

PATHOLOGY

The neuropathology of neurofibromatosis chiefly involves the study of its peripheral nerve tumors. The neurofibroma is the characteristic tumor type in NF. Although these tumors can arise anywhere along the peripheral nerve, they are characteristically found in the form of subcutaneous nodules involving terminal nerve twigs and as fusiform enlargements along the course of peripheral nerves.[34] They may be nodular and discrete or diffuse with extensive interdigitation with surrounding tissues.[27] Histologic study shows widely separated fusiform or stellate cells with wiry (nerve) cell processes separated by collagen bundles[35] [Fig.13–3]. Moreover, neurofibromas are composed of several cell types (excluding the nerve cell processes). These include the three main cells of the peripheral nerve sheath: fibroblasts (neurofibromas contain an abundant extracellular collagen matrix), Schwann cells (these cells show a distinct basal lamina on EM[34] and stain for S-100 by protein immunoperoxidase techniques), and perineurial cells (these cells demonstrate an elongated shape and poor reactivity for S-100 protein),[28] as well as mast cells (their role in neurofibromas is speculative). Just which of these cells is the principal tumor cell is a subject of some disagreement and will be considered shortly. Schwannomas tend to occur along peripheral nerve roots [Fig. 13–4].The tumor cell of the Schwannoma is the Schwann cell, as demonstrated by its conspicuous basal lamina on EM. Importantly, both of these tumors can occur in patients without the disease of neurofibromatosis, which has prompted investigators to seek to identify any characteristics which might distinguish the tumors occurring in NF patients from those in non-NF patients. Riccardi, however, holds that there are no apparent differences between NF-associated neurofibromas and those occurring in non-NF patients.[33]

Some authors classify plexiform neurofibroma as a separate lesion, distinct from other

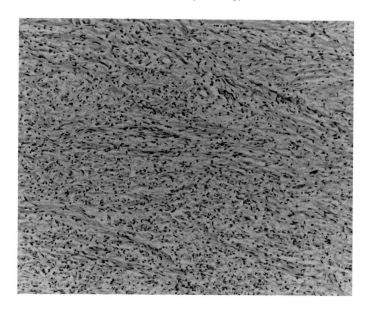

Fig. 13–3. Neurofibroma. The fusiform cells are arranged in loose streams separated by neurites and collagen bundles. H&E × 100.

neurofibromas. This tumor may range from a small cutaneous lesion to a large lesion growing toward the spinal cord, compressing and destroying tissue as it expands. The tumor grows within a nerve fascicle, causing the fascicles to twist upon themselves, eventually creating a lesion resembling a tangle of worms [Fig. 13–5]. Importantly, plexiform neurofibroma is considered by some to be found only in patients with NF although this is not universally accepted.[28]

The identity and nomenclature of the principal cell of the neurofibroma is a subject of some debate. As described earlier, the peripheral nerve sheath comprises three main cells: the fibroblast, the Schwann cell, and the perineurial cell. The name neurofibroma was originally given to this tumor because of the presence of nerve cell processes in an extensive collagen matrix believed to be produced by the fibroblasts. Nevertheless, the emphasis on the fibroblast fell into disfavor, especially after it was demonstrated that Schwann cells were also capable of producing collagen.[35] Consequently, the Schwann cell was considered paramount. Erlandson and Woodruff, however, demonstrated that the neoplastic elements of the neurofibroma lack features of differentiated Schwann cells. Histologically, the principal cell in the neurofibroma is "spindle-shaped with long and extremely thin bipolar cytoplasmic processes" and, on EM, "cell processes

bearing . . . numerous pinocytic vesicles—features more consistent with perineurial cells—are illustrated".[35] Thus, they conclude that the principal cell of the neurofibroma is the perineurial cell. Perineurial cells ensheathe the axons of unmyelinated fibers. What then is the relationship between the perineurial cell and the Schwann cell? This is not fully clear. Like Schwann cells, perineurial cells express the glycosphingolipid galactocerebroside, the major glycolipid of the myelin sheath; unlike Schwann cells, however, perineurial cells stain poorly for S-100 protein and express GFAP and certain other molecules not found on myelin-forming Schwann cells.[36] So the perineurial cell and the Schwann cell may be derived from a common precursor cell (hence, functional variants of the same cell). Because of this uncertainty the perineurial cell is sometimes referred to as a Schwann-like cell (SLC).

Neuropathologic study of the CNS neoplasms in NF patients shows that they do not differ histologically from the same tumors found in non-NF patients. With regard to the malformative lesions that may be found in the central nervous system of patients with neurofibromatosis, the cells of these lesions are noted to show an overly proliferative character. One example of this is subependymal gliofibrillary nodules. These consist of focal, cellular proliferations of fibrillated subependymal glial cells which give rise to well-defined nod-

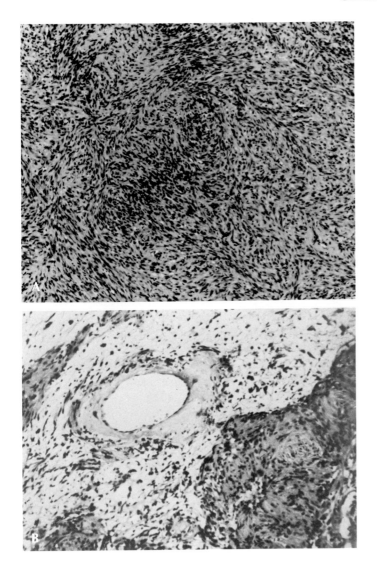

Fig. 13-4. Schwannoma. The tumor is composed of two parts intermingled yet different. The more solid portion, referred to as Antoni A, consists of cells arranged in sheaths or cords, sometimes with nuclei aligned in a pallisade (Fig. 13-4A). The other component of this tumor, named Antoni B consists of loosely arranged cells set in a meshwork of reticulin fibers and microcysts (Fig. 13-4B). H&E × 100.

ules or finger-like projections at various levels of the ventricular cavities.[24] When located along the Aqueduct of Sylvius, they may lead to aqueductal stenosis and consequently, hydrocephalus. Another example is intramedullary Schwannosis, foci of Schwann cells and reticulin fibers within the spinal cord. These are located adjacent to Schwannomas of the dorsal nerve root.[24] Their hyperproliferative nature raises the question if these lesions in fact represent normal reactive processes which have gone awry. This has led to the suggestion that such may be the case even with the neurofibroma. Pleasure et al. studied the response of cultured SLCs to mitogens in an effort to clarify this point.[37] They reason that if these

SLCs are normal cells, their mitosis-rate response to mitogens should be that of normal cells; conversely, if these cells are neoplastic, their baseline mitosis rate should be elevated. However, if the SLCs show a hyperproliferative response, their mitosis-rate response to mitogens will be elevated but their baseline rate will be normal. Thus far, the issue has not been fully clarified.

So far, we have seen that neurofibromatosis is characterized by a wide variety of clinical presentations. In addition, the disease demonstrates several different types of pathologic processes in the nervous system, encompassing neoplastic, proliferative, vascular, and developmental lesions. What pathogenetic

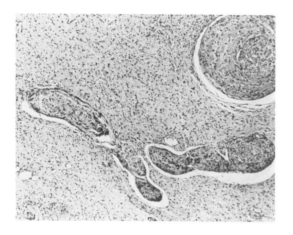

Fig. 13–5. Plexiform neurofibroma. Finger-like projections of the tumor (neurofibroma) invading a tumorous nerve fascicle. H&E × 100.

mechanism, then, might account for this heterogeneous disorder?

In 1974, Bolande put forth the neurocristopathy hypothesis, linking various dysgenetic, hamartomatous, and neoplastic conditions as being of cells which are of neural crest origin.[38] This theory notes that the cells of the neural crest—a transient embryonic structure—are migratory and initially pluripotential.[39] Moreover, neural crest cells are invasive, exhibiting invasive properties when transplanted ectopically into embryonic hosts,[40] and lack fibronectin at their surfaces.[37,38,41] (Transformed neoplastic cells also lack cellular fibronectin.[40]) Clinically, the complex neurocristopathies (of which NF is one) may show marked variability in their phenotypic expression and tend to be hereditable.[38] Pathologically, neurofibromatosis demonstrates several lesions composed of neural crest cells. Cafe-au-lait spots consist of heavily pigmented melanoblasts which are derived from the neural crest; the principal constituents of the neurofibroma are derived from the neural crest; and pheochromocytoma, a recognized complication of NF, may arise from the neuroblast, a primitive neural crest cell. Conversely, APUD cells which are not of neural crest origin do not seem to be involved in the neurocristopathies.[42]

Nevertheless, quite a few aspects of NF are not adequately explained by the neurocristopathy approach. As Riccardi notes, this approach does not explain the mental and motor milestone lags noted in NF patients, the association with NF of some tumors which are not composed of cells that are of neural crest origin (such as rhabdomyosarcoma, and possibly, Wilms' tumor), the role of trauma as a precipitant of tumor formation, or the effect of puberty and pregnancy on the disease.[23] Therefore, other perspectives on the disease are needed in order to gain a fuller understanding of its pathogenesis.

The cellular environment is an area of investigation receiving a good deal of attention. Perhaps the development of neurofibromas is induced by an alteration in the cell's surroundings rather than a product of a primary defect in (tumor) cell functioning. One mechanism by which this might occur is through abnormal hormonal communication between cells. Nerve growth factor (NGF) is a hormone that has been studied extensively in neurofibromatosis. It is curious that some NF patients have elevated levels of NGF cross-reacting protein by radioimmune assay yet the biologic activity of the hormone remains normal in these patients. This suggests that a structurally abnormal NGF molecule may be produced in some cases of NF.[29,41] Another finding suggestive of hormonal mediation is the association of pregnancy and puberty with exacerbation of neurofibromas. Finally, the malformative CNS lesions described earlier suggest a hyperproliferative response of an otherwise normal reactive process and raise the possibility of increased activity of cell growth factors in these patients.[24]

Another area to consider is the role of mast cells. They are an important component of neurofibromas yet their embryologic origin is obscure. The presence of mast cells in the tumors presumably represents a positive influence on the tumors' growth. Mast cell secretions can change local intercellular environments thereby altering cell functions and proliferation.[27] In addition, trauma as a precipitant of local cutaneous neurofibromas, and the attendant pruritus, suggest an association of neurofibroma formation with mast cells.

Returning to Bolande's neurocristopathy model, these lesions may thus arise due to abnormalities of the neural crest cell's microenvironment.[40] It is known that although neural crest cells are initially pluripotential, their ultimate differentiation depends, in part, upon local cell-cell interactions. For example, would-be vagal cells from the upper part of the body can be transplanted to the lower part where they become adrenergic cells.[41] So, it can be hypothesized that certain abnormalities in the neural crest cell's environment may induce neoplastic dedifferentiation in this invasive, pluripotential cell.

Cellular membrane abnormalities must also be considered in the pathogenesis of neurofibromas. A number of investigators proposed that dominant gene mutations involve structural protein genes and that some of these (abnormal) structural proteins are inserted into the cell membrane. Thus, hormonal (or other messenger) receptors on the cell membranes may be awry due to abnormalities of the receptors themselves or of the structure of the cell's plasma membrane.[43] This concept will also be discussed in connection with Huntington's disease.

HUNTINGTON'S DISEASE (See Chap. 7)

Huntington's disease is an inherited, degenerative disease of the brain. First described in 1872 by George Huntington, based upon observations of a family in his father's medical practice, this disease has enjoyed a renaissance of interest in the 1970s and 1980s. New concepts regarding its neuropathologic processes have been advanced and explorations into the disease's biochemical abnormalities have been made. In addition, determination of the gene's locus on chromosome 4 has contributed to the kindling of interest in genetic investigation of this disease.

CLINICAL MANIFESTATIONS

Clinically, Huntington's disease comprises a triad of autosomal dominant inheritance, dementia, and choreoathetosis. The mental and movement disorders need not develop simultaneously, and there is no general rule regarding which one will develop first. The mental disorder may evolve through several subtle states before dementia is apparent. These early stages may manifest as emotional alterations

of character or mood. Older medical writings reported that Huntington's disease families have a high incidence of psychopathy and sociopathy;[44] however, Adams and Victor do not concur.[45] The movement abnormality is, likewise, progressive. At first slight, with the patient considered fidgety, it becomes more pronounced until the entire musculature is involved. The usual age of onset is in the third, fourth, or fifth decade. Chandler et al. observed that in patients with late onset Huntington's disease (sixth and seventh decade) the choreiform movements and progressive dementia have their onset at nearly the same time while the emotional alterations are usually less prominent.[44]

PATHOLOGY

Neuropathologic investigation demonstrates that degenerative changes occur throughout the brain. In the first decades following Huntington's description, neuropathologic observations were interpreted as indicative of a chronic encephalopathy. The first reports which linked Huntington's disease to an alteration in the brain's structure were made early this century with the demonstration of caudate shrinkage in postmortem specimens.[46,47] Due to the gliotic appearance of the atrophied tissue, it was assumed that the observed atrophy was the result of an increase in the population of glial cells.

Recent work has demonstrated loss of neuronal as well as glial cells in the striatum of Huntington's disease brains. Furthermore, the neuronal loss has been shown to be related to cell size.[48] Morphometric studies by Lange et al. and others have revealed that the small to large neuron ratio of the striatum is normally around 175:1. This is reduced to 40:1 or less in Huntington's disease, the major loss being neurons which average 8.5 μm in diameter.[49] Moreover, quantitative studies have shown that glial cell loss also occurs in the striatum.[48] Thus, the gliotic appearance of the tissue—the changes in neurons and glia result in an increase of the normal neuron to glial cell ratio of 1:3.5 to 1:10—is chiefly produced by the relatively greater loss of neurons than glial cells.[49] Fibrillary hyperplasia of astrocytes undoubtedly occurs and is particularly intense in the subependymal tissues and around blood vessels, however, this must be interpreted as a defense reaction.[46] Neuronal and glial cell loss subseqeuntly leads to neostriatal shrinkage.

Loss of neuronal and glial cells occurs both in the putamen and caudate nucleus. At times, both are affected equally; at other times, one is more affected than the other. In addition, cell loss within either striatal nucleus is not evenly distributed. For example, the earliest changes seen in the caudate nucleus are in the medial paraventricular portions and the tail.[47] With regard to the neuronal cell loss distribution in the putamen in Huntington's disease, Roos et al. demonstrated that the ventral anterior portion was relatively spared (as compared with the other parts of the putamen).[50] The external segment of the globus pallidus shows depletion of large neurons; in some instances, so does the internal segment. Demyelination may affect the border between the pallidum and the internal capsule. In some cases, volume reduction of the globus pallidus may be similar to that of the striatum. The ansa and fasciculus lenticularis show pallor.[48]

In the diencephalon, the small internuncial neuron population in the ventrolateral basal thalamus is reduced by 50% with the macroneuronal population unaltered.[51] Neuronal hyperchromasia with shrinkage and loss in the supraoptic and ventromedial hypothalamic nuclei as well as cell loss in the lateral hypothalamic nuclei have been reported.[46] Study of the substantia nigra reveals that cell loss to some degree is present in many cases. Fibrillary gliosis is present particularly in the zona reticularis. Other changes which are found at times include loss of dentate nucleus cells and Purkinje cells of the cerebellum. According to Bruyn et al., there is severe involvement of the superior olivary, lateral vestibular, dorsal vagal, and hypoglossal nuclei of the brainstem.[46] The spinal cord regularly demonstrates pallor of the lateral and anterior tracts. The cerebral cortical mantle is reduced in thickness with neuronal loss and architectural disarrangement of the third and fifth (and also often the fourth) layers. The neuronal loss may be either diffuse or focal. The frontal lobes are usually most affected. Many remaining neurons are shrunken, show bizarre shapes, and are misaligned with respect to the cortical surface. Some are reduced to "ghost" cells. Many neurons and glial cells show accumulation of lipofuscin. Diffuse myelin loss with accumulation of lipopigment in astrocytes and perivascular histiocytes occurs in the white matter. The apparent increase in astrocytes is due to tissue shrinkage.

Ultrastructural analysis reveals abnormalities of both neuronal and glial cells. Striking with regard to neurons is the extent to which the membrane systems of these cells are disturbed. Using frontal cortex brain biopsy material, Tellez-Nagel et al. demonstrated irregularity and interruption of the nuclear envelope by numerous pores, proliferation of Golgi apparatus membranes, as well as disorganization of the rough endoplasmic reticulum in association with a relative increase in the number of smooth endoplasmic reticulum membranes.[52] Roos and Bots made a detailed examination of the nuclear membrane irregularities in the frontal cortex, caudate nucleus, and nucleus accumbens of Huntington's disease patients against age-matched controls.[53] They described a marked (6- to 7-fold) increase in the frequency of these nuclear membrane indentations in the caudate nucleus and nucleus accumbens of Huntington's disease patients; controls had a nearly 2-fold greater frequency of nuclear membrane indentations in the frontal cortex. (Interestingly, these groups of observers drew different conclusions regarding the implications of the nuclear membrane irregularities. The former group advocated that the general disturbance of the neuron in Huntington's disease was reflected most profoundly in a derangement of membrane structures, whereas the latter group maintained that membrane irregularities served a defensive role for the cell for they resulted in greater membrane surface area for protein synthesis.) Membrane abnormalities were also apparent at the mitochondrial level as the mitochondria were greatly enlarged with few cristae and dense, granular material occupied the matrix. These changes were noted in the mitochondria of neurons and astrocytes. Important to this discussion of Huntington's disease, these membrane irregularities may be the result of a genetic defect manifested as abnormal structural proteins.

Accumulation of lipopigment granules was

frequent in neurons and astrocytes. The glial lipofuscin granules were more varied in appearance. Some showed more abundant vacuolar portions, while others had a more abundant dense portion of the granule. Finally, the neurons presented clumping of nuclear chromatin into numerous small aggregates.

NEUROCHEMISTRY

Study of the biochemistry of Huntington's disease has attracted a great deal of attention since the early 1970s. In 1973, Perry et al. reported a decrease of GABA (gamma aminobutyric acid) in the substantia nigra, globus pallidus, and striatum of Huntington's disease patients as compared to normal subjects.[54] GABA is held to be the principal neurotransmitter involved in the mainly inhibitory output of the striatum to the globus pallidus and substantia nigra. Thus, accepting the combination of decreased GABA concentration with the loss of striatal small neurons as the cause of the choreic symptoms appeared seductive. Complicating the picture, however, further study has shown depletion of other neurotransmitters, including enkephalins, substance P, and dynorphin. These neurotransmitters, as well as GABA, are produced by a population of morphologically similar cells termed spiny neurons. What is more, Ferrante et al. have reported that the population of aspiny neurons in the neostriatum is selectively resistant to the degenerative process(es) of Huntington's disease.[55] The neurotransmitters identified with aspiny neurons include NADPH-d (nicotinamide adenine dinucleotide phosphate diaphorase), somatostatin, neuropeptide Y, and others. This differential cell loss has focused attention on the process(es) responsible for selective cellular degeneration in Huntington's disease.

Kanaic acid, a product isolated from Japanese seaweed, is a conformational analogue of L-glutamic acid and acts as a more potent excitant of CNS neurons than L-glutamic acid. Because a major input to the GABA-ergic cells of the striatum is from cerebral cortical cells which use glutamate as their neurotransmitter, it is hypothesized that striatal neuronal degeneration in Huntington's disease is due to a neurotoxic potential of glutamate-induced depo-

larization upon these cells.[56] Injection of kanaic acid into the striatum of rats produces a toxic effect which reproduces many of the morphologic features of Huntington's disease. For example, striatal neurons are lost, whereas bundles of myelinated axons (presumably internal capsule fibers) are preserved; however, the pattern of neuronal loss seen in kanaic acid injected striata is less selective than that seen in Huntington's disease.[57,58] More recently, quinolinic acid has been shown to induce neuronal, axon-sparing lesions in the rodent brain.[59] Quinolinic acid is an endogenous, neuroexcitatory metabolite of tryptophan. It is believed to act upon the N-methyl D-aspartate (NMDA) subgroup of glutamate receptors and its neurotoxic effects can be blocked by NMDA-receptor antagonists.[59] Beal et al. have demonstrated that quinolinic acid inflicts a pattern of neuronal loss in the striatum which is more specific than that seen with kanaic acid and more similar to the pattern of cell loss in the striatum seen in Huntington's disease.[58,60,61] Thus the concept of cellular degeneration due to excitatory neurotoxins has gained considerable currency. Why this cell loss is selective (to spiny neurons) remains to be explained. Current hypotheses include the observation that NADPH-d detoxifies quinone derivatives as well as the suggestion that NADPH-d-transmitting cells lack glutamate receptors and so are resistant to excitotoxins. Although they do not address certain issues, such as the role of the hereditary transmission of Huntington's disease, these toxic neuroexcitatory models serve as a promising base from which greater insights into the mysteries of Huntington's disease can be achieved.

Recently, a restriction fragment linked polymorphism (RFLP) has been associated with the Huntington's disease locus.[13] The RFLP is recognized by hybridization to a marker, called G8, which is a 17 kD (17,000 base pairs) fragment of DNA derived form the short arm of chromosome number 4 and is located approximately 10 million base pairs (more than 100 genes) from the actual Huntington locus.[62] At least 90% of those fated to experience Huntington's disease in one study had the characteristic Hind III restriction endonuclease fragment allele recognized by hybridization to the G8 marker, allowing for predictive determination analysis. This is because that particular RFLP is located near the Huntington locus and is co-inherited with the defective locus 90% of the time according to that study. Since the marker is not closer to or identical to the Huntington locus recombinations and there is a fixed possibility that other, as yet unappreciated loci, contribute to the Huntington's pathology, the accuracy of predictive diagnostic testing was limited to 90%. As markers closer (or identical) to the actual disease locus are discovered and more is understood about the genetics of Huntington's disease, the confidence in predictive testing will grow even further.

OLIVOPONTOCEREBELLAR ATROPHY

Concepts regarding the olivopontocerebellar atrophies (OPCA) have undergone a great deal of reworking since the term was introduced late last century. Dejerine and Thomas first used the term (l'atrophie olivopontocerebelleuse) in their study of two patients with a distinctive type of chronic progressive cerebellar degeneration appearing in middle age. The patients walked with a broad-based, ataxic gait. Additional features included minimal action tremor, slow, scanning speech and disturbance of ocular motility. Autopsy examination in one of the patients demonstrated a particular pattern of atrophy: in summary, symmetric atrophy of the cerebellar cortex with atrophy of the basis pontis and marked atrophy of the inferior olive. Thus was born the descriptive term "olivopontocerebellar atrophy" which served as the title of the published report.[63]

EPIDEMIOLOGY

Over the years, numerous reports of familial (principally autosomal dominant inheritance) ataxia associated with autopsy demonstrated atrophy of the inferior olive, basis pontis, and cerebellar cortex have been published. These included retrospective reflections upon cases in the literature which appeared prior to Dejerine and Thomas's work, such as Menzel's monograph of 1891. It became apparent that those conditions grouped together due to ataxia and this shared pattern of atrophy demonstrated many differences in their clinical presentations, even within a kindred.[64] In addition, differences in the pathologic condition

of other CNS structures among OPCA patients were observed. In an effort to impose order on this disparate group of patients, classification schemes based chiefly on clinical similarities and differences among patients were devised. Perhaps the schema of Konigsmark and Weiner is the best known.[65] Nevertheless, each schema has been challenged and no method of classifying the OPCAs is universally accepted.

CLINICAL MANIFESTATIONS

Progressive ataxia is the unifying clinical feature in these patients with several broad categories of associated findings. Disorders of ocular motility are frequently encountered; abnormality of saccadic movements in OPCA has been remarked upon since the latter part of the 19th century.[66] Optic atrophy and pigmentary retinal degeneration are described as well. Extrapyramidal, or Parkinsonian, symptomatology constitutes another group of associated findings. Sometimes, the extrapyramidal symptoms serve to mask the cerebellar syndrome, rendering the latter difficult to identify. As OPCA does not respond to L-DOPA therapy, L-DOPA failure in the absence of family history may lead to the mistaken diagnosis of striatonigral degeneration. Dementia may be seen as an associated finding in OPCA. It can appear in any phase of the disease, particularly in the middle to late period. When present early in the disease course, it may cause errors of diagnosis. Some other associated abnormalities reported include alteration in deep tendon reflexes (both increased and decreased stretch reflexes have been described), bulbar palsies, and autonomic nervous system dysfunction. This last abnormality, when it presents as the initial, prominent symptom may result in diagnostic confusion with other dysautonomic diseases such as the Shy-Drager syndrome. Harding (1982) and Berciano (1982), among others, give full discussions of the clinical features of these disorders.[64,66]

PATHOLOGY

Essentially, the term olivopontocerebellar atrophy represents a neuropathologic description. On gross examination, the cerebellum is small and the cisterna magna and ambient cistern are expanded. The dentate nuclei may re-

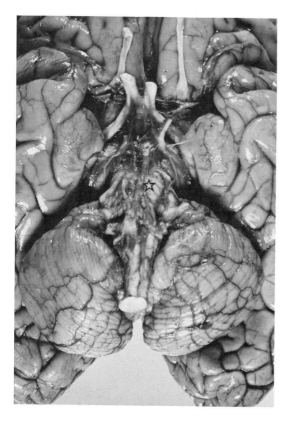

Fig. 13–6. Olivopontocerebellar atrophy. The star indicates the shrunken pons.

veal no abnormalities or may be poorly defined. The pons is diminished in size and the protuberance of the basis pontis is reduced [Fig. 13–6]. There is atrophy of the middle cerebellar peduncle. The basilar artery lies loose in the widened prepontine space. The bulge of the inferior olive may vary from shrunken to normal in size.

Light microscopic examination consistently reveals loss of Purkinje cells in the cerebellum. The remaining Purkinje cells may be unevenly distributed throughout the cerebellar cortex, although this does not obviously correlate with position in the folium or relationship to the vasculature.[67] Bergmann astrocytes become prominent. Silver staining techniques show well-formed ganglionic plexus axons surrounding the remaining Purkinje cells as well as encircling empty spaces where Purkinje cells presumably once had been.[68] Eosinophilic torpedoes—expansion of Purkinje cell axons—are variable in the granular layer. Neuronal loss and gliosis in the dentate nuclei is variable. Increased amounts of lipofuscin in the neurons of the dentate nuclei have been reported.[68] Sections of the pons display loss of pontine nuclei and transverse pontine fibers as well as replacement gliosis [Fig. 13–7]. Simi-

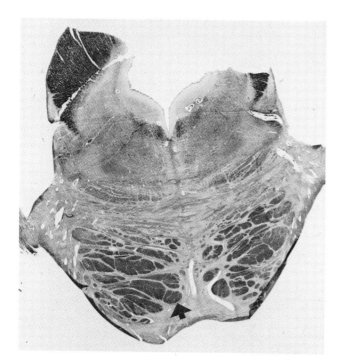

Fig. 13–7. Olivopontocerebellar atrophy. Pons. Myelin stained section showing normally myelinated pyramidal tract (arrow) surrounded by demyelinated (unstained) frontocerebellar tract.

larly, there is neuronal loss and reactive gliosis in the inferior olive. This neuronal loss ranges from minor to complete. In addition, periolivary fibers and fibers of the amiculum are reduced.[69]

Electron microscopy studies confirm that the Purkinje cells bear the brunt of neuropathologic change in the cerebellum. Ultrastructural studies have detailed an aberrant pattern of membrane organization in the Purkinje cells.[67] This comprises a paucity of RER and a concomitant increase in the number of free ribosomes, stacked cisternae (flattened membraneous stacks) in the perikaryon, dendritic arbor, and axon collateral plexus, as well as a proliferation of membraneous tubules. These findings are not pathognomonic of this disease. Increased amounts of lipofuscin and increased numbers of mitochondria were also noted in the Purkinje cells. The eosinophilic torpedoes noted on light microscopy are composed of randomly arranged, occasionally branching filaments measuring approximately 12 to 15 μm in diameter, with minute osmophilic particles, short profiles of ER, and mitochondria dispersed among them.[68] Crystalloid inclusions are observed in the cerebellar biopsy material of Landis et al. These structures appeared to be a lattice of roughly spherical particles 20 to 25 μm in diameter, packed in orthogonal array in one axis and in hexagonal array in another axis.[67] Marked changes in the fibers projecting to the cerebellum were noted on biopsy specimens, thereby identifying the neurons in the inferior olive and pons as major targets of the disease process.[68]

NEUROCHEMISTRY

Neurochemistry has opened up new vistas in our exploration of nervous system function. As it is not bound by the limits inherent in microscopy—morphologic descriptions of static states—neurochemical analysis has begun to open the door to a greater understanding of nerve cell interactions and disease processes. A broad literature is developing concerning the differing patterns of neurotransmitter abnormalities among patients with OPCA.

Deficiencies of glutamate, aspartate, GABA,

and taurine in the cerebellum of patients with OPCA have been described. In 1981, Perry measured amino acid contents in the brains of patients with OPCA from three different pedigrees. Despite clinical similarities—these patients were classifed as having the same clinical diagnosis—three biochemically distinct disorders were found.[70] Each disorder comprised a specific combination of amino acid deficiencies. One pedigree demonstrated decreased aspartate, glutamate, and GABA in the cerebellar cortex along with marked decrease of GABA in the dentate nucleus. The second family showed increased taurine in the cerebellar cortex along with the above findings. And the third pedigree revealed no biochemical abnormality of the cerebellar cortex with decrease of dentate nucleus GABA.[71] Similarly, in 1977, Perry et al. reported on the amino acid contents in the autopsied brains of two affected members of a pedigree afflicted with OPCA. These specimens demonstrated reduction of aspartic acid and GABA in the cerebellar cortex and dentate nucleus in addition to elevation of taurine content in the same brain regions; glutamate content was normal in the regions where aspartate was reduced.[72] The above findings suggest two interesting hypotheses. First, each combination of neurotransmitter deficiencies represents a unique disease entity, classifiable according to its amino acid deficiency profile. Second, these abnormalities imply loss or dysfunction of specific cerebellar neurons, i.e. those neurons which utilize the deficient amino acids as neurotransmitters.

Glutamic acid is considered to be the neurotransmitter of the parallel fibers of the granule cells. These cells innervate the Purkinje cells forming excitatory synapses. Glutamic acid is probably also the excitatory neurotransmitter of the population of mossy fibers. GABA is considered to be the inhibitory neurotransmitter of the Purkinje cells as well as of the Golgi and basket cell interneurons. The third category of cerebellar interneurons, the stellate cells, employs taurine as its inhibitory neurotransmitter. Aspartic acid acts as the neurotransmitter of the climbing fibers. As with the parallel fibers of the granule cells, the climbing fibers form excitatory synapses with the Purkinje cells.

Linking neurotransmitter abnormalities and selective neuronal loss with genetically determined phenomena in these inherited diseases has become a second field of research and imagination. With an eye toward the enzyme coding function of DNA, a good deal of work has been done regarding the enzyme glutamate dehydrogenase (GDH). GDH forms part of an enzymatic complex for transferring amino groups between alpha keto acids and their corresponding alpha amino acids. Deficiency of GDH (which can be measured in vitro in cultured skin fibroblasts and leukocytes) has been found in a limited subset of OPCA patients.[73] Duvoisin et al. identified 9 patients with GDH deficiency and pointed out that enzyme activity in these patients is not totally absent, but rather is reduced to about 40% of mean control values.[74] He explained this partial decrease as due to loss of a specific subpopulation of the GDH enzyme. Perhaps the residual activity accounts for the delay in the appearance of the disease until adult life.

Recently, the neurotoxic properties of excitatory neurotransmitters have been demonstrated. These observations have led to the hypothesis that altered neuroexcitatory mechanisms may be responsible for the selective neuronal degeneration that occurs in certain disorders. In the brain, GDH is thought to play a part in the catabolism of glutamate released at synapses as a neurotransmitter. Plaitakis hypothesizes that decreased catabolism of glutamate, causing accumulation of the amino acid at the Purkinje cell nerve terminal, could lead to toxic degeneration of the postsynaptic (Purkinje) neuron.[73] That glutamate levels in the brains of OPCA patients have been found to be either normal or diminished is explained by degeneration of the parallel fibers as a secondary event attributable to the disappearance of the Purkinje cell (transneuronal degeneration). Whether or not this mechanism proves to be correct,[75] it is a useful model because it explains a process of neuronal loss on the basis of a genetically determined phenomenon (i.e., the metabolism of glutamate).

Lately, the concept of olivopontocerebellar atrophy has come under increasing attack. As indicated earlier, the clinical presentation is quite varied and diagnosis is often mistaken. Furthermore, the constellation of pathologic features implied by the term olivopontocerebellar atrophy is rarely isolated; associated degenerative changes are the rule rather than the exception. Thus, OPCA is a pathologic description, "not specific to a single disease, but may be found in a number of disorders. . .".[75] What is emerging from studies of neurochemistry and molecular genetics is a new way to look at inherited, degenerative disorders of the nervous system. This new orientation is based upon the selective loss of one or more species of nerve cells. With this loss, the mode of communication—the neurotransmitter—of each lost species of cell is diminished. Symptoms are the product of this selective alteration of neurotransmitter input upon nerve cells downstream. The causes of selective neuronal degeneration remain undefined. The toxic neuroexcitatory model may in the future be confirmed as one mechanism. Be that as it may, mechanisms of selective neuronal degeneration in inherited disease will have to be explained with reference to genetically determined phenomena.

In the meantime, the appellation OPCA will continue to serve as a holding area for these diseases. As their genetic and biochemical bases are determined, they will be renamed accordingly and removed from the generic OPCA category. As an example, one type of OPCA has been mapped to a specific human chromosome and can be tracked, in part, with an RFLP marker. This inherited ataxia has been shown to be genetically linked to the major histocompatibility locus on chromosome 6.[77,78] Recently, a 7 generation kindred with this HLA-linked OPCA was studied to detect RFLPs that might more precisely locate the putative ataxia locus. These investigators report success and that an anonymous DNA marker derived from chromosome 6 does identify an RFLP located near (but not identical to) the OPCA locus.[79] Reliable predictive testing is not yet possible, since the RFLP is reasonably distant from the "defective" OPCA locus. There is now on the horizon, however, promise that objective criteria for classification of the olivopontocerebellar atrophies are forthcoming and that the beginnings of a molecular understanding of these varied disorders are now at hand.

MACHADO-JOSEPH DISEASE

Machado-Joseph disease is a hereditary disease with an autosomal dominant pattern of transmission which presents primarily as a progressive ataxia. Like the olivopontocerebellar atrophies, Machado-Joseph disease is an ataxia with associated multiple system degenerations; however, in contrast to the OPCAs, the cerebellar cortex and olivary nuclei are consistently spared. An early report of this entity was made in 1972 and was a study of 51 affected members of a family living in Massachusetts descended from one William Machado, a native of the Portuguese Azores. That report along with reports of ataxia associated with multiple system degeneration in other families of Portuguese ancestry (Thomas family of Massachusetts, 1972; Joseph family of California, 1976) led neurologists to the Azores in an effort to identify the disease there. This resulted in a unification of these maladies under the umbrella of one disease with separate but interrelated subtypes. The discovery of yet another similarly affected American family of Portuguese Azores descent led to the proposition to call the disease "Azorean disease of the Nervous System." However, subsequent reports of individuals affected with this disease but not of Azorean, or even Portuguese, ancestry rendered the concept of "Azorean disease" incorrect.[80,81] Thus, by convention, the eponym "Machado-Joseph disease" is used to designate these patients.

CLINICAL MANIFESTATIONS

With its associated multiple system degenerations and different severities of ataxia, Machado-Joseph disease demonstrates varied clinical presentations among patients, even within families. In addition to ataxia, other findings include progressive amyotrophy, pyramidal tract involvement, peripheral neuropathy, progressive external ophthalmoplegia, and dystonic posturing. Intelligence remains normal. The mode of inheritance is autosomal dominant with variable penetrance. In 1984, diagnostic criteria were established by the

Quebec Cooperative Study of Friedreich's Ataxia.[82]

PATHOLOGY

The neuropathology of Machado-Joseph disease has been reviewed by Coutinho et al. and by Sachdev et al.[83,84] Neuronal loss and gliosis are consistently noted in the substantia nigra and are usually observed in the dentate nucleus, pontine nuclei, anterior horns, and Clarke's column. Cranial nerve motor nuclei are at times involved as well. Loss of myelinated fibers is reported in the spinocerebellar tracts and middle cerebellar peduncle. The cerebellar cortex and inferior olives are decidedly normal. In summary then, the neuropathology of Machado-Joseph disease is a multi-system degeneration of the nervous system particularly affecting the dentate nucleus of the cerebellum, pontine nuclei, spinocerebellar tracts, and substantia nigra, while consistently sparing the cerebellar cortex and inferior olives.[84]

NEUROCHEMISTRY

Thus far, the primary biochemical defect in Machado-Joseph disease has not been identified.[85] In an effort to identify a physiologic marker, Hotson et al. have suggested that in certain oculomotor abnormalities of saccade and smooth pursuit a gain may lead to early confirmation of the disease.[86] However, their data indicate that such eye movement studies are in fact relatively insensitive.

The greatest promise to understanding the pathogenesis of Machado-Joseph disease lies in identifying the molecular genetic basis of the malady. Rosenberg and Grossman have recently described preliminary findings based upon restriction fragment length polymorphism studies in this disease.[87,88] Using leukocyte genomic DNA to obtain DNA polymorphisms on Southern blots, their data suggest that the primary mutation may reside on the short arm of chromosome 1, near the amylase gene locus (1p21). The authors admit, however, that these data are weak and efforts to look elsewhere for linkage should continue.

An issue of importance in the study of genetic diseases, especially those with autosomal dominant inheritance, is the observation of variable (or incomplete) penetrance. Theoretically, 50% of the children of a parent affected by an autosomal dominant disease should themselves be affected. However, Rosenberg and Grossman studied 164 families with a parent affected by Machado-Joseph disease and observed that only 38.3% of their children over 40 expressed the disease.[87] In an effort to put the phenomenon of variable penetrance onto a molecular genetic basis, these authors have proposed the presence of a modifier gene in Machado-Joseph disease. This modifier gene, located at a separate locus from the primary defect, has the ability to influence the expression of the disease. "An association of an electrophoretic form of erythrocyte acid phosphatase (ACP-1) and absence of clinical disease was seen in one of our Joseph disease families, so that the postulated modifier gene may be linked to the ACP-1 locus and cosegregate with it. This implies that those persons who inherit the modifier gene . . . and the mutant . . . disease gene will have minimal or no clinical disease."[87] The gene map location for ACP-1 is the short arm of chromosome 2 (2p23).

LATE ONSET FAMILIAL AMYLOIDOTIC POLYNEUROPATHY (FAP) (Transthyretin Neuropathy)

Familial amyloidotic polyneuropathy (FAP) is a group of autosomal dominant diseases characterized by the presence of amyloid, containing transthyretin (TTR) (or prealbumin) in peripheral nerves and in other organs.[89-93] The onset of all forms of FAP occurs usually between the ages of 25 and 55 and less frequently between 55 and 82. The average duration of the disease is 9 to 10 years. Late onset familial amyloidotic polyneuropathy (FAP) is the name given to the disease when the onset is after the age of 55; more often the onset is before the age of 55 but the patient consults the physician for the first time after the age of 55.[94]

BIOCHEMISTRY

FAP was first recognized by Andrade in the Santo Antonia Hospital in Oporto, Portugal in 1952.[89] There followed clinical descriptions of familial variants of FAP in other countries, mostly Japan, Sweden, and the United States.[95-111] Eventually the disease was subdivided into 5 main types, based on the clinical manifestations and their chronology, the age of onset, the distribution of organ involvement and the family history: Type I (Portuguese), Type II (Indiana), Type III (Iowa), Type IV (cranial neuropathy with corneal lattice dystrophy), Type V (familial oculoleptomeningeal amyloidosis). With the discovery by Costa and his colleagues in 1978[112] that TTR was associated with FAP, considerable work has been done in the structure and genetic characteristics of the variants of TTR involved in FAP.[113-119] TTR is a product of chromosome 18.[120,121]

TTR is a plasma protein with an anti-parallel beta-sheet conformation. RFLP markers have indicated different amino acid substitution in the TTR protein in different clinical forms of FAP.[103,111,122-127,143] Valine is replaced by methionine at position 30 of TTR in Type I FAP;[15,31] serine is substituted for isoleucine at position 84 in Type II FAP;[126] isoleucine is substituted for phenylalanine at position 33 in another case[124] and alanine is replaced by threonine at position 60 in yet another case.[125] These genetic studies have shown that a biochemical defect in FAP may be expressed by a particular clinical picture. Holmgren et al.[128] have reported that the near age onset of symptoms in 17 members of a Swedish family with Type I FAP (methionine for valine substitution) was 53 years of age, whereas it was 32 years in a Portuguese family,[98] 32 years in a Japanese family[127] and 40 years in a USA family of Swedish descent.[129]

EPIDEMIOLOGY

Type 1 (Portuguese) is the most common type and includes the elderly cases of the disease. The onset is usually after the age of 25 and it presents as a sensory neuropathy with eventual autonomic involvement and amyloid deposition in kidneys, ears, eyes, and skin. The first signs of the disease appeared after the age of 40 in 67 of the 483 patients registered at the Santo Antonia Hospital in Oporto.[98] Fifty-three of these patients corresponded to 46 family trees. In 12 of these families late onset cases were dominant and 6 of 3 families were composed exclusively of late onset cases (over 60). Andersson[7] described cases of FAP with onset at the average age of 55 for women and 45 for men; 10 of these patients were ages 60 to 70 when first examined. Hofer and Andersson[96] reported that the diagnosis of FAP was confirmed by biopsy in 18 patients between the ages of 60 and 75. Saraiva and his colleagues[108] described 31 individuals with FAP in 1 family with onset at ages 6 to 70 years in 3 generations. Tanaka and his colleagues[110] described a 47-year-old woman with FAP; her 81-year-old mother and 53-year-old sister were proved to be asymptomatic carriers of the TTR variant.

Type II FAP has been reported in 2 families in Indiana.[130-132] The earliest symptoms are pain and numbness in the hands, associated with a carpal tunnel syndrome in early middle life, followed eventually by generalized sensory and autonomic neuropathies and deposition of amyloid in the viscera. In type 2 there is a substitution of serine for isoleucine in position 84 of TTR.[126]

The clinical manifestations and evolution of the disease of Type III FAP (van Allen) resembles those of Type I, with a higher incidence of duodenal ulcer. Some authors consider Types I and III to be the same disease. Present studies of the chemical construction of TTR in the clinical variants will presumably clarify the situation.

Meretoja[133] reported 10 patients in 3 families with a generalized amyloidosis characterized by cranial neuropathy, lattice cornea, dystrophy, and skin laxity. The disease pattern here is referred to as Type IV FAP.

PATHOLOGY

The pathologic picture in all cases of FAP is that of deposition of masses of amyloid fibrils primarily around blood vessels and throughout the tissue [Fig. 13–8]. Besides the perivascular deposits of amyloid in the peripheral and autonomic nerves there are deposits in the perineurium, in the endoneurium, and in the endoneurial spaces where it mingles with the collagen fibers. Alkaline congo red and polarizing studies of this congo positive material (green) is an effective way of identifying the amyloid. Electron microscopy studies show the typical amyloid fibrils measuring 50 pm in width. The EM study also reveals a striking decrease in the number of unmyelinated fibers, varying degrees of loss of myelinated fibers of all sizes and masses of connective tissue interwoven among the fibers [Fig. 13–9]. There is some invasion of the Schwann cells by the amyloid.

The diagnosis of late onset FAP is based on the following factors: (1) The clinical manifes-

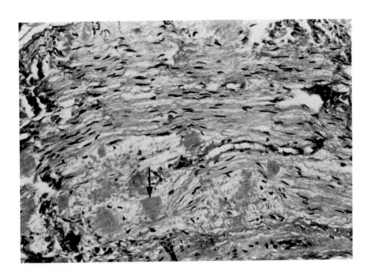

Fig. 13–8. FAP. Arrow indicates deposit of amyloid nerve fascicle. H&E × 100.

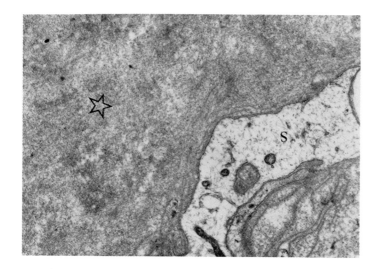

Fig. 13-9. Fibrillary amyloid deposit (star) situated near Schwann cell (s). × 7000.

tations, chronology of the disease and the family history. (2) The presence of amyloid around vessels and in the parenchyma of various organs, in particular peripheral nerves. For diagnostic purposes, the demonstration of amyloid in a biopsy of the skin suffices.[131] (3) Quantitation of TTR in blood and CSF can be of diagnostic help.[134-135] The electrophoretic pattern of blood serum usually does not show a TTR (pre-albumin) band and its presence is indicative of higher than normal TTR level, however, its absence does not exclude that diagnosis. The TTR band in the electrophoretic study of CSF is usually present.[136] (4) DNA analysis in which total genomic DNA is extracted from leukocytes and examined with hybridization probes for the presence of specific RFLP markers.[137]

ALZHEIMER'S DISEASE (See Chap. 4)

The pathogenesis of Alzheimer's Disease (AD) is being investigated with recently developed molecular biologic techniques which identify the proteins and genes which encode them. These techniques have been used to study the predominant histologic lesions in AD, amyloid deposits in senile plaques in the cerebral grey matter and around cerebral and meningeal blood vessels and cells containing bundles of argentophilic fibrils named neurofibrillary tangles (NFT).[138-140] Such lesions are also present but in lesser number in the brains of aging individuals, normal or presenting with neurologic disease other than AD.

PATHOLOGY

The senile plaque is a rounded structure, 10 to 200 μ in diameter, with a core of amyloid surrounded by a halo of cellular debris. Amyloid is a degenerative substance composed of protein fibrils 6 to 10 nm wide. X ray cristallography studies have shown that the fibrils have an anti-parallel sense beta-pleated structure. There are different types of amyloid but all typically stain red with Congo Red and have a green birefringence under the polarizing scope, show metachromasia with a number of dyes, and are fluorescent with thioflavin S. All types of amyloid are constituted of two components, the P component which represents 5% of the deposit and the protein fibrils mentioned above, which differ with the different types of amyloidotic diseases. The amyloid in the brain in AD and in Down syndrome has been isolated and named amyloid beta-peptide (ABP)[141,142] or A4.[143,144] Recently a peptide identical to ABP/A4 has been identified in amyloid deposits located in cerebral blood vessels in an autosomally transmitted cerebral vascular amyloidotic disease in middle-age individuals which causes fatal hemorrhages.[145,146] The cDNA clones which encode the ABP within a precursor protein (APP) have been isolated and sequenced.[147-150] The APP gene has been mapped to chromosome 21.[148,150-154] It has long been assumed that chromosome 21 plays a role in the development of NFT and senile plaques in the brain of adult cases of Down syndrome trisomy 21.[155] A debated speculation is that the Down syndrome may be caused by an overproduction of APP due to an extra dose of the gene.[156-160] The APP gene is expressed in kidney, heart, spleen, muscle[19-21,39,148-150,161] and in large neurons of certain regions in the brain such as the nucleus basalis of Meynert and the locus coerulens.[162-167]

Neurofibrillary tangles (NFTs) are bunches of helically intertwined filaments, 10 nm wide, named paired helical filaments (PHF). Much work was done to identify the components of PHF[168-173] and eventually it was discovered that many anti-PHF antibodies cross-reacted with the phosphorylated regions of tau proteins. Tau appears to be localized in the fuzzy outer coat of PHF. There are data which suggest that tau may have a role in microtubule polymerization and synthesis.[176-182]

The halo of senile plaques and NFTs in AD brains are stained by a monoclonal antibody Alz-50 which detects an antigen particularly abundant in AD but barely detectable in normal adult brain.[183-185]

Genetic linkage studies of large families presenting with AD (FAD) as an autosomal dominant trait have suggested important leads in the investigation of sporadic AD.[186-188] The disease phenotype of the clinical, pathologic and biochemical features of FAD is indistinguishable from that of AD.[189] This suggests that the identification of the primary defect in FAD may be at least similar to that of sporadic AD. The FAD gene in some families is located on the proximal half of chromosome 212 long arm.[161,190-192] The presence of the APP gene on chromosome 21 may be coincidence but it is a relationship which is being examined.[193-196]

There are important limits to the use of the genetic linkage study for the localization of the FAD gene; (1) too few FAD families to provide unequivocal proof of cosegregation between the marker and the disease gene, (2) the high rate of error (10%) in clinical diagnosis, (3) proven paternity, (4) the possibility that an FAD pedigree may be an assembly of sporadic

AD, and (5) lack of assurance in some parameters used in the statistical assessment of the linkage.[197]

REFERENCES

1. Mc Kusick, V.A.: Mapping and Sequencing the Human Genome. N. Engl. J. Med., 320(14):910, 1989.
2. Mc Kusick, V.A.: *Mendellian Inheritance in Man*: catalogs of autosomal dominant, autosomal recessive and x-linked phenotypes. 8th Ed., Baltimore, Johns Hopkins University Press, 1988.
3. Tanzi, R.E., St. George-Hyslop, H., and Gusella, J.F.: Molecular genetic approaches to Alzheimer's disease. TINS, 12(4):151, 1989.
4. Maniatis, T., Fritsch, D.F., and Sambrook, J.: *Molecular cloning, a Laboratory Manual.* Cold Spring Harbor, NY, Cold Spring Harbor Laboratory, 1982.
5. Southern, E.M.: Detection of specific sequences among DNA fragments separated by gel electrophoresis. J. Mol. Biol., 98:503, 1975.
6. Gusella, J.F.: DNA polymorphism and human disease. Ann. Rev. Biochem., 55:831, 1986.
7. St. George-Hyslop, P.H., et al.: The genetic defect causing familial Alzheimer's disease maps on chromosome 21. Science 235:885, 1987.
8. Holmgren, G., et al.: Diagnosis of familial amyloidotic polyneuropathy in Sweden by RFLP analysis. Clin. Genetics, 33:176, 1988.
9. Jackson, J., et al.: Genetic linkage and spinocerebellar ataxia. Adv. Neurol. 21:315, 1978.
10. Koeppen, A.H., et al.: Genetic linkage in hereditary ataxia. Lancet 2:92, 1980.
11. Watkins, P.C.: Restriction fragment length polymorphism (RFLP): Applications in human chromosome mapping and genetic disease research. Biotechniques, 6:310, 1988.
12. Cooper, D.N., and Schmidtka, J.: Diagnosis of genetic disease using recombinant DNA. Human Genet. 66:1, 1984.
13. Martin, J.B., and Gussella, J.F.: Huntington's Disease: Pathogenesis and management. N. Engl. J. Med., 315:1267, 1986.
14. Folstein, S.E., et al.: Huntington's Disease: Two families with differing clinical features show linkage to the G8 probe. Science, 229:1746, 1986.
15. Llewellyn, D.H., et al.: DNA polymorphism of human porphobilinogen deaminase gene in acute intermittent porphyria. Lancet, 2:706, 1987.
16. Fain, P.R., et al.: Genetic analysis of NF1: Identification of close flanking markers on chromosome 17. Genomics, 1:340, 1987.
17. Mulvihill, J.J., and Parry, D.M.: Closing in on the gene for von Recklinghauser neurofibromatosis (NF1) with DNA markers for chromosome 17. Genomics, 1:349, 1987.
18. Rouleau, G.A., et al.: Genetic linkage of bilateral acoustic neurofibromatosis to a DNA marker on chromosome 22. Nature, 329:246, 1987.
19. Egeland, J.A., et al.: Bipolar affective disorders linked to DNA markers on chromosome 11. Nature, 25:783, 1987.
20. Wilkie, P., Rich, S., Schut, L., et al.: Spinocerebellar ataxia: Localization of the autosomal dominant HLA-linked form between two markers on human chro-

mosome 6. HGM9 1987, Cytogenet. Cell Genet., *45*(1): 715, 1988.

21. Boue, J., et al.: First trimester prenatal diagnosis of adrenoleukodysystrophy by determination of very long chain fatty acid levels and by linkage analysis to a DNA probe. Human Genet., *69*:272, 1985.

22. Rubenstein, A.E.: *Neurofibromatosis: A Review of the Clinical Problem.* In Ann. New York Acad. Sci. (Eds.) A.E. Rubenstein, R.P. Bunge, and D.E. Housman. New York, The New York Academy of Sciences, 1986.

23. Riccardi, V.M., and Eichner, J.E.: *Neurofibromatosis.* Baltimore, The John Hopkins University Press, 1986.

24. Rubinstein, L.J.: The malformative central nervous system lesions in the central and peripheral forms of neurofibromatosis: A neuropathological study of 22 cases. In Ann. New York Acad. Sci. (Eds.) A.E. Rubenstein, R.P. Bunge, and D.E. Housman. New York, The New York Academy of Sciences, 1986.

25. Fountain, J.W., et. al.: Physical Mapping of a Translocation Breakpoint in Neurofibromatosis. Science, *244*:1085, 1989.

26. O'Connell, P., et al.: Two NF-1 Translocations Map Within a 600-Kilobase Segment of 17q11.2. Science, *244*:1087, 1989.

27. Riccardi, V.M.: Von Ricklinghausen neurofibromatosis. N. Engl. J. Med., *305*:1617, 1981.

28. Harkin, J.C.: *Pathology of Nerve Sheath Tumors.* In Ann. New York Acad. Sci. (Eds.) A.E. Rubenstein, R.P. Bunge, and D.E. Housman. New York, The New York Academy of Sciences, 1986.

29. Rubenstein, A.E., Mytilineoau, C., Yahr, M.D., et al.: Neurological aspects of neurofibromatosis. In: Adv. Neurol., Vol. 29. (Eds.) V.M. Riccardi, and J.J. Mulvihill. New York, Raven Press, 1981.

30. Deans, W.R., et al.: Arteriovenous fistula in patients with neurofibromatosis. Radiology, *144*:103, 1982.

31. Sobata, E., Ohkuma, H., and Suzuki, S.: Cerebrovascular disorders associated with von Recklinghausen's neurofibromatosis: A case report. Neurosurg., *22*:544, 1988.

32. Gebarski, S.S., Gabrielsen, T.O., Knake, J.E., et al.: Posterior circulation intracranial arterial occlusive disease in neurofibromatosis. AJNR, *4*:1245, 1983.

33. Riccardi, V.M.: Personal Communication.

34. Lott, I.T., and Richardson, Jr., E.P.: Neuropathological findings and the biology of neurofibromatosis. In: Adv. Neurol., Vol. 29. (Eds.) V.M. Riccardi, and J.J. Mulvihill. New York, Raven Press, 1981.

35. Erlandson, R.A., and Woodruff, J.M.: Peripheral nerve sheath tumors: An electron microscopic study of 43 cases. Cancer, *49*:273, 1982.

36. Mirsky, R., and Jessen, K.R.: The biology of non-myelin-forming Schwann cells. In: Ann. New York Acad. Sci. (Eds.) A.E. Rubenstein, R.P. Bunge, and D.E. Housman. New York, The New York Academy of Sciences, 1986.

37. Pleasure, D., et al.: Schwann-like cells cultured from human dermal neurofibromatosis: Immunohistological identification and response to Schwann cell mitogens. In: Ann. New York Acad. Sci. (Eds.) A.E. Rubenstein, R.P. Bunge, and D.E. Housman. New York, The New York Academy of Sciences, 1986.

38. Bolands, R.P.: Neurofibromatosis—The quintessential neurocristopathy: Pathogenetic concepts and relationships. In: Adv. Neurol., Vol. 29. (Eds.) V.M. Riccardi, and J.J. Mulvihill. New York, Raven Press, 1981.

39. Le Douarin, N.M.: Investigations on the neural crest: Methodological aspects and recent advances. In: Ann. New York Acad. Sci. (Eds.) A.E. Rubenstein, R.P. Bunge, and D.E. Housman. New York, The New York Academy of Sciences, 1986.

40. Weston, J.A.: The regulation of normal and abnormal neural crest cell development. In: Adv. Neurol., Vol. 29. (Eds.) V.M. Riccardi, and J.J. Mulvihill. New York, Raven Press, 1981.

41. Knudson, A.G.: A geneticist's view of neurofibromatosis. In: Adv. Neurol., Vol. 29. (Eds.) V.M. Riccardi, and J.J. Mulvihill. New York, Raven Press, 1981.

42. Johnston, M.C., Vig, K.W.L., and Ambrose, L.J.H.: Neurocristopathy as a unifying concept: Clinical correlations. In: Adv. Neurol., Vol. 29. (Eds.) V.M. Riccardi, and J.J. Mulvihill. New York, Raven Press, 1981.

43. Peltonen, J., et al.: Neurofibromatosis tumor and skin cells in culture: II. Structural proteins with special reference to the cytoskeletal and cell surface components. Acta Neuropath. (Berl), *63*:269, 1984.

44. Chandler, J.H., Reed, T.E., and DeJong, R.N.: Huntington's disease in Michigan. Neurology, *10*:148, 1960.

45. Adams, R.D., and Victor, M.: *Principles of Neurology* 3rd Ed., New York, McGraw-Hill Book Co., 1985.

46. Bruyn, G.W., Bots, G.T.A.M., and Dom, R.: Huntington's chorea: Current neuropathological status. In: Adv. Neurol. Vol. 23. (Eds.) T.N. Chase, N.S. Wexler, and A. Barbeau. New York, Raven Press, 1979.

47. Vonsattel, J.P., et al.: Neuropathological classification of Huntington's disease. J. Neuropath. Exp. Neurol., *44*:559, 1985.

48. Lange, H., Thorner, G., Hopf, A., et al.: Morphometric studies of the neuropathological changes in choreatic patients. J. Neurol. Sci., *28*:401, 1976.

49. Adams, J.H., Corsellis, J.A.N., and Duchen, L.W. (eds.): *Greenfield's Neuropathology,* 4th Ed., New York, John Wiley & Sons, 1984.

50. Roos, R.A.C. and Bots, G.T.A.M.: Nuclear membrane indentations in Huntington's chorea. J. Neurol. Sci., *61*:37, 1983.

51. Dom, E., Malfroid, M., and Baro, F.: Neuropathology of Huntington's disease: Cytometric studies of the ventrobasal complex of the thalamus. Neurology, *26*:64, 1976.

52. Tellez-Nagel, I., Johnson, A., and Terry, R.: Studies on brain biopsies of patients with Huntington's chorea. J. Neuropath. Exp. Neuro., *33*:308, 1974.

53. Roos, R.A.C., Pruyt, J.F.M., de Vries, J., et al.: Neuronal distribution in the putamen in Huntington's disease. J. Neurol. Neurosurg, Psy., *48*:422, 1985.

54. Perry, T.L., Hansen, S., and Kloster, M.: Huntington's chorea: Deficiency of aminobutyric acid in brain. N. Engl. J. Med., *288*:337, 1973.

55. Ferrante, R.J., et al.: Morphologic and histochemical characteristics of a spared subset of striatal neurons in Huntington's disease. J. Neuropathol. Exp. Neurol., *6*:12, 1987.

56. Coyle, J.T., London, E.D., Biziere, K., et al.: Kanaic acid neurotoxicity: Insights into the pathophysiology of Huntington's disease. In: Adv. Neurol., Vol. 23. (Eds.) T.N. Chase, N.S. Wexler, and A. Barbeau. New York, Raven Press, 1979.

57. McGeer, E.G., McGeer, P.L., Hattori, T., and Vincent, S.R.: Kanaic acid neurotoxicity and Huntington's disease. In: Adv. Neurol., Vol. 23. (Eds.) T.N. Chase, N.S. Wexler, and A. Barbeau. New York, Raven Press, 1979.

58. Beal, M.F., et al.: Replication of the neurochemical characteristics of Huntington's disease by quinolinic acid. Nature, 321:168, 1986.

59. Schwarcz, R., Whetsell, W., and Mangano, R.: Quinolinic acid: An endogenous metabolite that produces axon-sparing lesions in the rat brain. Science, 219:316, 1983.

60. Davies, S.W., and Roberts, P.J.: Model of Huntington's disease (Letter). Science, 241:474, 1988.

61. Beal, M.F., et al.: Model of Huntington's disease (Response). Science, 241:475, 1988.

62. Folstein, S.E., et al.: Huntington's disease: Two families with differing clinical features show linkage to the G8 probe. Science, 229:776, 1986.

63. Duvoisin, R.C.: An apology and an introduction to the olivopontocerebellar atrophies. In: Adv. Neurol. Vol. 41. (Eds.) R.C. Duvoisin and A. Plaitakis. New York, Raven Press, 1984.

64. Harding, A.E.: The clinical features and classification of the late onset autosomal dominant cerebellar ataxias. Brain, 105:1, 1982.

65. Konigsmark, B.W., Weiner, L.P.: The olivopontocerebellar atrophies: A Review. Medicine, 49:227, 1970.

66. Berciano, J.: Olivopontocerebellar atrophy: A review of 117 cases. J. Neurol. Sci., 53:253, 1982.

67. Landis, D.M.D., et al.: Olivopontocerebellar degeneration: Clinical and ultrastructural abnormalities. Arch. Neurol., 31:295, 1974.

68. Petito, C., Hart, M., Porro, R., et al.: Ultrastructural studies of olivopontocerebellar atrophy. J. Neuropath. Exp. Neurol., 32:503, 1973.

69. Koeppen, A., and Basson, K.: The neuropathology of olivopontocerebellar atrophy. In: Adv. Neurol., Vol. 41. (Eds.) by R.C. Duvoisin, and A. Plaitakis. New York, Raven Press, 1984.

70. Perry, T.L., Kish, S.J., Hansen, S., et al.: Neurotransmitter amino acids in dominantly inherited cerebellar disorders. Neurology, 31:237, 1981.

71. Perry, T.L.: Four biochemically different types of dominantly inherited olivopontocerebellar atrophy. In: Adv. Neurol. Vol. 41. (Eds.) R.C. Duvoisin, and A. Plaitakis. New York, Raven Press, 1984.

72. Perry, T.L., Currier, R.D., Hansen, S., et al.: Aspartate-Taurine imbalance in dominantly inherited olivopontocerebellar atrophy. Neurology, 27:257, 1977.

73. Plaitakis, A.: Abnormal metabolism of neuroexcitatory amino acids in olivopontocerebellar atrophy. In: Adv. Neurol. Vol. 41. (Eds.) R.C. Duvoisin, and A. Plaitakis. New York, Raven Press, 1984.

74. Duvoisin, R.C., Chokroverty, S., Lepore, F., et al.: Glutamate dehydrogenase deficiency in patients with olivopontocerebellar atrophy. Neurology, 33:1322, 1983.

75. Harding, A.: Degenerative ataxic disorders: Still perplexing (Letter). Br. Med. J., 295:1233, 1987.

76. Harding, A.E.: Commentary: Olivopontocerebellar atrophy is not a useful concept. In: Movement Disorders 2. (Eds.) C.D. Marsen, and S. Fahn. London, Butterworths, 1987.

77. Jackson, J.F., Currier, R.D., Terasaki, P.I., et al.: Spinocerebellar ataxia and HLA linkage: Risk prediction by HLA typing. N. Engl. J. Med., 296:1138, 1977.

78. Jackson, J.F., et al.: Genetic linkage and spinocerebellar ataxia. In: Adv. Neurol., Vol. 21. (Eds.) R.A.P. Kark, R.N. Rosenberg, and L. J. Schut. New York, Raven Press, 1978.

79. Wilkie, P., Rich, S., Schut, L., et al.: Spinocerebellar ataxia: Localization of the autosomal dominant HLA-linked form between two markers on human chromosome 6. Human Gene Map Workshop #9. Cytogen. Cell Genet., 45(1):715, 1988.

80. Healton, E.B., et al.: Presumably Azorean disease in a presumably non-Portugese family. Neurology, 30:1084, 1980.

81. Bharucha, N.E., Bharucha, E.P., and Bhabha, S.K.: Machado-Joseph-Azorean disease in India. Arch. Neurol. 43:142, 1986.

82. Barbeau, A., et al.: The natural history of Machado-Joseph disease: An analysis of 138 personally examined cases. Can. J. Neurol. Sci., 11:510, 1984.

83. Coutinho, P., Guimaraes, A., and Scaravilli, F.: The pathology of Machado-Joseph disease. Acta Neuropathol., 54:48, 1982.

84. Sachdev, H.S., Forno, L.S., and Kane, C.A.: Joseph disease: A multisystem degenerative disorder of the nervous system. Neurology, 32:192, 1982.

85. Grossman, A., Rosenberg, R.N., and Warmouth, L.: Glutamate and malate dehydrogenase activities in Joseph disease and olivopontocerebellar atrophy. Neurology, 37:106, 1987.

86. Hotson, J.R., Langston, E.B., Louis, A.A., et al.: The search for a physiologic marker of Machado-Joseph disease. Neurology, 37:112, 1987.

87. Rosenberg, R.N., and Grossman, A.: Molecular genetics of Joseph disease. In: The Molecular Biology of Neurological Disease. (Eds.) R.N. Rosenberg, and A.E. Harding. London, Butterworth, 1988.

88. Rosenberg, R.N.: Personal communication.

89. Andrade, C.: A peculiar form of peripheral neuropathy. Familial atypical generalized amyloidosis with special involvement of the peripheral nerves. Brain, 75:408, 1952.

90. Koeppen, A.H., et al.: Familial amyloid polyneuropathy. Muscle and Nerve, 8:733, 1985.

91. Sasaki, H., et al.: Diagnosis of familial amyloidotic polyneuropathy by recombinant DNA techniques. Biochem. Biophys. Res. Commun., 125:636, 1984.

92. Shoji, S., and Okano, A.: Amyloid fibril protein in familial amyloid polyneuropathy. Neurology, 31:186, 1981.

93. Skinner, M., and Cohen, A.S.: Prealbumin nature of amyloid protein in familial amyloid polyneuropathy. Biochem. Biophys. Res. Commun., 99:1326, 1981.

94. Bastos, Lima A., and Martins da Silva, A.: Clinical evaluation of late onset cases in type I (Andrade) amyloid polyneuropathy. In: Amyloid and Amyloidosis. (Eds.) G.G. Glenner, P. Costa, and A. Freitas. Amsterdam: Excerpta Medica, 1980, pp. 99.

95. Anderson, R.: Hereditary amyloidosis with polyneuropathy. Acta Med. Scand., 188:85, 1970.

96. Hofer, P.A., and Anderson, R.: Postmortem findings in primary familial amyloidosis with polyneuropathy. Acta Pathol. Scand., 83:309, 1975.

97. Kito, S., et al.: Studies on familial amyloid polyneuropathy in Ogawa village, Japan. Euro. Neurol., 90:141, 1980.

98. Coutinho, P., Martins da Silva, A., Kopes Lima, J., et al.: Forty years of experience with type I amyloid neuropathy. Review of 483 cases. (Eds.) G.G. Glenner, P. Costa, and A. Freitas. Excerpta Medica, 1980, pp. 88.

99. Tawara, S., et al.: Amyloid fibril protein in type I familial amyloidotic polyneuropathy in Japanese. J. Lab. Clin. Med., 98:811, 1981.

100. Steen, L., Wahlin, A., Bjerle, P., et al.: Renal function in familial amyloidosis with polyneuropathy. Acta Med. Scand., 212:233, 1982.

101. Steen, L., Ek, B.: Familial anyloidosis with polyneu-

ropathy, long-term follow-up of 21 patients with special references gastrointestinal symptoms. Acta Med. Scand., *214*:387, 1983.

102. Julien, J.C., et al.: Neuropathies amyloides familiales dans trois familles d'origine francaise. Rev. Neurol. (Paris). *139*:259, 1983.

103. Mita, S., et al.: Familial anyloidotic polyneuropathy diagnosed by cloned human prealbumin. Neurology, *36*:298, 1986.

104. Kametani, F., et al.: Variant prealbumin related low molecular weight amyloid fibril protein in familial amyloid polyneuropathy of Japanese origin. Biophys. Res. Commun., *125*:622, 1984.

105. Libbey, C.A., et al.: Familial amyloid polyneuropathy. Demonstration of prealbumin in a kinship of German/English ancestry with onset in the 7th decade. Am. J. Med., *76*:18, 1984.

106. Ueji, M., et al.: Genetic studies of familial amyloid polyneuropathy in the Arao district of Japan. III. Analysis of amyloid fibril protein. Jap. J. Hum. Gen., *29*:311, 1984.

107. Felding, P., et al.: Prealbumin in Swedish patients with systemic amyloidosis and familial amyloidotic polyneuropathy. Scand. J. Immunol. *21*:133, 1985.

108. Saraiva, M.J.M., Costa, P.P., and Goodman, D.S.: Genetic expression of a transthyretin mutation in typical and late onset Portuguese families with familial amyloidotic polyneuropathy. Neurology, *36*:1413, 1986.

109. Araki, S.: Familial amyloidotic polyneuropathy: review of the 20 years' study and prospective views. Clin. Neurol., *26*:1256, 1986.

110. Tanaka, M., et al.: Familial amyloidotic polyneuropathy without familial occurrence: carrier detection by the radioimmunoassay of variant transthyretin. J. Neurol., *51*:576, 1988.

111. Masamitsu, N., et al.: Structurally abnormal transthyretin causing familial amyloidotic polyneuropathy in Sweden. Clin. Chem. Acta, *167*:341, 1987.

112. Costa, P., Figueira, A.S., and Bravo, F.R.: Amyloid fibril protein related to prealbumin in familial amyloidotic polyneuropathy. Proc. Natl. Acad. Sci. (USA), *75*:4499, 1978.

113. Dalakis, M.C., and Engel, W.K.: Amyloid in hereditary amyloid polyneuropathy is related to prealbumin. Arch. Neurol., *38*:420, 1981.

114. Tawar, S.: Identification of amyloid prealbumin variant in familial amyloidotic polyneuropathy. Biochem. Biophys. Res. Commun., *116*:880, 1983.

115. Sariava, M., Costa, P.P., Birken, S., et al.: Presence of abnormal transthyretin in Portuguese patients with familial amyloidotic polyneuropathy. Trans. Assoc. Am. Physicians, *96*:261, 1983.

116. Nadazato, M., et al.: Identification of a prealbumin variant in the serum of a Japanese patient with familial amyloidotic polyneuropathy. Biochem. Biophys. Res. Commun., *122*:712, 1984.

117. Dwulet, F.E., and Benson, M.D.: Primary structure of amyloid prealbumin and plasma precursor in a heredofamilial polyneuropathy of Swedish origin. Proc. Natl. Acad. Sci. USA, *81*:694, 1984.

118. Husby, G., Ranlov, P.J., Sletten, K., et al.: The amyloid in familial amyloidotic cardiomyopathy of Danish origin is related to pre-albumin. Clin. Exp. Immunol., *60*:207, 1985.

119. Cornwell, III, G.G., Westermark, P., Kyle, R.A., et al.: Senile systemic amyloidosis. In: *Amyloidosis.* (Eds.) G.G. Glenner, E.F. Osserman, E.P. Benditt, E. Calkins, A.S. Cohen, and D. Zucker-Franklin. New York, Plenum Press, 1986.

120. Tsuzuki, T.S., et al.: Structure of the human prealbumin gene to chromosome 18. Biochem. Biophys. Res. Comm., *129*:753, 1985.

121. Wallace, M.R., et al.: Localization of the human prealbumin gene to chromosome 18. Biochem. Biophys. Res. Comm., *129*:753, 1983.

122. Pras, M., Prelli, F., Franklin, E.C., et al.: Primary structure of an amyloid prealbumin variant in familial polyneuropathy of Jewish origin. Proc. Natl. Acad. Sci. USA, *80*:539, 1983.

123. Saraima, M.J., Birken, S., Costa, P.P. et al.: Amyloid fibril protein in familial polyneuropathy of Portuguese type. Definition of molecular abnormality in transthyretin. J. Clin. Invest., *74*:104, 1984.

124. Nakazato, M., et al.: Revised analysis of amino acid replacement in a prealbumin variant associated with familial amyloidotic polyneuropathy of Jewish origin. Biochem. Biophys. Res. Commun., *123*:921, 1984.

125. Saraiva, M.J.M., Costa, P.P., and Goodmam, D.S.: Biochemical marker in familial amyloidotic polyneuropathy. Portuguese type. Family studies on the transthyretin (prealbumin)-methionine-30 variant. J. Clin. Invest., *76*:2171, 1985.

126. Benson, M.D., and Dwulen, F.E.: Identification of a new amino acid substitution in plasma prealbumin associated with hereditary amyloidosis. Clin. Res., *33*:590a (Abstr.), 1985.

127. Nakazato, M., et al.: Structurally abnormal transthyretin, causing familial amyloidotic polyneuropathy in Sweden. Clin. Chem. Acta, *167*:341, 1987.

128. Holmgren, G., et al.: Diagnosis of familial amyloidotic polyneuropathy in Sweden by RFLP analysis. Clin. Genet., *33*:176, 1988.

129. Benson, M.D., and Cohen, A.S.: Serum amyloid: a protein in amyloidosis, rheumatic and neoplastic disease. Arth. Rheum., *22*:36, 1979.

130. Falls, H.F., et al.: Ocular manifestations of hereditary primary systemic amyloidosis. Arch. Ophthalmol., *54*:660, 1955.

131. Rukavina, J.G., et al.: Primary systemic amyloidosis: a review and an experimental genetic and clinical study of 29 cases with particular emphasis on the familial form. Medicine (Balt.), *35*:239, 1956.

132. Mahloudji, M., et al.: The genetic amyloidosis with particular reference to hereditary neuropathic amyloidosis. Type II (Indiana or Rukavina type). Medicine (Balt.), *48*:1, 1969.

133. Meretoja, J.: Familial systemic paramyloidosis with lattice dystrophy of the cornea, progressive cranial neuropathy, skin changes and various internal symptoms. Ann. Clin. Res., *1*:314, 1969.

134. Nakazato, M., Kangawa, K., Miniamino, M., et al.: Radioimmunoassay for detecting abnormal prealbumin in serum for diagnosis of familial amyloidotic polyneuropathy. Biochem. Biophys. Res. Commun., *122*:719, 1984.

135. Nakazato, M., et al.: Diagnostic radioimmunoassay for familial amyloidotic polyneuropathy before clinical onset. J. Clin. Invest., *77*:1699, 1986.

136. Nakazato, M., et al.: Variant transthyretin in the cerebrospinal fluid of patients with familial amyloidotic polyneuropathy. J. Neurol. Sci. (in press).

137. Wallace, J., Dwulet, F., Conneally, M., et al.: Biochemical and molecular genetic characterization of a new variant prealbumin associated with hereditary amyloidosis. J. Clin. Invest., *78*:6, 1986.

138. Kidd, M.: Alzheimer's disease: An electron microscopical study. Brain, 87:307, 1964.
139. Terry, R.D.: The fine structure of neurofibrillary tangles in Alzheimer's disease. J. Neuropathol. Exp. Neurol., 22:629, 1963.
140. Duckett, S., and Galle, P.: Evidence of aluminum in senile plaques of Alzheimer disease: Castaing microprobe study. Comptes Rendus des Seances de l'Academie des Sciences (D), Paris, 282:295, 1976.
141. Glenner, G.G., and Wong, C.W.: Alzheimer's disease: Initial report of the purification and characterization of a novel cerebrovascular amyloid protein. Biochem. Biophys. Res. Commun., 120:885, 1984.
142. Glenner, G.G., and Wong, C.W.: Alzheimer's disease and Down syndrome: Sharing of a unique cerebrovascular amyloid fibril protein. Biochem. Biophys. Res. Commun., 122:1131, 1984.
143. Masters, C.L., et al.: Amyloid plaque core protein in Alzheimer's disease and Down syndrome. Proc. Natl. Acad. Sci. (USA), 82:4245, 1985.
144. Selkoe, D.J., Abraham, C.R., Podlisny, M.B., et al.: Isolation of low molecular weight proteins from amyloid plaque fibers in Alzheimer's disease. J. Neurochem., 146:1820, 1986.
145. Van Duinen, S.G., et al.: Hereditary cerebral hemorrhage with amyloidosis in patients of Dutch origin is related to Alzheimer disease. Proc. Natl. Acad. Sci., (USA), 84:5991, 1987.
146. Prelli, F., et al.: Different processing of Alzheimer's beta-protein precursor in the vessel wall of patients with hereditary cerebral hemorrhage of amyloidosis-Dutch type. Biochem. Biophys. Res. Commun., 151:1150, 1988.
147. Kang, J., et al.: The precursor of Alzheimer's disease amyloid A4 protein resembles a cell-surface receptor. Nature, 325:733, 1987.
148. Tanzi, R.E., et al.: The amyloid beta protein gene is not duplicated in brains from patients with Alzheimer's disease. Science, 238:666, 1987.
149. Golgaber, D., et al.: Characterization and chromosomal localization of a cDNA encoding brain amyloid of fibril protein. Science, 235:877, 1987.
150. Robakis, N.K., Ramakrishna, N., Wolfe, G., et al.: Molecular cloning and characterization of the cDNA encoding the cerebrovascular and the neuritic plaque amyloid peptides. Proc. Nat. Acad. Sci., (USA), 84:4190, 1987.
151. Blanquet, V., et al.: The beta amyloid protein (AD-AP) cDNA hybridizes in normal and Alzheimer individuals near the interface of 21q21 and q22.1. Anal. Genet., 30:68, 1987.
152. Graw, S., et al.: Irradiation-reduced human chromosome 21 hybrids. Somatic Cell Molec. Genet., 14:233, 1988.
153. Patterson, D., et al.: Mapping of the gene encoding the beta-amyloid precursor protein and its relationship to the Down syndrome region of chromosome 21. Proc. Natl. Acad. Sci., (USA), 85:8266, 1988.
154. Korenberg, J.R., West, R., and Pulst, S-M.: The Alzheimer protein precursor maps to chromosome 21 sub-bands q21.15q21.2. Neurology, 38(1):265, 1988.
155. Oliver, C., Holland, A.J.: Down Syndrome and Alzheimer's disease: a review. Psychol. Med., 16:307, 1986.
156. Delabar, J-M., et al.: Beta-amyloid gene duplication in Alzheimer disease and karyotypically normal Down syndrome. Science, 235:1390, 1987.
157. Yamada, R., et al.: Complimentary DNA for the mouse homolog of the human amyloid beta protein precursor. Biochem. Biophys. Res. Commun., 149:665, 1987.
158. Tanzi, R.E., Bird, E.D., Latt, S.A., et al.: The Amyloid beta protein gene is not duplicated in brains from patients with Alzheimer's disease. Science, 238:666, 1987.
159. St. George-Hyslop, P.H., et al.: The genetic defect causing familial Alzheimer's disease maps on chromosome 21. Science, 238:664, 1987.
160. Podisney, M.B., Lee, G., and Selkoe, D.J.: Gene dosage of the amyloid beta precursor protein in Alzheimer's disease. Science, 238:669, 1987.
161. Zimmerman, K., et al.: EMBO J., 7:362, 1988.
162. Bahmanyar, S., et al.: Localization of amyloid beta-protein messenger RNA in brains from patients with Alzheimer's disease. Science, 237:77, 1987.
163. Cohen, M.L., et al.: In Situ hybridization of nucleus basalis neurons shows increased beta-amyloid mRNA in Alzheimer disease. Proc. Natl. Acad. Sci. (USA), 85:1227, 1988.
164. Goedert, J.: Neuronal localization of amyloid beta protein precursor mRNA in normal human brain and Alzheimer's disease. EMBO J., 6:3627, 1987.
165. Higgins, G.A.: Differential regulation of amyloid beta-protein mRNA expression within hippocampal neuronal subpopulations in Alzheimer's disease. Prod. Natl. Acad. Sci. (USA), 85:1297, 1988.
166. Lewis, D.A., et al.: Distribution of the precursor of amyloid-beta-protein messenger RNA in human cerebral cortex: relationship to neurofibrillary. Proc. Natl. Acad. Sci. (USA), 85:1691, 1988.
167. Palmert, M., et al.: Amyloid protein precursor messenger RNAs: differential expression in Alzheimer's disease. Science, 241:1080, 1988.
168. Cork, L.C., et al.: Phosphorylated neurofilament antigens in neurofibrillary tangles in Alzheimer's disease. J. Neuropathol. Exp. Neurol., 455:56, 1986.
169. Gambetti, P., et al.: Alzheimer neurofibrillary tangles: an immunohistochemical study. In: Aging of the Brain. (Eds.) L. Amaducci, A.N. Davison, and P. Antuono. New York, Raven Press, 1980.
170. Ihara, Y., Nukina, N., Sugita, H., et al.: Staining of Alzheimer's neurofibrillary tangles with anti-serum against 200 K component of neurofilament. Proc. Jpn. Acad., 57:152, 1981.
171. Rasool, C.G., and Selkoe, D.J.: Alzheimer's disease: exposure of neurofilament immunoreactivity in SDS-insoluble paired helical filaments. Brain Res., 322:194, 1984.
172. Perry, G., Rizzuto, N., Autilio-Gambetti, L., et al.: Paired helical filaments from Alzheimer disease patients contain cytoskeletal components. Proc. Natl. Acad. Sci. (USA), 82:3916, 1985.
173. Brion, J.P., Couck, A.M., Passareiro, E., et al.: Neurofibrillary tangles of Alzheimer's disease: an immunohistochemical study. J. Submicrosc. Cytol., 17:89, 1985.
174. Ihara, Y., Abraham, C., and Selko, D.J.: Antibodies to paired helical filaments in Alzheimer's disease do not recognize normal brain proteins. Nature, 304:727, 1983.
175. Yen, S-H., Crowe, A., and Dickson, D.W.: Monoclonal antibodies to Alzheimer. Neurofibrillary tangles. Am. J. Pathol., 120:282, 1985.
176. Kosik, K.S., Joachim, C.L., and Selkoe, D.J.: The microtubule associated protein tau is a major antigenic component of paired helical filaments in Alzheimer's disease. Proc. Natl. Acad. Sci. (USA), 83:4044, 1986.
177. Gundke-Igbal, I., et al.: Microtubule-associated pro-

tein tau: a component of Alzheimer's pair filaments. J. Biol. Chem., *261*:6084, 1986.

178. Brion, J.P., van der Bosch de Aguilar, P., and Flament-durand, J.: Senile dementia of the Alzheimer type. In: Adv. Appl. Neurol. Sci. (Eds.) J. Traber, and W.H. Gispen. New York, Springer, 1985.

179. Nukina, N., and Ihara, Y.: One of the antigenic determinants of paired helical filaments is related to tau protein. Biochem., *99*:1541, 1986.

180. Wood, J.G., Mirra, S.S., Pollock, N.J., et al.: Neurofibrillary tangles of Alzheimer's disease share antigenic determinants with the axonal microtubule associated protein tau. Proc. Natl. Acad. Sci. (USA), *83*:4040, 1986.

181. Nukina, N., Kosick, K.S., and Selkoe, D.J.: Recognition of Alzheimer paired helical filaments by monoclonal antibodies is due to crossreaction with tau protein. Proc. Natl. Acad. Sci. (USA), *84*:3415, 1987.

182. Ksiesak-Reding, J., Dickson, D.W., Davis, P., et al.: Recognition of tau epitopes by anti-neurofilament antibodies that bind to Alzheimer neurofibrillary tangles. Proc. Natl. Acad. Sci. (USA), *84*:3410, 1987.

183. Wolozin, B.L., and Davies, P.: Alzheimer-related neuronal protein A68: Specificity and distribution. Ann. Neurol., *22*:521, 1987.

184. Wolozin, B.L., Prunchnicke, A., Dickson, D.W., et al.: A neuronal antigen in the brains of Alzheimer patients. Science, *232*:648, 1986.

185. Wolozin, B.L., Scicutella, B., and Davies, P.: Re-expression of a developmentally regulated antigen in Down syndrome and Alzheimer's disease. Proc. Natl. Acad. Sci. (USA), *85*:6202, 1986.

186. Nee, L.E., et al.: A family with histologically confirmed Alzheimer's disease. Arch. Neurol., *40*:203, 1983.

187. Foncin, J.F., et al.: Demence presenile d'Alzheimer transmise dans une famille etendue. Rev. Neurol. (Paris), *141*:194, 1985.

188. Goudsmit, J., et al.: Familial Alzheimer's disease in two kindreds of the same geographic and ethnic origin: A clinical and genetic study. J. Neurol. Sci., *49*:79, 1981.

189. Davies, P.: The genetics of Alzheimer's disease: a review and a discussion of the implications. Neurobiol. Aging, *7*:459, 1986.

190. Goate, A., et al.: Predisposing locus for Alzheimer's disease on chromosome 21. Lancet (in press).

191. David, F., and Lucotte, G.: Alz. Dis. Assoc. Dis., *2*:287, 1988.

192. van Broekhoven, C., et al.: The familial Alzheimer's disease gene is located close to the centromere of chromosome. Am. J. Hum. Genet., *43*:A205, 1988.

193. Tanzi, R.D., et al.: The genetic defect in familial Alzheimer's disease is not tightly linked to the amyloid B-protein gene. Nature, *329*:156, 1987.

194. van Broekhoven, C., et al.: Genetic defect in familial Alzheimer's disease is not tightly linked to the amyloid B-protein gene. Nature, *329*:153, 1987.

195. Schellenberg, G.D., et al.: Absence of linkage of chromosomes 21q21 markers to familial Alzheimer's disease. Science, *241*:1507, 1988.

196. Pericak-Vance, M.A., et al.: Anatomical and behavioral correlates of a xenograft medicated pupillary reflex. Exp. Neurol., *102*:271, 1988.

197. St. George-Hyslop, P.H., et al.: The Molecular Biology of Alzheimer Disease. In: *Current Communications in Molecular Biology.* (Eds.) C.E. Finch, and P. Davies, Cold Spring Harbor, NY., Cold Spring Harbor Laboratory, 1988.

14

Central Nervous System Trauma in the Elderly

EVERETT J. AUSTIN

Mechanical trauma to the central nervous system, although primarily affecting young people in Western, and undoubtedly other societies, remains an important cause of disability and mortality in the elderly and presents interesting age-related features. With increases in the proportion of older individuals in the population and decreases in the proportion of high-risk younger people, trauma, along with other geriatric conditions, will affect increasing numbers of older people.[1] The head-injured elderly, who currently comprise about 5 to 6% of the head-injured reported in the literature,[2] will constitute a much more important fraction of those recovering, permanently disabled, or dead from traumatic brain injuries. With modernization of medical care delivery systems and creation of regional trauma centers in wealthy countries such as the United States and United Kingdom, some attention is beginning to be focused on the outcome and even the appropriateness of treatment of the traumatized elderly.[2–13] It seems clear that a sig-

nificant proportion of our limited medical resources could easily be expended in this area.[1] For health care policy making and for guidance of physicians in treatment of individuals, detailed clinical and neuropathologic information regarding modes and mechanisms of injury, pathogenesis, outcome and prognostication must be available.

The study of central nervous system injury, especially head injury, on which this chapter will focus, is an old one. This is amply illustrated by Courville in the excellent historic introduction to his monograph *Commotio Cerebri*,[14] in which he points out that most then (and currently) accepted theories of brain injury are not new, but "rediscovered", even centuries-old. In this century, the neuropathology of head injury has been detailed and consolidated in terms of the human perhaps most importantly by Courville,[14,15] Lindenberg (and Freytag),[16,17] Strich,[18–20] and by Adams and colleagues,[21–27] with important clinical and analytical contributions by Symonds[28,29] and Russell.[30] Experimental clarification has come from Denny-Brown and Russell[31] and later from Ommaya, Gennarelli and Adams and co-workers.[32-36] The picture of head injury currently seems remarkably full. Treatment, on the other hand, though considerably advanced beyond the simple palpation of open skull lesions advocated in the Smith surgical papyrus, remains largely supportive and ameliorative,[37] with future developments perhaps to derive from progress in the growing field of neural regeneration.[38]

EPIDEMIOLOGY

As mentioned above, head injury is largely a plague affecting younger persons. Most studies indicate the vast majority of sufferers to be between 10 and 35 years of age,[39-42] peaking in the 14 to 24-year-old group, with a substantial decline in incidence with advancing age. Secondary peaks, however, occur in the very young and the very old.[41]

With the exception of certain densely populated urban areas, where assaults and firearm injuries predominate,[43,44] the major causes of head injury are road/transport accidents and accidental falls.[39-44] The etiologies of head injury differ in a noteworthy manner between age groups. Falling is probably most important in the young and in the elderly,[45] and traffic accidents involve the elderly in a high proportion as in any age group, but much more often as pedestrians than as drivers or passengers compared to other ages.[3,5,6,10]

The propensity of elderly persons to fall and injure themselves[3,4,9,46] may relate to various physiologic and pathologic accompaniments of aging which may be present, such as: decreased speed of muscular movement,[47] increased reaction time in the inactive elderly,[48] gait instability,[49] visual changes (cataract, glaucoma, macular degeneration),[50] and other less common contributors.[46]

NEUROPATHOLOGY

Traditionally, classifications of head injury have been dichotomous. Some are complementary and remain valid and informative, whereas others should be discarded, since they

TABLE 14-1. Head Injury Classifications

MISSILE vs NON-MISSILE HEAD INJURY
DIFFUSE and FOCAL BRAIN INJURY
FOCAL: Contusions Intracranial hemorrhage: extradural, intra/subdural, intracerebral Other (vascular, cranial nerve, pituitary/hypothalamic)
DIFFUSE: Diffuse Axonal Injury (DAI) Hypoxic Brain Damage Brain Swelling Multiple Petechial Hemorrhages
MILD, MODERATE AND SEVERE HEAD INJURY

are based on notions which have been essentially disproven. An example of the latter is the formerly much-disputed distinction between concussion, implying an absence of structural brain injury, and concussive brain damage with gross evidence of necrosis or hemorrhage. This distinction was rejected many years ago by Symonds,[28] who eloquently restated his position in 1962.[29] His position, that concussive head injury represents a continuum, appears now to be firmly supported.[30,51-55] This chapter will review several valid classifications which greatly facilitate the study and understanding of head injury both pathologically and clinically (Table 14-1.)

Although the neuropathology of head injury has been amply summarized in classical accounts[14-17,20] and by recent authors, to whom the reader is also referred,[25,27,39,56] the fundamentals will be treated here, since these are largely independent of age, and important age-dependent differences can be highlighted on this background.

MISSILE VERSUS NON-MISSILE HEAD INJURY

Only non-missile brain injuries will be further considered here. As mentioned above, firearm and other missile wounds are of relatively minor civilian importance, except in some urban areas, and primarily affect younger age groups. For their pathologic conditions, the reader is referred elsewhere.[16,17,27]

EXPERIMENTAL NON-MISSILE HEAD INJURY

From a scrutiny of experimental head injury research undertaken since the 1930s, it appears that these works were largely inspired by a desire to produce in the laboratory animal findings which had been well-described and reasonably accounted for theoretically in clinicopathologic observations on brain-injured humans. In particular, the clinicopathologic observations of Strich and others in the 1950s and 1960s clarified the nature of the predominantly white matter lesions responsible for the "severe dementia" (later variously referred to as the "apallic syndrome"[57] or "persistent vegetative state"[58]) of certain patients, persistently unresponsive after head injury, who had never had intracranial hematomas or extensive contusions.[18–20] This "shearing of nerve fibers" or "diffuse white matter injury", clearly identified by Strich and others, was later exhaustively studied in human autopsy material by Adams and colleagues,[22] but only relatively recently were similar lesions produced and identified in experimentally head-injured animals and dubbed "diffuse axonal injury" (DAI).[33] In the course of developing the "Penn 2" device used to produce DAI lesions in primates with single accelerations of the head, its proponents had initially used a device called "Penn 1", which inadvertently but reliably produced acute subdural hematomas and other types of acute focal brain lesions classically described in man (Table 14–1), completing the experimental mirror of human head injury.[27,34,35] Thus, although historically inverted, it makes sense to review these findings first for the sake of clarity.

Angular acceleration had been shown to produce concussion, whereas purely translational acceleration did not.[34] Purely compressive forces, slowly applied (crushing or compressing injury), may produce severe skull damage and even cerebral contusion, but consciousness may be preserved.[14] The Penn 1 device produced a short-duration, purely sagittal 60 degree angular acceleration of the subject's head.[34] Acute subdural hematomas (SDH), due to tearing of bridging veins, as well as contusional hemorrhages and hemorrhagic necroses, could be readily produced, but without

DAI. In contrast, the Penn 2 device, which applied angular acceleration at a lower rate and longer duration, and which varied the plane of rotation of the head,[27,34] could produce persistent coma and pathologically DAI, without SDH, though contusions could occur, especially with more severe insults. Furthermore, as the rotation plane was varied from purely sagittal through oblique to purely lateral (coronal), the tendency to produce white matter shearing lesions increased.[27,34] Furthermore, a spectrum of severity of DAI lesions was noted, corresponding clinically to the duration of post-traumatic coma, with a centripetal distribution as predicted by Ommaya and Gennarelli some years before, and with the same lesions characteristic of human DAI.[27,32] The milder lesions ("grade 1") showed axonal degeneration and glial scars in the cerebral white matter; more severely affected animals ("grade 2") had, in addition, shearing lesions in the corpus callosum; the most severely traumatized ("grade 3") also had focal lesions in the dorsolateral rostral brainstem. The callosal and brainstem lesions showed axonal shearing and microglial/astroglial scars, and frequently were hemorrhagic due to shearing of small blood vessels.[27]

In the human situation, the Penn 1 is analogous to the fall onto a hard surface or assault with a hard object, whereas the Penn 2 is analogous to the more prolonged, gradual accelerations occurring in traffic accidents. As Gennarelli[34] and Adams and colleagues[23,24] point out, assaults and most falls are associated with intracranial hematoma, such as SDH, and not DAI, whereas the converse is true of traffic accidents.

FOCAL BRAIN INJURY

Focal traumatic brain lesions, as listed in Table 14–1, are grossly visible lesions of classic description,[14–17,20,27,56] familiar to all pathologists and general physicians. Those resulting from primary impact are primarily intracranial hematomas and contusions, the latter term referring to areas of traumatic necrosis, usually hemorrhagic, and usually relatively superficial, especially involving gyral crests. Other impact lesions include cranial nerve injury (especially olfactory, facial, and auditory) through tearing

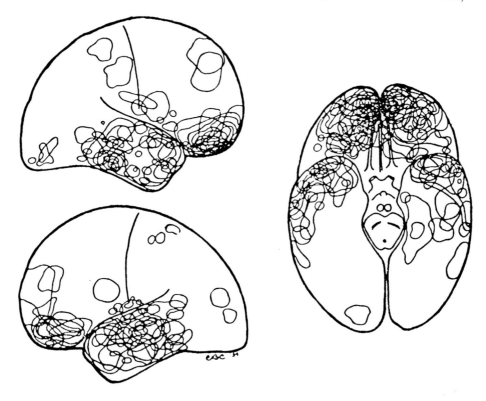

Fig. 14–1. Sites of cerebral contusions (from C.B. Courville's *Pathology of the Central Nervous System,* 3rd ed., Mountain View, Calif., Pacific Press Publ. Assoc., 1950, p. 305).

or skull fracture, tearing of the pituitary stalk and arterial tears and dissections involving cervical carotid or vertebral arteries or the intracavernous carotid artery. Secondary focal brain lesions are mainly consequences of brain shifts and herniations due to brain swelling or mass lesions.

CONTUSIONS

In the case of an assault with a blunt object, or other similar injury, focal contusions may well underly the site of the blow, often associated with a depressed skull fracture. In other cases of unilateral fracture, contusions may predominate ipsilaterally.[39] However, in most non-missile head injury in which the head is freely mobile, contusions of the frontal and temporal poles predominate, regardless of the site of impact, as shown in Figure 14–1 taken from Courville.[15] This is due to "swirling" movements of the brain in which the temporal and frontal poles contact the adjacent skull

and the orbitofrontal and inferior temporal surfaces move over the rough surfaces of the anterior and middle fossae, producing surface shear lesions,[39] or "gliding contusions".[27] Similar gliding contusions are also commonly seen in the cingulate gyri due to contact with the unyielding falx.[27] Coup and contrecoup contusions (lesions underlying and diagonally opposite an impact), when present, are thought to be associated with angular accelerations of the moving head and a lesser thickness of CSF "cushion" over the contre-coup site ("brain lag").[59] These can be typically seen in a short fall onto a hard surface.[59] All these considerations apply to the elderly as to any other age group.

INTRACRANIAL HEMATOMAS

SUBDURAL HEMATOMA

Acute subdural hematoma has been covered above in the context of experimental head injury, being associated with short-duration, sagittal accelerations of the head.[27,34,60,61] These lesions, due to tearing of bridging veins or to dural laceration,[60] may occur anywhere in association with the dura, but are most commonly convexity or interhemispheric. As in the experimental animal, they are markers of severe head injury and carry a grave prognosis.[27,34,62-64]

Chronic subdural hematomas are peculiar to the older population, due to the increased incidence of cerebral atrophy and the consequent ease with which cerebral bridging veins may be torn when the brain moves relative to the dura within the cerebrospinal fluid, even during trivial trauma, and for the same reason are frequently bilateral.[27,62,63,65-68] These may enlarge step-wise, due to repeated minor trauma, or may resolve spontaneously.[65] Pathologically, they are composed of hemorrhage of varying ages, bounded by membranes composed of granulation tissue.[16] Liquefaction of the gross clot may occur after 48 hours.[27] The evolution and nature of this "hematoma" may be followed clinically using CT and magnetic resonance imaging.

EXTRADURAL HEMATOMA

Extradural hematomas are unusual in the elderly.[69] These are classically due to arterial bleeding from the middle meningeal artery where it passes through a fracture in the temporal bone, and clinically, with brief loss of consciousness, followed by rapid deterioration as the extratemporal mass lesion expands.[27,70,71] An underlying cerebral contusion or laceration is usual.[69]

INTRACEREBRAL HEMATOMA

Intracerebral hematomas due to trauma typically occur in association with hemorrhagic contusions, and may be small or large and in that case act as mass lesions. Many of these probably take hours to days to develop, as indicated by serial cranial computed tomographic studies[72,73] and by magnetic resonance imaging.[74] In some cases these can lead to dramatic clinical deterioration: the so-called "delayed traumatic intracerebral hem-

orrhage".[72-74] Although plausible, it is not known whether the elderly trauma victim is at higher risk for intracerebral hemorrhage due to the greater incidence of arterioles made fragile by hypertensive or cerebral amyloid angiopathies.

OTHER PRIMARY IMPACT LESIONS

As enumerated above, cranial nerve, hypophyseal and vascular trauma are also known. The functional consequences of such lesions are obvious. A rare case of entrapment of the basilar artery in a clivus fracture producing the locked-in syndrome has even been reported.[75] This suggests an uncommon "exception" to the rule that traumatic brainstem lesions do not occur in isolation (see below): in fact, it is not, since this is a vascular and not a primary parenchymal lesion. None of these insults are peculiar to the aged.

DIFFUSE BRAIN INJURY

Adams[27] categorizes four types of diffuse brain injury which may occur in head trauma: diffuse axonal injury (see above), hypoxic brain damage, brain swelling, and multiple petechial hemorrhages. All may occur in the elderly head trauma victim. A certain variety of acute brain swelling occurs most readily in children,[76] but may also be seen in adults.[77]

DIFFUSE AXONAL INJURY

As discussed in the section on experimental head injury, DAI is a common cause of disability in closed head injury and its features in man and in experimental primates are identical. In order of increasing severity, the classical lesions are: axonal interruption (shearing) in the cerebral white matter, focal necroses in the corpus callosum, and focal necroses in the dorsolateral quadrants of the rostral brainstem.[27,34,78,79] This is the centripetal distribution of lesions with increasing severity of injury predicted by Ommaya and Gennarelli,[32] and which has also been confirmed in living patients by magnetic resonance imaging studies.[80] A corrolary rule, and subject of much prior debate,[81,82] is that primary brainstem lesions ("brainstem contusion") do not occur in the absence of cerebral white matter lesions in non-missile head injury. Despite a few notes of dissent, and a minority opinion that the brainstem lesions are vascular and not due to shearing forces,[57] this controversy appears largely settled.[22,23,25,27,81,83]

HYPOXIC BRAIN DAMAGE

Experimentally and in the field, hypoxia due to transient hypotension, asphyxia or apnea is a common occurrence and a theoretically preventable factor unfavorably affecting outcome.[27,34,37,72,84-86] As in other settings, the principal neuropathologic manifestations of hypoxic brain injury are ischemic neuronal changes preferentially affecting the hippocampal pyramidal cells, cerebellar Purkinje cells, and arterial boundary zones.[27,72,87]

BRAIN SWELLING

Vasogenic edema actually tends to occur multifocally around areas of contusion, due to increased permeability of injured capillaries.[25,27] An element of cytotoxic edema is contributed when neuronal damage is severe, but, as in hypoxic cerebral damage, would be likely to cause serious cerebral swelling by itself only if widespread irreversible cellular damage were present. As indicated above, a particular type of acute brain swelling can lead to serious consequences, with secondary brain lesions due to trantentorial and tonsillar herniations. This occurs most dramatically in children and appears to represent an acute increase in intracranial blood volume.[27,76] Thus, this phenomenon is actually a form of brain hyperemia or vascular congestion, rather than an edema in the usual sense.

MULTIPLE PETECHIAL HEMORRHAGES

This group of patients is set aside as a separate category of diffuse brain injury by Adams, as a subset with particularly severe insults who die essentially at impact, with diffuse cortical petechiae being found at autopsy.[27] Survival presumably would have

yielded more substantial multifocal hemorrhagic contusions.

SECONDARY LESIONS

Secondary lesions seen in association with primary impact lesions are of great interest clinically, as they are potentially preventable.[72,85] Brain swelling or expanding intra-axial or extra-axial hematomas may lead to increased intracranial pressure and brain shifts such as central or uncal transtentorial herniation (potentially proceeding to midbrain notching, Duret hemorrhage and compression of the occipital branches of the posterior cerebral artery against the tentorium), subfalcine cingulate herniation, or upward or downward cerebellar herniation. These processes are not specific to head injury, nor certainly to the elderly patient, and for a more detailed discussion the reader is referred to other sources.[16,17,39,71,88]

MILD, MODERATE, AND SEVERE BRAIN INJURY

In recent years, clinical and pathologic study of head injury has drawn more attention to mild and moderate injuries.[51-54,89-93] Previously, most attention was (and still is) focussed on severe head injury, because of the seriousness of the problem and the availability of ample material for clinicopathologic correlation. The mildly head injured patient, on the other hand, was the subject of much dispute, but mainly of a medicolegal nature, due to the difficulty in deciding whether a patient's symptoms were of an organic or psychogenic nature.[14,90] Currently, based on agreement between neuropsychologic, clinicopathologic, and experimental data, head injury can be regarded as a continuum of injuries with a common mechanism, from mild concussion to fatal impact.[31,54,91] This point of view was already clearly enunciated by Sir Charles Symonds,[28,29] who pointed out the distinction between reversible and obviously partially irreversible head injury as artificial and incorrect: "In the most severe degree of concussion there is widespread irreversible damage. In the slightest degree there may be rapid and complete recovery of cerebral function; but this does not necessarily exclude that a small number of neurones may have perished—a number so small as to be negligible at the time, but leaving the brain more susceptible as a whole to the effects of further damage of the same kind."[29] This statement is now amply supported in experiment and clinical experience. Detailed neuropsychologic studies of mildly head-injured individuals demonstrate defects in memory and other aspects of information processing: the recovery of these defects requires weeks to months following injury.[31,51,53,89,90,92,93] Importantly, as Symonds had suggested, the effects of recurrent head injury are cumulative,[52] indicating that recovery is not literally complete, but that restitution takes place at the expense of limited brain "reserves", as it were. Short-latency auditory-evoked potential studies have also suggested brainstem dysfunction even after "minor" head injury.[91,94-96] Combined findings on neuropsychologic outcome and magnetic resonance imaging have also shown parallel results, and imaging findings seemed to mirror expected neuropathologic lesions known from autopsy material.[97] Finally, in mildly head injured experimental subjects, milder degrees of axonal injury have been documented.[54,55,91] Unfortunately, the preponderant harmony of results seems discordant here, since in two reports the lesions were primarily located in the brainstem in moderately injured animals and essentially limited to the brainstem in mildly injured subjects.[55,91] This would seem to violate the centripetal theory of lesion distribution referred to above.[32] Jane and colleagues suggest on this basis that different mechanisms are at work,[91] but clearly an adequate explanation is not yet at hand in this relatively little-studied area.

No specific information regarding milder degrees of head injury in the elderly is readily available. Based on this data in younger persons and the known age-related worsening of outcome in more severe forms of head injury (see below), one would suspect that the elderly are more susceptible to lasting neuropsychologic sequelae, especially if one keeps in mind their special susceptibility to diffuse encephalopathy due to other forms of generalized brain insult.[71,98]

OUTCOME AFTER HEAD INJURY

The assessment of head-injured patients (e.g., Glasgow Coma Scale[39,99]) and prognostication of their outcomes is a large subject which cannot be fully reviewed here. Many variables must be addressed, including age, sex, mode of injury, degree and duration of neurologic dysfunction, specific brain lesions or conditions present (hematomas, contusions, raised intracranial pressure, etc.), transportation time, presence or absence of multiple trauma, cardiac arrest, hypoxia, etc.[2,3,7-13,23,25,26,37,39-45,53,80,83,86,89,90,97,100-104] Different measures of outcome also introduce additional complexities, since this can be looked at in terms of survival, neurologic function (level of consciousness, cognition, motor function), neuropsychologic function, social and emotional adjustment, development of post-traumatic epilepsy, and so on.[39,105-108] From the point of view of the elderly head trauma victim, however, the conclusions are fairly simple, insofar as they have been examined. In contrast to the generally good outcomes possible after head injury in children[45,101] and the intermediate results in the high risk young adult and moderate risk middle-aged populations, survival and neurologic outcomes appear to be uniformly worse with advanced age.[2,3,5,7,8,10,12,45,100,103,104] The occurrence of subdural or extradural hematomas, severe neurologic dysfunction, or coexistence of multiple trauma, hypotension, or hypoxia, confer a worse prognosis in the elderly as in other age groups.[45,100,102] Nevertheless, the rehabilitation potential of the elderly patient is considerable, and in the setting of the modern trauma center with adequate emergency support services, many older patients can return home and function near their previous level.[7,10,11]

ACKNOWLEDGMENTS

Arnulf H. Koeppen, MD, for reviewing the manuscript. Albany Veterans Administration Medical Center Medical Library, Albany, New York, for reference materials.

REFERENCES

1. Fischer, R.P. and Miles, D.L.: The demographics of trauma in 1995. J. Trauma, 27:1233, 1987.
2. Tamas, L.B., Dacey, R.G., Jr., and Winn, H.R.: Stud-

ies of severe head injury: an overview. In: *Trauma of the Central Nervous System.* (Ed) R.G. Dacey. New York, Raven Press, 1985.

3. Waller, J.A.: Injury in aged. New York State J. Med., 74:2200, 1974.
4. Gryfe, C.I., Amies, A., and Ashley, M.J.: A longitudinal study of falls in an elderly population: I. Incidence and morbidity. Age and Ageing, 6:201, 1977.
5. Händel, K.: Gefährdung älterer Menschen im Strassenverkehr. Z. Gerontologie, 14:313, 1981.
6. Zollinger, H.U.: Unfallursachen und Unfalltod im Alter. Z. Unfallmed. Berufskr., 75:207, 1982.
7. Oreskovich, M.R., Howard, J.D., Copass, M.K., and Carrico, J.: Geriatric trauma: injury patterns and outcome. J. Trauma, 24:565, 1984.
8. Karimi-Nejad, A., and Tritz, W.: Sequelae and prognosis of craniocerebral trauma in elderly people. Adv. Neurosurg., 12:212, 1984.
9. Udén, G.: Inpatient accidents in hospitals. J. Am. Geriatr. Soc., 33:833, 1985.
10. Marx, A.B., Campbell, R.B., and Harder, F.: Polytrauma in the elderly. World J. Surg., 10:330, 1986.
11. DeMaria, E.J., et al.: Aggressive trauma care benefits the elderly. J. Trauma, 27:1200, 1987.
12. Galbraith, S.: Head injuries in the elderly. Br. Med. J., 294:325, 1987.
13. Brocklehurst, G., Gooding, M., and James, G.: Comprehensive care of patients with head injuries. Br. Med. J., 294:435, 1987.
14. Courville, C.B.: *Commotio Cerebri. Cerebral Concussion and the Postconcussion Syndrome in their Medical and Legal Aspects.* Los Angeles, San Lucas Press, 1953.
15. Courville, C.B.: *Pathology of the Central Nervous System.* 3rd Ed., Mountain View, California, Pacific Press Publ. Assoc., 1950.
16. Lindenberg, R.: Trauma of meninges and brain. In: *Pathology of the Nervous System,* Vol. 2. (Ed) Minckler, J. New York, McGraw-Hill, 1971.
17. Lindenberg, R.: Forensic Neuropathology. In: *Pathology of the Nervous System,* Vol. 3. (Ed) Minckler, J. New York, McGraw-Hill, 1971.
18. Strich, S.J.: Diffuse degeneration of the cerebral white matter in severe dementia following head injury. J. Neurol. Neurosurg. Psychiatr., 19:163, 1956.
19. Strich, S.J.: Shearing of nerve fibers as a cause of brain damage due to head injury. Lancet, 2:443, 1961.
20. Strich, S.J.: Cerebral Trauma. In: *Greenfield's Neuropathology.* 3rd Ed. (Eds) Blackwood, W. and Corsellis, J.A.N., London, Arnold, 1976.
21. Graham, D.I. and Adams, J.H.: Ischemic brain damage in fatal head injuries. Lancet, 1:265, 1971.
22. Adams, J.H., Mitchell, D.E., Graham, D.I., et al.: Diffuse brain damage of immediate impact type. Its relationship to 'primary brain-stem damage' in head injury. Brain, 100:489, 1977.
23. Adams, J.H., Graham, D.I., Murray, L.S., et al.: Diffuse axonal injury due to nonmissile head injury in humans: an analysis of 45 cases. Ann. Neurol., 12:557, 1982.
24. Adams, J.H., Doyle, D., Graham, D.I., et al. Diffuse axonal injury in head injuries caused by a fall. Lancet, 2:1420, 1984.
25. Adams, J.H., Graham, D.I. and Gennarelli, T.A.: Contemporary neuropathological considerations regarding brain damage in head injury. In: *Central Nervous System Trauma Status Report 1985.* (Eds) Becker, D.P. and Povlishock, J.T. Washington, D.C., Na-

tional Institute of Neurological and Communicative Disorders and Stroke, National Institutes of Health, 1985.
26. Graham, D.I., Lawrence, A.E., Adams, J.H., et al.: Brain damage in non-missile head injury secondary to high intracranial pressure. Neuropath. Appl. Neurobiol., 13:209, 1987.
27. Adams, J.H.: Head injury. In: *Greenfield's Neuropathology.* 4th Ed., (Eds) Adams, J.H., Corsellis, J.A.N., and Duchen, L.W. London, Arnold, 1984.
28. Symonds, C.P.: Concussion and contusion of the brain. In: *Injuries of the Skull, Brain and Spinal Cord.* (Ed) by Brock, S. London, Baillière, 1940.
29. Symonds, C.P.: Concussion and its sequelae. Lancet, 1:1, 1962. Cited in *Studies in Neurology.* (Ed) by Sir Charles Symonds. London, Oxford University Press, 1970.
30. Russell, W.R. *The Traumatic Amnesias.* London, Oxford University Press, 1971.
31. Denny-Brown, D.E. and Russell, W.R.: Experimental cerebral concussion. Brain, 64:93, 1941.
32. Ommaya, A.K. and Gennarelli, T.A.: Cerebral concussion and traumatic unconsciousness. Correlation of experimental and clinical observations on blunt head injuries. Brain, 97:633, 1974.
33. Gennarelli, T.A., et al.: Diffuse axonal injury and traumatic coma in the primate. Ann. Neurol., 12:564, 1982.
34. Gennarelli, T.A.: Head injury in man and experimental animals: clinical aspects. Acta Neurochir., Suppl. 32:1, 1983.
35. Gennarelli, T.A., et al.: Diffuse axonal injury and traumatic coma in the primate. In: *Trauma of the Central Nervous System.* (Ed) Dacey, R.G., Jr. New York, Raven Press, 1985.
36. Thibault, L.E. and Gennarelli, T.A.: Biomechanics and craniocerebral trauma. In: *Central Nervous System Trauma Status Report* 1985. (Eds) Becker, D.P. and Povlishock, J.T. Washington, D.C., National Institute of Neurological and Communicative Disorders and Stroke, National Institutes of Health, 1985.
37. Trunkey, D.: Neural trauma: from the point of view of the general surgeon. In: *Trauma of the Central Nervous System.* (Ed) Dacey, R.G., Jr. New York, Raven Press, 1985.
38. Cotman, C.W., Nieto-Sampedro, M., and Gibbs, R.B.: Enhancing the self-repairing potential of the CNS after injury. Central Nervous System Trauma, 1:1, 1984.
39. Jennett, B. and Teasdale, G.: *Management of Head Injuries.* Philadelphia, F.A. Davis Co., 1981.
40. Frankowski, R.F., Annegers, J.F., and Whitman, S.: Epidemiological and descriptive studies part I: the descriptive epidemiology of head trauma in the United States. In: *Central Nervous System Trauma Status Report 1985.* (Eds) Becker, D.P. and Povlishock, J.T. Washington, D.C., National Institute of Neurological and Communicative Disorders and Stroke, National Institutes of Health, 1985.
41. Kraus, J.F.: Epidemiology of head injury. In: *Head Injury.* 2nd Ed., (Ed) Cooper, P.R. Baltimore, Williams & Wilkins, 1987.
42. Nestvold, K., Lundar, T., Blikra, G., and Lønnum, A.: Head injuries during one year in a central hospital in Norway: a prospective study. Epidemiologic features. Neuroepidemiol. 7:134, 1988.
43. Cooper, J.D., Tabaddor, K., and Hauser, W.A.: The epidemiology of head injury in the Bronx. Neuroepidemiol., 2:70, 1983.

44. Whitman, S., Coonley-Hoganson, R., and Desai, B.T.: Comparative head trauma experiences in two socioeconomically different Chicago-area communities. A population study. Am. J. Epidemiol., 119:570, 1984.

45. Luerssen, T.G., Klauber, M.R., and Marshall, L.F.: Outcome of head injury related to patient's age. A longitudinal prospective study of adult and pediatric head injury. J. Neurosurg., 68:409, 1988.

46. Wolfson, L.I. and Katzman, R.: The neurologic consultation at age 80. In: The Neurology of Aging, (Eds) Katzman, R. and Terry, R.D. Philadelphia, F.A. Davis Co., 1983, pp. 229-231.

47. Terävainen, H., and Calne, D.B.: Motor system in normal aging and Parkinson's disease. In: The Neurology of Aging, (Eds) Katzman, R. and Terry, R.D. Philadelphia, F.A. Davis Co., 1983, p. 91.

48. Terävainen, H., and Calne, D.B.: Motor system in normal aging and Parkinson's disease. In: The Neurology of Aging, (Eds) Katzman, R. and Terry, R.D. Philadelphia, F.A. Davis Co., 1983, p. 90.

49. Wolfson, L.I. and Katzman, R.: The neurologic consultation at age 80. In: The Neurology of Aging, (Eds) Katzman, R. and Terry, R.D. Philadelphia, F.A. Davis Co., 1983, pp. 225-229.

50. Wright, B.E. and Henkind, P.: Aging changes and the eye. In: The Neurology of Aging, (Eds) Katzman, R. and Terry, R.D. Philadelphia, F.A. Davis Co., 1983, pp 149-165.

51. Gronwall, D. and Wrightson, P.: Delayed recovery intellectual function after minor head injury. Lancet, 2:605, 1974.

52. Gronwall, D. and Wrightson, P.: Cumulative effect of concussion. Lancet, 2:995, 1975.

53. Hugenholtz, H., Stuss, D.T., Stethem, L.L., and Richard, M.T.: How long does it take to recover from a mild concussion? Neurosurgery, 22:853, 1988.

54. Povlishock, J.T., Becker, D.P., Cheng, C.L.Y., et al.: Axonal change in minor head injury. J. Neuropath. Exp. Neurol., 42:225, 1983.

55. Jane, J.A., Steward, O., and Gennarelli, T.A.: Axonal degeneration induced by experimental noninvasive minor head injury. J. Neurosurg. 62:96, 1985.

56. Hardman, J.A.: The pathology of traumatic brain injuries. Adv. Neurol., 22:15, 1979.

57. Jellinger, K.: Pathology and pathogenesis of apallic syndromes following closed head injuries. In: The Apallic Syndrome. (Eds) Ore, G.D., Gerstenbrand, F., Lucking, C.H., Peters, G., and Peters, U.H. Berlin, Springer, 1977.

58. Jennett, B. and Plum, F.: Persistent vegetative state after brain damage. Lancet, 1:734, 1972.

59. Dawson, S.L., Hirsch, C.S., Lucas, F.V., et al.: The contrecoup phenomenon. Reappraisal of a classic problem. Human Pathol., 11:155, 1980.

60. Gennarelli, T.A. and Thibault, L.E.: Biomechanics of acute subdural hematoma. J. Trauma, 22:680, 1982.

61. Ommaya, A.K. and Yarnell, P.: Subdural haematoma after whiplash injury. Lancet, 2:237, 1969.

62. Echlin, F.A., Sordillo, S.V.R., and Garvey, T.Q.: Acute, subacute and chronic subdural hematoma. JAMA, 161:1345, 1956.

63. McKissock, W.: Subdural haematoma. A review of 389 cases. Lancet, 1:1365, 1960.

64. Ramamurthi, B.: Acute subdural haematoma. In: Handbook of Clinical Neurology. Vol. 24. (Eds) Vinkin, P.J. and Bruyn, G.W. Amsterdam, North-Holland, 1976.

65. Bender, M.B., Christoff, N.: Nonsurgical treatment of subdural hematomas. Arch. Neurol., 31:73, 1974.

66. Potter, J.F. and Fruin, A.H.: Chronic subdural hematoma—the "great imitator". Geriatrics, 32:61, 1977.

67. Loew, F. and Kivelitz R.: Chronic subdural haematomas. In: Handbook of Clinical Neurology. Vol. 24. (Eds) Vinkin, P.J. and Bruyn, G.W. Amsterdam, North-Holland, 1976.

68. Spallone, A., Giuffrè, R., Gagliardi, F.M., et al.: Chronic subdural hematoma in extremely aged patients. Eur. Neurol. 29:18, 1989.

69. Andrioli, G.C., Zuccarello, M., Trinicia, G. et al.: Extradural hematomas in elderly. A statistical analysis of 58 cases. Adv. Neurosurg., 12:218, 1984.

70. Jamieson, K.G.: Epidural haematoma. In: Handbook of Clinical Neurology. Vol. 24. (Eds) Vinkin, P.J. and Bruyn, G.W. Amsterdam, North-Holland, 1976.

71. Plum, F. and Posner, J.: The Diagnosis of Stupor and Coma. 3rd Ed. Philadelphia, F.A. Davis Co., 1980.

72. Cooper, P.R.: Delayed brain injury: secondary insults. In: Central Nervous System Trauma Status Report 1985. (Eds) Becker, D.P. and Povlishock, J.T. Washington, D.C., National Institute of Neurological and Communicative Disorders and Stroke, National Institutes of Health, 1985.

73. Nelson, P.R., Rosenbaum, A.E., Moossy, J., et al.: Delayed deterioration in the syndrome of temporal lobe contusion: evaluation by computed tomography (CT). J. Trauma, 22:39, 1982.

74. Tanaka, T., et al.: MR imaging as predictor of delayed posttraumatic cerebral hemorrhage. J. Neurosurg., 69:203, 1988.

75. Shaw, C-M. and Alvord, E.C., Jr.: Injury of the basilar artery associated with closed head trauma. J. Neurol. Neurosurg. Psychiatr., 35:247, 1972.

76. Bruce, D.A., et al.: Diffuse cerebral swelling following head injuries in children: the syndrome of "malignant brain edema". J. Neurosurg., 54:170, 1981.

77. Reilly, P.L., Adams, J.H., Graham, D.I., et al.: Patients with head injury who talk and die. Lancet, 2:375, 1975.

78. Clifton, G.L., McCormick, W.F., and Grossman, R.G.: Neuropathology of early and late deaths after head injury. Neurosurg., 8:309, 1981.

79. Komatsu, S., et al.: Traumatic lesions of the corpus callosum. Neurosurg., 5:32, 1979.

80. Levin, H.S., et al.: Relationship of depth of brain lesions to consciousness and outcome after closed head injury. J. Neurosurg., 69:861, 1988.

81. Mitchell, D.E. and Adams, J.H.: Primary focal impact damage to the brainstem in blunt head injuries: does it exist? Lancet, 2:215, 1973.

82. Turazzi, S. and Bricolo, A.: Acute pontine syndromes following head injury. Lancet, 2:62, 1977.

83. Rosenblum, W.I., Greenberg, R.P., Seelig, J.M., et al.: Midbrain lesions: frequent and significant prognostic feature in closed head injury. Neurosurg., 9:613, 1981.

84. Editorial: Head injuries—from accident department to necropsy room. Lancet, 1:589, 1978.

85. Editorial: Preventing secondary brain damage after head injury. Lancet, 2:1189, 1978.

86. Anderson, I.D., Woodford, M., de Dombal, F.T., et al.: Retrospective study of 1000 deaths from injury in England and Wales. Br. Med. J., 296:1305, 1988.

87. Brierly, J.B. and Graham, D.I.: Hypoxia and vascular disorders of the central nervous system. In: Green-

field's Neuropathology. 4th Ed. (Eds) Adams, J.H., Corsellis, J.A.N., and Duchen, L.W. London, Arnold, 1984.

88. Miller, J.D. and Adams, J.H.: The pathophysiology of raised intracranial pressure. In: *Greenfield's Neuropathology.* 4th Ed. (Eds) Adams, J.H., Corsellis, J.A.N., and Duchen, L.W. London, Arnold, 1984.

89. Dacey, R.G., Jr. and Dikmen, S.G.: Mild head injury. In: *Head Injury.* 2nd Ed. (Ed) Cooper, P.R. Baltimore, Williams & Wilkins, 1987.

90. Alves, W.M. and Jane, J.A.: Mild brain injury: damage and outcome. In: *Central Nervous System Trauma Status Report 1985.* (Eds) Becker, D.P. and Povlishock, J.T. Washington, D.C., National Institute of Neurological and Communicative Disorders and Stroke, National Institutes of Health, 1985.

91. Jane, J.A., et al.: Minor and moderate head injury: model systems. In: *Trauma of the Central Nervous System.* (Ed) Dacey, R.G., Jr. New York, Raven Press, 1985.

92. Rutherford, W.H., Merrett, J.D., and McDonald, J.R.: Sequelae of concussion caused by minor head injuries. Lancet, 1:1, 1977.

93. Gronwall, D. and Wrightson, P.: Memory and information processing capacity after closed head injury. J. Neurol. Neurosurg. Psychiatr., 44:889, 1981.

94. Schoenhuber, R., et al.: Brain stem auditory evoked potentials in early evaluation of cerebral concussion. J. Neurosurg. Sci., 27:157, 1983.

95. Montgomery, A., Fenton, G.W., and McClelland, R.J.: Delayed brainstem conduction time in post-concussional syndrome (letter). Lancet, 1:1011, 1984.

96. Schoenhuber, R., Gentilini, M., and Orlando, A.: Prognostic value of auditory brain-stem responses for late postconcussion symptoms following minor head injury. J. Neurosurg., 68:742, 1988.

97. Wilson, J.T.L., et al.: Early and late magnetic resonance imaging and neuropsychological outcome after head injury. J. Neurol. Neurosurg. Psychiatr., 51:391, 1988.

98. Blass, J.P. and Plum, F.: Metabolic encephalopathies in older adults. In: *The Neurology of Aging,* (Eds) Katzman, R. and Terry, R.D. Philadelphia, F.A. Davis Co., 1983, p. 91.

99. Jennett, B.: Severity of brain damage—altered consciousness and other indicators. Prog. Neurol. Surg., 10:164, 1981.

100. Carlsson, C.-A., von Essen, C., and Löfgren, J.: Factors affecting the clinical course of patients with severe head injuries. J. Neurosurg., 29:242, 1968.

101. Bruce, D.A., et al.: Outcome following severe head injuries in children. J. Neurosurg., 48:679, 1978.

102. Gennarelli, T.A., et al.: Influence of the type of intracranial lesion on outcome from severe head injury. J. Neurosurg., 56:26, 1982.

103. Born, J.D., Albert, A., Hans, P., et al.: Relative prognostic value of best motor response and brainstem reflexes in patients with severe head injury. Neurosurg., 16:595, 1985.

104. Conroy, C. and Kraus, J.: Survival after brain injury. Neuroepidemiol., 7:13, 1988.

105. Jennett, B.: Posttraumatic epilepsy. Adv. Neurol., 22:137, 1979.

106. Editorial: Epilepsy after head trauma and fitness to drive. Lancet, 1:401, 1980.

107. Cooper, P.R. (Ed.): *Head Injury.* 2nd Ed. Baltimore, Williams & Wilkins, 1987.

108. Becker, D.P. and Povlishock, J.T. (eds.): *Central Nervous System Trauma Status Report 1985.* Washington, D.C., National Institute of Neurological and Communicative Disorders and Stroke, National Institutes of Health, 1985.

15

Infection of the Central Nervous System in the Elderly

MARK STACY and
DAVID ROELTGEN

Infectious organisms by direct and indirect processes produce an abundance of pathologic changes in the central (CNS) and peripheral (PNS) nervous system. In the elderly patient the diagnosis of these diseases becomes more difficult because many of the signs and symptoms are nonspecific and nonlocalizing (e.g. headache, confusion, dementia, delirium, anorexia). When physical findings do suggest an anatomic site, this is not always accurate in predicting etiology. With the aid of ancillary laboratory assessment diagnosis can be made much easier. Imaging, such as magnetic resonance imaging (MRI) or computed tomography (CT) scanning, arteriography, and traditional plane films will often facilitate localization. Isotope brain (SPECT) scanning may be helpful in some instances. The electroencephalogram (EEG) may provide anatomic information and demonstrate impairment of cerebral functioning. Evoked potentials, nerve conduction velocities (NCV), and electromyography (EMG) will at times be useful in the work-up of these patients. Often, lumbar puncture and tissue biopsy will be necessary to determine the infectious agent.

This chapter is an attempt to highlight the numerous etiologic possibilities concerning CNS or PNS infection in the aging population. Besides the traditional organisms infecting the nervous system, the immunocompromised host will also be discussed.

MENINGITIS

ACUTE BACTERIAL MENINGITIS

Bacterial infections of the nervous system in immunocompetent patients are most often confined to the CNS; specifically the meninges, brain parenchyma, and parameningeal spaces. Meningitis occurs most often and is a frequent cause for agitation, confusion, dementia, and headache. Although any bacterium may cause purulent meningitis, the majority of cases in the adult and the geriatric population are caused by three organisms: *Neisseria meningitidis, Streptococcus pneumoniae*, and *Hemophilus influenzae* type B.[1] In the past 20 years, however, the variety and frequency of uncommon meningeal pathogens has been increasing.[2,3]

Invasion of the subarachnoid space most commonly occurs via hematogenous spread, but also results from parameningeal foci, and direct innoculation. *N. meningitidis, S. pneumoniae*, and *H. influenzae* are normal flora of the nasopharynx. Colonization with new strains of these organisms, a continuing process, allows for a changing population of flora in the pharyngeal cavity[4-6] and introduction of a new subtype may predispose to infection. The ability of these organisms to reach the subarachnoid space may be related to a factor that allows crossing of the blood-brain barrier (BBB). In *H. influenzae* strains this factor may be lipo-oligosaccharide, a molecule shown to produce meningeal inflammation in the rabbit,[7] but further data are needed to clarify this hypothesis. Scheifele and others[8] have shown that meningitis results in primates from local inflammation after colonization with new strains of organisms when there is an associated bacteremia.

A number of pathologic lesions from bacterial meningitis have been described. These are largely due to inflammation in response to the purulent exudate in the subarachnoid space. Edema is produced in the CNS by several mechanisms.[9] Inflammatory exudate may block the arachnoid granulations at the cerebral convexities, leading to CSF outflow arrest and rapid increase in intracranial pressure. Eventually, CSF enters the periventricular white matter and may cause destruction of nerve fibers; host response to this process may cause further edema. Organismal disruption of endothelial tight junctions may lead to capillary leakage and parenchymal ischemia and infarction, thus causing further CNS edema. Although bacteria rarely invade brain parenchyma, tangential infarction may occur via toxins released from polymorphonucleocytes or in the case of gram-negative infection, endotoxin.

Bacteria survival is dependent on host response; a decrease in T-cells and monocytes have been shown to impair host survival.[1] Sande et al.[10] have reported decreased bacterial growth in the presence of fever, a normal response to microbiologic invasion in the nonimmunocompromised host, in some animals including man. This point is of interest in the context of infections in the elderly. It is known that elderly patients frequently develop less of a febrile reaction than younger patients. This may be one of the factors that increases host susceptibility to infection in the aging patients.

Increasing age predisposes to meningeal infection; this is believed to be, primarily, a function of cell mediated immunity.[1] Most patients diagnosed with meningitis will have headache, photophobia, and stiff neck; many will report fever. The headache typically is severe, holocephalic, and increases with movement. Nausea and vomiting may also be present. However, in the aging population these symptoms may not be present and only a change in behavior may be noted. Frequently, this is only drowsiness, but may progress to lethargy and coma. Increasing agitation and irritability are also seen. On physical examination ocular tenderness (pain with light pressure on a closed eye), Kernig's sign (pain with extension of the knee with hip flexed) and Brudzinski's sign (neck flexion producing knee and hip flexion) may be produced.[1]

Focal neurologic deficits can occur with meningitis; this is usually a result of increased intracranial pressure, but may rarely be secondary to vasculitic infarction. Oculomotility problems, facial weakness and deafness are reported as well as papilledema.[1] Generally, papilledema is thought to be rare in this condition, but in a recent review of neurologic infection Wood and Anderson[11] cite a 20% frequency. Seizures can also occur in the adult population, but this is felt to be an exception to the norm.[12]

Confirmation and identification of the etiologic agent of meningitis is dependent on the lumbar puncture. The common abnormalities present in the bacterial varieties include: CSF pleocytosis (usually PMNs), hypoglycorrhachea, and elevated protein (Table 15–1). Gram stain, bacterial culture, fungal culture, acid fast stain and culture, India ink and cryp-

TABLE 15–1.   Spinal Fluid Profiles in Infections*

Infection	Number	Cell Type	Protein mg/dl	Glucose mg/dl	Other
Bacterial meningitis	100–10,000 (89%)	PMN	45–1000 (90%)	<40 (80%)	+culture +Gram st +CIE
"Aseptic" meningitis	5–500	Lymphocyte	50–80	20–40/nl	
Mollaret's	50–1000	Lymphocyte	70–100	nl	
Fungal meningitis	10–500	Lymphocyte	50–500	10–40/nl	+culture +India +crypto
Carcinoma	0–500	Lymphocyte PMN	20–1200	<70	+cytology
Brain Abscess	0–500	Lymphocyte PMN	nl/>50	>40	(contraindicated)
Herpes simplex	50–1000	Lymphocyte	50–400	nl	
zoster	10–100	Lymphocyte	<100	nl/<70	
Tb	50–1000	Lymphocyte	100–500	<40	+AFB stain culture antigen
Syphilis	0–2000	Lymphocyte	50–100	<40 (45%)	+serology
Spinal epidural abscess	0–1000	Lymphocyte PMN	45–100	nl	

*Adapted from Roeltgen[16] and Fishman.[86]

tococcal antigen are also important. In addition there are now rapid tests available for serologic diagnosis. Counterimmunoelectrophoresis (CIE) can be completed usually within several hours and is a useful adjunct to the traditional studies. The sensitivity and specificity of identification of this test in bacterial meningitis are 85 to 90%.[1] CIE may also be used in the identification of Streptococcus b, *Escherichea coli,* and Listeria. Other methods for rapid identification of infectious organisms include ELISA, immunofluorescence, radioimmunoassay, enzyme immunoassay, and coagglutination. If gram-negative infection is suspected, the Limulus lysate test remains a useful means for identifying the presence of endotoxin.[13] Treatment of bacterial meningitis is dependent on antibiotic penetration of the BBB. Properties facilitating this transfer are lipid solubility at pH = 7.4, ionization, protein binding, and molecular size.[14] An analysis of BBB antibiotic penetration is continually updated by Sanford.[15] Recommended broad spectrum coverage for bacterial meningitis is:

Pneumococcus	Penicillin (PCN) G, 2.3 million units every 3 hours.
Meningococcus	PCN G, 2.3 million units every 3 hours.
Staphylococcus aureus	Methacillin, 3 million units every 4 hours.
Haemophilus influenzae	Ampicillin, 1 g every 4 hours or Chloramphenicol 1 g every 6 hours
Unknown organism	PCN G, 2.3 million units every 3 hours and Chloramphenicol 1/g every 6 hours.

Adapted from Roeltgen.[16]

CHRONIC MENINGITIS

Chronic meningeal infection usually develops over a period of several weeks to a month. Intermittent changes in behavior or consciousness, cranial nerve dysfunction, evidence of raised intracranial pressure, and gait abnormality are sometimes associated with this problem. More often, varying changes in behavior, giving rise to the diagnosis of dementia and headache are the only symptoms. Fungal infection is a common etiology in this condition; *Cryptococcus neoformans* occurs most frequently, but *Histoplasma capsulatum, Coccidioides immitis,* and *Candidia albicans* are also seen. Tuberculosis, spirochetal diseases (Treponema and Borrelia), and brucellosis must also be included in this differential. Other rare mycotic infections as well as some parasitic infestations (Toxoplasma and Cysticercosis) are also reported, but these are more common in the immunocompromised patient.

The occurrence of dementia as the presenting feature of chronic infection is the major reason CSF analysis is included as a diagnostic tool in the assessment of declining mentation. The hallmark of chronic meningitis is CSF lymphocytosis. Glucose can be reduced while protein is usually elevated (Table 15–1). Cultures, stains, serology, and immunologic studies are important in establishing a more definitive diagnosis. Carcinomatous meningitis, a common non-infectious cause for chronic meningitis, may be excluded with negative cytology on multiple spinal taps with 80% confidence.[17] However, Trump[18] reports a 13% coincidence of carcinomatous and infectious meningitis in one series of cancer patients. Other noninfectious causes, sarcoidosis and granulomatous angiitis, are much less common and CSF examination is rarely helpful.

Fungal Infection. Mycotic infection most often begins after these organisms are inhaled, but direct innoculation through broken skin can occur. Symptoms develop as a function of the amount of the innoculum, the virulence of the agent, and the integrity of the host defenses.[11] In the geriatric population, these infections are frequent, because many patients, by virtue of underlying illness or pharmacologic intervention, have depressed immune function.[1] With neutropenia candidiasis and aspergillosis often occur. T-cell dysfunction may also predispose a patient to candidiasis as well as Blastomycetes, Coccidioidomyces, Cryptococcus, and Histoplasma infection. Nocardia is seen in association with B-cell dysfunction. Disease states which predispose a patient to opportunistic fungal infection include: chronic steroid therapy, organ transplantation requiring immunosuppressive therapy,[19–22] leukemia and other lymphoproliferative diseases,[23,24] diabetes,[1] renal failure,[25] and AIDS.[26]

After aspiration of the infectious agent and lung colonization, the organism then migrates to the local lymph tissue. Replication and subsequent toxemia ensue. Reticuloendothelial system invasion precedes CNS infection. Pathologically, chronic fungal infection appears similar to other meningeal pathogens. Although the pathologic lesions do vary depending on the specific etiology, diffuse purulent exudates, microabcesses, granulomata and giant granulomata may all be seen.[27]

Treatment of fungal meningitis remains unsatisfactory. Early diagnosis and treatment will improve prognosis, but because adequate antimicrobial therapy cannot always be given and underlying disease is frequently present, the outlook for good recovery remains poor. In most cases involving treatment of cryptococcosis, candidiasis, histoplasmosis, and coccidiomycosis, a combined approach of intravenous and antibiotics and surgical removal of abscesses and granulomata are used. In some instances intrathecal antibiosisis is also used. Amphotericin B is the drug of choice, however, a significant number of patients are unable to tolerate this agent and ketoconazole must be sustituted. The duration of treatment varies, but should be continued for at least 6 weeks.[28]

Tuberculosis. *Mycobacterium tuberculosis* is a prolific pathogen that can cause damage to any human organ system. Though this disease no longer represents the threat to public health that it once did, tuberculosis (TB) is still endemic in the developing countries and in the poorer socioeconomic and overcrowded areas in industrialized nations.[29] TB is increasing in the nursing home community as a result of nosocomial exposure.[31] Primary CNS infection is thought not to occur, but nervous system involvement is found in 3 to 6% of all autopsied cases of adults diagnosed with TB prior to death.[32] TB meningitis is subacute to chronic in tempo and presents in the same fashion as described in the fungal infections. Besides advancing age, malnutrition, concurrent disease (AIDS, diabetes mellitis, neoplasm) and those receiving immunosuppressive therapy are at increased risk for developing clinical infection.[33]

CNS TB is secondary to infection elsewhere in the body, usually pulmonary or gastric varieties. At autopsy, meningeal tubercles are seen throughout the CNS, but predominate in the basal areas. Circumscribed casseous plaques and a greenish exudate are also seen. Microscopically, lymphocytes, plasma cells, and epithelial cells are seen. Fibrin deposition

TABLE 15–2.*

Drug	Dosage (adults)	Side effects
Isoniazid	5–10 mg/kg/day	peripheral, neuropathy, convulsions, encephalopathy, memory impairment, optic neuritis, liver disturbance, hypersensitivity, anemia, lupoid syndrome.
Rifampicin	600 mg/day 9 mg/kg/day	headache, fatigue, ataxia, confusion, weakness, optic neuritis, drug fever.
Pyrazinamide	25 mg/kg/day	hepatitis, arthralgia.
Ethambutol	25 mg/kg/day	optic neuritis.
Streptomycin	.75–1 g/day IM	VIII nerve damage, renal toxicity.

*Adapted from Sanford.[15]

and necrotic exudates predominate on the floor of the skull and tend to become more prominant with disease progression. The meningeal vessels as well as the internal carotid artery, vertebrobasilar artery, and the anastamoses forming the Circle of Willis often become narrowed, and may result in infarction.[32] In addition basal exudates may compromise the cerebral aqueducts and cause hydrocephalus.[9]

Tuberculomas are solid granulomas that initially begin as small necrotic tubercles, but eventually grow to form relatively avascular structures surrounded by a gelatinous gray capsule. The surrounding parenchyma shows a loss of neuronal and supporting cells, but an astroglial proliferation may occur. These masses are predominantly supratentorial in adults and are often multiple. Some series report a frequency of 10%.[30] Tuberculus spinal osteomyelitis may also produce neurologic symptoms secondarily by cord compression.[36] Extraparenchymal tuberculomas (scrofula) attached to the meninges and causing neural compression have also been reported.[35]

Symptoms and signs of CNS TB are myriad. In the elderly diagnosis is often difficult because the more typical systemic changes may not be seen.[29] Tuberculus meningitis patients have the common symptoms of chronic meningitis, but as a result of the large amount of basilar exudation other signs can be seen. Papilledema may result from CSF outflow obstruction or from arachnoid granulation obliteration. Frequently cranial nerve deficits (VII, VI, III) are seen. With vascular compromise more extensive brainstem and cortical deficits develop. In addition convulsions, particularly focal seizures, secondary to tuberculomas, may be seen in the adult population.[32]

Diagnosis of CNS TB is dependent on iso-

lation of the acid fast bacillus. Lumbar puncture will reveal CSF pleocytosis, elevated protein, and hypoglycorrhachia (Table 15–1). Ziehl-Neelson staining may identify the acid fast bacillus,[32] and culture of the organism may take as long as 8 weeks. CSF bromide-partition tests and adenosine deaminase levels have been proposed as possible adjuncts to aid in diagnosis, but some problems still exist with specificity.[37] If a tuberculoma is present on imaging, biopsy may be helpful in confirming the diagnostic suspicion. Culture and stain of sputum, urine, gastric secretions, chest x-ray and PPD may be helpful. Fundoscopic examination may also reveal characteristic changes.

Treatment of CNS TB involves three to four drugs initially; most often these are isoniazid, rifampin, pyrazinamide and either ethambutol or streptomycin. The former three are known to achieve high levels in the CSF.[30] As organism sensitivities to these medications are learned, therapy may be adjusted. The dosages and side effects to these antibiotics are listed in Table 15–2. With isoniazid therapy it is important to add pyridoxine to the regimen to avoid permanent peripheral neuropathy.[38] Duration of therapy varies, but can be as long as 2 years. Serial lumbar punctures with quantification of adenosine deaminase is a proposed method to follow treatment efficacy.[39]

Syphilis. The incidence of syphilis has been increasing in the last 5 years. Initially, this was thought to be secondary to unsafe sex practices in homosexual men, but some data exist to suggest a stronger interrelationship between syphilis and AIDS.[40] Transmission of the spirochete, *Treponema pallidum,* is via intimate contact and there are usually three phases. Primary syphilis, also known as chancre, is recognized as a single, indurated, painless skin lesion at the site of infection. Occasionally, regional lymphadenopathy is seen. This usually heals in several weeks. The development of secondary syphilis occurs with the development of a diffuse skin rash. At this time bacteremia has occurred and treponemal meningitis may result via hematogenous spread.[41] Interestingly, though the typical findings of a basilar meningitis can be seen, CSF serology is often negative, while the serum serology is positive. Spinal fluid shows the typical findings described in Table 15–1.

Tertiary syphilis occurs from 2 years after the initial infection. Merritt et al.[11] classified the symptoms of neurosyphilis into several categories: asymptomatic, meningeal, meningovascular, general paresis, tabes dorsalis, optic atrophy, and spinal parenchymal. Gumma, a mass lesion composed of spirochetal and inflammatory tissue, may also cause CNS compromise.[42]

Asymptomatic neurosyphilis is seen in neurologically normal patients with an abnormal spinal fluid examination. These patients should be treated to avoid neurologic decline. Meningeal neurosyphilis may occur acutely, subacutely or chronically. The chronic signs, symptoms, and pathologic findings closely resemble those of tuberculus meningitis, but serologic tests are positive. Meningovascular syphilis results from vasculitis of large and middle sized cerebral vessels. Symptoms vary with the location of thrombosis.

General paresis of the insane usually develops 10 to 20 years after primary infection. The decline is a result of parenchymal invasion of CNS parenchyma. Mental deterioration, behavioral changes, paralysis, tremor, ataxia, sensory disturbances, and incontinence can occur. Death is usually seen within 2 to 10 years. At autopsy, rod cells, a stereotypical lesion in neurosyphilis, may be seen.

Tabes dorsalis also occurs 10 to 20 years after infection and is a result of pathogen invasion of the dorsal roots of the spinal cord. From nerve root invasion lightning pains, ataxia, areflexia, and Argyll-Robertson pupils result. With loss of the sensory roots the patient is without pain, tactile, and proprioceptive sensation. As a result, patients are unaware of bodily trauma. Repeated insult often results in pressure ulcers and arthritic degeneration (Charcot joint). Optic atrophy via trep-

onemal invasion of the optic nerve is usually seen with tabes dorsalis and, if untreated, will result in blindness.

Despite increasing numbers of serologic and bacteriologic tests, neurosyphilis remains difficult to diagnose. *T. pallidum* invasion produces a number of host reactions; these result in the generation of antibody compounds—reagins.[43] Serologic testing has evolved to assess the presence of these compounds in the CSF and serum. The first of these, the Wasserman test, is the least sensitive and is no longer used. The Venereal Disease Research Laboratory (VDRL) uses a flocculation reaction, and is highly specific for the detection of treponemal antibodies,[44] but has poor sensitivity.[45] False-positives may also occur with traumatic lumbar puncture or any other condition that elevates the CSF protein.[43] However, the VDRL does remain a clinically useful test, because levels do correlate with disease activity.[46] CSF Fluid Treponemal Antibody (FTA) is reported to detect reaginic proteins 6 times more frequently than the VDRL,[47] and is now considered the diagnostic test for syphilis.[43] False-positives may also be seen with this study in similar circumstances as the VDRL.

When evaluating a patient for possible syphilis, the VDRL is often used as a screening test; if this is positive, a serum CSF-FTA should be obtained. A positive FTA-ABS indicates past infection with *T. pallidum*, but does not reflect active infection. If neurologic abnormalities are found, CSF examination is necessary. Positive CSF FTA-ABS with more than 5 leukocytes or protein greater than 40 mg/dl is consistent with neurosyphilis.[43]

Treatment for neurosyphilis is still penicillin (Table 15-3). This antimicrobial inhibits transpeptidase, an enzyme important in cell wall synthesis.[41] With decreasing cell wall stability, osmotic pressure increases and cytolysis ensues. Because the spirochete divides every 33 hours, prolonged treatment is required to assure adequate drug exposure to vulnerable di-

TABLE 15–3.   Treatment for Neurosyphilis*

PCN G, 4 million units IV every 4 hours for 21 days. Follow this with PCN G, 2.4 million units IM every week for 3 doses.
PCN G, 2.4 million units IM per day for 10 days and Probenicid 500 mg 4 times a day.

*Adapted from MMWR.[49]

viding cells. Panconesi et al.[48] have shown that blood levels from .1 to .4 μg/ml may allow microbe survival. Current recommendations by the World Health Organization suggest maintenance of blood levels above .08 μg/ml for 7 to 15 days for early syphilis and longer for late syphilis.[43] Several treatment protocols have been postulated to accomplish this.[43,49]

The treponeme is still quite sensitive to PCN, and, if no allergy exists, is the treatment of choice. If the patient is allergic to PCN, desensitization and treatment with this drug is now recommended.[49]

Lyme Disease. In 1975 a group of children living in the rural areas surrounding Lyme, Old Lyme, and East Hadden, Connecticut began to exhibit symptoms of monoarticular and oligoarticular joint pain. In adults a more systemic syndrome involving skin lesions, cardiac abnormalities, and neurologic signs was seen.[50] The skin lesion was identified as erythema chronicum migrans (ECM), an erythematous papule with a surrounding red annular lesion; this was first identified in the United States in a patient with a tick-associated illness.[51] A significant percentage of patients could remember tick bites prior to their symptoms, and the vector for this infection, *Ioxodes dammini*, was proposed in 1978.[52] Since then other vectors have been reported to transmit the infection agent.[54] *Borrelia burgdorferi* was identified as the microorganism responsible for Lyme disease in 1982.[54] Lyme neuroborreliosis is reported worldwide; in the United States there are three major endemic areas: Northeastern (Connecticut, Delaware, Maryland, Massachusetts, New Jersey, New York, Pennsylvania, and Rhode Island), Midwestern (Minnesota and Wisconsin), and Western (California, Nevada, Oregon, and Utah).[55] In their series of 38 patients Pachner and Steere[52] report an age range of 7 to 64 with a median age of 28 years.

Not unlike treponemal infection, Lyme disease produces a wide range of symptoms and may involve multiple organ systems.[56] Dermatologic lesions are seen early during this infection with the cardiologic, arthritic, and neurologic complications following shortly thereafter. There are several stages in the neurologic progression, but an overlap of these may be seen.[56]

Stage I of Lyme disease is characterized by dermal invasion and host inflammatory response; this is associated with ECM. As the organisms disperse, a viral syndrome (fever, headache, arthralgia, vomiting, and myalgia) may occur; during dissemination, invasion of any organ system may occur, but there may be a predilection for the reticuloendothelial system. The second stage of this illness occurs from a few weeks to a few months after initial infection. CSF pleocytosis occurs at this stage, and cranial nerve abnormalities, classically bilateral Bell's palsy, but also oculomotility disturbances, are reported. Perivascular mononuclear cell infiltrate and lymphocytic invasion of peripheral nerves are seen.[57] The late stage is associated with parenchymal invasion.[56] Spirochetes have been demonstrated in parenchymal nerve cells and perineurally. As the disease continues, vasculitis obliterans and focal demyelination can be seen. Both ischemia and conduction disturbance have been proposed as mechanisms for producing symptoms.[57] In addition, as with other spirochetsial infection, vasculitis,[58,59] peripheral neuropathy,[51,52] and myopathy[57] have been reported.

Lyme meningitis is of the acute lymphocytic variety with the patient exhibiting the usual signs and symptoms of this condition. History of skin rash, joint pain, and tick exposure are helpful in establishing the diagnosis. EKG should be done in suspected cases because 4 to 10% of patients will have A-V conduction block.[66]

Parenchymal involvement may be difficult to establish. These patients usually have a pleocytosis and elevated CSF IgG to *B. burgdorferi* antibody. Pachner[61] lists five criteria for the diagnosis of Stage III neuroborreliosis:

1. objective CNS involvement unexplained by other factors,
2. reproducible, high-titer Lyme serology,
3. other organ system involvement,
4. lymphocytic pleocytosis, and
5. positive response to IV antibiotics

Residence in an endemic area is also included in some protocols.[56]

As stated previously, *B. burgdorferi* is transmitted most often by the ixodid tick, however, this spirochete has been cultured from other arthropod vectors.[53] *I. damminis* infection with this organism occurs with ingestion of a blood meal and microorganismal proliferation continues through a complex life cycle; intermediate host (human) infection may be initiated via salival infection, midgut regurgitation, or fecal deposition by the vector on primary host.[53]

ACUTE LYMPHOCYTIC MENINGITIS

This condition, often termed "aseptic" because a sterile CSF and lymphocytosis and with lumbar puncture, has numerous causes; viral, rickettsial, spirochetsial, and partially treated bacterial meningitis are only a few. Many patients have complaints consistent with meningismus, and will often report a 1 to 2 week history of a prodromal illness. Spinal fluid examination reveals lymphocytosis, mildly elevated protein, and occasionally, a decreased glucose (Table 15–1).

The most common etiology for this condition is viral infection. The enteroviruses, polio, coxsackie, and ECHO, compromise a vast majority of the viral meningitides. Transmission of the enterovirus is mainly the oral-fecal route, but respiratory spread has been reported.[11] Ingestion of an inoculum is followed by replication of these DNA viruses in the lymphoid tissue surrounding the gut. After a brief viremia, dissemination to reticuloendothelial structures is seen. If a second viremia occurs, the now symptomatic patient may develop meningitis. It is not known how these organisms reach the subarachnoid space; both hematogenous and local invasion via pharyngeal lymph organs has been proposed.[62] Diagnosis may be obtained via antigenic determination or viral culture.

Other causes of viral meningitis, though unusual when beyond the pediatric ages, include mumps, lymphocytic choriomeningitis, Herpes simplex, cytomegalovirus, and arbovirus. Human immunodeficiency virus will be discussed in another section.

Another condition producing a lymphocytic pleocytosis with meningeal irritation is Mollaret's meningitis. This syndrome is characterized by recurrent meningitis lasting 4 to 5 days in which no other etiology is found. This condition is probably benign and usually resolves within 1 year.[63] Chemical lymphocytic meningitis as a result of NSAIAs and sulfonamides has also been described.[64] In addition multisystem disease, systemic lupus erythematosus, Behcet's, sarcoidosis, and Vogt-Koyanagi-Harada disease, are known to produce a lymphocytic meningitis. However, in the elderly population these syndromes rarely represent a diagnostic dilemma and will not be outlined here.

FOCAL INFECTIONS

BRAIN ABSCESS

The incidence of brain abscess, about 4 per million population per year, has remained constant despite the development of antibiotics. The greatest prevalence is in young males.[65] However, about 15% of all brain abscesses are diagnosed in those patients over 60 years of age.[66,67] In a recent review of the autopsied cases in the Medical Center of Vermont, Pendlebury et al.[69] found the incidence of CNS infection to be 4.4% (92/2,107) of consecutive autopsied patients. Of these 92 patients with neurologic infection eight were reported to have brain abscesses, and 35 were reported to have microabscesses. This frequency is much higher than reported in earlier series,[66,67] and may reflect the increasing frequency of immunocompromised patients in today's population. As with many CNS infections, leukemia, lymphoma, chronic steroid therapy, immunosuppressive therapy, and chronic disease predispose to this condition.[65] Encapsulated purulent material within brain parenchyma meet the requirement for brain abscess; they may vary in size from microscopic collections of inflammatory cells, so prevalent in the above study, or may enlarge to involve the majority of a cerebral hemisphere. Abscesses occur in the frontal, parietal, temporal, and occipital lobes as well as the cerebellum[68] and the brainstem.[70]

Brain abscesses arise either by direct extension from primary infection in the head and neck[72] or via hematogenous spread.[67] Suppuration of the middle ear and mastoid sinus usually spread to involve the temporal lobe or cerebellum, while the more rare infections of the ethmoid, sphenoid, maxillary and frontal sinus infections extend to involve the frontal lobe.[71] Metastatic abscesses reach the CNS via the bloodstream, and most commonly originate from the pleuropulmonary system but other primary infections have been reported.[65,70] Trauma also predisposes to abscess formation either by disrupting the integrity of the BBB or by direct penetrating injury.[67]

The predisposing lesion to microbial invasion in the brain is not known. Experimentally, an ischemic insult is necessary to produce abscess formation. Ischemic or necrotic tissue creates a microenvironment quite suited to anaerobic bacteria. Abscesses are seen most frequently in areas that are poorly vascularized; typically, the subcortical white matter and the grey-white junction.[65] The evolution from focal cerebritis to encapsulated abscess may take 2 to 4 weeks.

Experimental models have demonstrated four stages in the evaluation of brain abscess; early cerebritis, late cerebritis, early capsule formation, and late capsule formation.[27,73] Initially, perivascular cuffing by inflammatory cells is seen around a necrotic focus. With disease progression increased edema accompanies an enlarging necrotic center and fibroblast proliferation. At maturity a collagenous capsule surrounds a necrotic center and a peripheral zone of inflammatory cells. Externally, cerebritis and neovascularization continue, as well as reactive gliosis and cerebral edema. Capsule formation is more prominent cortically, away from the white matter; perhaps, this reflects the vascular supply to the lesion.

The composition of organisms in a bacterial abscess is quite varied.[67] In 10 to 25% of cases two or more organisms are isolated.[74] Streptococci of aerobic and anaerobic varieties are found in 60 to 70% of cases; Bacteroides, Fusobacteria, and Clostridium species are other anaerobic bacteria frequently found.[75] Other bacteria rarely reported in the adult population include Listeria[76] and M. tuberculosis.[77] In the immunocompromised host fungi are more frequently isolated from abscesses;[78] Aspergillus, Blastomyces, Candida, Coccidioides, Cryptococcus, and Histoplasma have been reported. In the Latin American countries and Asia cysticercosis is prevalent,[79] and the most common cause of cerebral abscess in the AIDS population is toxoplasmosis.[80,81]

Clinically, patients can have signs and symptoms referable to infection, increase in intracranial pressure, or with neurologic changes referable to the site of abscess formation, but usually headache and focal neurologic deficits are the initial features.[66] Focal and generalized seizures have also been noted.[65] Obviously, multiple abscesses will complicate the clinical picture. A rapid decline in the patient's level of consciousness indicates possible interventricular rupture of the abscess (if associated with increased temperature) or hemorrhage into the abscess.[82] Prognosis in these situations is quite guarded.

If cerebral abscess is suspected, CT scanning with and without contrast is the study of choice.[65,67,68] MRI is also useful, and some evidence exists to question CT superiority.[83] EEG will demonstrate focal, high-voltage delta activity in 50% of supratentorial lesions.[84] The hazards of lumbar puncture in these situations have been documented,[79,85] and this procedure should be stringently avoided. Fishman[86] reports increasing cell counts with cerebritis (> 500) and with ventricular rupture (>1000) (Table 15–1).

Therapeusis in these patients must be tailored to individual cases. Surgical treatment depends on several factors. Rapidity of disease progression, site of the lesion (superficial or deep), hemisphere involved (dominant vs. non-dominant), and the number of lesions all play a role.[82] If timely surgical intervention can be obtained, then antibiotic implementation should be delayed. Sanford[15] recommends the following for broad coverage in this population:

Non-traumatic	Penicillin G, 20 million units IV per day, Ceftazidime 2000 mg IV every 8 hours, and Metronidazole 15 mg/kg loading dose followed by 7.5 mg/kg IV every 8 hours.
Traumatic	Nafcillin 2000 mg every 4 hours IV and Ceftazidine 2000 mg IV every 8 hours.

In addition, if cerebral edema imposes increased risk to the patient, dexamethasone may be a necessary short term therapy.[87] However, since steroid therapy can interfere with the resolution of infection, this treatment modality should be limited.

Morbidity and mortality have improved since the advent of the CT scan.[68,88] With improved culture technique and refined antibiotic therapy prognosis is improving. Wood and Anderson[11] totaled several recent series of published brain abscess studies and found that of 47 patients, 40 survived without surgery, 4 required surgery, and 1 died from abscess related complications. Two other patients died of unrelated causes. These authors also report that of the survivors of brain abscess, about 50% will have seizures. Most will have seizure onset within 5 years, and it is seen more commonly in young patients with a previous history of epilepsy. In addition, focal neurologic deficit has been noted in 27 to 47% of patients.[11]

SPINAL EPIDURAL ABSCESS

Although rare, over one fourth of all patients having epidural abscess are over 60 years of age.[89] Prompt and accurate diagnosis is essential for favorable prognosis. Epidural infection may result from hematogenous spread, metastatic invasion, or local erosion from contiguous structures.[89] In adults intravenous drug addiction is the predominant risk factor.[90] In addition bladder infection and instrumentation, pelvic infection and infected intravenous lines have also been noted.[91] Abscesses tend to form in the mid- to low-thoracic regions and upper lumbar areas. Fat and the increased dorsal epidural space are thought to be possible factors in this association.[92] Staphylococcus aureus is the most frequently found organism, but with increased association of abscess formation and pelvic infection, gram-negatives (E. coli, Pseudomonas, and Proteus) are also seen.[91] In the immunocompromised population fungal infections may also occur.[93,94] Tuberculosis must also be considered as part of the differential.

Patients usually have back pain; this is frequently followed by paraspinous spasm, and later, radicular pain.[91] Paraparesis, sensory changes, and sphincter disturbance may follow as the suppuration increases.[89] Diagnosis is usually made by myelogram, but MRI is also useful in some settings. Gadolinium enhanced MRI is often better tolerated by the patient and has the advantage of being much less invasive. Acute cord compression is always an emergency, and requires neurosurgical intervention and appropriate antibiotic therapy.

ACUTE ENCEPHALITIS

Numerous organisms are reported to cause encephalitis. In the western hemisphere, the vast majority of cases of known etiology are viral and include the arboviruses, herpesviruses, lymphocytic choriomeningitis virus, and mumps virus. However, 74.3% of the 1441 cases reported to the CDC in 1978 were of indeterminate cause.[95] Initially, it may be quite difficult to distinguish these patients from the meningitis population, because both groups may complain of headache and show signs of fever, neck stiffness, and photophobia. However, with the onset of cerebral dysfunction the distinction will become clearer. Many patients will be lethargic, and abnormalities in language, thought patterns, and motor control are not uncommon; seizures and memory disturbance are also frequent.[12]

Viral organisms reach the CNS via hematogenous spread, direct invasion, and by neuronal spread.[95] Invasion of the brain parenchyma results in neuronal and glial destruction and inflammatory exudate. Initially polymorphonuclear cells are seen, but with disease progression lymphocytes and monocytes predominate. These microglia exhibit phagocytosis of the impaired neurons (neuronophagia). In addition, inclusion bodies may be seen with herpes, adenovirus, and measles infection. Negri bodies, a specific inclusion, are diagnostic of rabies encephalitis.[96]

HERPES ENCEPHALITIS

In the elderly, the most important cause of encephalitis is the Herpes simplex virus (HSV) Type 1.[95] The mechanism of cerebral infection has not been proved. Twomey et al.[97] suggests that transmission could occur nasally via viral passage through the cribriform plate. Another hypothesis proposes retrograde transport from the skin via the trigeminal nerve, followed by dura to temporal lobe transfer from the trigeminally innervated intracranial structures.[98] Pathologically, congested tissue and hemorrhagic necrosis are seen in the parenchyma, and peticheal hemorrhages are found tangentially. These changes occur most often in the frontal, cingulate, temporal and insular gyri.[96]

Diagnosis of encephalitis is dependent on lumbar puncture. However, in the instance of focal neurologic signs a CT scan should be done to rule out a significant mass lesion before CSF collection. The CSF profile is listed in Table 15-1. Identification of the specific agent is not always accomplished, but with culture and serology diagnostic accuracy is improving. Ancillary evaluation is also useful. Pulmonic infiltrates are seen on chest x-rays of patients with Chlamydial or Mycoplasmal infection and malaria or trypanosomiasis can be diagnosed with evaluation of the peripheral blood smear.[11]

For absolute diagnosis, brain biopsy is frequently necessary. However, the sensitivity of this procedure is not 100%,[101] and is not without risk.[99] For these reasons definitive therapy is often started without tissue diagnosis. The development of vidarabine and acyclovir have provided clinicians with effective therapeutic tools to treat viral encephalitis. Well-controlled clinical trials have shown acyclovir 10 mg/kg/8 hours to be the more effective of these agents.[100] Outcome is highly dependent on the age and level of consciousness prior to therapy.[102] Uniformly, all patients in coma prior to therapy did poorly.

Herpes Zoster (HZV) encephalitis is rare, but most often present in the geriatric immunocompromised population. The clinical presentation is similar to that of HSV infection, except dermatologic lesions frequently precede the neurologic changes. The frequency of encephalitis with HZV infection is about 1 per 1000 infected patients; prognosis is good and permanent sequelae are not common.[95] More detailed discussion of HZV infection will follow.

ARBOVIRAL ENCEPHALITIDES

Arboviral encephalitis accounted for 11% of diagnosed encephalitides in 1978.[95] St. Louis encephalitis (SLE), California encephalitis (CE), eastern equine encephalitis (EEE), and western equine encephalitis accounted for the vast majority of these cases. Infection is dependent on vector transmission and these illnesses have both seasonal and demographic factors influencing their frequencies; all are mosquito borne.[103,104] SLE is the most common in the United States. Symptomatic infection is most often seen in the aged and cases occur frequently in clusters. The disease produces neurologic symptoms similar to other encephalitides, but dysuria, pyuria, and SIADH are also seen.[95] EEE is the most severe of these infections with mortality rates approaching 50%. In a recent review Przelomski et al.[105] report 7 of 17 patients being older than 50 years. Three patients recovered with little neurologic sequelae, but 4 did not survive their illness. WEE is also predisposed to old and young patients, but the infection is less severe and fatality rates are only 2 to 3%. Permanent deficits are usually confined to the very young. The equine encephalitides are associated with similar outbreaks of illnesses in horses, but transmission from mammal to mammal is dependent on the arthropod vector. CE exhibits similar features as discussed above.

SLOW VIRUS INFECTIONS

Creutzfeldt-Jacob disease (CJD), Kuru, and Gerstmann-Straussler-Scheinker disease (GSS) comprise a group of rare dementing illnesses that are pathologically classified under the heading of subacute spongiform encephalopathy.[106,107] Symptoms most often appear in the 50s; a rapid course ensues with death usually occurring within 1 year.

With CJD patients may first have complaints of cognitive difficulties including impaired judgment, memory loss, acalculia, and depression, but often exhibit signs of more global neurologic dysfunction. Pyramidal and extrapyramidal deficits can be elicited and myoclonic jerks become a dominant feature. The myoclonus can often be seen in response to loud noises. With disease progression, seizures are often seen; serial EEGs will typically show periodic sharp wave complexes, but this is not present in all cases.[108]

CJD is a sporadic illness with an incidence of less than 1 per million[109] and it is suggested that the most common method of contact is through particle ingestion.[107] It has been proposed that CJD is caused by an infectious agent such as a viral particle (prion) or protein which requires a long incubation period prior to pathologic change.[107] Transmission has also been reported in 2 patients who received corneal transplant[110] and 7 patients who received growth hormone extracts from human pituitary glands.[112,113] No treatment is available, and absolute diagnosis is dependent on brain biopsy. However, abnormal protein associated with prion infection (PrP)[114] have been reported, and isolated from the CSF of these patients.[115]

Kuru and GSS often begin with cerebellar degeneration and ataxia is seen before cognitive decline is noted. Kuru, now rare, is associated with ritualized cannibalism practiced in New Guinea. GSS may represent a genetic form of prion disease[107] and a chromosomal anomaly predisposing patients with particle infection to spongioform change may be present. Recently, an Indiana kindred of patients with GSS has been described.[116] Autopsies from 2 affected patients reveal widespread neurofibrillary tangles in the cerebellum and the cerebrum, and amyloid plaques confined to the cortex.[117] The amyloid plaques did not react with the Alzheimer's disease amyloid A4 protein, but did show homology with PrP. These authors suggest the greater prevalence of neurofibrillary tangles is an indicator of genetic GSS; they also propose that this heritable illness may be a function of impaired cytoarchitecture.

Progressive multifocal leukoencephalopathy was first described by Astrom, Mancall, and Richardson[118] in patients with lymphoreticular disorders. Clinically, these patients have signs of mental disturbance, visual field deficits, hemiparesis, cognitive abnormalities, and disturbance of consciousness. Occasionally, seizures occur. The disease is progressive and the initially asymmetric difficulties become bilateral. Since the initial report, many other diseases associated with immunocompromise have been linked to this condition, most notably AIDS.[119] Pathologically, multiple foci of demyelination secondary to oligodendroglial destruction are seen.[118] Since the original description, virus-like particles resembling the papova virus[120] as well as the JC virus[121] and the SV40 particle[122] have been associated with this disease.

HERPES ZOSTER INFECTION

HZV infection occurs in 1.3 to 4.8 cases per 1000 person years,[124] and of these patients over 40% are 50 to 70 years of age. In those who have reached 80 years, the incidence will approach 10.1 per 1000 person years.[123] Age is also positively correlated with the duration and severity of the symptoms and the development of post herpetic neuralgia (PHN). Portenoy et al.[124] report the incidence of PHN to increase from 4.2% in those under 20 to 47.5% of patients over 70. The incidence of HZV is increased in those patients with impaired cellular immunity. This group includes patients with carcinoma, AIDS, and those on immunosuppressive therapy.[124]

VZV infection occurs spontaneously in all populations. Typically, patients will first complain of tingling or burning in a unilateral dermatomal distribution. The thoracic dermatomes are involved in 50% of affected patients, while cervical and lumbar lesions are seen in 3 to 20% and 10 to 20% respectively.[125,126] The most frequent nerve affected is the ophthalmic division of the trigeminal nerve[127] and with advancing age cranial involvement is seen more frequently.[125,126] Sensory change may precede the development of skin rash from 4 to 5 days. The rash begins as an erythematous area preceding to vesicular eruptions quite early in the course. The vesicles often begin proximally and may involve adjacent dermatomal segments. Rupture of vesicles occurs usually within 3 to 4 days and if secondary infection is avoided, the dermatologic changes may resolve within 5 weeks.[128] Occasionally, scattered vesicles may be seen in areas distant from the symptomatic dermatome, but this is not disseminated HZV. Systemic symptoms may accompany shingles, and most often consist of headache, malaise, fever, lymphadenopathy, nausea and vomiting.[128,129] Diagnosis is made by culture, identification of viral particles by electron micrograph, or by visualization of inclusion bodies from a specimen scraped from the base of a dermatologic lesion.

Acute varicella infection begins as a digestive or upper respiratory tract infection. With viremia, dissemination to the epidermis is seen.[129] Dorsal root ganglia colonization occurs via retrograde transport. Clinical HZV is seen with virus reactivation and centripetal migration via axonal transport to the skin, but also has been reported with reinfection from new serotypes.[130] Reactivation is often related to a pertubation of the immune status of the host.

The majority of patients recover without complication, but 15 to 20% of those affected may develop more serious problems. If the nasolacrimal branch of the fifth cranial nerve is involved, as it is in a large percentage of patients,[131] conjunctivitis, keratitis, uveitis, and irodocyclitis may result. This places patients at risk to lose vision. If the facial nerve is involved, facial palsy, ear pain, and dermatologic changes may be seen (Ramsay Hunt syndrome). There are also reports of vasculitic infarction of the brainstem and cerebral hemisphere with cranial and cervical HZ.[132-134]

Involvement of the motor roots has also been reported; usually the segment affected corresponds to the sensory distribution. If the cervical roots are affected, upper extremity involvement may result, while if the sacral roots are involved, sphincter disturbance will be seen. Atrophy, fasciculations and weakness will occur in the involved myotome.[11]

PHN is defined as a persistence of dermatomal pain beyond the dermatologic stage of the infection, and is seen in 12 to 20% of patients.[124] Burgdoon, et al.[126] report higher incidence and more severe symptoms in the elderly population. These patients complain of constant severe burning pain that is occasionally paroxysmal. Many also report changing sleep habits, anorexia, malaise, and depression. The pain usually resolves within 1 year, but more persistent symptoms are possible.[124]

Treatment strategies in HZV infection are designed to promote dermatologic resolution and to decrease the incidence and intensity of herpetic neuralgia. Many anecdotal remedies for treatment have been proposed, but their efficacy remains questionable.[124] Of the controlled pharmacologic trials, vidarabine,[101] acyclovir,[135,136] and topical idoxuridine[127] have shown improved response when compared to placebo. However, vidarabine therapy has many potential side effects and for this reason

acyclovir is preferred.[100,137] Good results have now been reported using oral acyclovir 300 mg every 6 hours.[138,139] In cancer patients human leukocyte interferon is helpful in treating the skin lesion, preventing dissemination, and avoiding PHN.[140]

Prolonged antiviral therapy for HZV infection has been postulated to delay and perhaps prevent the onset of PHN.[140] If pain does develop, a bimodal strategy is seen; amitriptyline seems most effective for the typical constant burning pain,[141] while carbamazepine appears to improve the paroxysmal component.[142] Eaglestein et al.[143] found in a double blind trial that triamcinolone administration produced marked decline in symptoms in patients over 60 years old. Subcutaneous corticosteroid injection has also shown good results.[124] Amantidine,[144] cimetidine,[145] and other drugs have also been proposed to decrease pain.

ACQUIRED IMMUNODEFICIENCY SYNDROME (AIDS)

In 1981 the first cases of what is now known as AIDS were reported, and in 1984 a retrovirus identified as HTLV III, now termed human immunodeficiency virus (HIV), was identified as the etiologic agent.[146] This illness, originally confined to homosexual males, intravenous drug abusers, and those receiving blood products by transfusion, has now spread to heterosexual segments of the population. It is not unreasonable to expect the prevalence of cases to increase in the elderly.

HIV is a lymphotrophic and neurotrophic retrovirus. This RNA virus infects CD4+ (helper) T-cells by binding to the CD4 glycoprotein and being internalized. Once in human cells reverse transcriptase, an HIV protein, catalyzes the production of DNA from its RNA genome; the DNA strand is then incorporated into the host genome. Increasing viral protein from the viral genome impairs cell function, and eventually leads to cell death.[147]

T-helper cells function in a complex cell mediated immunosurveillence system as an intermediary in the cascade of antigen destruction. Activated T-cells release interleukin-1, interleukin-2, gamma interferon, and macrophage activating factor. These molecules promote margination and activation of natural killer cells, B-cell clones and macrophages, the major cells involved with destruction of foreign compounds and cells. CD4+ cell depletion requires alternate and less efficient mechanisms to be employed in host protection. In addition, macrophages have also been shown to carry the CD4 glycoprotein.

Neurologic invasion occurs in an unknown fashion, but has been found to be as high as 75% in autopsy studies of AIDS patients; neurologic symptoms have been identified in 40 to 60% of patients in most series.[147] The literature is replete with reports of CNS and PNS involvement in patients infected with HIV. Neurologic pathology may result from direct neurotoxicity, opportunistic infection, or AIDS associated malignancy.[148]

A syndrome of viral meningitis correlates with seroconversion or the development of symptomatic HIV related disease. Besides the usual constellation of viral meningitic symptoms, patients will sometimes present with cranial nerve dysfunction, or pyramidal signs.[149] This illness is self limited, and requires no treatment. The most common sequelae seen in this population is the AIDS-Dementia complex.[150] Gradual decline in behavioral, cognitive and motor abilities is seen in 30 to 60% of patients.[147] On physical examination these patients will exhibit features consistent with multifocal degeneration of the CNS including dementia, cranial nerve abnormalities, weakness, tremor, and ataxia.[149] Postmortem studies suggest early involvement of the subcortical gray matter. White matter pallor, reactive astrocytosis and microgliosis are also seen.[150]

Vacuolar degeneration of the spinal cord is seen in 20 to 30% of AIDS patients. These changes, most prominent in the lateral and posterior columns, produce a gait disturbance with both sensory and motor components as well as incontinence.[148] However, an infection related demyelinating syndrome may mimic this picture, and must be ruled out.[151,152] Vasculitis has also been reported in one instance to produce an AIDS related CNS disturbance[147] and Englestrom[153] published a discussion of HIV vasculitis in transient ischemic attacks.

In the peripheral nervous system syndromes similar to chronic and acute inflammatory polyradiculopathy (Guillain-Barre syndrome),

and distal sensory-motor axonal polyneuropathies are often seen.[154,155] Polymyositis[156] nemaline rod myopathy,[157] and zidovidine induced myopathy[147] have all been reported.

Opportunistic infection is quite frequent in AIDS patients and multiple infections are frequently seen.[119,150,151,158,159] Of the viral pathogens, CMV, HSV, HZV are the most common.[147] PML also occurs.[119] Cryptococcosis and Toxoplasmosis are the most common nonviral pathogen,[81] but the list of possible etiologic agents in this setting is extensive.

Finally, primary CNS lymphoma, systemic lymphoma, and CNS Kaposi's sarcoma may all produce neurologic decline. Symptoms are referable to the size and location to the lesion.[147]

NEUROLOGIC SYMPTOMS CAUSED BY NON-CNS INFECTIONS

ENCEPHALOPATHY

An elderly patient often will exhibit signs similar to those of a patient with encephalitis when compromised by an otherwise silent infection remote from the CNS.[16] These symptoms may include headache, delirium, delusions, paranoia, hallucinations, anxiety, seizures, stupor, and coma. The severity of the primary infection will often be reflected in the intensity of the behavioral change. In the elderly the most common infections producing this condition are pneumonia, urinary tract infection, and nonspecific viral infection. Patients with unexplained changes in behavior should undergo EEG, CT scan of the head, and frequently, CSF analysis, besides general infection work-up to address the long differential for this problem.

LEGIONNAIRES' DISEASE

Legionnaires' disease was first described in 1976 during an American Legion Convention in Philadelphia; 29 deaths and 182 cases were reported.[160] *Legionella pneumophila* was eventually found to be the causative agent, and this organism has been implicated in up to 20% of pneumonias in the elderly in some institutions.[161] Most patients have fever, chills, malaise, diarrhea, and non-productive cough. On laboratory assessment electrolyte disturbances

bances and pulmonary infiltrates are frequently seen.[162] Neurologic deficits range from headache and confusion to delirium and coma. Focal findings are not common, but do occur. Those patients with a history of seizure, are likely to suffer convulsions during the acute phase of the illness.[162] Johnson et al.[163] reviewed the pathologic data in 183 patients, and found anatomic abnormality in only 15. This suggests that *L. pneumophila* is not neurotrophic and the cerebral symptoms are secondary to remote encephalopathy.

ENDOCARDITIS

Bacterial endocarditis is seen most often in older patients with valvular disease or valve replacement;[164] hospital based autopsy series reveal that 42 to 55% of endocarditis patients are over 60.[165] Infectious endocarditis will present usually in two ways, acutely and subacutely. Acute bacterial endocarditis results in a rapid decline in cardiopulmonary function; complications in other organ systems can also be seen. Subacute bacterial endocarditis, however, may be much more insidious and 30% of these patients will need evaluation of neurologic complaints.[164] Headache is the most frequent complaint. This may reflect meningitis, the most common infectious neurologic complication of endocarditis; but encephalitis and subarachnoid hemorrhage are also reported. Prompt attention is necessary in all of these settings because neurologic complications were reported in 70% of patients prior to antibiotic therapy.[166] Cerebral infarction and TIA from emboli are seen in 15 to 20% of patients.[167] Back pain as a result of disc space infection, spinal cord compression, or nerve root impingement also occurs.[164] General physical examination looking for a new or different cardiac murmur is essential. In addition erythrocyte sedimentation rate was found to be above 40 in 103 of 110 patients in one series.[164] Blood cultures are frequently positive in at least one of three sample sets.[165] Antibiotic treatment depends on the cultured agent, and in some instances valve replacement will be required. Staphylococci and streptococci are isolated in 89% of patients.[165] Anticoagulation is not felt to be effective in these patients, but should not be stopped in the prosthetic valve group.[167]

SUMMARY

Neurologic infection represents a difficult diagnostic problem in the elderly patient. Because of a relative decline in immune function, the usual systemic signs of toxemia are not often present. Many of these patients have some deficit in cell-mediated immunity, and are predisposed to atypical infections. However, they also are more prone to the usual pathogens in our environment. A disciplined approach is important to avoid potential complications from treatment delay.

REFERENCES

1. Benson, C.A., Harris, A.A., and Levin, S.: Acute bacterial meningitis: general aspects. In: *Handbook of Clinical Neurology*, (Ed) A.A. Harris. Amsterdam. Elsevier Science Publications BV, *8 (3)*:1, 1988.
2. Massanari, R.M.: Purulent meningitis in the elderly: When to suspect an unusual pathogen. Symp. Geriatrics, *33*:55, 1977.
3. Fraser, D.W., Henke, C.E., and Feldman, R.A.: Changing patterns of bacterial meningitis in Olmsted County, Minnesota, 1935–1970. J. Infect. Dis., *128*(3):300, 1973.
4. Robbins, J.B., Schneerson, R., Argamann, M., et al.: Haemophilus influenzae type b: Disease and immunity in humans. Ann. Intern. Med., *78*:259, 1973.
5. Greenfield, S., Sheehe, P.R., and Feldman, H.A.: Meningococcal carriage in a population of "normal" families. J. Infect. Dis., *123*(1):67, 1971.
6. Suhs, R.H. and Feldman, M.: Pneumococcal types detected in throat cultures from a population of "normal" families. Am. J. Med. Sci., *250*:424, 1965.
7. Mustafa, M.M., et. al.: Induction of meningeal inflammation by outer membrane vesicles of *Haemophilus influenzae* type b. J. Infect. Dis., *159*(5):917, 1989.
8. Scheifele, D.W., et al.: Haemophilus influenzae bacteremia and meningitis in infant primates. J. Lab. Clin. Med., *95*(3):450, 1980.
9. Fishman, R.A.: Brain Edema. NEJM, *293*(14):706, 1975.
10. Sande, M.A.: The influence of fever on the development of experimental streptococcus pneumoniae meningitis. J. Infect. Dis., *156*(5):849–850, 1987.
11. Wood, M. and Anderson, M: *Neurological Infection*. Philadelphia, W.B. Saunders Co., 1988.
12. Annegers, J.F., et al.: The risk of unprovoked seizures after encephalitis and meningitis. Neurology, *38*:1407, 1988.
13. Roth, R.I., Levin, J., and Behr, S.: A modified limulus ameocyte lysate test with increased sensitivity for detection of bacterial endotoxin. J. Lab. Clin. Med., *114*(3):306, 1989.
14. Barling, R.W.A., and Selkon, J.B.: The penetration of antibiotics into cerebrospinal fluid and brain tissue. J. Antimicrobial Chemotherapy, *4*:203, 1978.
15. Sanford, J.: *Guide to Antimicrobial Therapy*. Bethesda, MD., Antimicrobial therapy Inc., 1989.
16. Roeltgen, D.P.: Infections and the nervous system in the elderly. Geriatrics, *38*(2): 105, 1983.

17. Olson, M.E., Chernik, N.L., and Posner, J.: Infiltration of the leptomeninges by systemic cancer. Arch. Neurol., *30*:122, 1974.
18. Trump, D.L., Grossman, S.A., Thompson, G., et al.: CSF infections complicating the management of neoplastic meningitis. Arch. Intern. Med., *142*:583, 1982.
19. Conti, D.J. and Rubin, R.H.: Infection of the central nervous system in organ transplant recipients. Neurol. Complic. Transplants, *6*(2):241, 1988.
20. Johnson, R.B., et al.: Isolated cardiac aspergillosis after bone marrow transplantation. Arch. Intern. Med., *147*:1942, 1987.
21. Montero, C.G., and Martinez, A.J.: Neuropathology of heart transplantation: 23 cases. Neurology, *36*:1149, 1986.
22. Patchell, R.A., et al.: Neurologic complications of bone marrow transplantation. Neurology, *35*:300, 1985.
23. Kimmel, D.W., Hermann, R.C., Jr., and O'Neill, B.P.: Neurologic complications of hairy cell leukemia. Arch. Neurol., *41*:202, 1984.
24. Hooper, D.C., Pruitt, A.A., and Rubin, R.H.: Central nervous system Infection in the chronically immunosuppressed. Medicine: *61*(3):166, 1982.
25. Raskin, N.H. and Fishman, R.A.: Neurologic disorders in renal failure. N. Engl. J. Med., *294*(4):204, 1976.
26. Levy, R.M., Bredesen, D.E., and Rosenblum, M.L.: Opportunistic central nervous system pathology in patients with AIDS. Ann. Neurol., *23* (suppl):S7, 1988.
27. Harriman, D.G.F.: In: *Greenfields Neuropathology*. 4th ed. (Eds) J.H. Adams, J.A.N. Corselias and L.W. Duchen. New York, Wiley Medical, 1984.
28. Sabetta, J.R. and Andriole, V.T.: Cyptococcal infection of the central nervous system. Med. Clin. No. Am., *69*(2):333, 1985.
29. Church, J.M., Blanchet, N.B., and Wai, L.K.: A neglected disease: tuberculosis. Canadian J. Public Health, *80*:73, 1989.
30. Tandon, P.N., Bhatia, R., and Bhargava, S.: Tuberculous meningitis. In: *Handbook of Clinical Neurology*. (Ed) Harris, A.A., Amsterdam, Elsevier Science Publisher AV. *8*(52):195, 1988.
31. Stead, W.W.: Pathogenesis of tuberculosis: clinical and epidemiologic perspective. Reviews Infect. Dis., *11* (suppl):S366, 1989.
32. Molavi, A. and LeFrock, J.L.: Tuberculous meningitis. Med. Clin. No. Am., *69*(2):315, 1985.
33. Dannenberg, A.M.: Immune mechanisms in the pathogenesis of pulmonary tuberculosis. Reviews Infect. Dis., *11*(2) (suppl):S369, 1989.
34. Rich, A.R. and McCordock, H.A.: The pathogenesis of tuberculous meningitis. Bull. Johns Hopkins Hosp. *52*:5, 1933.
35. Glass, J.D., Becker, P.S., Moses, H., et al.: Dural scrofula. Neurology, *39*(12):1123, 1989.
36. Omari, B., Robertson, J.M., Nelson, R.J., et al.: Potts disease: A resurgent challenge to the thoracic surgeon. Chest, *95*:145, 1989.
37. Daniel, T.M.: New approaches to the rapid diagnosis of tuberculous meningitis. Infect. Dis., *155*(4):599, 1987.
38. Ochoa, J.: Isoniazid neuropathy in man: quantitative electron microscope study. Brain, *93*:831, 1970.
39. Ribera, E., et al.: Activity of adenosine deaminase in cerebrospinal fluid for the diagnosis and follow-up of tuberculous meningitis in adults. J. Infect. Dis., *155*(4): 603, 1987.
40. Hook, III, E.W.: Syphilis and HIV infection. J. Infect. Dis., *160*(3):530, 1989.
41. Goodman, L.J. and Karakusis, P.H.: Neurosyphilis. In: *Handbook of Clinical Neurology*. (Ed) A.A. Harris. Amsterdam, Elsevier Science Publishers, *8*(52):273, 1988.
42. Curie, J.N., Coppeto, J.R., and Lessell, S.: Chronic syphilitic meningitis resulting in superior orbital fissure syndrome and posterior fossa gumma. J. Clin. Neuropathol., *80*:145, 1988.
43. Jordan, K.G.: Modern neurosyphilis-A critical analysis. West J. Med., *149*:47, 1988.
44. Hart, G.: Syphilis tests in diagnostic and therapeutic decision making. Ann. Intern. Med., *104*:368, 1986.
45. Burke, J.M. and Schaberg, D.R.: Neurosyphilis in the antibiotic era. Neurology, *35*:1368, 1985.
46. Miller, J.N.: Value and limitations of nontreponemal and treponemal tests in the laboratory diagnosis of syphilis. Clin. Obstet Gyn, *18*(1):191, 1975.
47. Escobar, M.R., Dalton, H.P., and Allison, M.J.: Fluorescent antibody tests for syphilis using cerebrospinal fluid: clinical correlation in 150 cases. Am. J. Clin. Path., *53*:886, 1970.
48. Panconesi, E., Zuccati, G., and Cantini, A.: Treatment of syphilis: A short critical review. Sex Trans Dis, *8*(4):321, 1981.
49. Sexually transmitted diseases treatment guidelines. MMWR, *38*(S-8): 94, 1989.
50. Andriole, V.T.: Introduction Rev. Infect. Dis., *11*(suppl. 6):S1433, 1989.
51. Finkel, M.F.: Lyme disease and its neurologic complications. Arch. Neurol., *45*:99, 1988.
52. Pachner, A.R., and Steere, A.C.: The triad of neurologic manifestations of Lyme Disease: Meningitis, cranial neuritis, and radioculoneuritis. Neurology, *35*:47, 1985.
53. Burgdorfer, W., Hayes, S.F., and Corwin, D.: Pathophysiology of the Lyme Disease spirochete, *Borrelia burgdorferi*, in ixodid ticks. Rev. Infect. Dis. *11*(suppl. 6):S1442, 1989.
54. Burgdorfer, W., et al.: Lyme Disease—a tick-borne spirochetosis? Science, *216*:1317, 1982.
55. McKenna, D.F.: Lyme Disease: a review for primary health care providers. Nurse Practitioner, *14*(3):18, 1989.
56. Pachner, A.R.: Neurologic manifestations of Lyme Disease, the new "great Imitator". Rev. Infect. Dis., *11*(suppl. 6):S1482, 1989.
57. Duray, P.H.: Clinical pathologic correlations of Lyme Disease. Rev. Infect. Dis., *11*(suppl. 6):S1487, 1989.
58. Midgard, R. and Hofstad, H.: Unusual manifestations of nervous system *Borrelia burgdorferi* infection. Arch. Neurol., *44*:781, 1987.
59. Veenendaal-Hilbers, J.A., et al.: Basal meningovasculitis and occlusion of the basilar artery in two cases of *Borrelia burgdorferi* infection. Neurology, *38*:1317, 1988.
60. McAlister, M.B., et al.: Lyme carditis: An important cause of reversible heart block. Ann. Intern. Med., *110*:339, 1989.
61. Pachner, A.R., Duray, P. and Steere, A.C.: Central nervous system manifestations of lyme disease. Arch. Neurol., *46*:790, 1989.
62. Ratzan, K.R.: Viral meningitis. Med. Clin. No. Am., *69*(2):399, 1985.
63. Frederick, J., and Bruyn, G.W.: In: *Handbook of Clinical Neurology*. (Eds) Vinken, P.J., Bruyn, G.W. and Klawans, H. Amsterdam, Elsevier/North-Holland Inc. *34*:545, 1978.

64. Ewert, B.H.: Resident Article: Ibuprofen-associated meningitis in a woman with only serologic evidence of a rheumatologic disorder. Am. J. Med. Sci., 297(5):326, 1989.

65. Kaplan, K.: Brain abscess. Med. Clin. No. Am., 69(2):345, 1985.

66. Brewer, N.S., MacCarty, C.S., and Wellman, W.E.: Brain Abscess: a review of recent experience, Ann. Intern. Med., 82:571, 1975.

67. Yang, S-Y.: Brain abscess: a review of 400 cases. J. Neurosurg., 55:794, 1981.

68. Rosenblum, M.L., et al.: Decreased mortality from brain abscesses since advent of computerized tomography. J. Neurosurg., 49:658, 1978.

69. Pendlebury, W., Perl, D.P., and Munoz, D.G.: Multiple microabscesses in the central nervous system: a clinicopathologic study. J. Neuropath. Exp. Neurol., 48(3):290, 1989.

70. Samson, D.S. and Clark, K.: A current review of brain abscess. Am. J. Med., 54:201, 1973.

71. Nelson, D.A., et al.: Neurological syndromes produced by sphenoid sinus abscess. Neurology, 17:981, 1967.

72. Kaplan, R.J.: Neurological complications of infections of the head and neck. Otolaryngol. Clin. No. Am., 9(3):729, 1976.

73. Britt, R.H., Enzmann, D.R., and Yeager, A.S.: Neuropathological and computerized tomographic findings in experimental brain abscess, J. Neurosurg., 55:590, 1981.

74. Mathisen, G.E., et al.: Brain abscess and cerebritis. Rev. Infect. Dis., 6(Suppl.) 136:S101, 1984.

75. DeLouvois and Hurley, R.: Inactivation of penicillin by purulent exudates. Br. Med. J. 1:998, 1977.

76. Crocker, E.F. and Leicester, J.: Cerebral abscess due to Listeria monocytogenes. Med. J. Aust., 1:90, 1976.

77. Whitener, D.R.: Tuberculous brain abscess. Arch. Neurol., 35:148, 1978.

78. Chernik, N.L., Armstrong, D., and Posner, J.B.: Central nervous system infections in patients with cancer. Medicine, 52(6):563, 1973.

79. Nash, T.E. and Neva, F.A.: Recent advances in the diagnosis and treatment of cerebral cysticercosis. N. Engl. J. Med., 311(23):1492, 1984.

80. Alonso, R., Heiman-Patterson, T., and Mancall, E.L.: Cerebral toxoplasmosis in acquired immune deficiency syndrome. Arch. Neurol., 41:321, 1984.

81. Navia, B.A., et al.: Cerebral toxoplasmosis complicating the acquired immune deficiency syndrome: clinical and neuropathological findings in 27 patients. Ann. Neurol., 19:224, 1986.

82. Molavi, A. and Dinubile, M.J.: Brain abscess. In: Handbook of Clinical Neurology. (Ed) Harris, A.A. Amsterdam, Elsevier Science Publ. BV 8(52):143, 1988.

83. Schroth, G., et al.: Advantage of magnetic resonance imaging in the diagnosis of cerebral infections. Neuroradiology, 29:120, 1987.

84. Neidermyer, E., and Lopez da Silva, F. Electroencephalography, Basic Principles, Clinical Applications and Related Fields. 2nd ed., Baltimore. Urban and Schwarzenberg, 1987.

85. Carey, M.E., Chou, S.N., and French, L.A.: Experience with brain abscesses. J. Neurosurg., 36:1, 1972.

86. Fishman, R.A.: Cerebrospinal Fluid in Disease of the Central Nervous System. Philadelphia, W.B. Saunders Co., 1980.

87. Yildizhan, A., Pasaoglu, A., and Kandemir, B.: Effect of dexamethasone on various stages of experimental brain abscess. Acta. Neurochir., 96:141, 1989.

88. Haimes, A.B., et al.: MR imaging of brain abscesses. AJR, 152:1073, 1989.

89. Kaufman, D.M., Kaplan, J.G., and Litman, N.: Infectious agents in spinal epidural abscesses. Neurology, 30:844, 1980.

90. Koppel, B.S., et al.: Epidural spinal infection in intravenous drug abusers. Arch. Neurol., 45:1331, 1988.

91. Verner, E.F. and Musher, D.M.: Spinal epidural abscess. Med. Clin. No. Am., 69(2):375, 1985.

92. Dandy, W.E.: Abscesses and inflammatory tumors in the spinal epidural space (so-called pachymeningitis externa). Arch. Surg., 13:477, 1926.

93. Chee, Y.C. and Poh, S.C.: Aspergillus epidural abscess in a patient with obstructive airway disease. Postgrad. Med. J., 59:43, 1983.

94. Wesselius, L.J., Brooks, R.J., and Gall, E.P. Vertebral coccidioidomycosis presenting as Pott's disease. JAMA, 238(13):1397, 1977.

95. Ho, D.D. and Hirsh, M.S.: Acute viral encephalitis. Med. Clin. No. Am., 69(2):415, 1985.

96. Okazaki, H.: Fundamentals of Neuropathology, 1st ed., New York. Igaku-Shoin, 1983.

97. Twomey, J.A., et al.: Olfactory mucosa in herpes simplex encephalitis. JNNP, 42:983, 1979.

98. Davis, L.E. and Johnson, R.T.: An explanation for the localization of herpes simplex encephalitis? Ann. Neurol., 5:2, 1979.

99. Kaufmann, H.H. and Catalano, L.W. Diagnostic brain biopsy: a series of 50 cases and a review. Neurosurgery, 4:129, 1979.

100. Whitley, R.J., et al.: Vidarabine versus acyclovir therapy in herpes simplex encephalitis. N. Engl. J. Med., 314(3):144, 1986.

101. Whitley, R.J., et al.: Herpes simplex encephalitis. JAMA. 247(3):317, 1982.

102. Whitley, R.J., et al.: Herpes simplex encephalitis. N. Engl. J. Med., 304(6):313, 1981.

103. Laboda, M. and Kozuch, O.: Amplification of arborvirus transmission by mosquito intradermal probing and interrupted feeding. Acta. Virol. 33:63, 1989.

104. Sellers, R.F. and Maarouf, A.R. Impact of climate on western equine encephalitis in Manitoba, Minnesota and North Dakota, 1980–1983. Epidem. Inf., 101:511, 1986.

105. Przelomski, M.M., O'Rouke, E., Grady, G.F., et al. Eastern equine encephalitis in Massachusetts: A report of 16 cases, 1970–1984. Neurology, 38(1):736, 1988.

106. Nevin, S., et al.: Subacute spongiform encephalopathy—a subacute form of encephalopathy attributable to vascular dysfunction (spongiform cerebral atrophy). Brain, 83:519, 1960.

107. Prusiner, S.B.: Prions and neurodegenerative diseases. N. Engl. J. Med., 317(25):1571, 1987.

108. Zochodne, D.W., et al.: Creutzfeldt-Jakob disease without periodic sharp wave complexes: a clinical, electroencephalographic, and pathologic study, Neurology, 38:1056, 1988.

109. Brown, P., et al.: Potential epidemic of Creutzfeldt-Jakob disease from human growth hormone therapy. N. Engl. J. Med., 313(12):728, 1985.

110. Duffy, P., Wolf, J., and Collins, G.: Possible person-to-person transmission of Creutzfeldt-Jakob disease. N. Engl. J. Med., 290(12):692, 1974.

112. Brown, P.: The decline and fall of Creutzfeldt-Jakob

disease associated with human growth hormone therapy. Neurology, 38(7):1135, 1988.

113. Gibbs, C.J., et al.: Creutzfeldt-Jakob disease (spongiform encephalopathy): transmission to the chimpanzee. Science, 161:388, 1968.

114. Bockman, J.M., et al.: Creutzfeldt-Jakob disease prion proteins in human brains. N. Engl. J. Med., 312(2):73, 1985.

115. Harrington, M.G., et al.: Abnormal proteins in the cerebrospinal fluid of patients with Creutzfeldt-Jakob disease. N. Engl. J. Med., 315(5), 279, 1986.

116. Farlow, M.R., et al.: Gerstmann-Straussler-Scheinker disease. I. Extending the clinical spectrum. Neurology, 39(11):1446, 1989.

117. Ghetti, B., et al.: Gerstmann-Straussler-Scheinker disease. II. Neurofibrillary tangles and plaques with PrP-Amyloid coexist in an affected family. Neurology, 39(11):212, 1989.

118. Anstrom, K-E, Mancall, E.L., and Richardson, Jr., E.P.,: Progressive multifocal leukoencephalopathy. A hitherto unrecognized complication of chronic lymphatic leukaemia and Hodgkin's disease. Brain, 81:93, 1958.

119. Miller, J.R., et al.: Progressive multifocal leukoencephalopathy in a male homosexual with T-cell immune deficiency. N. Engl. J. Med., 307:1436, 1982.

120. Zu Rhein, G.M. and Chou, S-M.: Particles resembling papova viruses in human cerebral demyelinating disease. Science, 148:1477, 1965.

121. Padgett, B.L., et al.: Cultivation of papova-like virus from human brain with progressive multifocal leucoencephalopathy. Lancet, 1. 1257, 1971.

122. Weiner, L.P., et al.: Isolation of virus related to SV40 from patients with progressive multifocal leukoencephalopathy. N. Engl. J. Med., 286(8):385, 1972.

123. Hope-Simpson, R.E.: The nature of herpes zoster: a long-term study and a new hypothesis. Proc. Royal Soc. Med., 58:9, 1965.

124. Portenoy, R.K., Duma, C., and Foley, K.M.: Acute herpetic and postherpetic neuralgia: clinical review and current management. Ann. Neurol., 20(6):651, 1986.

125. Brown, G.R.: Herpes zoster: correlation of age, sex, distribution, neuralgia, and associated disorders. South. Med. J., 69(5):576, 1976.

126. Burgoon, C.F., Burgoon, J.S., and Baldridge, G.D.: The natural history of Herpes Zoster. JAMA, 164(3):265, 1957.

127. Wildenhoff, K.E., et al.: Treatment of trigeminal and thoracic zoster with idoxuridine. Scand. J. Infect. Dis., 13:257, 1981.

128. Balfour, H.H.: Varicella zoster virus infections in immunocompromised hosts. Am. J. Med., 85(suppl. 2A):68, 1988.

129. Straus, S.E., et al.: Varicella-zoster virus infections. Ann. Intern. Med., 108:221, 1988.

130. Gershon, A.A., et al.: Clinical reinfection with varicella-zoster virus. J. Infect. Dis., 149(2):137, 1984.

131. Cobo, M.: Reduction of the ocular complications of herpes zoster ophthalmicus by oral acyclovir. Am. J. Med., 85(suppl. 2A):90, 1988.

132. MacKenzie, R.A., Forbes, G.S., and Karnes, W.E.: Angiographic findings of Herpes arteritis. Ann. Neurol., 10:1458, 1981.

133. Snow, B.J. and Simcock, J.P.: Brainstem infarction following cervical Herpes Zoster. Neurology, 38:1331, 1988.

134. Joy, J.L., Carlo, J.L., and Vertez-Borias, J.R.: Cerebral infarction following Herpes Zoster: The enlarging clinical spectrum. 39:1640, 1989.

135. Bean, B., Braun, C., and Balfour, Jr., H.H.: Acyclovir therapy for acute herpes zoster. Lancet, 2:118, 1982.

136. Peterslund, N.A.: Acyclovir in Herpes Zoster. Lancet, 2:827, 1981.

137. Shepp, D.H., Dandliker, R.N. and Meyers, J.D.: Current therapy of varicella zoster virus infection in immuno-compromised patients. Am. J. Med., 85(2A):96, 1988.

138. Wood, M.J., et al.: Efficacy of oral acyclovir treatment of acute herpes zoster. Am. J. Med., 85(suppl. 2A):79, 1988.

139. Huff, J.C., et al.: Therapy of herpes zoster with oral acyclovir. Am. J. Med., 85(suppl. 2A):84, 1988.

140. Merigan, T.C., et al.: Human leukocyte interferon for the treatment of herpes zoster in patients with cancer. NEJM, 298(18):981, 1978.

141. Max, M.D., et al.: Amitriptyline, but not lorazepam, relieves postherpetic neuralgia. Neurology, 38:1427, 1988.

142. Swerdlow, M. and Cundill, M.B.: Anticonvulsant drugs used in the treatment of lancinating pain. A comparison. Anaesthesia, 36:1129, 1981.

143. Eaglestein, W.H., Katz, R., and Brown, J.A.: The effects of early corticosteroid therapy on the skin eruption and pain of herpes zoster. JAMA, 211(10):1681.

144. Galbraith, A.W.: Treatment of acute herpes zoster with amantadine hydrochloride (symmetrel). Br. Med. J., 4:693, 1973.

145. Mavligit, G.M. and Talpaz, M: Cimetidine for herpes zoster. N. Engl. J. Med., 310(5):318, 1984.

146. Elder, G.A. and Sever, J.L.: AIDS and neurological disorders: an overview. Ann. Neurol., 23(suppl.):S4, 1988.

147. Kieburtz, K. and Scheffer, R.B. Neurologic manifestations of human immunodeficiency virus infection. Neurologic Clinics, 7(3):447, 1989.

148. Petito, C.K.: Review of central nervous system pathology in human immunodeficiency virus infection. Ann. Neurol., 23(suppl.):S54, 1988.

149. Gabuzda, D.H. and Hirsch, M.S.: Neurologic manifestations of infection with human immunodeficiency virus. Ann. Intern. Med., 107:383, 1987.

150. Navia, B.A. and Price, R.W.: The acquired immunodeficiency syndrome dementia complex as the presenting or sole manifestation of human immunodeficiency virus infection. Arch. Neurol., 44:65, 1987.

151. Britton, C.B., et al.: A new complication of AIDS: thoracic myelitis caused by herpes simplex virus. Neurology, 35:1071, 1985.

152. Tucker, T., et al.: Cytomegalovirus and herpes simplex virus ascending myelitis in a patient with acquired immune deficiency syndrome. Ann. Neurol. 18:74, 1985.

153. Englestrom, J.W., Lowenstein, D.H. and Bredesen, D.E.: Cerebral infarctions and transient neurologic deficits associated with acquired immunodeficiency syndrome. Am. J. Med., 86:528, 1989.

154. Parry, G.J.: Peripheral neuropathies associated with human immunodeficiency virus infection. Ann. Neurol., 23(suppl.):S49, 1988.

155. Eidelberg, D., et al.: Progressive polyradiculopathy in acquired immune deficiency syndrome. Neurology, 36:912, 1986.

156. Dalakas, M.C., et al.: Polymyositis associated with AIDS retrovirus. JAMA, 256(17):2381, 1986.

157. Dalakas, M.C. and Pezeshkpour, G.H.: Neuromus-

cular diseases associated with human immunodeficiency virus infection. Ann. Neurol., *23*(suppl.):S38, 1988.

158. Cuadrado, L.M., et al.: Cerebral mucormycosis in two cases of acquired immuno-deficiency syndrome. Arch. Neurol., *45*:109, 1988.

159. Laskin, O.L., Stahl-Bayliss, C.M., and Morgello, S.: Concomitant herpes simplex virus type 1 and cytomegalovirus ventriculoencephalitis in acquired immunodeficiency syndrome. Arch. Neurol., *44*:843, 1987.

160. Fraser, W., et al.: Legionnaires' disease: description of an epidemic pneumonia. N. Engl. J. Med., *197*:1189, 1977.

161. Yu, V.L., et al.: Legionnaires' disease: new clinical perspective from a prospective pneumonia study. Am. J. Med., *73*:357, 1982.

162. Davis, J.P., et al.: Recently recognized central nervous system infections: legionellosis, toxic shock syndrome, lyme disease and kawasaki disease. In: *Hand-*

book of Clinical Neurology. (Ed) by A.A. Harris. Amsterdam, Elsevier Science Publications, *81*:253, 1988.

163. Johnson, J.D., Raff, M.J. and Van Arsdall, J.A.: Neurologic manifestations of Legionnaires' disease. Medicine, *63*(5):303, 1984.

164. Jones, Jr., H.R. and Siekert, R.G.: Neurologic complications of infective endocarditis (bacterial endocarditis). In: *Handbook of Clinical Neurology.* (Ed) by A.A. Harris. Amsterdam, Elsevier Science Publications, *8*(52):289, 1988.

165. Terpenning, M.S., Buggy, B.P., and Kauffman, C.A.: Infective endocarditis: clinical features in young and elderly patients. Am J. Med., *83*:626, 1987.

166. Salgado, A.V., et al.: Neurologic complications of endocarditis: a 12-year experience. Neurology, *39*:173, 1989.

167. Cerebral Embolism Task Force: Cardiogenic brain embolism: the second report of the cerebral embolism task force. Arch. Neurol., *46*:727, 1989.

16

Peripheral Neuropathy

CLAUDE VITAL and
ANNE VITAL

Individuals 55 to 75 years constitute the largest group of any age afflicted with a peripheral neuropathy (PN) according to recorded clinical information and documented nerve biopsies in the United States, France, and Australia.[1-4] Diabetes and malignancy are the most common causes in the elderly, followed by alcohol, drugs, acute and chronic demyelinating neuropathies, autoimmune diseases and nutritional diseases. In cases where the diagnosis is not clinically evident, nerve biopsies may be useful.

Peripheral nerves contain nerve fibers that are long, thin processes from motor, sensory, and autonomic neurons. Peripheral nerves may be damaged at the neuronal or axonal levels. The definition of the degree of such damage and of its origin has been the introduction of numerous new morphologic techniques and sophisticated laboratory tests during the past 30 years. A thorough re-evaluation of 205 cases reported previously as unclassified peripheral neuropathies (PN) enabled Dyck et al.[5,6] to classify 76% of these patients. In a series of 519 patients with PN and nerve biopsies investigated by Mc Leod et al.,[7] 67 patients (13%) remained undiagnosed. The age of onset of symptoms in these 67 patients was 12 to 73 years (mean 50.6 years). Aging in itself appears to be responsible for a progressive loss of and damage to nerve fibers with great variations from patient to patient.

The examination of the human peripheral nerve obtained at biopsy is suitably done by light and electron microscopy, immunopathology and quantitative techniques. These methods show the nature and extent of damage to axons or myelin and surrounding tissues. In a few cases a specific cause of the nerve damage can be seen on paraffin embedded nerve fragments; for example, when there are amyloid deposits, necrotizing vasculitis, or certain cellular infiltrates. In certain cases of PN, anti-IgM serum binds to the myelin sheaths as demonstrated by immunopathologic study and such cases usually display a specific myelinic alteration on ultrastructural examination. Specific Schwann cell inclusions may be disclosed in cases of PN due to certain drugs. However, most peripheral nerve biopsies do not display any specific lesion and the diagnosis is made by correlation with clinical investigations (leading sometimes to the diagnosis of inherited disorders) or with biologic and radiologic studies.

MATERIAL AND METHODS

The sural nerve or the superficial peroneal nerve are usually biopsied for study. Portions of muscle tissue[8] may be removed through the same incision for diagnostic purposes at the time of the biopsy, particularly in vascular disease which is common in elderly people. Nerve fragments taken at autopsy are of limited use because of autolytic modifications, but can be examined by light microscopy.[9,10] The length of nerve removed should ideally be 2 to 3 cm length, according to the clinical and bio-

logic setting, and divided into two or three fragments. The first is embedded in paraffin for standard histologic techniques. The second is frozen and sections stained with antigen to IgA, IgG, IgM kappa and lambda light chains are processed for direct immunofluorescence. The third fragment is immediately fixed in 2.5% glutaraldehyde and postfixed in 1% osmium tetroxide. Plastic embedded semithin and ultra-thin sections are prepared for light and electron microscopic examinations. Another portion of this postfixed third fragment is prepared for examination of isolated nerve fibers by teasing. Dyck et al.[14,15] have simplified a classification which is now widely used: A = normal; B = myelin wrinkling; C = demyelination; D = demyelination and remyelination; E = axonal degeneration; F = remyelination; G = focal myelin reduplication; H = myelin debris adjacent to axonal regeneration [Fig. 16–1].

Quantitative study of myelinated fibers is usually performed by a semi-automatic method on transverse semithin sections stained with toluidine blue or paraphenylene-

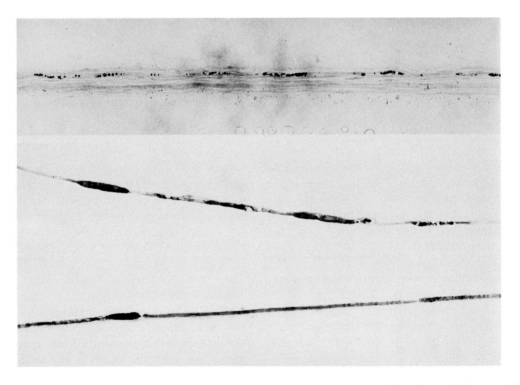

Fig. 16–1. Teased fibers. Top: A row of ovoids is seen along a degenerated myelinated fiber. Middle: axonal degeneration. Bottom: segmental remyelination.

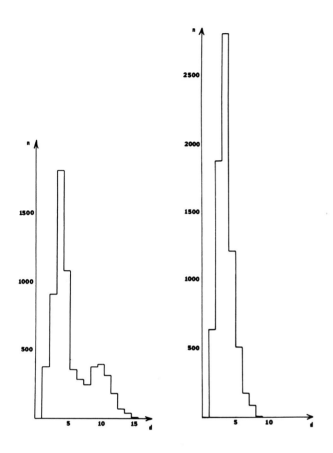

Fig. 16-2. Histograms. Left: Normal bimodal distribution. Right: unimodal distribution due to loss of large myelinated fibers.

diamine. Normally the average number of myelinated fibers is 7,000 to 10,000/mm^2. Their distribution according to diameter size is bimodal, with a first peak corresponding to small fibers and a second lower peak corresponding to large fibers. In such a bimodal type histogram at least 25% of myelinated fibers have a diameter greater than 7 μm. Three other types of histogram may be observed according to the distribution of small and large myelinated fibers. In the unimodal type no myelinated fiber has a diameter over 7 μm. In the unbalanced distribution type less than 25% of myelinated fibers have a diameter over 7 μm. In the dramatic loss type, the number of myelinated fibers is less than 3,000/mm$_2$ and there is a decrease in both small and large myelinated fibers [Figs. 16–2 and 16–3].

ELEMENTARY LESIONS[13–18]

Two main pathologic processes affect the peripheral nerve: axonal degeneration and primary demyelinating disorders. A mixture involving both axonal degeneration and demyelination is usually found for most chronic neuropathies. Thus, demyelination follows as a Schwann cell response to primary axonal degeneration, and in severe or sustained primary demyelination, nerve fiber loss often occurs.

AXONAL DEGENERATION

Axonal degeneration has been thoroughly studied experimentally and has been reviewed recently in the light of clinical applications.[19] Morphologic variations are now better understood, as well as the ensuing demyelination.[20] Several types of axonal degeneration are now recognized.

1. Wallerian degeneration is the result of acute axonal damage. It is typically induced by transection of a peripheral nerve and was first described by Waller.[21] More detail on this process has come from ultrastructural studies.[16,22] Twelve hours after a crush lesion, the distal axons begin to show signs of degeneration with a paranodal accumulation of mitochon-

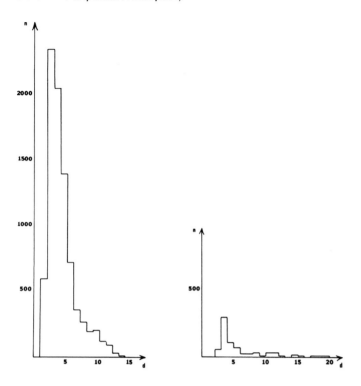

Fig. 16–3. Histograms. Left: Unimodal pattern with unbalanced distribution. Right: dramatic loss of myelinated fibers.

dria. After 24 hours, axoplasmic density is increased. The myelin splits at the interperiod line and lamellae peel off at the nodes. After 3 days there is extensive breakdown of myelin in the Schwann cell cytoplasm. Large ovoids consisting of myelin debris and disrupted axons are then observed [Fig. 16–4]. Some macrophagic histiocytes containing lipid debris are seen in the vicinity of the severely damaged fibers which are sometimes invaded by macrophagic histiocytes. During Wallerian degeneration the basement membrane surrounding the Schwann cells remains in place and forms tubes within which the Schwann cells proliferate to form columns referred to as bands of Bungner. In cross section Schwann cell processes can be seen containing various presentations of degenerated myelin, homogeneous lipid droplets, vacuoles, smooth and granular endoplasmic reticulum, Golgi complexes, microtubules, filaments, and glycogen. Regenerating axonal sprouts appear at about the fifth day and grow within the tubes derived from the Schwann cell basement membrane. The axons separate from each other to form the classic clusters which contain several rounded

axons. The growing axons stay close together although a few intervening collagen fibers can be observed. Some of these axons remyelinate, and are surrounded by a myelin sheath which is too thin in relation to the axonal diameter [Figs. 16–5 to 16–7].

2. The technique of permanent axotomy enabled Dyck et al.[23,24] to study the retrograde effects of the axonal section: axonal atrophy, myelin remodeling and degeneration.

3. Distal axonopathy corresponds to distal axonal degeneration that spreads in a progressive manner towards the cell body as the disease evolves. Such neuropathies have been characterized by Cavanagh[25,26] as being of the "dying-back" type. The phenomenon has been studied in greater detail by Spencer and Schaumburg[27,28] in hexacarbon induced neuropathy. This gives rise to multifocal preterminal axonal swellings with neurofilamentous accumulations. These swellings are situated on the proximal sides of several consecutive or nonconsecutive nodes of Ranvier, and the process then spreads sequentially to more and more proximal nodes. Other axoplasmic organelles may be aggregated. Axonal swelling is

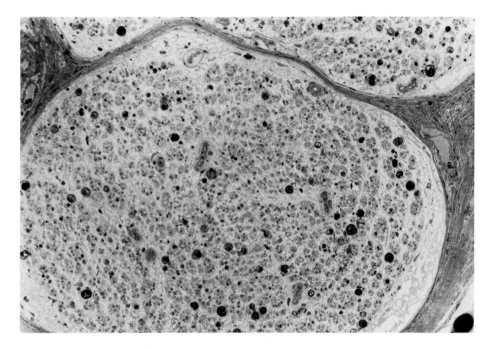

Fig. 16–4. Mononeuropathy multiplex and essential mixed cryoglobulinemia. Semi-thin section, toluidine blue. There is a dramatic loss of myelinated fibers and there are several ovoids (× 370).

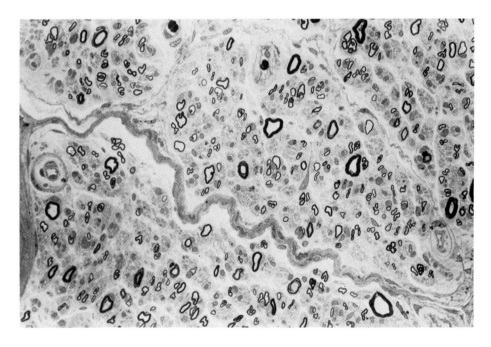

Fig. 16–5. Long-standing PN in a 77-year-old woman. Semi-thin section, toluidine blue. There are numerous clusters of regenerating myelinated fibers (× 430).

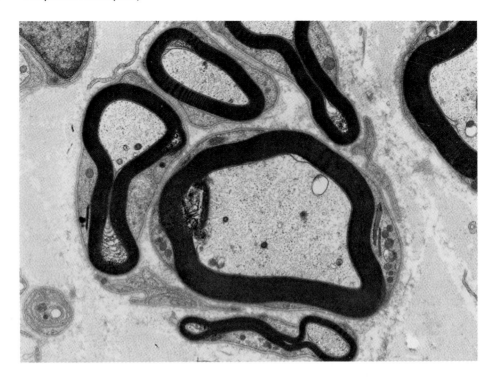

Fig. 16–6. Guillain-Barré syndrome in a 65-year-old man. There is a characteristic cluster composed of five myelinated fibers (× 13,900).

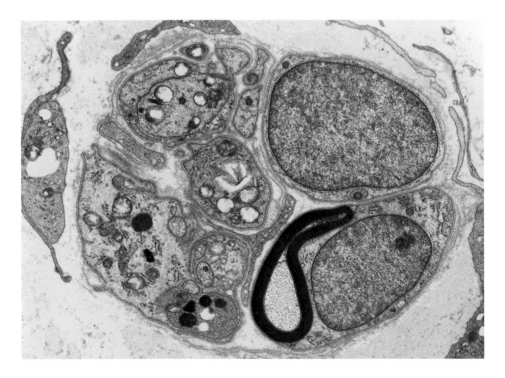

Fig. 16–7. Guillain-Barré syndrome in a 65-year-old man. In this cluster of regenerating fibers, there is only one remyelinating (× 12,500).

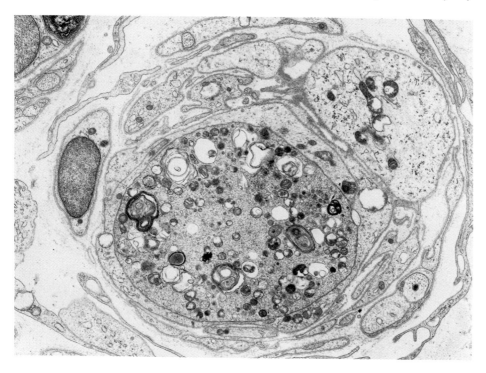

Fig. 16–8. PN in a 74-year-old man with benign IgM MG. This axon is swollen and packed with abnormal mitochondria and vesicular structures (× 18,000).

associated with thinner myelin sheaths and the myelin may disappear leaving a large naked axon.

4. According to Lampert and Schochet,[14] axonal dystrophy corresponds to most of the axonopathies that are not secondary to a nerve section. In human pathology, biopsies from various cases of polyneuropathy show intra-axonal accumulation of filaments, mitochondria and membranous bodies [Fig. 16–8]. Experimental peripheral nerve ischemia is a good example of axonal dystrophy,[29–32] which can lead to axonal swelling with aggregates of organelles.[32]

5. In the early stages of acute neuropathy, unmyelinated axons appear enlarged and have a watery appearance due to dissolution of axoplasmic organelles. The enlarged axons then collapse, leaving flattened Schwann cell columns. In chronic neuropathies, some unmyelinated axons are moderately enlarged and filled with mitochondria and vesicular structures. Other axons become flattened [Fig. 16–9] but most axons disappear, leaving empty bands of Schwann cells. Some fibers show flattened axons and collagen pockets [Fig. 16–10].

Regeneration takes place in the form of miniature axonal sprouts with Schwann cell cytoplasm rich in organelles.[33–38]

SEGMENTAL DEMYELINATION

Segmental demyelination was first described in experimental lead neuropathy by Gombault[39] and in experimental diphtheritic neuropathy.[40,41] The initial changes are widening at the node of Ranvier by retraction of the myelin paranodal loop, followed by myelin breakdown and accumulation of myelin debris in the paranodal Schwann cell cytoplasm. In some internodes this process results in complete removal of the myelin sheath. Segmental demyelination stimulates Schwann cell division resulting in multiple Schwann cells arranged along the demyelinated internodes. Some of these daughter Schwann cells are remyelinated. On transverse semi-thin sections the new remyelinated fibers have a myelin sheath too thin for the axonal diameter [Fig. 16–11]. Teased fiber preparations show that the new remyelinated internodes are shorter and more variable in length than the original

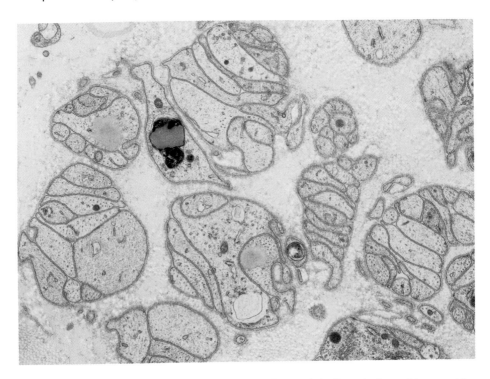

Fig. 16–9. Mononeuritis multiplex and mixed essential cryoglobulinemia in a 64-year-old man. No myelinated fiber is visible and certain unmyelinated axons are flattened (× 14,000).

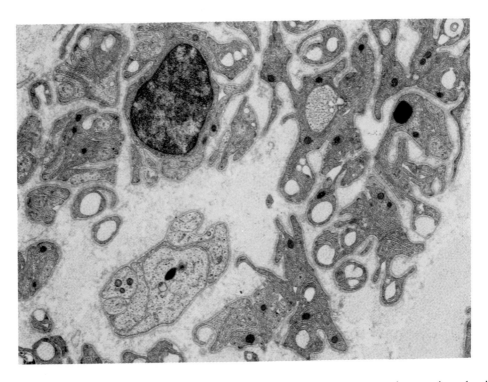

Fig. 16–10. PN and IgG k multiple myeloma in an 82-year-old woman. Several examples of collagen pockets are present and most axons are flattened or have disappeared (× 14,000).

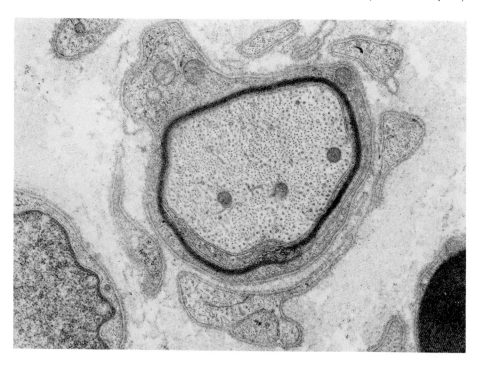

Fig. 16–11. PN and benign IgM MG in a 72-year-old man. An isolated nerve fiber is remyelinating and there are only a few myelin lamellae encircling the axon (× 33,700).

internode [Fig. 16–1]. Active demyelination will be described in the section concerning inflammatory demyelinating polyneuropathies. Atypical periodicity in myelin will be dealt with in the section on polyneuropathies associated with monoclonal gammopathy. Onion bulb formations which are formed by concentric flattened Schwann cell processes [Figs. 16–12 and 16–13] are believed to be secondary to successive episodes of de- and remyelination. Such formations can also develop after demyelination secondary to axonal degeneration

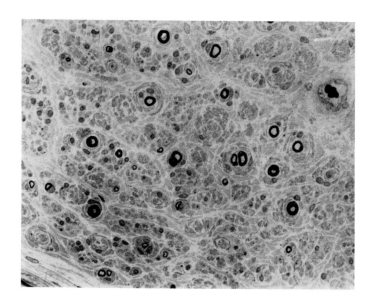

Fig. 16–12. Nerve biopsy from a 61-year-old man with a type I HMSN. Semi-thin section, toluidine blue. Several onion bulb formations are seen around myelinated and demyelinated fibers. Two clusters of regenerating myelinated fibers are also visible. (× 430).

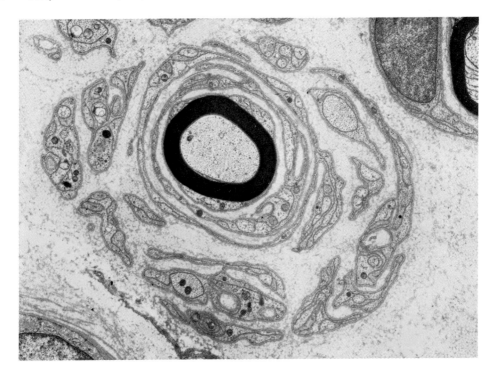

Fig. 16–13.   PN and benign IgM MG in a 74-year-old man. An onion bulb formation is present around a myelinated fiber (× 11,700).

and are sometimes [Fig. 16–14] difficult to differentiate from clusters of regenerating myelinated fibers at ultrastructural examination.[18]

INTERSTITIAL LESIONS

1. Pathology of endoneurial and perineurial capillaries, venules and arterioles will be discussed below in the light of the disease concerned.

2. Cellular infiltrates may be inflammatory or tumoral. Various immunoperoxidase methods permit the identification of lymphomatous infiltrates which display a monotypic lymphocytic population.

3. Endoneurial amorphous deposits of amyloid may indicate familial amyloidosis or be secondary to plasma cell dyscrasia. These deposits must not be confused with Renaut bodies which are normal structures of the endoneurium[13] but which are more frequent in people over 80[13,42–44] [Fig. 16–15].

4. The perineurium may appear thickened in various PN. On ultrastructural examination hyperplastic perineurial lamellae can be seen to encase collagen fibers and a few unmyelinated fibers.[18]

PERIPHERAL NEUROPATHIES IN ELDERLY PEOPLE

NEUROPATHIES DUE TO VASCULAR DISEASES

Ischemia of the peripheral nerve may be due to microvasculitis, necrotizing vasculitis or large artery damage.

1. Microvasculitis affects vessels less than 50 μm in diameter sometimes present in the endoneurium but mainly seen in the epineurium. Various amounts of mononuclear cells, mainly lymphocytes, are arranged in a perivascular cuff [Fig. 16–16] but no vessel wall necrosis is seen. Such cellular reactions can occur in a paraneoplastic process,[45,46] systemic lupus erythematosus,[13] Sjogren syndrome,[47] or essential mixed cryoglobulinemia.[13,48,49] In this last disorder one may identify type II as mixed cryoglobulins with a monoclonal component or type III as mixed polyclonal cryoglobulins.[49]

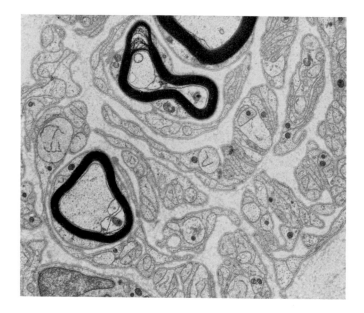

Fig. 16–14. Long-standing PN in a 75-year-old man. A cluster of regenerating myelinated fibers is surrounded by elongated Schwann cell processes containing small unmyelinated axons (× 14,000).

These two types of cryoglobulins can cause hypersensitivity vasculitis, the patients presenting with multifocal or symmetrical PN. Most of these patients have had episodes of vascular purpura of both legs. Cases with multifocal neuropathy usually show features of acute myelino-axonal degeneration with nu-

merous ovoids seen on semithin sections. Cases with symmetrical PN frequently display a dramatic loss of myelinated fibers on semithin sections. In certain cases numerous endoneurial capillaries display swollen endothelial cells and red blood cells and hemosiderin deposits can be seen within endoneurial mac-

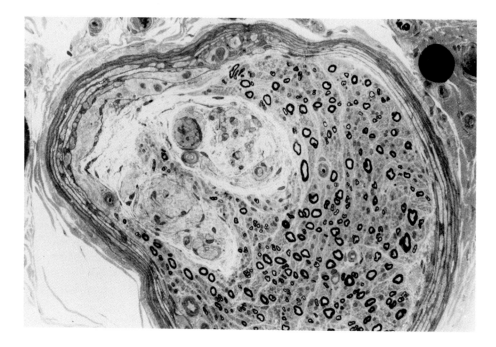

Fig. 16–15. Mononeuritis multiplex in 62-year-old man. Semi-thin section, toluidine blue. Characteristic Renaut bodies are present in the endoneurium.

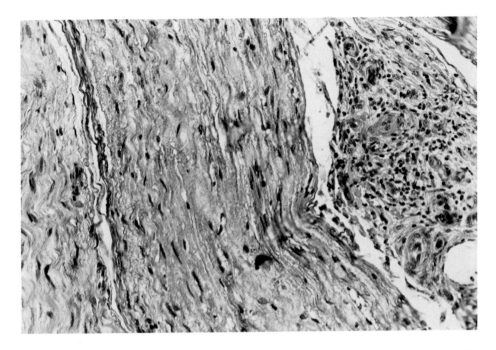

Fig. 16–16.   PN in a 63-year-old woman. Paraffin-embedded fragments. H.E.S. Lymphocytic infiltrates are seen around small epineurial vessels.

rophages. This endoneurial purpura may be considered to be the equivalent of the vascular purpura present in the dermis of such patients.[49] The presence of cryoglobulin in the serum can be suspected when endoneurial purpura is associated with numerous ovoids displaying features of severe axonal damage and tubulovesicular disruption of the myelin sheath [Fig. 16–17].[50] Recently, Sobue et al.[51] reported a case of chronic progressive sensory ataxic PN in a 63-year-old woman who had polyclonal gammopathy without any cryoglobulinemia. Small perivascular infiltrates were seen in peripheral nerves taken at autopsy. In a few biopsies microvasculitis is present in peripheral nerves without any precise cause.[52]

2. Necrotizing vasculitis combines segmental necrosis of the wall of epineurial arterioles and transmural inflammatory cell infiltration.[32,53] The inflammatory cells are mainly lymphocytes, mixed with a few plasma cells, histiocytes and polymorphonuclear leucocytes [Fig. 16–18]. Elderly people are particularly sensitive to necrotizing angiopathy: 29 out of 42 were more than 60 years old in three se-

ries.[54–56] Apart from occasional cases of rheumatoid arthritis,[56] cryoglobulinemia[48] or systemic lupus erythematosus,[10] most cases of necrotizing angiopathy correspond to classic polyarteritis nodosa (P.A.N.). Certain cases seem to be restricted to the peripheral nervous system and have been reported as nonsystemic vasculitic neuropathy by Dyck et al.[57]

3. Large artery diseases correspond mainly to arteriosclerosis; we know of no explicit case of PN reported in this setting. We have only observed in the muscle biopsy cholesterol embolism with P.N., the characteristic intraluminal embolus being sometimes surrounded by inflammatory cellular infiltrates with macrophagic histiocytes. We have not found these characteristic features in biopsied nerve fragments, but such a lesion has probably been illustrated by Dyck et al.[12,58] in their studies on diabetic PN. We have studied peripheral nerve damage in two series of patients suffering from severe arteriosclerosis severe enough to require amputation of the leg. The first series concerned 25 arteriosclerotic diabetic patients who were all more than 60 years old,[59] and the second series concerned 12 arteriosclerotic non-

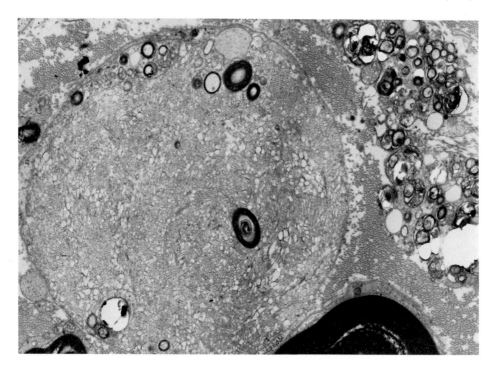

Fig. 16–17.   Mononeuritis multiplex with essential mixed cryoglobulinemia in a 70-year-old woman. The axon is totally destroyed and there is vesicular disruption of the myelin sheath (× 11,100).

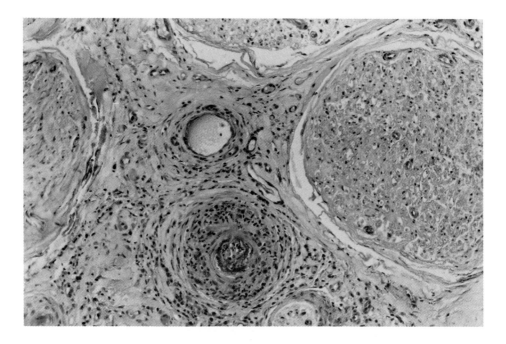

Fig. 16–18.   PN in a 78-year-old woman. Paraffin-embedded fragments. H.E.S. The media of an epineurial arteriole is necrotized and invaded by inflammatory cells (× 230).

diabetic patients of whom 9 were more than 60 years old.[60] The nerve fiber lesions were generally more severe in the diabetic patients, highlighting the role of diabetic macroangiopathy, as will be seen in the following section.

Experimental[29,30] and human[42,54] studies have demonstrated the relative resistance of peripheral nerve to ischemia owing to a profuse collateral circulation and reported that the center of a nerve fascicle seems to be more sensitive to ischemia than the periphery. However, after microsphere embolization of nerve capillaries in the rat, Nukada and Dyck[31] demonstrated that the "ischemic core" may also assume a wedge shape. The severe modifications in one fascicle and the sparing of adjacent fascicles suggest an ischemic mechanism.[13] Harati and Niakan[61] found selective neurofascicular degeneration in sural nerve biopsies of 8 patients age 45 to 72 years (mean, 58 years) out of 250 consecutive biopsies. In 6 cases this degeneration was associated with angiopathic changes. The selective sensitivity to ischemia of myelinated fibers according to their size is still debated. From our own experience in humans[49,54] it appears that myelinated fibers of all sizes are equally affected by ischemia. Wallerian-like degenerative changes are prevalent in neuropathies due to vascular disease, especially in acute ischemic processes, such as PAN. Swollen axons with accumulation of various organelles have been reported in experimental ischemic neuropathy[30–32] as well as in humans[54,59,62] in whom we suspect ischemic mechanism.

NEUROPATHIES RELATED TO SYSTEMIC METABOLIC DISORDERS

1. Diabetes mellitus commonly causes PN, especially in the elderly. There are several syndromes:

(a) Distal sensory-motor PN is most common, affecting 22 of 39 patients who were 60+ years old in two series.[63,64] The pathology of diabetic PN was first described as a mixture of segmental demyelination and myelino-axonal degeneration which seemed to proceed independently of each other.[63,65,66] Schwann cell hypertrophy was a prominent feature in certain cases of PN.[67] However, axonal lesions have more recently been considered to be the

major pathologic modification,[68,69] as confirmed by morphometric and teased fiber studies[12,58] showing evidence that fiber loss is primary and that demyelination and remyelination with or without onion bulb formation is secondary. The spatial distribution of fiber loss is both diffuse and multifocal.[70] However, certain features of primitive demyelination in diabetic PN have been reported in the past few years[71,72] and onion-bulb formations are seen in certain biopsies [Fig. 16–19].

(b) The second major finding in diabetic patients is the presence of microangiopathy in the endoneurial capillaries.[73] The high frequency of endoneurial microangiopathy was established in four series of 16 to 65 patients.[62,64,74,75] We think that the main lesion of diabetic microangiopathy is the thickening of basal lamina corresponding to several concentric lamellae [Fig. 16–20]. In certain capillaries there are also swollen endothelial cells which sometimes almost occlude the lumen.[12,18,58,62,75] Dyck et al. concluded that diabetic PN is of ischemic origin[12,58,75] in view of the association of myelinated fiber modifications and the frequency of capillary closure. Two characteristic modifications prominent in certain cases of ischemic PN were not mentioned in these diabetic patients: the presence of crescent shaped or centrofascicular areas in the most severely damaged fibers and of axons swollen by normal and abnormal organelles.[18,32,54,59,62] Damage to the peripheral nerve is less severe in arteriosclerotic patients without diabetes[70] than in those with diabetes.[59] This highlights the role of microangiopathy in nerve fiber lesions observed in diabetic patients. Exchanges across the blood-nerve-barrier may vary according to the stage of microangiopathy, and hyperpermeability or hypopermeability may play a role in other cases. Johnson[76] emphasized the marked thickening of perineurial basement membranes in diabetic patients. In any event, an ischemic mechanism is likely in certain cases of proximal motor neuropathy.[76,77] Ischemia plays a role in cases of distal PN in which epineurial arterioles are obliterated by fat deposits.[12,58] This finding underlines the need to differentiate diabetic patients with patent arteriosclerosis from those who have sound arteries in the lower limbs. PN occurring in the latter patients probably have a more

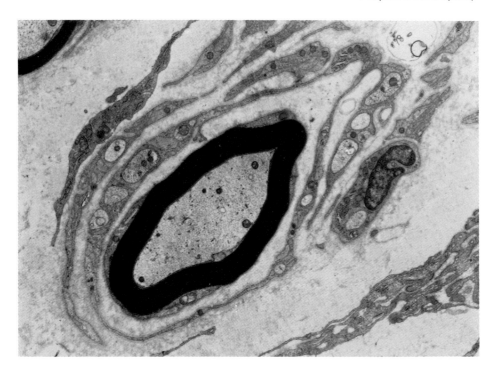

Fig. 16-19. PN in a 74-year-old diabetic patient. An onion bulb formation is seen around a myelinated fiber (× 12,200).

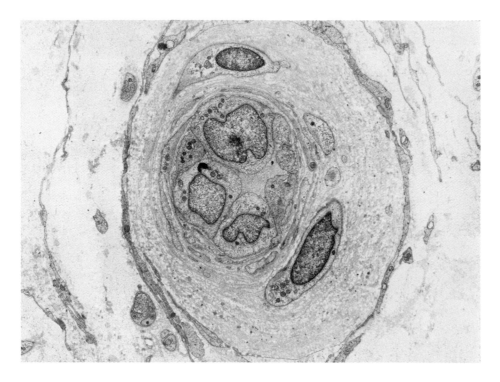

Fig. 16-20. In the same patient, a characteristic feature of diabetic microangiopathy is present in the endoneurium. Several layers of basal lamina are encasing hypotrophic pericytes (× 6,200).

complex mechanism than ischemia alone or a single metabolic disturbance, as suggested before. Recently, Low[78] suggested successive mechanisms, including hypoxia at various steps of nerve fiber damage. We agree with Johnson,[82] who favors a multiplicity of pathogenic mechanisms according to the heterogeneity of diabetic neuropathy. Other clinical presentations of diabetic neuropathy are:

(c) Acute painful neuropathy was described recently in diabetic patients by Archer et al.[79] This form is associated with severe weight loss and concerns mainly middle-aged people.[80] Only 1 out of 9 of their patients was 61 years old, but this patient did not have a nerve biopsy. In the biopsies from three other patients there was evidence of active degeneration of myelinated fibers and also degeneration of unmyelinated axons. The vasa nervorum were not modified and there were no inflammatory infiltrates.[79]

(d) Inflammatory demyelinating polyradiculoneuropathy in a diabetic patient can display unusual myelinic lesions. In a case of Guillain-Barré syndrome in a 72-year-old diabetic patient we observed features of active demyelination and also numerous features of vesicular disruption of the myelin sheath, which was present in 22% of the myelinated fibers.[81] This peculiar mode of myelin disruption is most frequent in animals with experimental allergic neuritis provoked by intraneural injection of experimental allergic serum.[82] Although the endoneurial capillaries of this patient were hardly modified, we suggest that their excessive permeability brought harmful serum factors into contact with the myelin sheaths.

2. Hypothyroidism is sometimes associated with a distal symmetric sensorimotor PN, which recovers with the treatment of the hypothyroidism. A few cases have occurred in elderly people.[83–85] The nerve biopsy from a 61-year-old woman[84] displayed features mainly consisting of segmental demyelination and onion-bulb formations. The density of myelinated nerve fibers was slightly low, 6133/mm^2. The electron microscopic study revealed the presence of glycogen accumulations in the axons and in the Schwann cell cytoplasm. Evidence of segmental demyelination and remyelination was seen in teased fiber preparations of axonal disorders.[83] Two of the 4 cases reported by Meier and Bischoff were over 60 years old and their nerve biopsies showed features of axonal degeneration.[85]

3. Uremic PN as described by Asbury et al.[86] is mainly observed in young and middle aged patients. The oldest patient in the series of Said et al. was 50 years old.[87] Various lesions were seen on peripheral nerve biopsies: acute axonal neuropathy, progressive axonal neuropathy with secondary segmental demyelination and a predominantly demyelinative neuropathy. Dyck et al.[20] described segmental demyelination secondary to axonal degeneration. Uremic PN develops less frequently now, possibly because of progress in hemodialysis.[5]

4. Polyneuropathies due to nutritional deficiencies can develop in elderly people under various conditions such as socioeconomic difficulties or mental impairment. Thiamine deficiency can produce PN in patients with beri beri characterized by axonal degeneration with secondary demyelination.[88] Vitamin B$_1$ deficiency may be difficult to differentiate from alcoholic PN in some patients. Moreover, both conditions give rise to axonal modifications without characteristic lesions.[16] The large series of alcoholic PN studies by Behse and Buchtal[89] and Said[90] mainly concerned patients under 60 years, but 2 patients over 60 years have been reported. Vitamin B$_{12}$ deficiency is mainly known to produce myelopathy, as in subacute combined degeneration. A few cases of PN have been reported with features of axonal degeneration.[92] Vitamin E deficiency can cause spinocerebellar syndrome developing in the sixth and seventh decade without fat malabsorption.[93] The sural nerve biopsy of a 62-year-old patient showed a moderate loss of large myelinated fibers and dense deposits in Schwann cells and between myofibrils of quadriceps fragments.[93]

5. PN can occur in each form of porphyria, often provoked by certain drugs, particularly barbiturates. A patient reported recently by Pellissier et al.[94] was 72 years old and had features of axonal degeneration.

6. Sjogren's syndrome is sometimes associated with joint manifestations. Nerve biopsies exhibited vasculitis and myelinoaxonal degeneration of nerve fibers in 3 cases reported by Kaltreider and Talal.[47]

7. Rheumatoid arthritis is sometimes associ-

ated with PN. Features of vasculitis are often present in epineurial vessels. Weller et al.[56] reported lesions of Wallerian-like degeneration.

8. Severe motor and sensory PN were described in critically ill patients: severe by Bolton et al.[95] Five cases were reported, one 66 years old. In 3 of 4 patients studied in Bordeaux, the ages ranged from 60 to 66.[96] In both series all patients had prolonged intensive care and nutritional factors may have played a role, especially since the patients improved with total parenteral nutrition. Hypoxia may have also played a role, especially at the peak of their critical illness. Moreover, 2 patients had suffered from chronic hypoxemia for years before their stay in the intensive care unit.[96] All nerve biopsies showed severe and acute axonal damage.[95,96]

POLYNEUROPATHIES ASSOCIATED WITH PLASMA CELL DYSCRASIA

These conditions are encountered with significant frequency in the elderly. Most concern benign or malignant IgM monoclonal gammopathies (MG) but neuropathies associated with other forms of dysglobulinemia occur.

(a) Polyneuropathy Associated with IgM Monoclonal Gammopathy. PN associated with IgM MG have been extensively studied in recent years.[18,97-104] Although Waldenstrom's macroglobulinemia (WM) and benign IgM monoclonal gammopathy (BMMG) are two conditions of different prognosis, peripheral nerves are damaged similarly.[18] Peripheral neuropathy associated with WM was described by Garcin,[105] and those related to BMMG by Forssman et al.[106] Typically, patients have a long-standing history of sensorimotor PN. In most cases, the neuropathy is demyelinating in type, with widening of some myelin lamellae (WML) at ultrastructural examination. Immunopathologic study shows IgM binding to peripheral nerve myelin and immunoblot analysis of the serum shows antibody binding to myelin associated glycoprotein (MAG). In a personal study of 31 patients suffering from PN associated with IgM MG,[104] 25 were more than 60 years old. Four patients had WM, and 21 had BMMG. In this series, features of WML were observed in 20 cases: 2 WM and 18 BMMG [Figs. 16–21 and 16–22].

This characteristic and almost specific WML has been reported in cases of WM[107-112] and in cases of BMMG.[111,112] WML has been extensively studied by King and Thomas,[113] and was present in a nerve biopsy from a patient with polyradiculoneuritis who developed an IgM MG a few months later. "Onion bulb" formations [Fig. 16–23] are sometimes associated with features of WML. Direct immunopathologic examination shows that in certain cases anti-IgM and anti-kappa or lambda or light chain serum fixes on myelin sheaths [Fig. 16–24].[108,109,110,114,115]

In a recent study, Dubas et al.[102] presented 12 personal cases and reviewed the literature, showing the good correlation between the presence of WML at ultrastructural examination and IgM binding to nerve myelin at immunopathologic examination. We also found a good correlation in our series: however, 5 cases had features of WML but with no IgM fixation on the myelin sheaths on direct immunofluorescence study. In fact, in these 5 cases the widening was restricted to the outermost myelin lamellae of only a few fibers [Fig. 16–25]. Moreover, in our series, apart from 1 case, all patients who had WML at ultrastructural examination had anti-MAG activity in their serum.[104] Abrams et al.[116] were the first to demonstrate that serum from some patients with PN and IgM MG binds to myelin sheaths from the human peripheral nerve, and Braun et al.[117] were the first to evoke MAG as a possible antigen. It has been confirmed that in this type of neuropathy lesions are mainly due to factors directed against myelin components, principally MAG. However, there are some cases in which the monoclonal immunoglobulin does not have anti-MAG activity. Latov et al.[118] and Steck et al.[103] reported the major antibody activities of human monoclonal IgM found in patients with various peripheral nerve disorders.

Other nonspecific but significant pathologic aspects include hypermyelination[119] and axonal damage. Hypermyelination of an internode is often associated with axonal swelling and intra-axonal organelle accumulation. These latter features may cause a slowing of axoplasmic flow and be secondary to axonal constriction at the level of hypermyelination. PN associated with IgM MG present in 8 pa-

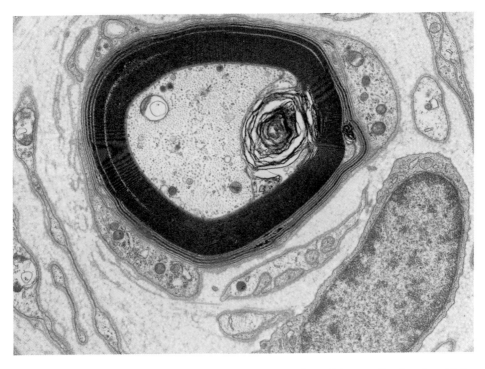

Fig. 16–21.   PN with IgM MG in a 74-year-old man. Outer lamellae of the myelin sheath exhibit a typical widening ($\times$ 14,200).

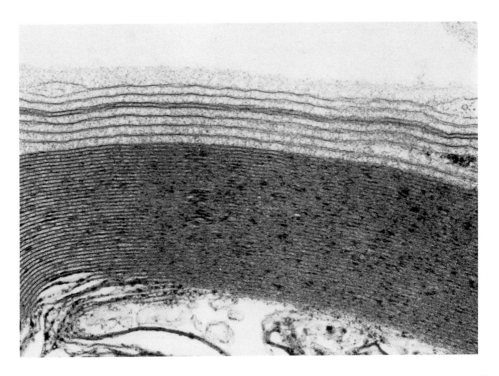

Fig. 16–22.   In the same case, there are other characteristic features of widened myelin lamellae ($\times$ 14,200).

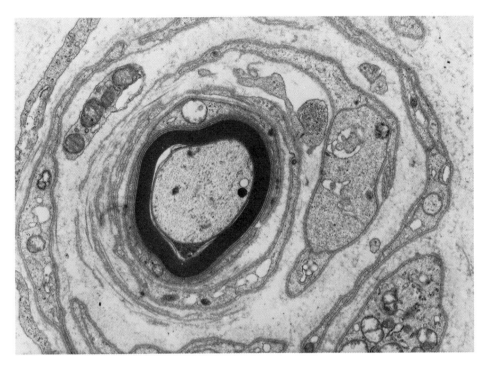

Fig. 16–23.   In the same case, an onion bulb formation is seen around a myelinated fiber exhibiting characteristic features of widened myelin lamellae (× 13,700).

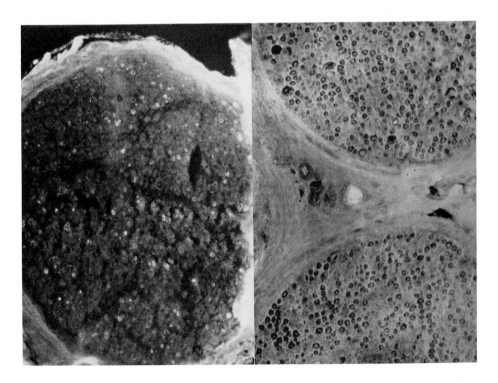

Fig. 16–24.   Direct immunopathologic examination. Left: PN and benign IgM MG in a 76-year-old woman. Anti-kappa light chain serum fixes on myelin sheaths. Right: Guillain-Barré syndrome: no fixation is visible with an anti-IgG serum (× 230).

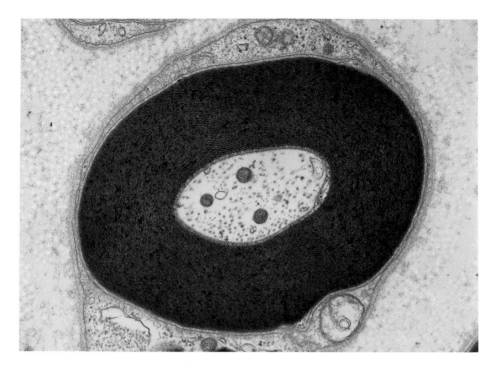

Fig. 16–25.   PN and benign IgM MG in a 74-year-old man. Only the outermost lamella shows a characteristic widening (× 21,000).

tients with marked loss of axons (less than 3000 myelinated fibers per mm²).[104] Endoneurial microangiopathy has been reported in some cases of PN with IgM MG. It may be a swelling of endothelial cells,[107] a thickening by reduplication of the vascular basement membrane,[98,120] or intracytoplasmic microfilament accumulation in endothelial cells.[121] Some cases of PN associated with IgM MG should be considered separately because the lesions are different from those usually observed. These cases are characterized by the presence of IgM deposits in the endoneurium of the peripheral nerve visualized on immunopathologic study. They appear as granular or sometimes microfibrillar deposits on ultrastructural examination. These immunoglobulin deposits not only compress nerve fibers, often erasing their basement membrane [Fig. 16–26], but also thicken the walls of endoneurial capillaries [Fig. 16–27]. Such interstitial deposits of IgM have been reported in a few cases of WM[122,125] and in cases of BMMG.[99,102–103] In a few cases plasma cells are dispersed in the endoneurium. Julien et al.[126] reported a case with a few atypical lymphocytes in the endoneurium, but this case

was unusual in that the IgM serum peak could be detected only 4 years after the WML was observed at peripheral nerve biopsy when the patient was 67 years old. Julien et al.[127] reported a case of PN with biclonal gammopathy in a 60-year-old man. The nerve biopsy exhibited both amyloid deposits related to an IgG-lambda light chain MG and the characteristic WML related to an IgM-kappa light chain MG. Busis et al.[128] reported PN with high serum IgM in mother and son. The PN began when the mother was 66 years old and at 53 in her only child. A nerve biopsy in the son exhibited characteristic WML. The authors suggested a familial disorder of immune regulation with antibody-mediated PN or a familial PN with a secondary immune response.

(b) Multiple Myeloma.   PN are classic in this setting and biopsies display features of chronic axonal degeneration without characteristic features.[110,129] In a few cases there are endoneurial amyloid deposits [See below].

(c) Osteosclerotic Myeloma and POEMS Syndrome.   The POEMS syndrome corresponds to the association of polyneuropathy, organomegaly, endocrinopathy, M-compo-

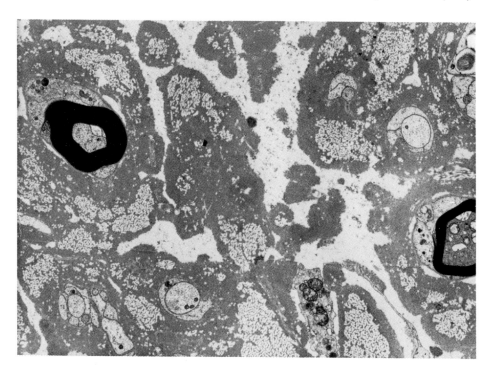

Fig. 16–26.   P.N. with benign IgM MG in an 84-year-old man. Abundant granular deposits are present in the endoneurium and there is a dramatic loss of myelinated fibers (× 6,900).

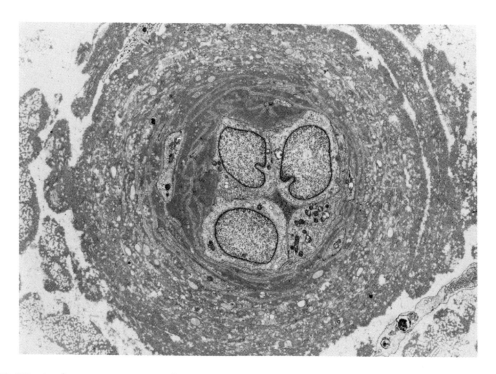

Fig. 16–27.   In the same case, granular deposits are pushing aside the basal lamina of an endoneurial capillary (× 6,900).

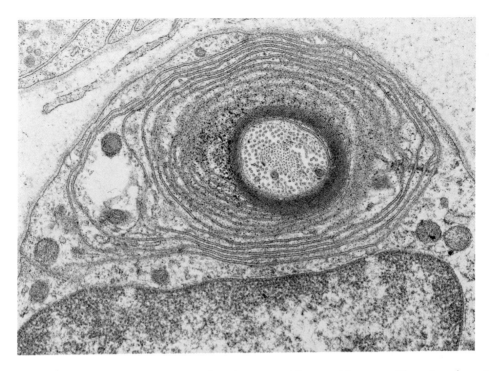

Fig. 16–28. PN and non-secreting malignant lymphoma in a 69-year-old woman. There is a characteristic feature of uncompacted myelin lamellae: the outer lamellae are not joined together ($\times$ 21,000).

nent and skin abnormalities. Frequent in Japan, it is sometimes called Crow-Fukase syndrome and is frequently associated with an osteosclerotic myeloma. Three recent cases, one of whom was 75 years old, have been studied with electron microscopy.[130] Some myelinated fibers showed features of myelino-axonal degeneration and others a more peculiar abnormality of the myelin sheath, described by Ohnishi and and Hirano[131] as "uncompacted myelin lamellae" (UML) in which the lamellae are not joined together as in a normal myelin sheath. This modification is frequently seen on the inner part of the sheath. UML must be differentiated from widened myelin lamellae,[18,113,131–133] but their features are usually quite different. Moreover, DIPE is negative in cases with UML. This peculiar myelin abnormality has been described in 3 patients, 2 of whom probably had a POEMS syndrome.[131] However, UML can also be seen in cases of nonsecretory plasma cell lymphoma[132] [Fig. 16–28] and in cases of inflammatory demyelinating polyradiculoneuritis.[134] At this time, no reported cases of POEMS syndrome have

been associated with endoneurial amyloid or immunoglobulin deposits.

(d) Other Benign Monoclonal Gammopathies. A few cases of IgG MG have been reported including an 84-year-old woman who had characteristic features of UML on her nerve biopsy.[132]

(e) Cryoglobulinemia, Type I. This features an isolated IgG or IgM MG and is rarely associated with PN. In a 53-year-old patient, Vallat et al.[135] demonstrated closely packed tubular structures in the endoneurium as well as in the lumen and wall of endoneurial capillaries. These structures were identical to the cryoprecipitate which the authors extracted from the serum. The essential mixed cryoblobulins are studied in the chapter on vascular disorders.

MALIGNANT LYMPHOMAS

They may invade the peripheral nerves in a few cases. A T-cell lymphoma caused a relapsing PN in a 63-year-old woman.[136] In the su-

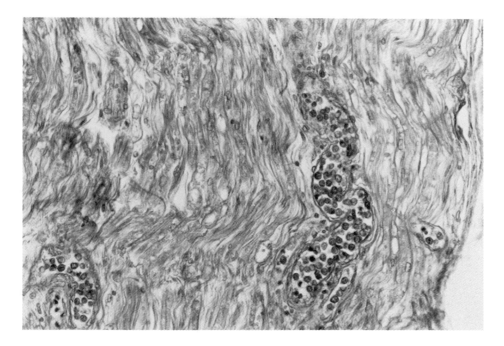

Fig. 16–29.   Acute mononeuritis of the leg in a 62-year-old woman. Paraffin-embedded fragments. H.E.S. Round tumoral cells are plugging the lumen of endoneurial capillaries ($\times$ 370).

perficial peroneal nerve abnormal lymphocytes were invading the endoneurium and especially the epineurium in a perivascular pattern. A 67-year-old woman investigated for a T-cell lymphoma had similar infiltrates in a nerve biopsy and in the peroneus brevis muscle.[18] Certain cases of malignant lymphoma invade the peripheral nervous system in unusual ways (as in the following 2 cases). In a case of IDPRN, a 75-year-old patient with chronic lymphoid leukemia had large lymphocytic infiltrates in the epineurium. Tumoral lymphocytic cells with unusual pseudopodia and intracytoplasmic filaments had invaded the myelinated fibers and destroyed the myelin sheath.[18,137] Intravascular malignant lymphomatosis can also appear as vascular disease in the central nervous system.[138] Epineurial vessels of both lateral popliteal nerves have been reported to be occluded.[139] Recently, we had the opportunity to study the superficial peroneal nerve biopsy from a 62-year-old woman who had an acute mononeuropathy of the leg. Fragments of muscle and nerve biopsies showed tumoral cells in the lumen of most small blood vessels [Fig. 16–29]. Tumoral

markers showed a lymphomatous origin of the B type.

AMYLOID PN

Amyloid PN (APN) may be of hereditary origin (familial amyloid polyneuropathy, FAP): or secondary to a plasma cell dyscrasia. Both conditions can be observed in elderly patients. In a series of 31 cases[140] the mean age was 63 years, with a range of 52 to 81. Certain familial forms have a late onset in countries like U.S.A.,[141] Japan,[142] and Ireland.[143] In 4 cases out of 7 studied in Ireland[143] the age at onset was 61 to 66 years. In a large Japanese series of 45 patients, 4 female patients had their first symptoms when they were over 60.[142] Elderly people are prone to present monoclonal gammopathy and APN can develop in the setting of a multiple myeloma[144–146] and in the course of Waldenstrom macroglobulinemia.[149] APN developing in the course of a benign MG is rare.[127]

The amyloid origin of a neuropathy can be strongly suspected when amyloid deposits are evidenced in another site of the body, usually

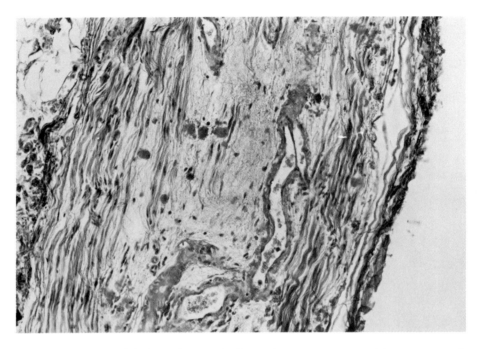

Fig. 16-30. PN and IgG-lambda light chain multiple myeloma in a 60-year-old woman. Paraffin-embedded fragments. H.E.S. Round amyloid deposits are seen in the endoneurium and the capillary walls are thickened by amyloidosis (× 230).

in a rectal biopsy, but sometimes the nerve damage is secondary to extraneural deposition with nerve compression. This is classically observed in some cases of carpal tunnel syndrome.[13] Thus, APN can truly be assessed when typical amyloid deposits are seen within endoneurial areas. There are round amorphous acidophilic deposits in the endoneurium, and some endoneurial capillaries' walls are thickened by the same deposits [Fig. 16–30]. Such deposits are not to be confused with Renaut bodies: amyloid deposits stain orange with congo red and display typical dichroic birefringence with polarized light. On ultrastructural examination there is a more or less severe nerve fiber loss with features of Wallerian-like degeneration. Some cases present more severe lesions of unmyelinated and small myelinated fibers.[150,151] Segmental demyelination is absent or rare. The amyloid deposits are fibrillar structures [Fig. 16–31] entangled at random or more rarely bundled in parallel.[148] The basal membrane of Schwann cells is often erased by amyloid deposits. In 2 out of 30 cases examined in our laboratory the diagnosis of APN was made only at ultrastructural examination,

which disclosed a few small deposits located in the vicinity of endoneurial capillaries [Fig. 16–32]. These minute deposits were not visible on the corresponding semithin sections.

Immunopathologic examination makes it possible to differentiate the origin of amyloid deposits. In familial cases anti-prealbumin serum, more appropriately called "anti-transthyretin", fixes on the deposits, whereas in cases of plasma cell dyscrasia specific anti-light chain serum marks the deposits.[152,153] In a personal case of APN and multiple myeloma, anti-IgG and anti-lambda light chain sera fixed only on the thickened walls of endoneurial capillaries. It is likely that in the large endoneurial deposits lambda light chain was transformed into amyloid.[110,147]

INFLAMMATORY POLYNEURITIS

The peripheral nerve can be involved in inflammatory processes:

(a) Lepromatous PN is mainly observed in young adults and biopsies of peripheral nerves reveal a wide variety of lesions.[13,16] The lepromatous form is characterized by large clear

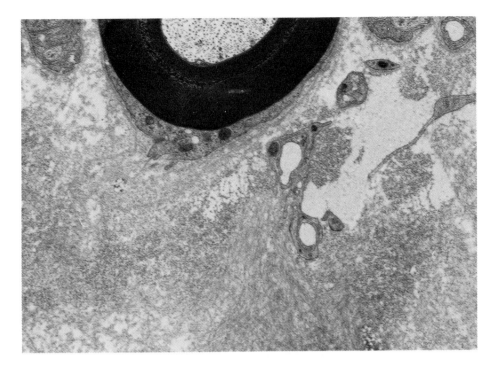

Fig. 16–31.   PN and IgG-kappa light chain multiple myeloma in an 82-year-old woman. Fibrillar deposits, characteristic of amyloidosis, are seen close to the nerve fibers (× 16,500).

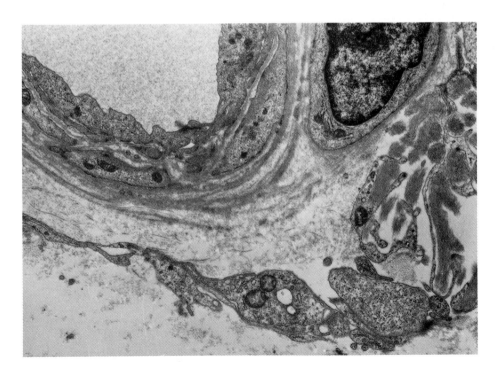

Fig. 16–32.   PN in a 60-year-old man. A few small bundles of amyloid fibrils are present in a perivascular location (× 18,000).

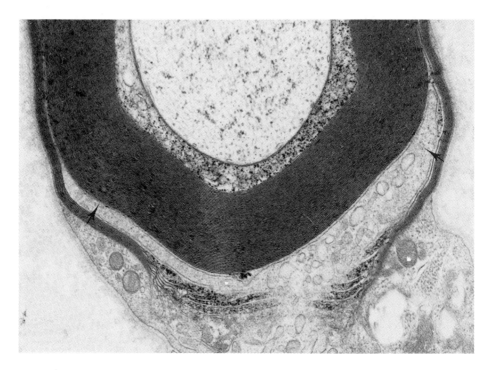

Fig. 16-33. Guillain-Barré syndrome in a 65-year-old woman. Elongated processes from an invading macrophage are peeling away myelin lamellae in a paranodal location ($\times$ 28,500).

histiocytes containing numerous acid fast leprosy bacilli. Ultrastructural examination discloses round electron dense bacilli surrounded by clear zones; these are numerous in histiocytes and in the Schwann cell cytoplasm of unmyelinated fibers. Occasionally they can be seen in the cytoplasm of myelinated fibers and even in an intra-axonal location.[18] In 4 cases of leprous neuropathies, Jacobs et al.[154] found several examples of "loose myelin". One of us, with Vallat, has already illustrated this myelinic modification in this setting, without suggesting any mechanism. In tuberculoid leprosy the endoneurium contains granulomas composed of epithelioid cells, lymphocytes and a few giant cells. Necrotic areas may be present in certain granulomas. Leprosy bacilli are absent or rare. However, osmiophilic bacilli can be detected on ultrastructural examination of nerves presenting tuberculoid lesions.[155] Mycobacterium leprae antigen can be demonstrated in these nerves using anti-bacille Calmette-Guerin by the PAP method.[155] In borderline forms, lepromatous and tuberculoid lesions may be seen in adjacent areas.

(b)   Tick-bite   meningo-radiculoneuritis (Barnwerth or Lyme disease) is suspected in patients with painful radiculoneuropathy, chronic lymphocytic meningitis, and erythema chronica migrans spreading from the bitten area. In the series of Vallat et al.[156] the 10 patients ranged from 48 to 80 years. Nerve biopsies showed infiltrates of lymphocytes and plasma cells around endoneurial and perineurial vessels without necrosis of the vessel walls. There was a significant loss of myelinated fibers and features of axonal degeneration.

(c) Inflammatory demyelinating polyradiculoneuritis (IDPRN) are generally thought to have an autoimmune mechanism that damages the peripheral nervous system in various ways. The acute form[157] is the classic Guillain-Barré syndrome (GBS) and this is the most frequent form in a global population. Sixty-five cases of GBS were investigated in Bordeaux during the past 12 years.[134] We also observed 10 patients with chronic cases of IDPRN, 5 of whom were over 60 years of age. There were two relapsing cases with intervals of 2 and 12 years between the two episodes, two recurrent cases and a subacute monophasic case. How-

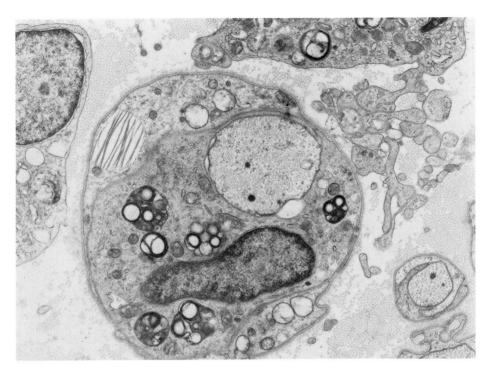

Fig. 16–34.   Guillain-Barré syndrome in 66-year-old man. A histiocyte is visible inside the Schwann cell cytoplasm and the axon is totally naked. Another macrophagic histiocyte is present in the endoneurium (× 6,600).

ever, this predominance of elderly people in chronic forms of IDPRN has not been present in other series with only 6 out of 35 cases reported.[158–160] The 5 patients' ages reported by Pollard et al.[161] ranged from 19 to 43. It is interesting to note that in 2 patients who consistently responded to plasma exchange, the main pathologic finding was segmental demyelination without prominent onion bulb formation.[161]

Paraffin embedded fragments of peripheral nerve biopsies taken from cases of GBS display only occasional and minimal endoneurial infiltrates of mononuclear cells. In our series of biopsies we have never seen the impressive features of inflammatory cells infiltrating the peripheral nervous system as reported by Asbury et al.[162] and Asbury and Johnson[13] on fragments from spinal roots and sciatic nerves taken at autopsy. Perivascular lymphocytic infiltrates have also been reported by Dyck and Arnason[163] in cases of chronic IDPRN. Direct immunofluorescence is disappointing, immunoglobulin deposits having been observed in

only one case.[134,164] In fact, ultrastructural examination is an excellent means to obtain the characteristic feature of IDPRN, i.e., "active demyelination".[9,13,18,134,158,165] In the endoneurium a few histiocytes may be clustered around a myelinated fiber, even invading the Schwann cell cytoplasm. Moreover, flattened and elongated processes from the invading histiocyte are peeling away certain myelin lamellae, whereas the axon remains normal or almost normal. This feature of active demyelination is specific in human pathology for IDPRN and has never been reported in any other condition apart from one exceptional finding in a thorough ultrastructural study of nerve biopsies from 17 patients with peroneal muscular atrophy[166] and in this case an additional inflammatory process may have developed.[167] Active demyelination has been reported in experimental allergic neuritis[168,169] and in GBS[162] [Figs. 16–33 and 16–34].

There are other anomalous changes observed with electron microscopy such as vesicular disruption of the myelin sheath, loose my-

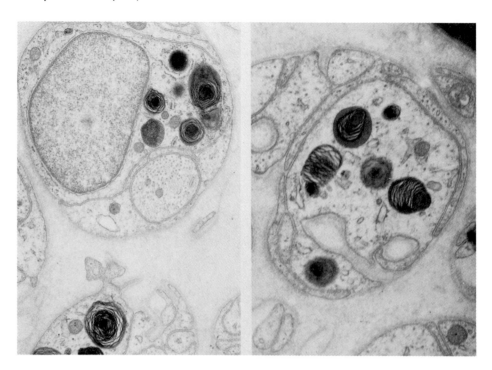

Fig. 16–35.   Chloroquine PN in a 72-year-old man. Typical multi-lamellar inclusions are seen in the cytoplasm of these unmyelinated fibers (× 22,000).

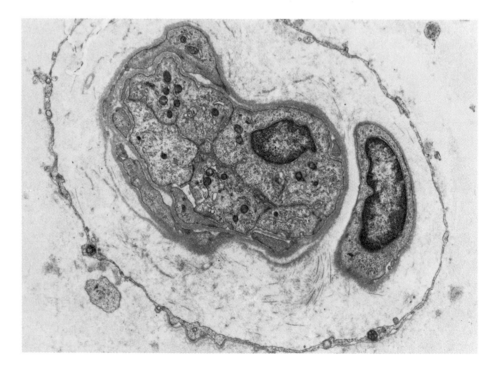

Fig. 16–36.   PN in an 87-year-old woman. This endoneurial capillary exhibits an almost normal basal lamina and is surrounded by a flattened fibroblastic process (× 11,000).

elin lamellation, and uncompacted myelin lamellae described in dysglobulinemic polyneuropathies and in experimental allergic neuritis.[170]

In summary, "active demyelination" is the hallmark of IDPRN Sometimes, it can be suspected on semi-thin sections, but ultrastructural examination is mandatory to affirm its existence and to check for good preservation of the axon. Axonal degeneration was the main modification in 5 patients described recently as an "acute axonal form of Guillain-Barré polyneuropathy", of whom 2 out of 5 patients were over 60 years old.[171] Similarly, a recurrent case and a subacute monophasic case we observed in Bordeaux exhibited only features of acute myelino-axonal degeneration without lesions of segmental demyelination. A few cases of IDPRN have been reported in acquired immunodeficiency syndrome with biopsies exhibiting infiltration of the endoneurium by various inflammatory cells, but these cases have concerned only young adults.[172]

PARANEOPLASTIC NEUROPATHIES

These are classic PN of sensory[173] and sensorimotor type.[174] Peripheral nerve biopsy studies have been reported, including that of elderly patients.[175-177] The primary pathology is axonal with secondary demyelination.[177] Two 63-year-old patients with oat cell carcinoma of the lung[45] and another 61-year-old man with an epidermoid carcinoma of the lung[46] displayed features of vasculitis in the peripheral nerve. Using immunoelectron microscopy, endoneurial immune deposits have been noted in paraneoplastic neuropathies.[178]

TOXIC PN

1. PN due to environmental agents are mainly observed in factory workers and thus are rare in elderly people. However, they can be observed in particular situations.[179]

a. Ingestion of adulterated rapeseed oil in Spain a few years ago resulted in a toxic epidemic with neuromuscular disorders and various visceral and cutaneous disorders. Ricoy et al.[179] investigated 145 patients aged 9 to 67 years. Seventy-three sural nerve biopsies were studied. Initially lymphocytic infiltrates were seen in the epineurium, followed by severe perineuritis with focal degeneration of myelinated axons.

b. The neurotoxic effect of arsenic on peripheral nerve is axonal degeneration and loss of myelinated fibers.[18] Recently, Donofrio et al.[181] reported 4 cases of arsenic neuropathy, 3 of whom were over 60 years. They presented as progressive polyradiculoneuropathy; no biopsy was performed.

2. Iatrogenic PN are, on the other hand, relatively frequent in elderly people.[179,182]

a. Antineoplastic drugs

i. The toxic effects of vincristine have been known for more than 20 years. The first ultrastructural examinations of nerve biopsies disclosed axonal degeneration.[183,184,185] We have studied the biopsies of nerves of three such cases:[18] one case had numerous axonal modification, a second case showed a few unmyelinated axonal modifications and the third case showed numerous glycogen accumulations in the axons, Schwann cell cytoplasm and even endothelial cells of endoneurial capillaries. The last case had nerve fiber modifications which were similar to glycogen accumulations reported by Dyck and Lambert[83] in a case of PN associated with hypothyroidism. VP 16 had been incriminated with a possible enhancement of vincristine PN in 4 patients over 60 years. However, the myelin modifications reported on nerves removed at autopsy were probably of autolytic origin.[186]

ii. The effect of cisplatin on peripheral nerves has been described in two reports concerning 11 patients ranging in age from 47 to 71 years[187] and 7 patients of whom one was 67 years old.[188] Most of these patients had been treated for ovarian adenocarcinoma and all developed distal sensory PN. Morphologic studies performed on sural nerve biopsies exhibited axonal degeneration and secondary myelin breakdown.[187,188]

Platinum concentrations were assessed in 3 autopsied patients and were similar in tumor, sural nerve, and spinal ganglia, but lower in the brain.[187]

b. Drugs acting on the cardiovascular or pulmonary system:

i. Amiodarone is widely used in the treatment of cardiac arrythmias and angina pectoria. There may be a loss of myelinated fibers of all sizes and unmyelinated fibers show frequent features of regeneration[189–191] but segmental demyelination predominates in certain cases. Unusual inclusions are present in Schwann cells, fibroblasts, vessel walls, and perineurial cells. At ultrastructural examination one notes that most of these inclusions are round and contain concentric membranous lamellae.

ii. Perhexiline maleate has produced the same endoneurial inclusions associated with features of segmental demyelination and occasionally axonal degeneration.[192,193]

iii. Almitrine is a new drug and only one report provides detailed results of nerve biopsy.[194] Eight patients were studied in which almitrine had been prescribed for chronic obstructive pulmonary disease in 6 and for chronic cerebral vascular insufficiency in 2. Axonal damage affecting the large myelinated fibers was the most striking abnormality. In 5 biopsies endoneurial capillaries showed thickened basement membranes. The mechanism of this PN which is associated with a recent weight loss is not well understood.

c. Antibiotics and antiparasitics

i. Isoniazid in patients treated for tuberculosis can produce a motor and sensory PN. After interruption of isoniazid therapy, patients progressively recover. An electron microscopy study was done by Ochoa[195] on 9 patients, of whom 6 were over 60. Wallerian degeneration is the main pathologic process; myelinated and unmyelinated fibers were damaged in

all cases and there were relatively numerous fibers undergoing active axonal degeneration; features of regeneration were frequent and there was also degeneration of some fibers which had regenerated.

ii. Metronidazole therapy may lead to axonal degeneration without specific features.[18]

d. Other drugs

i. Thalidomide PN is rarely observed. Schroder and Gibbels[196] reported results of sural nerve biopsy from 4 patients, 3 of whom were over 60 years old. There were numerous features of axonal sprouting, as well as loss of large myelinated fibers.[196]

ii. Disulfiram PN has been observed in a recent case.[197] Neurofilament accumulation in enlarged axons was present. However, all these patients were under 60 years of age.

iii. Chloroquine may cause a PN in patients treated for malaria prophylaxis [Fig. 16–35], but in our experience such PN are mainly observed in patients treated for rheumatoid arthritis. The inclusions are identical to those observed in amiodarone therapy.[198,199] Three out of 4 patients reported recently had features of segmental demyelination and remyelination. The axonal degeneration observed in the fourth case was thought to be of rheumatoid origin.[199]

iv. Gold PN can be observed in patients with rheumatoid arthritis and is often associated with focal or generalized myokymia. Katrak et al.[200] performed an electron microscopic study on the sural nerve biopsy from 3 patients, 1 of whom was 65 years old. There was both axonal degeneration and segmental demyelination with remyelination.[200]

v. Colchicine PN may occur in patients with gout who have altered renal function.[201] These patients have mainly a proximal myopathy and the PN may go undetected. The recent report of Kuncl et al.[201] concerned 12 patients, of whom 4 were studied in detail. A sural nerve biopsy was performed in an 86-year-old man and showed moderate damage with occasional acute degeneration of myelinated fibers. The muscle biopsy performed in 6 patients exhibited features of vacuolar myopathy marked by accumulation of lysosomes and autophagic vacuoles. Fifteen patients with chronic idiopathic ataxic PN thought to be caused by pyridoxine abuse or doxorubicin administration were reported.

STORAGE DISORDERS AND PN

Certain storage disorders produce PN, but this occurs mainly in pediatric pathology and occasionally in young adults. We have found only two examples in patients over 60 years.

(a) Tangier disease is characterized by high density lipoprotein deficiency. Pietrini et al.[203] reviewed 19 cases with PN which were reported in the literature, 2 of whom were over 60 years of age.[203-205] Pollock et al.[206] reported the case of a 61-year-old man and Marbini et al.[207] the case of a man age 64 years with Tangier disease. Gibbels et al.[208] classified the PN of Tangier disease in three types: (1) Transient or relapsing, often asymmetrical syndromes, (2) slowly progressing symmetrical PN most marked in the lower extremities, and (3) slowly progressing symmetrical PN with a syringomyelia-like syndrome. On semi-thin sections clear vacuoles are seen in the Schwann cell cytoplasm, especially numerous in certain longitudinally cut fibers. At electron microscopy there are clear round vacuoles, sometimes with an osmiophilic rim.[199-201] Gibbels et al.[204] found that these vacuoles lacked a limiting structure. The production of these vacuoles is still discussed.

(b) Polyglucosan body (P.G.B.) disease has been described by Robitaille et al.[209] in 4 patients whose age ranged from 59 to 67 years. There was a massive involvement of central neuronal processes. Several P.G.G. were present in a single axon on the sural nerve of the fourth patient. Vos et al.[210] reported the case of 2 women under 60 who had numerous P.G.B. in their myelinated axons and a few in unmyelinated fibers. The diabetic patient reported by Mancardi et al.[211] was considered to have nonspecific changes. P.G.B. can be observed occasionally in nerve biopsies from aged patients without any specific correlation.[13,18,204] They are probably more frequent in intramuscular nerve twigs.[13]

HEREDITARY NEUROPATHIES

(a) A classification of the hereditary motor and sensory neuropathies (HMSN) has been proposed by Dyck et al.[212] Types I and II (HMSN) may occur in elderly humans.[213-215] In type I cases Schwann cell proliferation is the main modification. Concentric flattened Schwann cell processes surround an axon, creating "onion bulb" formations [Fig. 16–12]. The axon may be demyelinated or in the process of remyelination.[13,18,166,212,216] The demyelination appears to be secondary to the primary axonal atrophy. In type II, also called the neuronal form, demyelination and hypertrophic changes are rare or absent.[18,212]

(b) Hereditary sensory and autonomic neuropathy type I:[217,218]

This type of neuropathy sometimes begins as late as the fourth decade. Peripheral nerve biopsies show a marked nerve fiber loss. In the nerve biopsy of a 71-year-old woman, few small myelinated fibers were seen as well as flattened axons and Schwann cell cytoplasm of unmyelinated fibers.[18] Guimaraes et al.[218] found marked loss of myelinated fibers in 6 sporadic cases.[91]

(c) Hereditary pressure sensitive neuropathy is characterized by focal sausage shaped thickening of the myelin sheaths. This condition was described by Behse et al.[219] and the myelin thickening was called "tomaculae" by Madrid and Bradley.[220] Recently, Pellissier et al.[221] reported 10 cases and reviewed the literature. Though the age of onset is generally under 50, there are some patients over 60.[221] Focal myelin thickenings are seen on teased fibers and Pellissier et al.[221] found them in more than 25% of internodes. At ultrastructural examination hypermyelination exhibits various patterns: regular coilings of lamellae, internodal or external redundant loops. These modifications were studied in detail by Madrid and Bradley.[220] Other internodes can show demyelination or the onset of remyelination. The density of myelinated and unmyelinated fibers is normal but there is a loss of large myelinated fibers thought to be secondary to myelinic modifications.

THE AGING HUMAN PERIPHERAL NERVE

Changes during aging of the human peripheral nervous system have been reviewed by Schaumburg et al.[222] Clinical signs of peripheral nervous system dysfunction in the elderly are deterioration of most sensory modalities in the distal extremities, muscle wasting, decline in strength, and absence or decrease of tendon reflexes. We have had the opportunity of studying the superficial peroneal nerve biopsies of 46 patients from 70 to 95 years old;[223] like most elderly people, these patients displayed evidence of peripheral nervous system dysfunction, but they were not suffering from any affection known to alter the peripheral nerve. In a prospective study, Hessel et al.[3] found that in elderly patients, 20% of peripheral neuropathies are apparently idiopathic and the aim of our own study was to consider morphologic alterations as the human peripheral nerve ages. Lascelles and Thomas[224] and Jacobs and Love[225] noticed in humans that over the age of 60, irregularities of internodal length were common on isolated fibers from the sural nerve. The authors considered these modifications to be the result both of segmental demyelination and remyelination, and of regeneration after complete degeneration of nerve fibers. Ochoa and Mair[34] in a study of the normal sural nerve in man have described the increase with age of myelinated fiber degeneration; however, these authors have also pointed out aspects of myelinated fiber regeneration, and they insist on the fact that unmyelinated fibers are affected more markedly than the myelinated ones. Our study confirmed the possibility that myelinated fibers regenerate in elderly patients, and also underlined the large extent of unmyelinated fiber damage. Our study also showed that segmental demyelination was relatively rare, as was Wallerian-like degeneration and axonal organelle accumulation. Tohgi et al.[226] studied quantitative changes with age in normal human

sural nerves, and noticed that myelinated fibers decreased with advancing age, and that the ratio of small to large myelinated fibers increased with age. We also found in our cases that myelinated fiber loss predominated in the large diameter group, but several patients presented a high number of small myelinated fibers, which in fact correspond to clusters of regenerating fibers. The cause of the degeneration and decrease of peripheral nerve fibers with age is uncertain, although chronic mechanical trauma or vascular changes with age have been suggested. As reported by Jacobs and Love,[225] reduplication of the vascular basement membrane was noticed in nerves from our cases, but thickening was moderate. In fact, thickening of endoneurial capillary walls seen on semi-thin sections correspond frequently to accumulation of collagen fibers encased by a thin fibroblastic process [Fig. 16–36]. Therefore, the ultrastructual features are quite different from those observed in diabetic microangiopathy [Fig. 16–20]. Tohgi et al.[226] reported that after 60 years there was a greater reduction of large myelinated fibers, when the stenosis of vasa nervorum was more pronounced.

Thus, apart from neuropathies of known etiologies, the human peripheral nerve presents morphologic lesions due to aging. These consist mostly of chronic axonal lesions concerning both myelinated and unmyelinated fibers, and with coexistence of regeneration.

REFERENCES

1. Huang, C.Y.: Peripheral Neuropathy in the Elderly: A Clinical and Electrophysiologic Study. American Geriatrics Society, *XXIX*(2):49, 1981.
2. George, J., and Twomey, J.A.: Causes of Polyneuropathy in the Elderly. Age and Ageing, *15*:247, 1986.
3. Hessel, L., Corvisier, N., Vallat, J.M., et al.: Etiologies des neuropathies peripheriques chez les personnes ages. Med. et Hyg., *44*:1354, 1986.
4. Baruch, J.K.: Periphral neuropathy in elderly population (65 years and above). (Abstract) Neurology, *29*(1):208, 1989.
5. Dyck, P.J., Oviatt, K.F., and Lambert, E.H.: Intensive evaluation of referred unclassified neuropathies yields improved diagnosis. Ann. Neurol., *10*:222, 1981.
6. Dyck, P.J.: The causes, classification and treatment of peripheral neuropathy. N. Engl. J. Med., *307*:283, 1982.
7. Mc Leod, J.G., et al.: Chronic polyneuropathy of undetermined cause. J. Neurol. Neurosurg. Psychiatry, *47*:530, 1984.

8. Fardeau, M., Tome, F.M.S., Guimaraes, A., et al.: Role de la microscopie electronique en pathologie nerveuse peripherique. Arch. Anat. Cytol. Path., 26:283, 1978.

9. Prineas, J.W.: Pathology of the Guillain-Barre Syndrome. Ann. Neurol. Suppl 9:6, 1981.

10. Hirano, A.: Some postmortem structural changes in peripheral myelinated fibers. In: *The Pathology of Myelinated Axon.* (Eds.) M. Adachi, A. Hirano, and S.M. Aronson. New York, Igaku-Shoin, 1985.

11. Dyck, P.J., et al.: Pathologic alterations of the peripheral nervous system of humans. In: *Peripheral Neuropathy II.* (Eds.) P.J. Dyck, et al. Philadelphia, W.B. Saunders Co., 1984.

12. Dyck, P.J., et al.: Fiber loss is primary and multifocal in sural nerves in diabetic polyneuropathy. Ann. Neurol., 19:425, 1986.

13. Asbury, A.K., and Johnson, P.C.: *Pathology of Peripheral Nerve.* Philadelphia, W.B. Saunders Co., 1978.

14. Lampert, P.W., and Schochet, S.S.: Ultrastructural changes of peripheral nerve. In: *Diagnostic Electron Microscopy.* (Ed) Trump. New York, John Wiley & Sons, 1979.

15. Schaumburg, H.H., Spencer, P.S., and Thomas, P.K.: *Disorders of Peripheral Nerves.* Philadelphia, F.A. Davis Co., 1983.

16. Thomas, P.K., Landon, D.N., and King, R.H.M.: Diseases of the peripheral nerves. In: *Greenfield's Neuropathology.* (Eds.) by J.H. Adams, J.A.N. Corsellis, and L.W. Duchen. London, Edward Arnold, 1984.

17. Powell, H.C., and Myers, R.R.: Pathology of the peripheral myelinated axon. In: *The pathology of the Myelinated Axon.* (Eds.) M. Adachi, A. Hirano, and S.M. Aronson. New York, Igaku-Shoin, 1985.

18. Vital, C., and Vallat, J.M.: *Ultrastructural Study of the Human Diseased Peripheral Nerve.* 2nd Ed., New York, Elsevier, 1987.

19. Griffin, J.W., and Watson, D.F.: Axonal transport in neurological diseases. Ann. Neurol., 23:3, 1988.

20. Dyck, P.J., Johnson, W.J., Lambert, E.H., et al.: Segmental demyelination secondary to axonal degeneration in uremic neuropathy. Mayo Clin. Proc., 46:400, 1971.

21. Waller, A.: Experiments on the section of the glossopharyngeal and hypoglossal nerves of the frog and observations of the alterations produced thereby in the structure of their primitive fibres. Philos. Trans. R. Soc., 14:423, 1850.

22. Ballin, R.H.M., and Thomas, P.K.: Changes at the nodes of Ranvier during Wallerian degeneration: An electron microscope study. Acta Neuropathol., 14:237, 1969.

23. Dyck, P.J., et al.: Permanent axotomy, a model of axonal atrophy and secondary segmental demyelination and remyelination. Ann. Neurol., 9:575, 1981.

24. Dyck, P.J., Nukada, H., Lais, A.C., et al.: Permanent axotomy: A model of chronic neuronal degeneration preceded by axonal atrophy, myelin remodeling and degeneration. In: *Peripheral Neuropathy I.* (Eds.) P.J. Dyck, P.K. Thomas, E.H. Lambert, and R. Bunge. Philadelphia, W.B. Saunders Co., 1984.

25. Cavanagh, J.B.: The significance of the "dying-back" process in experimental and human neurological disease. Int. Nat. Rev. Exp. Pathol., 7:219, 1964.

26. Cavanagh, J.B.: The dying-back process: A common denominator in many naturally occuring and toxic neuropathies. Arch. Pathol. Lab. Med., 103:659, 1979.

27. Spencer, P.S., and Schaumburg, H.H.: Central peripheral distal axonopathy: The pathology of dying-back polyneuropathies. In: *Progress in Neuropathology III.* (Ed) H.M. Zimmerman, New York, Grune & Stratton, 1976.

28. Spencer, P.S., and Schaumburg, H.H.: Ultrastructural studies of the dying-back process: III. The evolution of experimental peripheral giant axonal degeneration. J. Neuropathol. Exp. Neurol., 35:276, 1977.

29. Korthals, J.K., and Wisniewski, H.M.: Peripheral nerve ischemia. Part 1. Experimental model. J. Neurol. Sci., 24:65, 1975.

30. Korthals, J.K., Korthals, M.A., and Wisniewski, H.M.: Peripheral nerve ischemia. Part 2. Accumulation of organelles. Ann. Neurol., 4:487, 1978.

31. Nukada, H., and Dyck, P.J.: Microsphere embolization of nerve capillaries and fiber degeneration. Am. J. Pathol., 115:275, 1984.

32. Nukada, H., and Dyck, P.J.: Acute ischemia causes axonal stasis, swelling, attenuation, and secondary demyelination. Ann. Neurol., 22:311, 1987.

33. Thomas, P.K.: The ultrastructural pathology of unmyelinated nerve fibers. In: *New Development in Electromyography and Clinical Neurophysiology.* (Ed) J.E. Desmedt. Basel, Karger, 1973.

34. Ochoa, J., and Mair, W.G.P.: The normal sural nerve in man I. Ultrastructure and numbers of fibers and cells. Acta Neuropathol., 13:197, 1969.

35. Ochoa, J., and Mair, W.G.P.: The normal sural nerve in man II. Changes in the axons and Schwann cells due to aging. Acta Neuropathol., 13:217, 1969.

36. Ochoa, J.: Electron microscope observation on unmyelinated fibers in normal and pathological human nerves. In: *Proceedings Sixth International Congress of Neuropathology.* Paris, Masson, 1970.

37. Ochoa, J.: Recognition of unmyelinated nerve fiber disease: Morphologic criteria. Muscle & Nerve, 1:375, 1978.

38. Behse, R., Buchthal, F., Carlse, F., et al.: Unmyelinated fibers and Schwann cells of sural nerve in neuropathy. Brain, 98:493, 1975.

39. Gombault, A.: Contribution a L'etude anatomique de la nevrite parenchymateuse subaigue et chronique: Nevrite segmentaire peri-axile. Arch. Neurol., 1:117, 1880.

40. Webster, H., de Spiro, F.D., Waksmann, B.H., and Adams, R.D.: Phase and electron microscopic studies of experimental demyelination I. Schwann cell changes in guinea pig sciatic nerves during experimental diphteritic neuritis. J. Neuropathol. Exp. Neurol., 20:5, 1961.

41. Weller, R.O.: Diphteric neuropathy in the chicken: An electron-microscope study. J. Pathol. Bacteriol., 89:591, 1965.

42. Dyck, P.J., Conn, D.L., and Okazaki, H.: Necrotizing angiopathic neuropathy: Three dimensional morphology of fiber degeneration related to sites of occluded vessels. Mayo Clin. Proc., 47:461, 1972.

43. Asbury, A.K.: Renaut bodies: A forgotten endoneurial structure. J. Neuropathol. Exp. Neurol., 32:334, 1973.

44. Bergouignan, F.X., and Vital, C.: Occurrence of Renaut's bodies in a peripheral nerve. Arch. Pathol. Lab. Med., 108:330, 1984.

45. Johnson, P.C., Rolak, L.A., Hamilton, R.H., et al.: Paraneoplastic vasculitis of nerve: A remote effect of cancer. Ann. Neurol., 5:443, 1979.

46. Vallat, J.M., et al.: Acute pure sensory paraneoplastic neuropathy with perivascular endoneurial inflam-

mation: Ultrastructural study of capillary walls. Neurology, *36*:1395, 1986.

47. Kaltreider, H.B., and Talal, N.: The neuropathy of Sjogren's syndrome: Trigeminal nerve involvement. Ann. Intern. Med., *70*:751, 1969.

48. Chad, D., et al.: The pathogenesis of cryoglobulinemic neuropathy. Neurology, *32*:725, 1982.

49. Vital, C., et al.: Peripheral neuropathy with essential mixed cryoglobulinemia; Biopsies from 5 cases. Acta Neuropathol., *75*:605, 1988.

50. Thomas, P.K., and Sheldon, H.: Tubular arrays derived from myelin breakdown during Wallerian degeneration of peripheral nerve. J. Cell Biol., *22*:725, 1964.

51. Sobue, G., Yanagi, T., and Hashizume, Y.: Chronic progressive sensory ataxic neuropathy with polyclonal gammopathy and disseminated focal perivascular cellular infiltrations. Neurology, *38*:463, 1988.

52. Vincent, D., et al.: Microvasculites nerveuses et musculaires: 50 cas. Rev. Neurol., *141*:440, 1985.

53. Kissel, J.T., Slivka, A.P., Warmolts, J.R., et al.: The clinical spectrum of necrotizing angiopathy of the peripheral nervous system. Ann. Neurol., *18*:251, 1986.

54. Vital, A., and Vital, C.: Polyarteritis nodosa and peripheral neuropathy: Ultrastructural study of 13 cases. Acta Neuropathol., *67*:136, 1985.

55. Schroder, J.M.: Proliferation of epineurial capillaries and smooth muscle cells in angiopathic peripheral neuropathy. Acta Neuropathol., *72*:29, 1986.

56. Weller, R.O., Bruckner, F.E., and Chamberlain, M.A.: Rheumatoid neuropathy: A histological and electrophysiological study. J. Neurol. Neurosurg. Psychiatry, *33*:592, 1970.

57. Dyck, P.J., et al.: Nonsystemic vasculitic neuropathy. Brain, *110*:843, 1987.

58. Dyck, P.J.: Pathology. In: *Diabetic Neuropathy*. (Eds.) P.J. Dyck, et al. Philadelphia, W.B. Saunders Co., 1987.

59. Vital, C., et al.: Ultrastructural study of peripheral nerve in arteritic diabetic patients. Acta Neuropathol., *61*:225, 1983.

60. Vital, A., et al.: Quantitative, histological and ultrastructural studies of peripheral nerve in arteriosclerotic non-diabetic patients. Clin. Neuropathol., *5*:224, 1986.

61. Harati, Y., and Niakan, E.: Clinical significance of selective nerve fascicular degeneration on sural nerve biopsy specimen. Arch. Pathol. Lab. Med., *110*:195, 1986.

62. Vital, C., Le Blanc, M., Coquet, M., et al.: A study of peripheral nerve in diabetic patients. In: *Biochemistry and Pathology of Basement Membranes*. (Ed.) L. Robert. Basel, Karger, 1979.

63. Vital, C., et al.: Les neuropathies peripheriques du diabete sucre: Étude ultrastructurale de 12 cas biopsies. J. Neurol. Sci., *18*:381, 1973.

64. Powell, H.C., Rosoff, J., and Myers, R.R.: Microangiopathy in human diabetic neuropathy. Acta Neuropathol., *68*:295, 1985.

65. Thomas, P.K., and Lascelles, R.G.: The pathology of diabetic neuropathy. Quart. J. Med., *35*:489, 1966.

66. Behse, F., Buchthal, F., and Carlsen, F.: Nerve biopsy and conduction studies in diabetic neuropathy. J. Neurol. Neurosurg. Psychiatry, *40*:1072, 1977.

67. Ballin, R.H.M., and Thomas, P.K.: Hypertrophic changes in diabetic neuropathy. Acta Neuropathol., *11*:93, 1968.

68. Sidenius, P.: The axonopathy of diabetic neuropathy. Diabetes, *31*:356, 1982.

69. Brown, M.J., and Asburg, A.K.: Diabetic neuropathy. Ann. Neurol., *15*:2, 1984.

70. Dyck, P.J., et al.: The spatial distribution of fiber loss in diabetic polyneuropathy suggests ischemia. Ann. Neurol., *19*:440, 1986.

71. Ohnishi, A., et al.: Segmental demyelination and remyelination in lumbar spinal roots of patients dying with diabetes mellitus. Ann. Neurol., *13*:541, 1983.

72. Said, G.: Neuropathies metaboliques I. Neuropathies diabetiques. Rev. Neurol., *141*:683, 1985.

73. Bischoff, A.: Die diabetische Neuropathie. Praxis, *24*:723, 1965.

74. Vital, C., et al.: Etude ultrastructurale du nerf peripherique chez 16 diabetiques sans neuropathie clinique: comparaisons avec 16 neuropathies diabetiques. Acta Neuropathol., *30*:63, 1974.

75. Yasuda, H., and Dyck, P.J.: Abnormalities of endoneurial microvessels and sural nerve pathology in diabetic neuropathy. Neurology, *36*:20, 1987.

76. Johnson, P.C.: Diabetic neuropathy. In: *The Pathology of the Myelinated Axon*. (Eds.) M. Adachi, A. Hirano, and S.M. Aronson. New York, Igaku-Shoin, 1985.

77. Asbury, A.K.: Focal and multifocal neuropathies of diabetes. In: *Diabetic Neuropathy*. (Eds.) P.J. Dyck, et al.: Philadelphia, W.B. Saunders Co., 1987.

78. Low, P.A.: Recent advances in the pathogenesis of diabetic neuropathy. Muscle & Nerve, *10*:121, 1987.

79. Archer, A.G., et al.: The natural history of acute painful neuropathy in diabetes mellitus. J. Neurol. Neurosurg. Psychiat., *46*:491, 1983.

80. Thomas, P.K., and Brown, M.J.: Diabetic polyneuropathy. In: *Diabetic Neuropathy*. (Eds.) P.J. Dyck, et al.: Philadelphia, W.B. Saunders Co., 1987.

81. Vital, C., et al.: Acute inflammatory demyelinating polyneuropathy in a diabetic patient: predominance of vesicular disruption in myelin sheaths. Acta Neuropathol., *67*:337, 1985.

82. Saida, K., et al.: Antiserum-mediated demyelination in vivo: a sequential study using intraneural injection of experimental allergic neuritis serum. Lab. Invest., *39*:449, 1978.

83. Dyck, P.J., and Lambert, E.H.: Polyneuropathy associated with hypothyroidism. J. Neuropathol. Exp. Neurol., *29*:631, 1970.

84. Shirabe, R., Tawara, S., Terao, A., et al.: Myxoedematous polyneuropathy: A light and electron microscopic study of the peripheral nerve and muscle. J. Neurol. Neurosurg. Psychiatry, *38*:241, 1975.

85. Meier, C., and Bischoff, A.: Polyneuropathy in hypothyroidism. Clinical and nerve biopsy study of four cases. J. Neurol., *215*:103, 1977.

86. Asbury, A.K., Victor, M., and Adams, R.D.: Uremic polyneuropathy: A clinicopathologic study. Neurology, *33*:567, 1983.

87. Said, G., et al.: Different patterns of uremic polyneuropathy: A clinicopathologic study. Neurology, *33*:567, 1983.

88. Ohnishi, A., et al.: Beriberi neuropathy: Morphometric study of sural nerve. J. Neurol. Sci., *45*:43, 1979.

89. Behse, F., and Buchthal, F.: Alcoholic neuropathy: Clinical, electrophysiological, and biopsy findings. Ann. Neurol., *2*:95, 1977.

90. Said, G.: A clinicopathologic study of acrodystrophic neuropathies. Muscle & Nerve, *3*:491, 1980.

91. Tredici, G., and Minazzi, M.: Alcoholic neuropathy:

An electron-microscopic study. J. Neurol. Sci., 25:333, 1975.

92. Mac Combe, P.A., and Mac Leod, J.G.: The peripheral neuropathy of vitamin B_{12} deficiency. J. Neurol. Sci., 66:117, 1984.

93. Yokota, T., et al.: Adult onset spinocerebellar syndrome with idiopathic vitamin E deficiency. Ann. Neurol. 22:84, 1987.

94. Pellissier, J.F., Serratrice, G., and Toga, M.: Pathologie de la neuropathie porphyrique. Arch. Anat. Cytol. Path., 35:173, 1987.

95. Bolton, C.F., Gilbert, J.J., Hahn, A.F., et al.: Polyneuropathy in critically ill patients. J. Neurol. Neurosurg. Psychiatry, 47:1223, 1984.

96. Barat, M., et al.: Polyneuropathies au cours de sejours prolonges en reanimation. Rev. Neurol., 143:823, 1987.

97. Latov, N., et al.: Plasma cell dyscrasia and peripheral neuropathy with a monoclonal antibody to peripheral nerve myelin. N. Engl. J. Med., 303:618, 1980.

98. Smith, I.S., et al.: Chronic demyelinating neuropathy associated with benign IgM paraproteinaemia. Brain, 106:169, 1983.

99. Mc Leod, J.G., Walsh, J.C., and Pollard, J.D.: Neuropathies associated with paraproteinemias and dysproteinemias. In: Peripheral Neuropathy II. (Eds.) P.J. Dyck, et al.: Philadelphia, W.B. Saunders Co., 1984.

100. Meier, C.: Polyneuropathy in paraproteinaemia. J. Neurol., 232:204, 1985.

101. Mendell, J.R., et al.: Polyneuropathy and IgM monoclonal gammopathy: Studies on the pathogenetic role of anti-myelin-associated glycoprotein antibody. Ann. Neurol., 17:243, 1985.

102. Dubas, F., Pouplard-Barthelaix, A., Delestre, F., et al.: Polyneuropathies avec gammapathie monoclonale IgM. 12 cas. Rev. Neurol., 143:670, 1987.

103. Steck, A.J., et al.: Peripheral neuropathy associated with monoclonal IgM autoantibody. Ann. Neurol., 22:764, 1987.

104. Vital, A., et al.: Polyneuropathy associated with IgM monoclonal gammopathy. Immunological and pathological study in 31 patients. Acta Neuropathol. (Berl.), 79:160, 1989.

105. Garcin, R., Mallarme, J., and Rondot, P.: Forme nevritique de la macroglobulinemie de Waldenstrom. Bull. Mem. Soc. Med. Hop. Paris, 74:562, 1958.

106. Forssman, O., Bjorkman, G., Hollender, A., et al.: IgM producing lymphocytes in peripheral nerve in a patient with benign monoclonal gammopathy. Scand. J. Haematol., 11:332, 1973.

107. Vital, C., et al.: Les neuropathies peripheriques de la maladie de Waldenstrom: Etude histologique et ultrastructurale de cinq cas. Ann. Anat. Pathol., 20:93, 1975.

108. Propp, R.P., et al.: Waldenstrom macroglobulinemia and neuropathy: Deposition of M-component in myelin sheaths. Neurology, 25:980, 1975.

109. Julien, J., et al.: Polyneuropathy in Waldenstrom's macroglobulinemia: Deposition of M-component on myelin sheath. Arch. Neurol., 35:423, 1978.

110. Vital, C., et al.: Peripheral nerve damage during multiple myeloma and Waldenstrom's macroglobulinemia: An ultrastructural and immunopathologic study. Cancer, 50:1491, 1982.

111. Melmed, C., et al.: Peripheral neuropathy with IgM Kappa monoclonal immunoglobulin directed against myelin-associated glycoprotein. Neurology, 33:1397, 1983.

112. Steck, A.J., et al.: Demyelinating neuropathy and monoclonal IgM antibody to myelin associated glycoprotein. Neurology, 33:19, 1983.

113. King, R.H.M., and Thomas, P.K.: The occurrence and significance of myelin with unusual large periodicity. Acta Neuropathol., 63:319, 1984.

114. Chazot, G., et al.: Manifestations neurologiques des gammapathies monoclonales: Formes neurologiques pures. Etude en immunofluorescence. Rev. Neurol., 132:195, 1976.

115. Takatsu, M., et al.: Immunofluoresence study of patients with neuropathy and IgM M-Proteins. Ann. Neurol., 18:173, 1985.

116. Abrams, G.M., et al.: Immunocytochemical studies of human peripheral nerve with serum from patients with polyneuropathy and paraproteinemia. Neurology, 32:821, 1982.

117. Braun, P.E., Latov, N.T., and Frail, D.E.: MAG is the antigen for a monoclonal IgM in polyneuropathy. Trans. Amer. Soc. Neurochem., 13:230, 1982.

118. Latov, N.: Peripheral neuropathy and antibodies to the myelin associated glycoprotein. In: Proceedings of the International Symposium on Peripheral Neuropathies. (Ed) I. Sobue. Tokyo, Excerpta Medica, 1984.

119. Vital, C., et al.: Hypermyelinisation dans un cas de neuropathie peripherique avec gammapathie monoclonale benigne a IgM. Rev. Neurol., 141:729, 1985.

120. Nemni, R., et al.: Polyneuropathy in non-malignant IgM plasma cell dyscrasia: A morphological study. Ann. Neurol., 14:43, 1983.

121. Powell, H.C., Rodriguez, M.M., and Hugues, R.A.C.: Microangiopathy of vasa nervorum in dysglobulinemic neuropathy. Ann. Neurol., 15:386, 1984.

122. Iwashita, H., Argyrakis, A., Lowitzch, K., et al.: Polyneuropathy in Waldenstrom's macroglobulinemia. J. Neurol. Sci., 21:341, 1974.

123. Meier, C., et al.: Polyneuropathy in Waldenstrom's macroglobulinemia: Reduction of IgM deposits after treatment with chlorambucil and plasmapheresis. Acta Neuropathol., 64:307, 1984.

124. Vital, C., et al.: Waldenstrom's macroglobulinemia and peripheral neuropathy: Deposition of M-component and kappa light chain in the endoneurium. Neurology, 35:603, 1985.

125. Lamarca, J., Casquero, P., and Pou, A.: Mononeuritis multiplex in Waldenstrom's macroglobulinemia. Ann. Neurol., 22:268, 1987.

126. Julien, et al.: Chronic demyelinating neuropathy with IgM producing lymphocytes in peripheral nerve and delayed appearance of "benign" monoclonal gammopathy. Neurology, 34:1387, 1984.

127. Julien, J., et al.: IgM demyelinative neuropathy with amyloidosis and biclonal gammopathy. Ann. Neurol., 15:395, 1984.

128. Busis, N.A., et al.: Peripheral neuropathy, high serum IgM, and paraproteinemia in mother and son. Neurology, 35:679, 1985.

129. Ohi, T., Kyle, R.A., and Dyck, P.J.: Axonal attenuation and secondary segmental demyelination in myeloma neuropathies. Ann. Neurol., 17:255, 1985.

130. Bergouignan, F.X., et al.: Uncompacted lamellae in three patients with P.O.E.M.S. syndrome. Eur. Neurol., 27:173, 1987.

131. Ohnishi, A., and Hirano, A.: Uncompacted myelin lamellae in dysglobulinemic neuropathy. J. Neurol., Sci., 51:131, 1981.

132. Vital, C., et al.: Uncompacted myelin lamellae in two

cases of peripheral neuropathy. Acta Neuropathol., 60:252, 1983.

133. Ohnishi, A.: Segmental demyelination and remyelination of myelinated axons in dysglobulinemic neuropathy. In: *The Pathology of the Myelinated Axon.* (Eds.) M. Adachi, A. Hirano, and S.M. Aronson, New York, Igaku-Shoin, 1985.

134. Brechenmacher, C., et al.: Guillain-Barre syndrome: An ultrastructural study of peripheral nerve in 65 patients. Clin. Neuropathol., 6:19, 1987.

135. Vallat, J.M., et al.: Cryoglobulinemic neuropathy: A pathological study. Ann. Neurol., 8:179, 1980.

136. Gherardi, R., et al.: T-cell lymphoma revealed by a peripheral neuropathy. A report of two cases with an immunohistologic study of lymph node and nerve biopsies. Cancer, 58:2710, 1986.

137. Vital, C., et al.: Polyradiculonevrite au cours d'une leucemie lymphoide chronique: Etude ultrastructurale d'une biopsie de nerf peripherique. Acta Neuropathol., 32:169, 1975.

138. Wick, R.R., et al.: Reassessment of malignant "angioendotheliomatosis". Evidence in favor of its reclassification as "intravascular lymphomatosis". Am. J. Surg. Pathol., 10:112, 1986.

139. Krieger, C., Robitaille, Y., Jothy, S., et al.: Intravascular malignant histiocytosis mimicking central nervous system vasculitis: An immunopathological diagnostic approach. Ann. Neurol., 12:489, 1982.

140. Kelly, J.J., Kyle, R.A., O'Brien, P.C., et al.: The natural history of peripheral neuropathy in primary systemic amyloidosis. Ann. Neurol., 6:1, 1979.

141. Koeppen, A.H., et al.: Familial amyloid polyneuropathy. Muscle & Nerve, 8:733, 1985.

142. Ikeda, C.I., et al.: Hereditary generalized amyloidosis with polyneuropathy. Brain, 110:315, 1987.

143. Staunton, H., et al.: Hereditary amyloid polyneuropathy in North West Ireland, Brain, 110:1231, 1987.

144. Davies-Jones, G.A.B., and Esiri, M.M.: Neuropathy due to amyloid in myelomatosis. Br. Med. J., 2:444, 1971.

145. Neundorfer, B., Meyer, J.G., and Volk, B.: Amyloid neuropathy due to monoclonal gammopathy: A case report. J. Neurol., 216:207, 1977.

146. Verghese, J.P., Bradley, W.G., Nemni, R., et al.: Amyloid neuropathy in multiple myeloma and other plasma cell dyscrasias. J. Neurol. Sci., 59:237, 1983.

147. Vital, C., et al.: Amyloid neuropathy and multiple myeloma: Ultrastructural and immunopathological study of two cases. Eur. Neurol., 22:106, 1983.

148. Vital, A., and Vital, C.: Amyloid neuropathy: Relationship between amyloid fibrils and macrophages. Ult. Pathol., 7:21, 1984.

149. Bajada, S., Mastaglia, F.L., and Fisher, A.: Amyloid neuropathy and tremor in Waldenstrom's macroglobulinemia. Arch. Neurol., 37:240, 1980.

150. Dyck, P.J., and Lambert, E.H.: Dissociated sensation in amyloidosis: Compound action potential, quantitative histologic and teased fiber, and electron-microscopic studies of sural nerve biopsies. Arch. Neurol., 20:490, 1969.

151. Thomas, P.K., and King, R.H.M.: Peripheral nerve changes in amyloid neuropathy. Brain, 97:395, 1974.

152. Linke, R.P.: Immunohistochemical identification and cross reactions of amyloid fibril proteins in senile heart and amyloid familial polyneuropathy: Lack of reactivity with cerebral amyloid in Alzheimer's disease. Clin. Neuropathol., 1:72, 1977.

153. Dalakas, M.C., and Cunningham, G.: Characteriza-tion of amyloid deposits in biopsies of 15 patients with "sporadic" (non-familial or plasma cell dyscrasic) amyloid polyneuropathy. Acta Neuropathol., 69:66, 1986.

154. Jacobs, J.M., Shetty, V.P., and Antia, N.H.: Myelin changes in leprous neuropathy. Acta Neuropathol., 74:75, 1987.

155. Barros, U., Shetty, V.P., and Antia, N.H.: Demonstration of mycobacterium leprae antigen in nerves of tuberculoid leprosy. Acta Neuropathol., 73:387, 1987.

156. Vallat, J.M., et al.: Tick-bite meningoradiculoneuritis: Clinical, electrophysiologic, and histologic findings in 10 cases. Neurology, 37:749, 1987.

157. Arnason, B.G.W.: Acute inflammatory demyelinating polyradiculoneuropathies. In: *Peripheral Neuropathy* II. (Eds.) P.J. Dyck, et al.: Philadelphia, W.B. Saunders Co., 1984.

158. Prineas, J.W., and Mac Leod, J.G.: Chronic relapsing polyneuritis. J. Neurol. Sci., 27:427, 1976.

159. Sluga, E., and Poewe, W.: Chronic idiopathic polyneuritis. Clin. Neuropathol., 2:31, 1983.

160. Rizzuto, N., et al.: Chronic relapsing polyneuritis: A light and electron microscopic study. Acta Neuropathol., 56:179, 1982.

161. Pollard, J.D., Mc Leod, J.G., Gatenby, P., et al.: Prediction of response to plasma exchange in chronic relapsing polyneuropathy. J. Neurol. Sci., 58:269, 1983.

162. Asbury, A.K., Arnason, B.G., and Adams, R.D.: The inflammatory lesion in idiopathic polyneuritis: Its role in pathogenesis. Medicine, 48:173, 1969.

163. Dyck, P.J., and Arnason, B.: Chronic inflammatory demyelinating polyradiculoneuropathy. In: *Peripheral Neuropathy II.* (Eds.) P.J. Dyck, et al.: Philadelphia, W.B. Saunders Co., 1984.

164. Luijten, J.A.F.M., Baart de la Faile-Kuyper, E.H.: The occurrence of IgM and complement factors along the myelin sheaths of peripheral nerves: An immunohistochemical study of the Guillain-Barre syndrome. J. Neurol. Sci., 15:219, 1972.

165. Prineas, J.W.: Acute idiopathic polyneuritis: An electron-microscope study. Lab. Invest., 26:133, 1972.

166. Madrid, R., Bradley, C.G., and Davis, D.J.F.: The peroneal muscular atrophy syndrome: Clinical, genetic, electrophysiological and nerve biopsy studies: Part 2. Observations and pathological changes in sural nerve biopsies. J. Neurol., Sci., 32:91, 1977.

167. Mitchell, G.W., Bosch, E.P., and Hart, M.N.: Response to immunosuppressive therapy on patients with hereditary motor and sensory neuropathy and associated dysimmune neuromuscular disorders. Eur. Neurol., 27:188, 1987.

168. Lampert, P.W.: Mechanism of demyelination in experimental allergic neuritis. Lab. Invest., 20:127, 1969.

169. Wisniewski, H., Prineas, J., and Raine, C.S.: An ultrastructural study of experimental demyelination and remyelination: Acute experimental allergic encephalomyelitis in the peripheral nervous system. Lab. Invest., 21:269, 1969.

170. Raine, S., and Bornstein, M.B.: Experimental allergic neuritis: Ultrastructure of serum induced myelin aberrations in peripheral nervous system cultures. Lab. Invest., 40:423, 1079.

171. Feasby, T.E., et al.: An Acute axonal form of Guillain-Barre polyneuropathy. Brain, 109:1115, 1986.

172. Cornblath, D.R., et al.: Inflammatory demyelinating

peripheral neuropathies associated with human T-cell lymphotropic virus type III infection. Ann. Neurol., 21:32, 1987.

173. Denny-Brown, D.: Primary sensory neuropathy with muscular changes associated with carcinoma. J. Neurol. Neurosurg. Psychiat., 11:73, 1948.

174. Wyburn-Masson, R.: Bronchial carcinoma presenting as polyneuritis. Lancet, 1:203, 1948.

175. Schlaepfer, W.W.: Axonal degeneration in the sural nerves of cancer patients. Cancer, 34:371, 1974.

176. Graus, F., Ferrer, I., and Lamarca, J.: Mixed carcinomatous neuropathy in patients with lung cancer and lymphoma. Acta Neurol. Scand., 68:40, 1983.

177. Lamarche, J., and Vital, C.: Carcinomatous neuropathy. An ultrastructural study of ten cases. Ann. Pathol., 7:98, 1987.

178. Ongerboer de Visser, B.W., Feltkamp Vroom, T.M., and Feltkamp, C.A.: Sural nerve immune deposits in polyneuropathy as a remote effect of malignancy. Ann. Neurol., 14:261, 1983.

179. Jacobs, J.M., and Le Quesne, P.: Toxic disorders of the nervous system. In: Greenfields' Neuropathology, 4th ed., (Eds.) J.H. Adams, J.A.N. Corsellis, and L.W. Duchen, London, Edward Arnold, 1984.

180. Ricoy, J.R., Cabello, A., Rodriguez, J., et al.: Neuropathological studies on the toxic syndrome related to adulterated rapeseed oil in Spain. Brain, 106:817, 1983.

181. Donofrio, P.D., et al.: Acute arsenic intoxication presenting as Guillain-Barre-like syndrome. Muscle & Nerve, 10:114, 1987.

182. Le Quesne, P.M.: Neuropathy due to drugs. In: Peripheral Neuropathy II. (Eds.) P.J. Dyck, et al.: Philadelphia, W.B. Saunders Co., 1984.

183. Bradley, W.G., Lassman, L.P., Pearce, G.W., et al.: The neuromyopathy of vincristine in man. J. Neurol. Sci., 10:107, 1970.

184. Vallat, J.M., et al.: Neuropathie peripherique a la vincristine: Etude ultrastructurale d'une biopsie du muscle et du nerf peripherique. Rev. Neurol., 129:365, 1973.

185. Wulfhekel, U., and Dullman, J.: Ein licht und elektronenophthischer: beitrag zur vinca alkaloid polyneuropathie. Virchows Arch. Abt. A. Pathol. Anat., 357:163, 1972.

186. Thant, M., et al.: Possible enhancement of vincristine neuropathy by VP-16, Cancer, 49:859, 1982.

187. Thompson, S.W., et al.: Cisplatin neuropathy. Clinical, electrophysiologic, morphologic, and toxicologic studies. Cancer, 54:1269, 1984.

188. Gastaut, J.L., and Pellissier, J.F.: Neuropathie au cisplatine. Etude clinique, electrophysiologique et morphologique. Rev. Neurol., 141:614, 1985.

189. Meier, C., Kauer, B., Muller, U., et al.: Neuromyopathy during chronic amiodarone treatment: A case report. J. Neurol. Sci., 63:251, 1984.

190. Pellissier, J.F., et al.: Peripheral neuropathy induced by amiodarone chlorhydrate. A clinico-pathological study. J. Neurol., Sc., 63:251, 1984.

191. Jacobs, J.M., and Costa-Jussa, F.R.: The pathology of amiodarone neurotoxicity II. Peripheral neuropathy in man. Brain, 108:753, 1985.

192. Mussini, J.M., Hauw, J.J., and Escourolle, R.: Etude en microscopie electronique des lesions nerveuses, musculaires et cutanees determinees par le maleate de perhexiline. Acta Neuropathol., 38:53, 1977.

193. Said, G.: Perhexiline neuropathy: A clinicopathological study. Ann. Neurol., 3:259, 1978.

194. Gherardi, R., Baudrimont, M., Gray, F., et al.: Almitrine neuropathy. A nerve biopsy study of 8 cases. Acta Neuropathol., 73:202, 1987.

195. Ochoa, J.: Isoniazid neuropathy in man: Quantitative electron microscope study. Brain, 93:831, 1970.

196. Schroder, J.M., and Gibbels, E.: Marklose nervenbasern im senium und im spatstadium der thalidomid-polyneuropathie: Quantitative elektronen-mikroskopiche untersuchungen. Acta Neuropathol., 39:271, 1977.

197. Bergouignan, F.X., Vital, C., Henry, P., et al.: Disulfiram neuropathy. J. Neurol., 235:382, 1988.

198. Pages, M., and Pages, A.M.: Lesions du nerf peripheral dans la neuromyopathie a la chloroquine, Ann. Pathol., 4:289, 1984.

199. Tegner, R., et al.: Morphological study of peripheral nerve changes induced by chloroquine treatment. Acta Neuropathol., 75:253, 1988.

200. Katrack, S.M., et al.: Clinical and morphological features of gold neuropathy. Brain, 103:671, 1980.

201. Kuncl, R.W., et al.: Colchicine myopathy and neuropathy. N. Engl. J. Med., 316:1562, 1987.

202. Dalakas, M.C.: Chronic idiopathic ataxic neuropathy. Ann. Neurol., 19:545, 1986.

203. Pietrini, V., et al.: Neuropathy in Tangier disease: A clinicopathologic study and a review of the literature. Acta Neurol., Scand., 72:495, 1985.

204. Dyck, P.J., Ellefson, R.D., Yao, J.K., et al.: Adult-onset of Tangier disease I. Morphometric and pathologic studies suggesting delayed degradation of neutral lipids after fiber degeneration. J. Neuropathol. Exp. Neurol., 37:119, 1978.

205. Yao, J.K., et al.: Peripheral neuropathy in Tangier disease. Brain, 106:911, 1983.

206. Pollock, P., et al.: Peripheral neuropathy in Tangier disease. Brain, 106:911, 1983.

207. Marbini, A., et al.: Tangier disease. A case with sensorimotor distal polyneuropathy and lipid accumulation in striated muscle and vasa nervorum. Acta Neuropathol., 67:121, 1985.

208. Gibbels, E.: Severe polyneuropathy in Tangier disease mimicking syringomyelia or leprosy. Clinical, biochemical, electrophysiological, and morphological evaluation, including electron microscopy of nerve, muscle, and skin biopsies. J. Neurol., 232:283, 1985.

209. Robitaille, Y., Carpenter, S., Karpati, G., et al.: A distinct form of adult polyglucosan body disease with massive involvement of central and peripheral neuronal processes and astrocytes. Brain, 103:315, 1980.

210. Vos, A.J.M., Joosten, E.M.G., and Gabreels-Festen, A.A.W.: Adult polyglucosan body disease: Clinical and nerve biopsy findings in two cases. Ann. Neurol., 13:440, 1983.

211. Mancardi, G.L., et al.: Polyglucosan bodies in the sural nerve of a diabetic patient with polyneuropathy. Acta Neuropathol., 66:83, 1985.

212. Dyck, P.J.: Inherited neuronal degeneration and atrophy affecting peripheral motor, sensory and autonomic neurons. In: Peripheral Neuropathy II. (Eds.) P.J. Dyck, et al. Philadelphia, W.B. Saunders Co., 1984.

213. Lapresle, J., and Salisachs, P.: Onion bulbs in a nerve biopsy specimen from an original case of Roussy-Levy disease. Arch. Neurol., 29:346, 1973.

214. Behse, F., and Buchthal, F.: Peroneal muscular atrophy and related disorders. Part 2., Histological findings. Ann. Neurol., 2:95, 1977.

215. Smith, T.W., Bhawan, J., Keller, R.B., et al.: Charcot-

Marie-Tooth disease associated with hypertrophic neuropathy: A neuropathologic study of two cases. J. Neuropath. Exp. Neurol., 39:420, 1980.

216. Nukada, H., Dyck, P.J., and Karnes, J.L.: Thin axons relative to myelin spiral length in hereditary motor and sensory neuropathy. type I. Ann. Neurol., 14:648, 1983.

217. Dyck, P.J.: Neuronal atrophy and degeneration predominantly affecting peripheral sensory and autonomic neurons. In: *Peripheral Neuropathy II.* (Eds.) P.J. Dyck, et al. Philadelphia, W.B. Saunders Co., 1984.

218. Guimaraes, A., Hauw, J.J., and Escourolle, R.: Etude quantitative et en microscopie electronique du nerf dans sept cas de neuropathie sensitive idiopathique sporadique. Acta Neuropathol., 46:133, 1979.

219. Behse, F., Buchthal, F., Carlsen, F., et al.: Hereditary neuropathy with liability to pressure palsies: Electrophysiological and histological aspects. Brain, 95:777, 1972.

220. Madrid, R., and Bradley, W.G.: The pathology of neuropathies with focal thickening of the myelin

sheath (tomaculous neuropathy): Studies on the formation of the abdominal myelin sheath. J. Neurol. Sci., 25:415, 1975.

221. Pellissier, J.F., et al.: Neuropathie tomaculaire. Etude histopathologique et correlations electrocliniques dans 10 cas. Rev. Neurol., 143:263, 1987.

222. Schaumburg, H.H., Spencer, P.S., and Ochoa, J.: The aging human peripheral nervous system. In: *The Neurology of Aging.* (Eds.) R. Katzman, and R.D. Terry. Philadelphia, F.A. Davis Co., 1983.

223. Vital, A., et al.: Morphological study of the aging human peripheral nerve. Clin. Neurophathol. 9:10, 1990.

224. Lascelles, R.G., and Thomas, P.K.: Changes due to age in internodal length in the sural nerve in man. J. Neurol. Neurosurg. Psychiat., 29:40, 1966.

225. Jacobs, J.M., and Love, S.: Qualitative and quantitative morphology of human sural nerve at different ages. Brain, 108:89, 1985.

226. Tohgi, H., Tsukagoshi, H., and Toyokura, Y.: Quantitative changes with age in normal sural nerves. Acta Neuropathol., 38:213, 1977.

17

Pathology of the Sympathetic Nervous System

ROBERT E. SCHMIDT

The mean age of the population of the United States is increasing steadily. The combination of the postwar baby boom, increased interest in preventative health measures, and improving medical technology are expected to triple the number of elderly people ($\geq$65 years old) in the next few years. Considering the public health significance of the problems of an aging populace and realizing that aging is a problem common to all races and cultures, surprisingly little is known of the effects of age on the nervous system, with the possible exception of the recently burgeoning field of Alzheimer's disease research.

The autonomic nervous system is charged with the maintenance and integration of visceral functions and is the substrate upon which more complex human behavior is based. Age-related autonomic nervous system dysfunction may result in clinical disease per se or may be subclinical, diminishing the safety factor upon which additional insults

may be superimposed, culminating eventually in functional autonomic neuropathy. The functional status of the autonomic nervous system, particularly its sympathetic component, may be challenged iatrogenically, for example, by sympatholytic antihypertensive drugs, to which the elderly may be unusually sensitive,[1] or by intensive insulin therapy for diabetes resulting in episodic hypoglycemia.

This review will focus on age-dependent pathologic condition in the sympathetic autonomic nervous system and on autonomic dysfunction in both experimental animals and humans. Much of the literature concerning this topic is contradictory and rarely involves corroboration with complementary methods. In this review I have attempted, when possible, to distill the flavor of the subject without its detail. In addition, the recent results of our systematic neuropathologic investigation of aging sympathetic autonomic ganglia in an autopsy series are discussed.

AGE-RELATED AUTONOMIC PATHOPHYSIOLOGY IN A CLINICAL SETTING

It is generally thought that autonomic nervous system function is impaired with age [2-6] in human subjects. Evidence, much of it subjective, has been accumulated for a variety of age-dependent autonomic dysfunctions; however, few areas of supposed autonomic dysfunction have undergone detailed investigation and, thus, the precise level of the central or peripheral nervous systems at which the various reflex paths are interrupted is generally unknown.

IMPAIRED THERMOREGULATION

Diminished vasoconstriction in response to experimental cooling has been reported in "normal" elderly and may result in abnormal thermoregulation.[6-8] Significant numbers of hospital admissions for hypothermia are reported in aged patients, often after minimal exposure to cold.[6] The potential central and peripheral nervous system sites at which thermoregulation may be interrupted are numerous and, at this time, the precise site of damage in aged subjects remains unknown.

CARDIOVASCULAR DYSFUNCTION

An increased incidence of orthostatic hypotension[2,9-13] and diminished beat to beat variation of heart rate (respiratory sinus arrhythmia[14,15]) has been reported in otherwise normal elderly subjects. In one large study of 494 patients of 65 years of age and older, fully 24% demonstrated a significant ($\geq$ 20 mm Hg) orthostatic decrease in blood pressure.[11] Other studies[16] have denied a high prevalence of orthostatic hypotension in the elderly. In one study[17] the increased prevalence of postural hypotension was ascribed to an age-associated increase in supine systolic blood pressure rather than to sympathetic hypofunction. The simple view of loss of postganglionic sympathetic neurons as an explanation for diminished postural control of blood pressure must be interpreted cautiously in the light of consistent findings that resting plasma norepinephrine concentration, a marker of baseline peripheral sympathetic tone, is increased in normal elderly[18-21] although diminished cardiac responsiveness to sympathetic stimulation has been reported.[5] In addition, the imposition of various stressors in a controlled laboratory setting typically results in the increased release of norepinephrine in the elderly suggesting a hyperadrenergic, not hypoadrenergic, response.[5,21-24]

In addition to the sympathetic ganglia and postganglionic nerves[18] other portions of the autonomic nervous system and its end-organs may also be involved in sympathetic nervous system dysfunction. For example, a given decrease in blood pressure results in a smaller increase in heart rate in the elderly, which is thought to reflect decreased baroreflex sensitivity to lower body negative pressure.[3] The response of the heart rate to the beta adrenergic agonist isoproterenol decreases with age which suggests abnormal postsynaptic sympathetic function.[25] Although the number of beta receptors on myocardial cells and lymphocytes is unaltered in the elderly, the agonist affinity of lymphocytic beta adrenergic receptors is reduced.[26] The pathophysiologic mechanism immediately underlying the abnormal postsynaptic adrenergic response is as yet unclear, however, the suggestion, often disputed, is made that diminished adrenergic receptor number with age is the result of, rather than the cause of, increased circulating norepinephrine levels.[12] The adrenal medulla, which contributes to the maintenance of blood pressure, does not show a consistent increase or decrease in activity in the normal aging population.[27]

In summary, evidence has accumulated to establish that regulation of cardiovascular reflexes is abnormal in aging subjects; however, it would appear that regulation and integration of sympathetic cardiovascular function are affected to a greater degree than simple loss of postsynaptic sympathetic neurons.

GASTROINTESTINAL COMPLAINTS

Alimentary dysfunction, frequently chronic constipation complicated by laxative abuse, represents a common complaint of the aged[6,28,29] and may reflect a variety of involved sites and several potential mechanisms (see[28,30] for review). Esophageal manometry has identified evidence of disordered motility including increased numbers of nonpropulsive contractions as well as diminished amplitude and duration of contractions. Small bowel motility is the least thoroughly studied of the alimentary age-related abnormalities probably as a result of the degree of invasiveness and cooperation required for testing. The migrating motor complex (MMC), an electrophysiologic monitor of small bowel motility, is replaced immediately after meals by frequent intermittent contractions which are followed by the return of the MMC 4 to 6 hours later.[31] Healthy elderly (although all were female in one study[31]) show no abnormality of baseline motility index, frequency, mean amplitude, or velocity of propulsion of selected phases of peristalsis; however, after a meal the motility index and frequency of contractions were decreased in otherwise normal elderly compared to healthy young adults.[29,31] Gastrointestinal symptoms were not described in any of these patients. In one large series of elderly patients admitted for a variety of medical emergencies 27% exhibited "major gastrointestinal dysfunction" prompting the claim that lesions of the digestive system are an important cause of morbidity and mortality in the elderly.[28] The frequent complaint of chronic constipation in the elderly is a well-recognized, if poorly documented, complaint. There is little objective data on this subject, its definition and incidence, and some studies which contradict this stereotype suggest that the problem may be overstated. Although available data suggest autonomic dysfunction is common in the aging alimentary tract, no definitive data establish the problem as sympathetic in origin. Such observations on alimentary dysfunction in aging subjects, however, lay the groundwork for correlation of abnormalities of alimentary function with neuropathologic findings in human and experimental animal studies.

The human sympathetic nervous system does not lend itself easily to detailed biochemical and neuropathologic analysis in living subjects using acceptably non-invasive methods. Therefore, in order to characterize age-related autonomic nervous system alterations, a variety of studies of aged experimental animals have been employed to determine the nature of age-related neuropathologic histologic findings in the sympathetic nervous system and to identify possible anatomic sites for analysis in humans, with the long range goal of developing and testing pathogenetic mechanisms underlying the development of age-dependent sympathetic autonomic neuropathy.

BIOCHEMICAL AND PHYSIOLOGIC STUDIES OF THE AGING SYMPATHETIC NERVOUS SYSTEM OF EXPERIMENTAL ANIMALS

Diminished sympathetic function has been demonstrated in aging rats. A decrease in heart rate and mean arterial blood pressure has been reported in aged (24 to 33 months) rats.[32] The reported decrease in norepinephrine in renal,[33] carotid,[34] and femoral[33] arteries, aorta,[34] spleen,[35,36] heart,[37] and small bowel[38] appeared consistent with a generalized decrease in sympathetic innervation of endorgans in the aged rat. However, study of additional vascular beds in the same animals showed that the result was not consistent from one vascular territory to another or from one laboratory to another, showing no change or, even an increase, in the norepinephrine content of superior mesenteric,[33,39] renal,[39] coronary,[34] and carotid[33] arteries, portal, mesenteric and renal veins,[39] heart,[34] and iris.[38] Examination of endorgan NE turnover is typically a better indicator of sympathetic activity than absolute endorgan NE content. Male rats failed to show an age related decrease in NE turnover in heart, liver, kidney, spleen, or pancreas.[40,41] Tyramine administration, which releases endogenous norepinephrine from the noradrenergic sympathetic nerve terminal stores, resulted in a decreased amount of cardiac NE released in aged rat heart,[42] which, however, may relate to prejunctional neuronal uptake mechanisms[42] rather than to the simple release of NE. Sympathetic nervous system function is dependent on endorgan response to NE and signal transduction as well as on the noradrenergic neuron itself. Claims for age related dysfunction in receptor metabolism have been described including decrease in pineal beta adrenergic receptors[43,44] but not those in myocardium, lung, and lymphocytes.[45] In summary no single theme characterizes the distribution of changes in norepinephrine content, turnover, or receptor metabolism from endorgan to endorgan in aging rats. Some results may differ due to the differences in biochemical or histochemical methods of measurement, however, in most cases the disparity remains unexplained.

In some cases baseline sympathetic functions are well maintained in aged animals, however, superimposition of additional stresses results in dysfunction as though a threshold has been exceeded. Immersion stress of aged Fischer 344 rats induced an abnormal sympathoadrenal response which developed more slowly but continued for a longer interval than in younger adults.[46] Reserpine-induced depletion of catecholamines was followed by resynthesis which lagged behind in aged animals.[47,48] The increase in beta adrenergic receptor number induced by reserpine administration was markedly blunted in aged rats.[43] Fasting decreased NE turnover in selected endorgans of young rats but not in aged animals suggesting abnormal integration of sympathoadrenal function.[40] Immobilization stress failed to increase heart rate and blood pressure in elderly rats compared to young rats.[49] Mechanical or toxin-induced damage to the terminal portion of postganglionic noradrenergic sympathetic axons is followed by terminal axonal sprouting and regeneration, a response which is decreased progressively as rats age (from 3 to 30 months),[50] particularly in males.[51] Sympathetic ganglia explanted to culture responded by increasing the substance P content of principal sympathetic neurons.[52] This alteration, which has an uncertain role in the ganglionic response to injury, is absent in explanted sympathetic ganglia of aged rats[52] suggesting decreased plasticity. This series of observations suggests that the aged sympathetic nervous system may be able to maintain baseline or resting autonomic functions but has little residual capacity when subjected to additional stressors. Superimposition of diabetes, for instance, on a borderline sympathetic reserve might exceed the threshold resulting in clinical dysfunction.

Various biochemical measurements have been used in the sympathetic ganglia of aging animals as monitors of ganglionic health. Formaldehyde induced fluorescence, which is a measure of norepinephrine content, is markedly decreased in aged rat hypogastric[53] and celiac/superior mesenteric ganglia (C/SMG) but not in superior cervical ganglion (SCG).[48,54–55] However, surprisingly, in most studies the activity of tyrosine hydroxylase, the rate limiting enzyme in norepinephrine biosynthesis, does not diminish with age in C/SMG or in other selected tissues;[47] conversely, in the rat SCG and adrenal, TOH activity actually increased substantially with age.[47,56,57] The activity of dopamine-beta-hyroxylase (DBH), another major enzyme in the norepinephrine biosynthetic pathway, shows little alteration in activity in sympathetic ganglia with increasing age.[47,56,57] Thus, the biosynthetic machinery for norepinephrine synthesis is present in neurons which purportedly lack perikaryal NE. These apparently conflicting findings are currently unresolved, but provide little support for major biochemical disruption of aged sympathetic autonomic ganglia.

The activity of choline acetyltransferase, an enzyme generally localized to presynaptic cholinergic elements in sympathetic ganglia, is variously reported as increased[47,57] or decreased[56] in aged rat SCG. The content of met-enkephalin, a presynaptic inhibitory neurotransmitter in sympathetic ganglia, has been reported to decrease 60% in the celiac and SCG of aged rats.[58] The few metabolic studies in aged rat sympathetic ganglia suggest a 30 to 40% increase in glucose utilization of paravertebral and prevertebral sympathetic ganglia;[32] conversely, studies of succinate dehydrogenase, an important enzyme involved in oxidative phosphorylation, have shown a decrease in the aged sympathetic nervous system.[59]

SUMMARY

A large number of biochemical, pharmacologic and physiologic observations have been made in aged humans and experimental animals, chiefly rats, suggesting a variety of abnormalities in sympathetic nervous system function with age but without the emergence of a single consistent theme. In most studies there has not been a concerted effort to develop a step by step investigation intended to identify and test pathogenetic mechanisms of sympathetic nervous system damage. Much of the work is mutually contradictory usually without an attempt being made to resolve the possible misinterpretations of the various disparate findings. It is necessary to recognize that the sympathetic nervous system is not homogeneous and the separation of pre- and paravertebral ganglia and their functions are necessary. It is, however, clear that a large number of observations of dysfunction have been made in aged humans and experimental animals sufficient to merit detailed investigation of possible underlying pathology in the various sympathetic ganglia, an area which has previously been neglected.

NEUROPATHOLOGIC ALTERATIONS IN THE SYMPATHETIC NERVOUS SYSTEM OF AGED EXPERIMENTAL ANIMALS

Although comparative neuron counts between various sympathetic ganglia of selected ages are generally not available, the neuronal packing density, a coarse measure of neuron number, is reported to decrease between 6 and 24 months in rat C/SMG.[32,60] In aging rat SCG significant neuron loss was reported to develop only after 18 months of age[60] or not to develop at all to 30 to 33 months.[32]

The structural alterations described in most previous studies of aging animal sympathetic ganglia are heterogeneous, sometimes subtle, and may be of uncertain pathologic significance. Neuronal cell bodies have been reported to: (1) contain distended perikaryal mitochondria,[54] (2) show disarrangement, irregularity, and dilatation of the rough endoplasmic reticulum and Golgi,[54] (3) accumulate axonal "residual bodies",[54] and (4) show increased somal area.[60]

Presynaptic elements represent a potential substrate for plasticity in the nervous system and alterations in this function may represent a significant mechanism for autonomic dysfunction. The number of axosomatic synaptic junctions/neuron and the average axon diameter increased approximately 50% from 6-month-old rat to 30-month-old rat.[61] Synaptic rearrangement of presynaptic elements has been examined in the dendrites in the SCG of living mice by examining the same vital-dye stained neuron at several intervals.[62] Dendritic length and complexity increased with age, suggesting dendritic remodeling with terminal elongation and retraction.[62]

In a study of aging rats in our laboratory,[63] we identified distinctive axonal abnormalities involving presynaptic terminal elements in selected sympathetic ganglia of male and female Sprague-Dawley and male Fischer 344 rats as a function of increasing age. Markedly dilated preterminal axons and synapses contained a variety of unusual subcellular organelles (tubulovesicular elements, paracrystalline membranous aggregates, tubular rings, layered loops, normal and degenerating subcellular organelles and neurofilaments) identical to the appearance of neuroaxonal dystrophy as seen in a variety of human inherited and metabolic diseases. Dystrophic axons were located immediately adjacent to the perikarya and primary dendrites of principal sympathetic neurons. Neuroaxonal dystrophy was infrequent within the first year of life, but increased rapidly afterwards. Although the prevertebral celiac and superior mesenteric ganglia developed lesions with age, the paravertebral superior cervical ganglia of the same animals showed approximately 10-fold fewer lesions. Extrapolation of these investigations to 12 to 15-month-old Chinese hamsters[64] and to aged 24-month-old mice (unpublished findings) have shown generally comparable results. Examination of subpopulations of presynaptic elements in Chinese hamster C/SMG using neuropeptide immunohistochemistry provided evidence for the selective involvement of subpopulations of presynaptic elements. Dystrophic preterminal axons and synapses contained substance P and gastrin releasing peptide (GRP/bombesin) in aged control hamsters and particularly in aged diabetics. Neuroaxonal dystrophy did not involve other subpopulations of presynaptic elements (VIP, met-enkephalin, Dynorphin-B).

Neuroaxonal dystrophy develops in aging sympathetic ganglia as well as in several other non-sympathetic sites (chiefly sensory terminals in the gracile and cuneate nuclei of the medulla,[65]) as a function of age in humans and in a variety of experimental animals (see [66] for review), suggesting the general sensitivity of terminal axons to the aging process. The long-held contention, for which there is little experimental confirmation, is that neuroaxonal dystrophy is the morphologic equivalent of aberrant synaptic remodeling,[67] an extension of the normal process of synaptic turnover and regeneration.[68,69] Terminal portions of many types of axons show ongoing cycles of degeneration and regeneration.[69] It is known, for example, that neuromuscular junction size, complexity and tortuosity increases with age in the rat.[70–72] These processes, which appear to represent some of the more consistent features of synaptic metabolism, may underlie synaptic plasticity in many sites.[69,73]

Auerbach's myenteric ganglia, one site of peripheral projection of sympathetic C/SMG, are reported to lose 40 to 60% of their neurons from 6 to 24 months of age.[74] The density of noradrenergic nerve terminals in the intrinsic myenteric ganglia showed a 75% decrease in number between 12 and 18 months of age.[38] The frequency of varicosities along the course of the axon, the sites of neurotransmitter release, diminished significantly over that time.[38] Loss of neurons in the Auerbach's myenteric alimentary ganglia might affect the neurons giving rise to its noradrenergic innervations, which are located in the C/SMG, as a retrograde transneuronal event. The decreased small bowel transit time reported in aged rats bears an uncertain, if any, relationship to noradrenergic gut innervation[75] but may reflect loss of intrinsic myenteric neurons. Extensive degeneration of sympathetic nerves in the cardiac atria, characterized by vacuolation of nerve terminals and empty mitochondria, were reported in rats beginning at 12 months of age and increasing in frequency to 24 months of age.[42] Degenerating and regenerating but not dystrophic sympathetic axons have been described in the heart[42,76] and ciliary muscle[73] of otherwise normal aging animals.

The results of animal studies have been valuable in identifying the type and distribution of neuroaxonal dystrophy in normal aging. Our subsequent human studies, detailed in the next section, represent the direct extrapolation of these findings to human subjects.

NEUROPATHOLOGIC ALTERATIONS IN THE AGING HUMAN SYMPATHETIC NERVOUS SYSTEM

An early study by Kuntz[77] described increased arborization of dendrites, short dendrites ending in club-shaped enlargement and some decrease in nuclear size and amount of Nissl substance in aged human sympathetic ganglia. Other early studies claimed a decrease in sympathetic neuron numbers[78,79] or size[79] or ongoing degeneration involving the majority of celiac ganglion neurons.[79] An increase in neuronal pigment(s),[80–85] consisting of lipofuscin and neuromelanin, was a consistent finding in aging sympathetic ganglia. A number of studies of paravertebral sympathetic "chain" ganglia removed surgically for vascular insufficiency exhibit diminished formaldehyde induced catecholamine fluorescence;[80,84,85] hypertrophy of dendritic processes;[80] neuroaxonal dystrophy;[80] mitochondria filled axonal swellings admixed with neurofilaments, glycogen and dense core vesicles;[86] laminar or "myelin" bodies;[82,87] and mitochondrial inclusions.[82] Neuronal perikarya contained filamentous bundles,[80] mitochondrial accumulation and a variety of inclusion bodies.[80] Interestingly, in one study 2 patients with Alzheimer's disease were claimed to show cytoskeletal elements which resembled neurofibrillary tangles.[80,87] An apparent decrease in preganglionic sympathetic neurons located in the intermediolateral column was described in aged patients.[88] A series of 23 patients 22 to 98 years old showed no decrease in packing density or neuronal dimensions in the paravertebral ganglia,[89] although there was a decrease in the proportion of neurons innervated by preganglionic enkephalin containing elements suggesting preferential involvement of subpopulations of sympathetic neurons within selected sympathetic ganglia. Segmental demyelination and Wallerian degeneration of myelinated axons have been described in aging human sympathetic paravertebral ganglia,[6] presumably involving preganglionic projections.

Previous studies of human aged sympa-

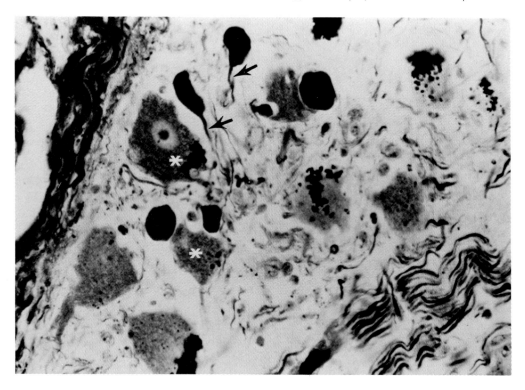

Fig. 17–1.   Light microscopic appearance of neuroaxonal dystrophy in aged human superior mesenteric ganglion. Multiple large dystrophic axons arise from axons of normal dimensions (arrows) and are located immediately adjacent to principal sympathetic neurons (*). Multiple dystrophic axons often cluster around individual perikarya. (magnification 800×)

thetic ganglia have: (1) concentrated on pathologically subtle "lesions", some questionably artifactual or of uncertain pathologic significance, (2) used qualitative methods alone often without application of corroborative techniques, (3) failed to address the possible contribution of age-related disease processes, patient sex and race, and (4) did not examine both prevertebral and paravertebral sympathetic ganglia, which respond differentially to a variety of insults.[90]

In order to address these deficiencies, we have systematically examined the prevertebral superior mesenteric (SMG) and paravertebral superior cervical (SCG) sympathetic ganglia of an autopsy series of 56 non-diabetic adults (> 15 years old) selected irrespective of underlying chronic disease(s) or cause of death. None of the patients had clinically documented autonomic neuropathy.

Routine hematoxylin and eosin stained SMG of aged patients showed variable numbers of spherical structures which were located immediately adjacent to the perikarya of principal sympathetic neurons or within the adjacent neuropil. These axonal lesions were not accompanied by significant neuron loss or ongoing perikaryal degeneration. Silver stains confirmed the presence of markedly swollen axons (5 to 30 μm in diameter) with a filamentous agyrophilic content and, frequently, focal origin from the terminal portion of an otherwise normal axon (Fig. 17–1, arrows) immediately adjacent to principal sympathetic neurons (*, Fig. 17–1). Multiple swollen axons often clustered around the circumference of individual neuronal perikarya. Lesions were never found to originate directly from primary dendrites or recurrent axons. Ultrastructural studies (Fig. 17–2 A to C) showed displacement of perikarya by swollen axons containing a central sheaf of disoriented neurofilaments surrounded by a subaxolemmal collection of marginated dense core granules. Other axons

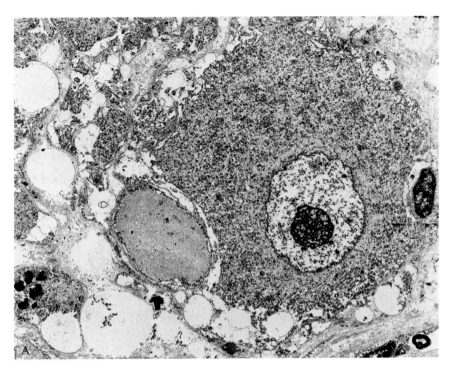

Fig. 17-2.   Ultrastructural appearance of neuroaxonal dystrophy in aging human superior mesenteric ganglion. A dystrophic axon immediately adjacent to the perikaryon of principal sympathetic neuron contains large numbers of neurofilaments. (magnification 3100×)

had the more classical ultrastructural appearance of neuroaxonal dystrophy, a distinctive type of axonal injury which characterizes aging rat sympathetic ganglia. Immunohistochemical localization of neuropeptide in presynaptic elements demonstrated the selective involvement of subpopulations of axons, specifically those containing neuropeptide tyrosine (NPY) while sparing those containing a variety of other neuropeptides (VIP, substance P and gastrin releasing peptide/bombesin). Many of the dystrophic swellings also stained for tyrosine hydroxylase, identifying them as likely projections from other sympathetic neurons. Since neuroaxonal dystrophy was not exclusively limited to the SMG of aged patients but could be found in qualitatively smaller numbers in younger subjects, it was necessary to quantitate the numbers of lesions in individual patients. We found that lesions were infrequent in patients before the age of 60 and were

increased in frequency thereafter. Detailed statistical analysis failed to document a disease state which explained the frequency of NAD independent of an age effect, although we had intentionally separated diabetic patients from the remaining subjects at the outset of this study. Statistical analysis demonstrated that older men had nearly twice as many lesions as women of the same age. As in experimental animals, the same patients whose superior mesenteric ganglia were markedly involved by neuroaxonal dystrophy showed minimal numbers of lesions in the superior cervical ganglia.

SUMMARY

Examination of aging rat, hamster, mouse and, most recently, human subjects have shown that neuroaxonal dystrophy of presynaptic elements is a reproducible neuropathologic hallmark of aging in the sympathetic autonomic nervous system. In addition, immu-

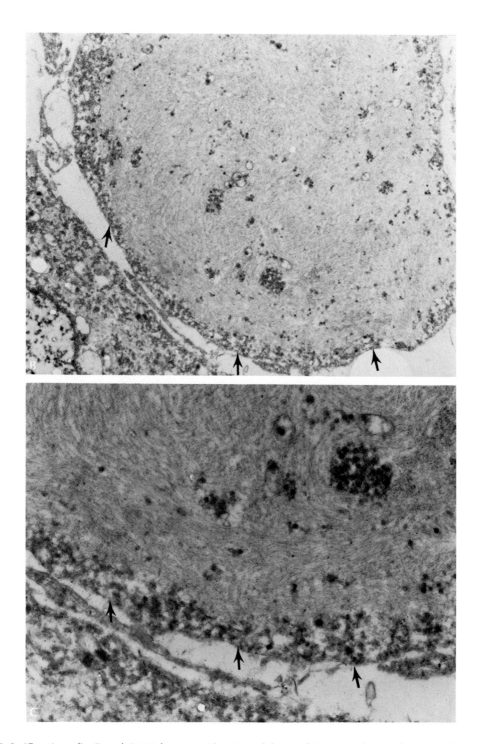

Fig. 17–2. *(Continued)*   B and C, Higher magnification of dystrophic axons shows a large number of dense core vesicles which form peripheral subaxolemmal halos (arrows). (magnification: B, 9300X; C, 25,500×)

nohistochemical localization of neuropeptides in presynaptic elements has shown that certain subpopulations of sympathetic terminals are affected in the presence of other uninvolved subpopulations. This observation argues against a diffuse field effect, ganglionic ischemia for instance, involving all intraganglionic terminals. The histologic resemblance between dystrophic alterations involving aging synapses and the neuritic elements of senile plaques of Alzheimer's disease may suggest potential shared pathogenetic mechanisms. Such terminal pathologic conditions may have significant, protean functional consequences, particularly for integrated nervous function. The selective involvement of subpopulations of axons might be expected to have more significant consequences than expected for loss of only a small percentage of the total number of synapses. The difficulty with which the aged nervous system responds to forced regeneration in a variety of animal systems suggests plasticity related synaptic remodeling could represent a preferential, highly susceptible target of the aging process. Understanding synaptic turnover and its frustration may have far ranging significance for understanding some of the most complex and critical processes in the peripheral and central nervous systems. Remodeling of terminal axons and synaptic sites is a common theme in neurobiology and we may be able to offer new insights into its pathogenesis using the age-related alterations in sympathetic autonomic ganglia.

REFERENCES

1. Heinsimer, J.A. and Lefkowitz, R.J.: The impact of aging on adrenergic receptor function: Clinical and Biochemical Aspects. J. Am. Geriatr. Soc. 33:184, 1985.
2. Vargas E. and Lye M.: The assessment of autonomic function in the elderly. Age Aging 9:210, 1980.
3. Collins K.J., Exton-Smith A.N., James, M.H. et al.: Functional changes in autonomic nervous responses with aging. Age Aging 9:17, 1980.
4. Christensen, N.J.: Sympathetic nervous activity and age. Eur. J. Clin. Invest. 12:91, 1982.
5. Rowe J.W. and Troen, B.R.: Sympathetic nervous system and aging in man. Endocrine Rev. 1:167, 1980.
6. Brocklehurst, J.C.: Ageing in the autonomic nervous system. Age Aging 4(Suppl):7, 1974.
7. Gorgy et al: Vasomotor tone in the aged. Arch. Neurol. 29:439, 1973.
8. Collins, K.J. et al.: Accidental hypothermia and impaired temperature homeostasis in the elderly. Br. Med. J. 1:353, 1977.
9. Wollner, L.: Postural hypotension in the elderly. Age Aging 7(Suppl.):112, 1978.
10. Johnson, R.H. et al: Effect of posture on blood-pressure in elderly patients. Lancet 1:731, 1965.
11. Caird, F.I., Andrews, G.R., and Kennedy, R.D.: Effect of posture on blood pressure in the elderly. Br. Heart J. 35:527, 1973.
12. Linares O.A. and Halter, J.B.: Sympathochromaffin system activity in the elderly. J. Am. Geriatr. Soc. 35:448, 1987.
13. Lipsitz, L.A.: Orthostatic hypotension in the elderly. N. Engl. J. Med. 321:952, 1989.
14. Hellman, J.B. and Stacy, R.W.: Variation of respiratory sinus arrhythmia with age. J Appl. Physiol. 41:734, 1976.
15. Davies, H.E.F.: Respiratory change in heart rate, sinus arrhythmia in the elderly. Geront. Clin. 17:96, 1975.
16. Mader, S.L., Josephson, K.R., and Rubenstein, L.Z.: Low prevalence of postural hypotension among community-dwelling elderly. JAMA 258:1511, 1987.
17. Harris, T., et al.: Is age or level of systolic blood pressure related to positional blood pressure change? Gerontologist 26 Suppl.:59 (abst.), 1986.
18. Pfeifer, M.A. et al.: Differential changes of autonomic nervous system function with age in man. Am. J. Med. 75: 249, 1983.
19. Ziegler, M.G., Lake, C.R., and Kopin, I.J.: Plasma noradrenaline increases with age. Nature 261:333, 1976.
20. Rubin, P.C., Scott, P.J.W., McLean, K., et al: Noradrenaline release and clearance in relation to age and blood pressure in man. Eur. J. Clin. Invest. 12:121, 1982.
21. Barnes, R.F., Raskind, M., Gumbrecht, G., et al: The effects of age on the plasma catecholamine response to mental stress in man. J. Clin. Endo. Metab. 54:64, 1982.
22. Young, J.B., et al.: Enhanced plasma norepinephrine response to upright posture and oral glucose administration in elderly human subjects. Metabolism 29:532, 1980.
23. Palmer, G.J., Ziegler, M.G., and Lake, C.R.: Response of norepinephrine and blood pressure to stress increases with age. J. Gerontol 33:482, 1978.
24. Liorica, V.: Plasma norepinephrine levels of elderly men on a controlled sodium intake diet. J. Am. Geriatr. Soc. 32:576, 1984.
25. Lakatta, E.G.: Age-related alterations in the cardiovascular response to adrenergic mediated stress. Fed. Proc. 39:3173, 1980.
26. Feldman, R.D.: Alterations in leukocyte beta-receptor affinity with aging: A potential explanation for altered beta-adrenergic sensitivity in the elderly. N. Engl. J. Med. 310:815, 1984.
27. Hill, T.J., et al.: Effect of age on epinephrine kinetics in humans. Clin. Res. 34:1000 (Abst.), 1986.
28. Geboes, K. and Bossaert, H.: Gastrointestinal disorders in old age. Age Ageing 6:197, 1977.
29. Anuras S and Loening–Baucke V.: Gastrointestinal motility in the elderly. J. Am. Geriatric Soc. 32:386, 1984.
30. Texter, E.C. (ed.): The aging gut Pathophysiology, Diagnosis and Management. New York, Masson Publishing USA, 1983.
31. Anuras, S. and Sutherland, J.: Small intestinal manometry in healthy elderly subjects. J. Am. Geriatr. Soc. 32:581, 1984.
32. Partanen, M., London, E.D., and Rapoport, S.I.: Glucose ultilization in sympathetic ganglia of male Fi-

scher-344 rats at different ages. J. Auton. Nerv. Syst. 5:391, 1982.

33. Dhall, V., Cowen, T., Haven, A.J., et al: Perivascular noradrenergic and peptide-containing nerves show different patterns of changes during development and ageing in the guinea pig. J. Auton. Nerv. Syst. 16:109, 1986.

34. Santer, R.M.: Fluorescence histochemical observations on the adrenergic innervation of the cardiovascular system in the aged rat. Brain Res. Bull. 9:667, 1982.

35. Martinez, J.L., et al.: Age-related changes in the catecholamine content of peripheral organs in male and female F344 rats. J.Gerontol. 36:280, 1981.

36. Felten, S.Y., et al.: Decreased sympathetic innervation of spleen in aged Fischer 344 rats. Neurobiol. Aging 8:159, 1987.

37. Frolkis, V.V., et al.: Catecholamines in the metabolism and functions regulation in aging. Gerontologia 16:129, 1970.

38. Baker, D.M. and Santer, R.M.: A quantitative study of the effects of age on the noradrenergic innervation of Auerbach's plexus in the rat. Mech. Ageing Devel. 42:147, 1988.

39. Mione, M.C., et al.: Age-related changes of noradrenergic innervation of rat splanchnic blood vessels: A histofluorescence and neurochemical study. J. Auton. Nerv. Syst. 25:27, 1988.

40. Rapoport, E.B., Young, J.B., and Landsberg, L.: Impact of age on basal and diet induced changes in sympathetic nervous system activity of Fischer rats. J. Gerontol 36:152, 1981.

41. Avakian, E.V. and Horvath, S.M.: Influence of aging and tyrosine hydroxylase inhibition on tissue levels of norepinephrine during stress. J. Gerontol. 37:257, 1982.

42. Goldberg, P.B., Kreider, M.S., McLean, M.R., et al.: Effects of aging at the adrenergic cardiac neuroeffector junction. Federation Proc. 45:45, 1986.

43. Weiss, B., Greenberg, L., and Cantor, E.: Age-related alterations in the development of adrenergic denervation supersensitivity. Federation Proc. 38:1915, 1979.

44. Greenberg, L.H.: Regulation of brain adrenergic receptors during aging. Federation Proc. 45:55, 1986.

45. Scarpace, P.J.: Decreased beta-adrenergic responsiveness during senescence. Federation Proc. 45:51, 1986.

46. McCarty, R.: Sympathetic-adrenal medullary and cardiovascular responses to acute cold stress in adult and aged rats. J. Auton. Nerv. Syst. 12:15, 1985.

47. Partanen, M., Waller, S.B., London, E.D., and Hervonen, A.: Indices of neurotransmitter synthesis and release in aging sympathetic nervous system. Neurobiol. Aging 6:227, 1985.

48. Santer, R.M.: Fluorescence histochemical evidence for decreased noradrenaline synthesis in sympathetic neurones of aged rats. Neurosci. Lett. 15:177, 1979.

49. Chiueh, C.C., Nespor, S.M., and Rapoport, S.I.: Cardiovascular, sympathetic and adrenal cortical responsiveness of aged Fischer-344 rats to stress. Neurobiol. Aging 1:157, 1980.

50. Scheff, S.W., Bernardo, L.S., and Cotman, C.W.: Decrease in adrenergic axon sprouting in the senescent rat. Science 202:775, 1978.

51. Milner, T.A. and Loy, R: Interaction of age and sex in sympathetic axon ingrowth into the hippocampus following septal afferent damage. Anat. Embryol. 161:159, 1980.

52. Adler, J.E., and Black, I.B.: Plasticity of substance P in

mature and aged sympathetic neurons in cultures. Science 225:1499, 1984.

53. Partanen, M., Santer, R.M., and Hervonen, A.: The effect of ageing on the histochemically demonstrable catecholamines in the hypogastric (main pelvic) ganglion of the rat. Histochem. J. 12, 527, 1980.

54. Santer, R.M., Partanen, M., and Hervonen, A.: Glyoxylic acid fluorescnece and ultrastructural studies of neurones in the coeliac-superior mesenteric ganglion of the aged rat. Cell Tissue Res. 211:475, 1980.

55. Hervonen, A., et al.: The sympathetic neuron as a model of neuronal aging. Neurohistochemistry: Modern Methods and Applications. (Eds.) Panula, P., Paivarinta, H., and Soinila, S. New York, Alan R. Liss, 1986, 569–586.

56. Giacobini, E.: Aging of autonomic synapses. Adv. Cell. Neurobiol. 3:173, 1982.

57. Reis, D.J., Ross, R.A., and Joh, T.H.: Changes in the activity and amounts of enzymes synthesizing catecholamines and acetylcholine in brain, adrenal medulla, and sympathetic ganglia of aged rat and mouse. Brain Res. 136:465, 1977.

58. Govoni, S., et al.: Decreased content of met-enkephalin-like peptides in superior cervical and coeliac ganglia of aged rats. Neurobiol. Aging 4:147, 1983.

59. Baker, D.M. and Santer, R.M.: Quantitative succinate dehydrogenase activity of prevertebral sympathetic neurons: variations with age. J. Anat. 146:252 (Abst.), 1986.

60. Baker, D.M. and Santer, R.M.: Morphometric studies on pre- and paravertebral sympathetic neurons in the rat: Changes with age. Mech. Age Devel. 42:139, 1988.

61. Kokabadze, S.A. and Teplyakova, N.P.: Ultrastructure of axosomatic junctions on neurons of the rat sensomotor cortex and celiac ganglia from the age aspect. Bull. Exp. Biol. Med. 91:395, 1981.

62. Purves, D., Hadley, R.D., and Voyvodic, J.T.: Dynamic changes in the dendritic geometry of individual neurons visualized over periods of up to three months in the superior cervical ganglion of living mice. J. Neurosci. 6:1051, 1986.

63. Schmidt, R.E., Plurad, S.B., and Modert, C.W.: Neuroaxonal dystrophy in the autonomic ganglia of aged rats. J. Neuropathol. Exp. Neurol. 42:376, 1983.

64. Schmidt, R.E., et al.: Ultrastructural and immunohistochemical characterization of autonomic neuropathy in genetically diabetic Chinese hamsters. Lab. Invest. 61:77, 1989.

65. Fujisawa, K. and Shiraki, H.: Study of axonal dystrophy. I. Pathology of the neuropil of the gracile and cuneate nuclei in ageing and old rats: a stereological study. Neuropathol. Appl. Neurobiol. 4:1, 1978.

66. Jellinger, K.: Neuroaxonal dystrophy: Its natural history and related disorders. Prog. Neuropathol. 36:129, 1973.

67. Sotelo, C. and Palay, S.L.: Altered axons and axon terminals in the lateral vestibular nucleus of the rat. Possible example of axonal remodeling. Lab. Invest.25:653, 1971.

68. Barker, P. and Ip, M.C.: Sprouting and degeneration of mammalian motor axons in normal and deafferented skeletal muscle. Proc. Roy. Soc. Lond., Ser. B 163:538, 1966.

69. Cotman, C.W., Nieto-Sampedro, M., and Harris, E.W.: Synapse replacement in the nervous system of adult vertebrates. Physiol. Rev. 61:684, 1981.

70. Fagg, G.E., Scheff, S.W., and Cotman, C.W.: Axonal

sprouting of the neuromuscular junction of adult and aged rats. Exp. Neurol. 74:847, 1981.

71. Gutmann, E., Hanzlikova, V., and Jakoubek, B.: Changes in the neuromuscular system during old age. Exp. Gerontol. 3:141, 1968.

72. Robbins, N. and Fahim, M.A.: Progression of age changes in mature mouse motor nerve terminals and its relation to locomotor activity. J. Neurocytol. 14:1019, 1985.

73. Townes-Anderson, E. and Raviola, G.: Degeneration and regeneration of autonomic nerve endings in the anterior part of rhesus monkey ciliary muscle. J. Neurocytol. 7:583, 1978.

74. Santer, R.M. and Baker, D.M.: Enteric neuron numbers and sizes in Auerbach's plexus in the small and large intestine of adult and aged rats. J Auton. Nerv. Syst. 25:59, 1988.

75. Varga, F.: Transit time changes with age in the gastrointestinal tract of the rat. Digestion 14:319, 1976.

76. McLean, M.R., Goldberg, P.B., and Roberts, J.: An ultrastructural study of the effects of age on sympathetic innervation and atrial tissue in the rat. J. Mol. Cell. Cardiol. 15:75, 1983.

77. Kuntz, A.: Histological variation in autonomic ganglia and ganglion cells associated with age and disease. Am. J. Pathol. 14:783, 1938.

78. Amprino, R.: Modifications de la structure des neurons sympathetiques pendant l'accrousement et la senescence recherches sur le ganglion cervical superior. C.R. Assoc. Anat. 33:3, 1938.

79. Botar, J.: Qualitative und quantitative untersuchung der nervenzellen des ganglion coeliacum im alter. Alterserscheinungen der sympathischen nervenzellen. Acta Anat. 28:157, 1956.

80. Hervonen, A.: Age related neuropathological changes in human sympathetic ganglia. Soc. Neurosci. Abst. 10:451, 1984.

81. Koistinaho, J., Sorvaniemi, M., Alho, H., et al.: Microspectrofluorometric quantitation of autofluorescent lipopigment in the human sympathetic ganglia. Mech. Ageing Devel. 37:79, 1986.

82. Hopfner, C., Caulet, T., and Adnet, J.J.: Etude ultrastructurale du neurone sympathique de l'homme age. Virchows Arch. Abt. B Zellpath. 5:326, 1970.

83. Hervonen, A., et al.: Age related heterogeneity of lipopigments in human sympathetic ganglia. Mech. Ageing Devel. 35:17, 1986.

84. Hervonen, A., et al.: Effects of ageing on the histochemically demonstrable catecholamines and acetylcholinesterase of human sympathetic ganglia. J. Neurocytol. 7:11, 1978.

85. Andrew, W.: Structural alterations with aging in the nervous system. J. Chronic Dis. 3:575, 1956.

86. Helen, P., Zeitlin, R., and Hervonen, A.: Mitochondrial accumulations in nerve fibres of human sympathetic ganglia. Cell Tiss. Res. 207:491, 1980.

87. Helen, P.: Fine-structural and degenerative features in adult and aged human sympathetic ganglion cells. Mech. Ageing Devel. 23:161, 1983.

88. Dyck, P.J.: Reconstruction of motor, sensory, and autonomic neurons based on morphometric study of sampled levels. Muscle & Nerve 2:399, 1979.

89. Jarvi, R., et al.: Age-related changes of enkephalinergic innervation of human sympathetic neurons. Mech. Ageing Devel. 44:143, 1988.

90. Schmidt, R.E., et al. Differential sensitivity of prevertebral and paravertebral sympathetic ganglia to experimental injury. Brain Res. 260:214, 1988.

18

Drugs and the Aging Brain

MICHAEL GORDON and
HAROLD G. PREIKSAITIS

Modern medical practice now includes a vast array of potent pharmaceutical agents that are available to treat a large number of illnesses experienced by older individuals. The elderly often have multiple medical problems occurring simultaneously that may require numerous medications. Because of changes in handling and distribution of drugs, the older individual is more susceptible to untoward reactions, especially those drugs which can have a negative impact on mental function. Careful review of medications should be part of the assessment of any older individual having mental decline.

The aging brain is particularly susceptible to the deleterious effects of certain drugs. A physician's evaluation of cognitive impairment or altered personality and mental function in older individuals must always include a careful review of all medications (prescriptions and over-the-counter), as these may be the sole or contributing—and potentially reversible—factor in the mental changes that have occurred.

Adjusting drug dosages in elderly patients, who are often taking many medications simultaneously, necessitates an understanding of drug pharmacodynamics and drug interactions, if therapeutic goals in prescribing medications are to be achieved. This overview focuses on problems of mental dysfunction common in elderly patients on multiple drug regimens and is intended as a practical guide to diagnosis and, if needed, dosage adjustment when elderly patients present with mental dysfunction.

Three case histories are presented to illustrate commonly seen clinical situations with this patient group.

Case 1. D.F., a 79-year-old woman living in her own home, was admitted to a general hospital with septicemia secondary to a urinary tract infection. Although her infection eventually responded to intravenous antibiotics, she became agitated and was given haloperidol 3 mg daily. She was unable to return home because of a decline in her mental function and was discharged to a nursing home several weeks later.

One year later she was assessed by the behavioral neurology unit at Baycrest Hospital because of continued decline in general and mental function. She had lost 40 pounds, was not eating well, and was poorly motivated. Examination revealed a thin woman with bradykinesia, cogwheel rigidity, a shuffling gait, tardive dyskinesia, akathisia, and minimal cognitive impairment.

Haloperidol was discontinued and, over the ensuing weeks of hospitalization, she made a slow but steady recovery, with improved gait and mental performance and weight gain. She did not tolerate carbidopalevodopa because of the development of an acute confusional state. At follow-up 6 months later, the patient was receiving no medications and had a good mental function and minimal gait disturbance.

Case 2. An 80-year-old man was brought for evaluation by his family because of a 7-month history of gradually increasing confusion, to the point that his wife was concerned about leaving him home alone. He had a 3-year history of angina pectoris and had been hospitalized 3 months previously because of a myocardial infarction. Hospitalization was complicated by confusion and disorientation. Other medical problems included parkinsonism, for which he received carbidopa/levodopa 25/100 3 times daily. He was also receiving enteric coated aspirin 650 mg twice daily; diltiazem 60 mg 4 times daily; hydrochlorothiazide with amiloride, 1 tablet every other day; digoxin 0/125 mg daily; nitropaste 4 times daily; ranitidine 150 mg at night; and diazepam 0.125 mg twice daily prn.

The main positive findings on examination were mild cognitive impairment and parkinsonian features. Laboratory results revealed mild azotemia, hyperkalemia, and digoxin toxicity. During a period of several weeks of careful office monitoring, the diazepam and hydrochlorothiazide/amiloride were discontinued and the dose of enteric coated ASA and diltiazem decreased. The digoxin was withheld for 3 days and reinstituted at 0.0625 mg daily. By the end of 2 weeks there was already marked improvement in physical and mental function. Azotemia disappeared, as did hyperkalemia and digoxin toxicity. With the discontinuation of the diuretic there was no need to give allopurinol, which was also discontinued without any rise of uric acid levels.

It was concluded that this patient suffered from polypharmacy with both psychoactive and nonpsychoactive drugs which affected his metabolic state, thus producing CNS malfunction.

Case 3. J.R., an 82-year-old woman residing in a nursing home, was admitted to an acute general hospital with pulmonary edema secondary to rapid atrial fibrillation. She had a previous history of ischemic heart disease and paroxysmal atrial fibrillation which, in the past, caused heart failure. She also suffered from angina pectoris which was treated with long-acting nitrates and sublingual nitroglycerin.

At the time of admission to the general hospital she was receiving, in addition to the nitrates, digoxin 0.125 mg daily, furosemide 40 mg daily, and a potassium supplement. She was discharged back to the nursing home on digoxin 0.25 mg daily, verapamil 80 mg 3 times daily, and furosemide 80 mg daily, in addition to the nitrates and potassium supplement.

Within 2 days of return to the nursing home she developed an acute confusional state. Investigations proved that she was azotemic and digoxin toxic. The furosemide was withheld for 3 days and restarted at the lower pre-hospitalization dose, the digoxin was withheld for 4 days and reintroduced at 0.125 mg daily, and the verapamil was discontinued and reinstituted after her digoxin level had returned to the lower end of the therapeutic scale. Her confusional state cleared, her heart failure was controlled, her sinus rhythm was maintained, and the azotemia was reversed.

This patient's symptoms were due to decreased digoxin clearance induced by azotemia which occurred when the furosemide was increased. The symptoms were further aggravated by the introduction of verapamil, which may interact with digoxin.[1] Modification of her drugs controlled her cardiac symptoms and allowed the deleterious effects on her mental function to subside.

PROBLEMS OF TARGETED PRESCRIBING

Drugs are prescribed for ailments affecting all organ systems. The organ that is targeted for a medication's beneficial effect may not be the same as the organ that is harmed by the drug's adverse affect. For example, aminoglycoside antibiotics used in the treatment of urinary tract infections may cause renal damage and can also have deleterious effects on the labyrinthine system, especially in older persons.

EFFECT ON MENTAL FUNCTION

Many drugs prescribed for organ systems other than the central nervous system can have a deleterious effect on mental function. Some medications—tranquilizers, anti-depressants, opiates—are clearly recognized as having psychoactive effects. Other drugs affecting the brain, such as anti-emetics, antihypertensives, cimetidine and anticholinergics, may not immediately be thought by some physicians as being "psychoactive," but in fact can be.

A basic understanding of the pharmacologic principles involved in drug handling is necessary to avoid CNS side effects in the elderly.[2,3] Surveys of practicing physicians reveal serious deficiencies in knowledge of geriatric pharmacotherapy.[4]

ACHIEVING A DELICATE BALANCE

The effect of a drug on the target organ depends on the body's ability to achieve and maintain adequate tissue levels of the drug for a sufficient period of time, so that the drug will have its full effect on the target tissue receptor or agent (i.e., microorganism). The combined effects of the drug or drugs—absorption (which depends on the mode of administration), penetration into various organs and tissues, specific effect on the organ, and excretion—must be balanced. In the elderly these factors may interact in such a way that drug prescribing techniques which are valid and effective for younger individuals may not be suitable.

Basic prescribing errors frequently occur. "Start low and go slow" is an invaluable clinical maxim which roughly allows for the altered disposition and distribution of drugs in the elderly. In addition, problems related to compliance, adverse drug reactions, and polypharmacy must be considered as of equal (and in some cases greater) importance.

PHARMACOKINETIC CHANGES WITH AGING

Pharmacokinetics include the absorption, distribution, and elimination of drugs. If the sum total of pharmokinetic changes that exist

in a given individual receiving a psychoactive drug is such that the brain tissue drug level is elevated, impairment of mental function may result. When dosage or dosage interval is appropriately modified, a decrease in CNS drug levels often occurs resulting in a reversal of the impaired mental function.

DRUG ABSORPTION

Drug absorption does not normally change significantly with age. Age-related changes in gastrointestinal function, such as decreased gastric acid secretion, motility, and reduced active transport processes, have little or no effect on drug absorption.[3]

Pathologic changes in the gastrointestinal function may, however, have profound effects on the absorption of certain drugs:

- mucosal edema of the gut can significantly impair the absorption of furosemide and other cardioactive agents;[5]
- malabsorption disorders or surgery affecting sites of drug absorption may impair absorption of certain medications; and
- loss of stomach acid following ulcer surgery might impede the absorption of oral iron.

If there is a problem with the oral absorption of a drug because of age-associated illness or a serious or urgent medical problem, parenteral administration of the drug might be necessary.[5]

DRUG DISTRIBUTION

The distribution of drugs within the body does not change significantly due to age alone.[3] The decrease in lean body mass and the increase in adipose tissue that occur with aging can change the distribution of certain drugs. Fat-soluble psychoactive drugs, such as diazepam and phenothiazines, have an increased volume of distribution, whereas drugs that are more water soluble have a decreased volume of distribution. For most drugs, however, such changes in distribution probably do not have a significant effect.

Age-related changes in protein binding usually do not have a significant effect on drug efficacy. However, changes in distribution due to drug binding interactions (as may occur with digoxin and verapamil or quinidine) can have a deleterious therapeutic effect warranting special consideration in this age group.[1]

These kinetic changes have no major effect on the steady state concentration, but they do affect the rate at which the steady state is attained. Such factors determine the optimum time to monitor drug levels or reassess therapy. For example, haloperidol, a highly lipid-soluble compound with a half-life of up to 35 hours, may produce profound extrapyramidal symptoms weeks after intiation because once fat stores are saturated, serum levels increase dramatically, thereby causing unanticipated cumulative CNS effects. Similarly, the recovery period after withdrawing medication may be much longer in the elderly (Case 1).

DRUG ELIMINATION

The elimination of medications in older patients is an important issue. Changes in renal and hepatic clearance of drugs can be both age-related and due to illnesses that occur more commonly in older persons.[2,3] The normal age-associated physiologic decline in renal function can lead to serious drug toxicity for renally excreted drugs such as digoxin.[6,7]

PHARMACODYNAMIC CHANGES

The change in pharmacodynamics that occurs with aging often causes drugs to have deleterious effects on the brain. The aging brain may be more sensitive to certain drug actions due to increased pharmacologic effects, even though the actual tissue drug levels may not be excessive. Benzodiazepines, commonly prescribed for the elderly, have significant CNS depressive effects.[8] It is known that there may be difficulties in weaning older individuals off these drugs after they have taking them for prolonged periods.[9] Such psychoactive drugs may increase the risk of falls and hip fractures.[10-12]

COMPLIANCE

Compliance (including over- or under-medication, whether accidental or intentional) is an important factor which may cause problems with drug usage in the elderly. Approximately 30 to 50% of patients of all ages fail to comply with their physician's prescription instructions, a problem that physicians largely underestimate.[13] Poor drug compliance has been identified as one of the significant factors precipitating hospital admission in many instances.[14]

Elderly patients are no better or worse than younger patients in this regard. However, the factors that lead to non-compliance in the geriatric population are unique: aside from aging itself, identified risk factors include living alone, multiple diagnoses, and general debility.[15]

An additional factor is the occasional problem of errors in prescribing and dispensing that occur despite the shared concerns of physicians and pharmacists about appropriate drug delivery for the elderly. Multiple generic and brand name preparations of drugs that may look alike may lead to confusion as well. If performed in the office by the physician, a careful review of all drugs in their original bottles may help avoid this problem. Methods of improving drug compliance have been suggested which include the cooperation of patient, family and a combination of health care professionals.[16,17]

AVOIDING ADVERSE DRUG REACTIONS

Adverse drug reactions (ADRs), which include any undesirable reaction caused by medication, result because of exaggeration of the intended therapeutic response, an unrelated toxic effect, or an interaction with a second therapeutic agent. In addition to contributing to patient non-compliance, ADRs also have been estimated to play a significant role in over 10% of geriatric hospital admissions, and they occasionally represent the sole reason for admission.[14,18]

Because many diseases can have atypical presentations in the elderly, ADRs may be more difficult to identify in this age group.[19] Drugs must always be considered in the etiology of a change in cognitive function, affect, or behavior. When ADRs are not recognized, more drugs, such as psychotropic agents for

TABLE 18–1.   Practical Recommendations to Avoid CNS Side Effects of Drugs:

Make an accurate diagnosis.

Check all other drugs used (prescription and OTC) before prescribing a new drug.

Modify dosage of drugs for older persons. Start with low dosages and gradually increase the dose until the therapeutic effect is achieved, hopefully without causing side effects.

Modify dosage of drugs for older persons. Start with low dosages and gradually increase the dose until the therapeutic effect is achieved, hopefully without causing side effects.

Monitor older patients for CNS side effects of drugs, i.e., change in sleep pattern, mood, personality, memory, mental function, etc.

Decrease the usually recommended dosage and increase dosage intervals for most non-urgent and some urgent drugs.

Consider the possibility of CNS effects of all drugs, including those not specifically known to be psychoactive.

Stop the drug altogether (unless absolutely life-saving) and reassess the patient when in doubt about CNS side effects.

Periodically examine all drugs in their bottles to make sure that drugs are not being duplicated or that drugs already discontinued are not being taken. Immediate disposal of unnecessary drugs can be accomplished at this time.

Avoid the assumption that mental decline in the elderly is due to age. Evaluate all drugs that a patient is taking and stop all drugs that are not absolutely essential and then reassess mental function.

Source: Prepared for Geriatrics by the authors.

drug-induced agitation, may be prescribed when the appropriate treatment is withdrawal of the offending agent [Table 18–1].

In the older patient, the consequences of ADRs may be more severe and recovery may be less complete. Consider, for example, the morbidity and mortality associated with falls in the elderly, a condition in which ADRs have been strongly implicated.[10,11] Extrapyramidal disorders which may be aggravated by the use of phenothiazines can cause serious disability (Case 1).

The incidence of ADRs in hospitalized patients over 80 years of age was found to be twice that of patients under 60.[20] The reasons for these differences include the existence of multiple medication use. Evidence suggests that there is a "threshold" number of drugs [1,5,6] above which the number of ADRs increases significantly. Many ADRs involve cardiovascular or psychotropic agents and 75% of nursing home residents receive at least one of these agents.[3]

DISCONTINUATION NOT INEVITABLE

Identifying an ADR does not always necessitate discontinuing the agent. Risks must be weighed against benefits. Mild dryness of the mouth may be tolerable in order to experience the beneficial effects of a tricyclic antidepressant, and mild extrapyramidal symptoms may be a worthwhile cost for improved function and mental comfort in a severely agitated, paranoid individual.

Although it is usually ill-advised to attempt to ameliorate an ADR by the addition of a second drug, in some circumstances this is acceptable—e.g., the use of anticholinergic agents to counteract severe extrapyramidal effects of phenothiazines, or the addition of potassium supplements for severe hypokalemia that occurs after essential diuretics are administered for heart failure.

POLYPHARMACY: THE IMPORTANCE OF REASSESSMENT

The number of medications used increased in proportion to the incidence of illness and disease that occurs with advancing age. This can have a major impact on the aging brain, because many of the drugs have a primary psychotropic effect and others have a secondary psychotropic effect as part of an ADR (analgesics, anti-emetics, H_2-antagonists, etc.). In addition psychotropic drugs initiated for brain disorders (depression, agitation, insomnia, anxiety) may cause adverse CNS reactions such as agitation, hallucinations, mental confusion, depression, or somnolence.

When patients receiving multiple medications are assessed, the question often arises whether polypharmacy is warranted. Medical histories may be inadequate or unavailable, and some patients or families cannot recall details of the medical past. Since compliance decreases and the incidence of ADRs increases with the number of drugs taken, reduction in drug usage can sometimes significantly improve the patient's general well-being and dramatically improve mental function (Case 2).

DISCONTINUATION AND TAPERING OF MEDICATIONS

A patient's drug regimen may include a number of medications that are not being taken regularly and hence may be discontinued immediately. Other medications, including some psychotropic agents, are best tapered with close monitoring of symptoms; the rapid discontinuation of benzodiazepines can cause withdrawal reactions that can be minimized when the medication is decreased gradually.[9]

Many antihypertensive agents that are traditionally given 4 times daily are as effective when administered once or twice daily. For example, beta-blockers and ACE-inhibitors often are as effective in once- or twice-daily doses when used as antihypertensives. Avoidance of long-acting preparations sometimes prevents prolonged periods of unwanted side-effects.

Some drug-related problems require admission to a hospital for close monitoring of the effects of discontinuing or changing drugs or their dosages. Such a move can be counterproductive, because the environmental changes accompanying hospitalization may lead to an aggravation of confusional states. Visits to a geriatric day hospital or outpatient program or frequent office assessments may be a more appropriate and safer way of dealing with this problem (Case 2). In fact hospitalization frequently results in the prescription of more, rather than fewer, medications (Case 3).

SUMMARY

The aging brain is more sensitive to the potentially deleterious effects of drugs used to treat common geriatric disorders. The atypical presentation of medical conditions can lead to inaccurate diagnoses and inappropriate drug prescribing.[21] Working from a knowledge of general principles of geriatric pharmacokinetics and pharmacodynamics, the clinician will be better attuned to the problems of prescribing for the elderly, so as to maximize beneficial therapeutic effects without compromising mental function. The potential detrimental impact of medications on the aging brain must always be considered when older patients with mental dysfunction are being evaluated.

REFERENCES

1. Gordon, M., and Goldenberg, L.M.C.: Clinical digoxin toxicity in the aged in association with co-administered verapamil: a report of two cases and review of the literature. J. Am Geriatr. Soc., 34:659, 1986.
2. Schmucker, D.L.: Drug disposition in the elderly: a review of the critical clinical factors. J. Am. Geriatr. Soc., 32:144, 1984.
3. Greenblatt, D.J., et al.: Drug disposition in old age. N. Engl. J. Med., 306:1081, 1982.
4. Ferry, M.E., Lamy, P.P., and Becker, L.A.: Physicians' knowledge of prescribing for the elderly: a study of primary care physicians in Pennsylvania. J. Am. Geriatr. Soc., 33(9):616, 1985.
5. Vasco, M.R., et al.: Furosemide absorption altered in decompensated congestive heart failure. Ann. Intern. Med., 102:314, 1985.
6. Lamy, P.P.: The elderly and drug interactions. J. Am. Geriatr. Soc., 34:586, 1986.
7. Stults, B.M.: Digoxin use in the elderly. J. Am. Geriatr. Soc., 30:158, 1982.
8. Reidenberg, M.M., et al.: Relationship between diazepam dose, plasma level and central nervous system depression. Clin. Pharmacol. Ther., 20:371, 1978.
9. Busto, U., et al.: Withdrawal reaction after long-term therapeutic use of benzodiazepines. N. Engl. J. Med., 14:854, 1986.
10. Ray, W.A., et al.: Psychotropic drug use and the risk of hip fracture. N. Engl. J. Med., 316:363. 1987.
11. Kelsey, J.L., and Hoffman, S.: Risk factors for hip fracture. N. Engl. J. Med., 316:404, 1987.
12. Tenitis, M. E., Speechley, M., and Ginter, F.: Risk factors for falls among elderly persons living in the community. N. Engl. J. Med., 319:1701, 1988.
13. Roth, H.P., and Caron H.S.: Accuracy of doctors' estimates and patients' statements on adherence to a drug regimen. Clin. Pharmacol. Ther., 23:361, 1978.
14. Grymonpre, R.E., et al.: Drug-associated hospital admissions in older medical patients. J. Amer. Geriatr. Soc., 36:1092, 1988.
15. Schwartz, D., et al.: Medication errors made by elderly, chronically ill patients. Am. J. Public Health, 52:2018, 1962.
16. Morrow, D., Leirer, V., and Sheikh, J.: Adherence and medication instructions. J. Amer. Geriatr. Soc., 36:1147, 1988.
17. Kazis, L.E., and Friedman, R.H.: Improving medication compliance in the elderly: Strategies for the health care provider. J. Amer. Geriatr. Soc., 36:1161, 1988.
18. Williamson, J., and Chopin, J.M.: Adverse reactions to prescribing drugs in the elderly: a multicentre investigation. Age Ageing 9:73, 1980.
19. Clark, B.G., and Vestal, R.E.: Adverse drug reactions in the elderly: case studies. Geriatrics 39:53, 1984.
20. Hurwitz, N.: Predisposing factors in adverse reactions to drugs. Br. Med. J. 1:556, 1969.
21. Gordon, M.: Differential diagnosis of weakness—a common geriatric symptom. Geriatrics 41:75, 1986.

19

Clinical Neurochemistry of Brain Disorders in Aging

CHRISTER ALLING

The role of clinical neurochemistry in the diagnosis of neurologic diseases of the elderly population is increasing rapidly in importance as a result of recent advances in methodology and instrumentation.[1-3] As biopsies from living individuals are generally not available for the diagnosis of brain disorders, biologic markers must be sought in the body fluids. The objective of this review is to demonstrate the value of biochemical measurements and their limitations. The pathologic conditions to be discussed concern vascular disorders, in particular stroke and infarcts, immunologic diseases, and the dementias. The different dementias will be identified as described elsewhere in this volume.

CEREBROSPINAL FLUID MEASURES

PLASMA DERIVED PROTEINS

More than 90% of the protein content of CSF originates from blood plasma and enters the CSF through the choroid plexus after ultra-filtration through choroid plexus microvessels.[4] The concentration of such proteins is correlated roughly with their concentrations in blood plasma and is inversely related to their molecular size.

Total Protein Concentrations and Electrophoretic Patterns. A rapid estimate of the concentration of total proteins in CSF can be obtained by one of several colorimetric methods. Different methods, however, vary in accuracy[5] and information from such assays is of limited value and should be used only for screening purposes.

Agarose and cellulose acetate electrophoresis have been widely used to obtain information about the protein patterns in CSF. This technique is primarily applied to the study of abnormal immunoglobulin concentrations and compositions.

A new approach was taken by Wikkelso et al.,[8,9] who separated the majority of plasma derived proteins from CSF enriched proteins by affinity chromotography. The two groups of proteins were isoelectrically focused and patients with Alzheimer's dementia and senile dementia of the Alzheimer's type revealed characteristic patterns among the CSF-specific proteins.[10]

Albumin and IgG-Index. A great advance occurred with the introduction of electroimmunoassays for individual proteins.[11] The concentrations of albumin and IgG in CSF can now be obtained with high accuracy and precision and the contribution of an abnormal local subarachnoid IgG production can be estimated.[12] The ratio between the albumin concentration in CSF and that in blood plasma is a measure of the function of the blood-brain barrier. The amount of IgG in CSF in relation to the albumin concentration is a precise indicator of pathologic immunoglobulin production in the brain. Reference values for different age groups have been worked out by Link and co-workers.[13-15] Improvement of the characterization of increased concentrations of IgG has been obtained by isoelectric focusing in agarose, double-antibody peroxidase labeling and avidinbiotin amplification.[16]

IgG Increase and Oligoclonal Banding. Patients with multiple sclerosis almost always have an increased concentration of IgG in the CSF. In a study of 1000 patients from neurologic wards,[6] it was found that 93% of patients with clinically definite multiple sclerosis demonstrated abnormal oligoclonal bands and in patients with possible multiple sclerosis such a finding was present in 31%. The value of such a technique for diagnostic purposes in other degenerative disorders of the brain is limited. Even improvement of the electrophoretic technique comprising high resolution, two-dimensional, polyacrylamide gel electrophoresis gives no further information. Alafuzoff et al.[7] applied this technique to the study of multi-infarct dementia and Alzheimer's disease and found no differences in comparison to age-matched non-demented individuals. Assuming that the volume of CSF is about 140 ml and is replaced about 3.5 times per day, it has also been possible to construct a formula to estimate the amount of IgG synthesized per day by the central nervous system in immunopathologic disorders.[24,25] Patients with systemic lupus erythematosus, sarcoidosis, and brain infections also demonstrate IgG increases and oligoclonal banding.[26] Patients

with dementia have been studied with regard to IgG abnormalities. No changes were found in patients with Alzheimer's diesase but 4 out of 28 patients with vascular dementia had slightly elevated IgG levels and 3 of them also showed oligoclonal banding.[27]

Blood-Brain-Barrier Damage. Cerebral hemorrhage with bleeding into the subarachnoid space (cerebrospinal fluid) produces an increased concentration of albumin.[17] More conflicting results are obtained in other forms of cerebral vascular disease, such as infarcts and transient ischemic attacks (TIAs). One study[18] revealed no albumin increase with either small or large infarcts and found no relationship to the localization of infarcts or between the time interval from the onset of infarction to the time of lumbar puncture and the albumin concentration. Other studies[17,19] showed significantly increased concentrations of albumin in patients with acute non-embolic and embolic infarcts compared to controls and patients with old infarcts. Patients with NAD had higher albumin concentrations than those with infarcts and a high level of CSF albumin was associated with poor short-term prognosis.[20]

Increased albumin concentrations within CSF have been demonstrated in patients with dementia.[21] When 53 patients with vascular dementia were compared with 50 healthy controls, the former group had a 30% higher level. Since the albumin concentration was not related to individual clinical vascular factors, it was suggested that the altered blood brain barrier was a consequence of a small vessel disorder rather than an indicator of the presence of infarcts. Patients with Alzheimer's disease also showed a higher albumin concentration, as compared to controls, which was related to vascular factors assumed to co-exist with Alzheimer's disease because in Alzheimer patients without vascular factors no significant increase in albumin was found.[22] Prealbumin (transthyretin) has also been suggested to correlate with the degree of dementia (see Chap. 3).[23]

BRAIN-SPECIFIC PROTEINS

Individual proteins that only exist in the central nervous system and proteins that predominantly occur in the central nervous system as well as those whose presence in CSF can be proved to originate from the nervous system, are usually named brain specific proteins. These include myelin basic protein, neuron-specific enolase, glial fibrillary acid protein, S-100 protein and cystatin C.

Myelin Basic Protein. By raising antibodies to myelin basic protein (MBP) it has been possible to design a radioimmunoassay for MBP.[28] It has been shown to be a valuable index of active demyelination with great importance for the diagnosis of multiple sclerosis. Radioimmunoassay of MBP can be used for objective evalution of disease activity since the levels of MBP in CSF correlate well with the clinical behavior of MS and other diseases in which there is an acute breakdown of myelin (e.g. severe anoxia, necrosis due to radiation, leukodystrophies, neurosurgical conditions, and stroke). MBP is a well-characterized protein with a molecular weight of 18400. However, in CSF the protein seems to be degraded and different fragments of the protein react with the antibodies.[29] In post-traumatic brain disorders and after surgery for brain tumors, the MBP level is increased for periods up to 3 weeks but it is high and it gradually returns to normal. Repeated measurements of myelin basic proteins in CSF seem to be useful for assessing the healing rate of brain tissue after trauma and other types of brain damage.[30] Increased levels of MBP are found in patients with stroke.[17] Patients with cerebral infarction and hemorrhage have increased concentrations of MBP, but those with TIAs have virtually normal levels. The amount of MBP also correlates significantly with the visibility of cerebral lesions on CT scan and the short-term outcome of patients. The amount of MBP is usually correlated with the extent of the tissue damage of the brain and high values indicate a poor short-term prognosis for the patient.[31] Recent studies in MS patients have indicated that 84% of patients have increased levels of MBP and that there exists a significant correlation between the concentration of MBP in CSF and relapse severity in patients seen within 4 weeks after the onset of symptoms, suggesting that the detection of MBP may indicate subclinical demyelination.[32]

Neuron-Specific Enolase. This protein is a glycolytic enzyme localized in neurons. Neuron-specific enolase appears to be a good marker of cell loss or of a decrease in neuronal functional activity. Significantly lower levels were found in 30 patients with Alzheimer's disease compared to 13 controls.[33] Lamour et al.[34] found, however, no difference in CSF levels between patients with Alzheimer's disease and healthy elderly controls of the same age range, and there was no correlation between neuron-specific enolase and severity of cognitive deficits. Similarly, negative findings resulted from another study.[35] These authors found that in patients with multi-infarct dementia without recent vascular events, the level of this brain-specific brain protein was lower than in controls or in Alzheimer patients.

Glial Fibrillary Acidic Protein (GFAP). This protein originates from astroglial cells and has been used as a marker for gliosis and gliomas.[36] The level in CSF is increased remarkably in acute cases of intracerebral hemorrhage and in some cases of subarachnoid hemorrhage and cerebral infarction.[37] The cellular localization can be demonstrated histologically.

S-100 Protein. This protein has higher concentrations in oligodendrocytes and astrocytes than in neurons. It is usually not detectable in normal healthy controls in CSF but was increased in 13 out of 18 patients with multiple sclerosis and might be a candidate for an index of active cell injury.[38] An effective histologic method is available for the demonstration of S-100.

Cystatin C. This is a basic microprotein. The tissue localization and amino acid sequence have been established.[39] This protein is involved in genetic vascular disorders of the central nervous system[40] and studies of this protein have opened up a new field of molecular biology for the diagnosis of disorders in the central nervous system.[41]

ANTIBODIES DIRECTED AGAINST NEURONS

In a recent series of publications, McRae-Degueurce and co-workers have reported that CSF from patients with Parkinson's disease and Alzheimer's disease contains antibodies that recognize neurons in cholinergic and dopaminergic areas in the rat brian.[42] These findings may open up a new test procedure for CSF. In a pilot study they found that IgG in the CSF of a patient with the clinical syndrome of parkinsonism recognized neurons in a dopamine cell-rich area of rat mesencephalon.[42] In a more extended series of patients they found that 2 patients out of 7 with Parkinson's disease demonstrated marked labeling of dopaminergic neurons in the substantia nigra of rat brain.[43] Sera from other patients were weakly positive or negative. CSF from Alzheimer disease patients contains antibodies that recognize specific neuronal populations in the rat central nervous system.[44] Not all CSF from Alzheimer patients demonstrated this finding, indicating that it holds true for a subgroup of patients with this disease. Interestingly, the antibodies recognized acetylcholine-like epitopes in cholinergic neurons. Some of these patients had CSFs that also recognized thyroglobulin in an ELISA assay and this antithyroglobulin recognized the same cholinergic neurons in the rat brain.[45] These results indicate that in a subgroup of Alzheimer disease patients autoimmune mechanisms may play a role in the pathogenesis of dementia and that disturbances in the handling of thyroid hormone in the CNS may be involved in the disease process. Another research group has found antibodies to cholinergic neurons by studying serum of patients with Alzheimer's disease,[46] also supporting the hypothesis that autoimmune mechanisms may operate in the pathogenesis of Alzheimer's disease.

BIOGENIC AMINES

Low quantities of intact biogenic amines leak into the CSF. Their metabolites on the other hand, occur in substantial amount and can be assayed biochemically. One of the few methods that permits the study of the neurotransmission in man is the measurement of levels of amine metabolites in lumbar spinal fluid.

For the purpose of measuring CSF metabolite levels in healthy and diseased patients it is important to standardize the procedures.[47] The site of lumbar puncture determines the levels of monoamine metabolites.[48] Higher concentrations are obtained if the fluid is obtained at

L_{3-4} compared to L_{4-5} or L_5-S_1. This is explained by the gradient of monoamine metabolites that exists within the subarachnoid compartments which has been amply demonstrated when consecutive portions of CSF are drawn and the concentrations determined in these fractions.[49] Other factors that influence the concentrations in CSF are motor activity, diet, circadian variation, seasonal variation, age, sex, body height, and drug treatment.[50] The analytic methods usually include a combination of gas chromatography mass spectrometry and high performance liquid chromatography with electrochemical detection.

The levels of the metabolites of biogenic amines are assumed to indicate the activity of the noradrenergic, dopaminergic, and serotonergic systems. But to what extent such a correlation between central neurotransmission and CSF amine metabolites holds true for humans is still a matter of debate. A study by Stanley et al.[51] included measurements of 5-hydroxyindole acetate [5-HIA] in lumbar CSF and in the cerebral cortex obtained simultaneously from 48 individuals at autopsy. A strong correlation ($r = 0.78$; $p < 0.0001$) between the two parameters shows that lumbar CSF levels of 5-HIA reflect brain levels.

A number of studies have addressed the question of whether neurotransmitter changes in dementia are revealed by studies of CSF. The major metabolite of norepinephrine in CSF, 3,5 methoxy-4-hydroxyphenylglycol (MHPG), has been found to be increased in two studies of Alzheimer disease patients.[52,53] In other studies, however, no differences between Alzheimer patients and controls were found and the usefulness of MHPG assays in dementia patients seems to be limited in view of these inconclusive and conflicting results.

The serotonin metabolite 5-hydroxyindoleacetate (5-HIA) and the major metabolite of dopamine, homovanillic acid (HVA) are the two compounds that can be measured to demonstrate a more or less deranged function of the two transmitter systems. (For review see [2].) A consistent finding is that HVA is significantly reduced in patients with Alzheimer's disease when compared to age-matched controls. Also, 5-HIA is significantly reduced. However, this reduction seems to be less evident. The dopamine and serotonin systems are morphologically interconnected and their metabolites normally correlate consistently with one another. It has also been demonstrated that HVA and 5-HIA co-variate in patients with Alzheimer's disease before and after treatment with a variety of antidepressant drugs.[54] The stability of the metabolites in CSF in individual patients seems to be rather stable over time.[55] However, the predictive value of these assessments for Alzheimer's disease has not yet been settled. Patients with extrapyramidal signs seem to have more pronounced diminution of HVA, which holds true also when patients are matched for age and severity of dementia.[56] These findings indicate that Alzheimer patients with extrapyramidal signs may form a distinct subgroup with evidence of a special central monoamine dysfunction.

Attention has also been paid to the relation between a reduced concentration of HVA and clinical symptoms. The predominant finding is a negative correlation between the degree of dementia and the concentration of HVA in CSF, but lack of such correlation has also been reported. Soininen et al.[57] found that both HVA and 5-HIA were significantly reduced in the most severely demented patients compared with less severely demented patients. These findings have been confirmed in recent studies applying psychobehavioral tests for intellectual and emotional deterioration.[58,59] Wester et al.[60] also found that the decreased levels of HVA were most obvious in a subgroup of dementia patients clinically characterized by asymmetry of neurologic signs, inceased neurolateral tonus, and stepwise progression. Obviously, detailed clinical assessment will reveal distinct patterns of abnormalities among the monoamine metabolites in the CSF of demented patients.

ACETYLCHOLINE

Markers for acetylcholine activity in the central nervous system include acetylcholinesterase, butylcholinesterase, choline acetyltransferase, and choline.

Several studies[61-66] have reported a reduction in CSF of acetylcholinesterase activity in dementias of Alzheimer type. Other have found no changes (for review see [2]). The pos-

sible reasons for these contrasting results seem to be related to differences in diagnostic criteria and the assessment of acetylcholinesterase activity. In a recent study[60] it was found that the degree of dementia as assessed by global deterioration score and activity of daily life status as well as symptoms like dyspraxia and dysphasia in Alzheimer patients was associated with low activities of acetylcholinesterase in CSF. Kaye et al.[67] studied different groups of dementias and found that acetylcholinesterase was significantly reduced but not significantly different between groups. Kumar et al.[68] found that choline levels were significantly higher in dementia of the Alzheimer type than in age-matched controls. Choline acetyltransferase activity is difficult to assay and no positive findings have been reported. Due to the involvement of acetylcholine in dementia further careful studies of the enzymes related to this transmitter will be worthwhile.

NEUROPEPTIDES

In the past 15 years numerous peptides found in the central nervous system have been proposed as putative neurotransmitters. Nearly all of these have been measured by radioimmunoassay in human CSF. The origin of these peptides in CSF are not precisely known. It has been suggested that there are four possible routes by which neuropeptides may reach the CSF:

1. Via random diffusion from the neuronal site of release through the interstitial space of the nervous system to CSF.
2. By a direct release of the peptide into the CSF from a neuron.
3. From the peripheral blood through the blood-brain barrier in areas with a relatively permeable barrier (median eminence, pineal gland, subforniceal organ, subcommisural organ, and area prostrema).
4. From the portal vessel blood to the third ventricle.

The stability of the neuropeptides in CSF is not fully elucidated, but it is generally assumed that many of them are sufficiently stable to allow valid radioimmunoassays to establish their concentrations in human CSF. Studies have now documented abnormalities of peptide concentrations in degenerative diseases of the brain. For review see Black,[69] Sagar et al.,[70] Jackson,[71] Berrettini et al.,[72] and Widerlov.[73]

Two studies with carefully selected control subjects have found decreased concentrations of corticotropin-releasing factor in CSF from patients with Alzheimer's disease.[74,75] Also, thyrotropin-releasing factor[76] and gonadotropin-releasing factor[77] have been found to be decreased in Alzheimer's disease. Facchinetti et al.[78] have measured the CSF content of ACTH and beta-endorphin in demented patients and age-matched healthy controls. They found substantially lower ACTH levels in demented patients, whereas the beta-endorphin levels were essentially the same in the two groups. The findings of a reduced level of ACTH, a normal level of cortico-tropin-releasing factor (CRF),[79] may indicate that the processing of the POMC precursor molecule is altered in demented states.

In non-demented patients with Parkinson's disease the levels of diazepam-binding inhibitor-like immunoreactivity (DSIP) were increased in a subgroup of depressed disturbances, whereas no differences were observed in the non-depressed cases.[80] Significantly lower levels have, however, also been reported for Alzheimer dementia, multi-infarct dementia, Parkinson's disease, vascular disease and communicating hydrocephalus.[81]

Somatostatin levels have been found to be reduced in almost all CSF studies of demented patients (for review see [2]). Whether these findings indicate a primary neurodegenerative process or alterations secondary to brain damage remains to be investigated. Atack et al.[82] found a significantly lower concentration of somatostatin in Alzheimer patients which was unrelated to dementia severity and did not change significantly during the progression of the disease. In a recent study[83] it was found that a low level of somatostatin in demented patients was significantly elevated when these patients were subjected to a 3-month program with integrity promoting care resulting in improved psychomotor functions compared to a control group.

Neuropeptide Y has also been studied in dementia but CSF levels did not differ significantly from age-matched controls.[82]

BLOOD MEASURES

Blood samples are more easily obtained than cerebrospinal fluid from patients. In spite of extensive research less conclusive findings have emerged from studies of blood. The causal relationship between blood abnormalities and disorders of the brain is far more complex than that of CSF. The great advantages of assays in blood plasma refer to monitoring drug therapy for brain disorders like anti-convulsive drugs and other neuropharmacologic regimens. Other areas of importance are assays for essential nutrients such as amino acids, trace elements, minerals, vitamins, platelet monoamine oxidase, and neuropeptides.

VITAMIN B$_{12}$

There are indications that vitamin B$_{12}$ has an etiologic role in the genesis of dementia and the findings have been described as a demyelinating subacute degeneration.[84,85] Low vitamin B$_{12}$ levels in serum are also known to be quite common in patients with senile dementia with confusion even in the absence of hematologic changes.[86] Also, values within normal limits have been reported.[87] In a recent study,[88] 5 out of 10 patients with Alzheimer's presenile disease and 13 out of 56 patients with senile dementia of the Alzheimer type had vitamin B$_{12}$ concentrations below the lower limit of the reference value. The findings indicate that there is a subgroup of patients with late onset dementia that has low vitamin B$_{12}$ blood concentrations.

Determinations of pepsinogen-I and gastrin in demented patients revealed that those with low vitamin B$_{12}$ levels also had concentrations of these peptides which were significantly lower compared to demented patients with normal B$_{12}$ levels. These findings indicate that the vitamin B$_{12}$ reaction mainly is determined by gastric mucosal atrophy.[89]

PLATELET MONOAMINE OXIDASE

Monoamine oxidase (MAO) is a key enzyme in the degradation of monoamines. It occurs in two different forms, MAO-A and MAO-B which have different substrate and inhibitor specificities. In human platelets MAO-B is assayed as an indicator of central MAO activity. A slow increase of MAO activity is associated with normal aging.[90,91]

In patients suffering from primary degenerative dementias of the Alzheimer type, platelet MAO activity has been found to be increased.[91–93] Comparing different varieties of dementia—vascular dementia, confusion, Alzheimer's disease and senile dementia—no differences between these subgroups were found but there might be a subgroup of patients with late onset dementia in which the MAO increase is more obvious.

NEUROENDOCRINE CHALLENGE TESTS

The recent and rapid development of research on neuropeptides in aging is obviously just beginning and findings with regard to degenerative brain disorders are still poorly understood. Most studies so far have used radioimmunologic assays (RIA) and these can still be substantially improved by using one or several well-characterized sequence specific antisera. New neuropeptides are continuously discovered and the sensitivity of the assays is improved by applying new techniques.

PROLACTIN

Prolactin secretion in blood is regulated by dopaminergic neurons in the brain which exert a tonic inhibitory influence on prolactin release. High serum concentrations of prolactin reflect possible damage to the region in the tubero-infundibular system which contains high numbers of dopamine neurons. Agnoli et al.[94] found high basal serum concentrations of prolactin in patients with severe Parkinson's syndrome. Thyrotropin hormone can challenge the prolactin response and is inhibited by dopamine. States of dopaminergic hypofunction may thus result in both higher baseline prolactin levels and high prolactin response to thyrotropin-releasing hormone challenge. Such a blunted prolactin response has been demonstrated in Parkinson's disease[95] and may be related to an enhanced dopaminergic tone in the tubero-infundibular system along with a selective nigrostriatal dopamine deficiency.

Balldin et al.[96] assayed basal prolactin levels in demented patients but found that the concentrations were the same as in controls indicating that dopamine neurons involved in prolactin regulation are not severely affected in dementing disorders.

CORTISOL

Dexamethasone suppresses cortisol secretion and indicates a disturbance in the hypothalamus-pituitary-adrenal axis. Originally designed as a laboratory test in patients with melancholia, it has subsequently been applied to patients with dementia and 50 to 70% of such patients have been reported as non-suppressors, i.e. they do not demonstrate the normal suppression of serum cortisol concentration after a dexamethasone load. Although most studies have excluded dementia patients who demonstrate depressive symptoms, the findings have been debated. However, the test-retest reliability is found to be high in dementia patients if environmental stress factors are controlled.[97] McAllister and Hays[98] also found that patients with primary degenerative dementia have a high percentage of dexamethasone suppression tests which paralleled a thyrotropin-releasing hormone test, indicating a hypothalamic-pituitary dysfunction in these patients.

THYROTROPIN

A challenge with thyrotropin-releasing hormone (TRH) increases the plasma level of thyrotropin (TSH). This test has been used in patients with dementia disorders.[99–102] Results from these studies are conflicting regarding differences between dementia patients and an age-matched population. The most prevailing finding is, however, that the response is blunted, indicating abnormalities in the hypothalamic-pituitary-thyroid (HPT) axis. Further research is required to evaluate the predictive value of this test in degenerative disorders of brain.

GROWTH HORMONE

The norepinephrine agonist clonidine is known to stimulate the secretion of growth hormone and the maximum growth hormone response can be considered as a marker for postsynaptic norepinephrine sensitivity. Balldin et al.[103] found that clonidine did not stimulate growth hormone in demented patients but depressed blood pressure levels. This might indicate a change in the alpha$_2$-receptor sensitivity but no changes in those receptors which regulate blood pressure.

REFERENCES

1. Hollander, E., Mohs, R.C., and Davis, K.L.: Antemortem markers of Alzheimer's disease. Neurobiol. Aging, 7:367, 1986.
2. Cutler, N.R.: In vivo markers in Alzheimer's disease and related dementias. In: *Psychopharmacology: The Third Generation of Progress.* (Ed) H.Y. Meltzer. New York, Raven Press, 1987.
3. Gottfries, C.G.: Diagnosis and treatment of senile dementia: early diagnosis and differential diagnosis. Diag. Treat. Senile Dement., 18:1, 1988.
4. Wood, J.H.: Technical aspects of clinical and experimental cerebrospinal fluid investigations. In: *Neurobiology of Cerebrospinal Fluid.* (Ed) J.H. Wood. New York, Plenum Press, 1980.
5. Karlsson, B., and Alling, C.: A comparative study of three approaches to the routine quantitative determination of spinal fluid total proteins. Clin. Chim. Acta, 105:65, 1980.
6. Ebers, G.C., and Paty, D.W.: CSF electrophoresis in one thousand patients. Can. J. Neurol. Sci., 7:275, 1980.
7. Alafuzof, I., et al.: Isoelectric focusing and two-dimensional gel electrophoresis in plasma and cerebrospinal fluid from patients with dementia. Eur. Neurol., 25:285, 1986.
8. Wikkelso, C., Blomstrand, C., and Ronnback, L.: Separation of cerebrospinal fluid specific proteins— A methodological study, Part I. J. Neurol. Sci., 44:247, 1980.
9. Wikkelso, C., et al.: Separation of cerebrospinal fluid-enriched proteins. A methodological study, Part 2. J. Neurol. Sci., 60:419, 1983.
10. Wikkelso, C., and Blomstrand, C.: Cerebrospinal fluid "specific proteins" in various degenerative neurological diseases. Acta Neurol. Scand., 66:199, 1982.
11. Laurell, C-B.: Composition and variation of gel electrophoretic fractions of plasma, cerebrospinal fluid and urine. Scand. J. Clin. Lab. Invest., 29:(124):71, 1972.
12. Ganrot, K., and Laurell C-B.: Measurement of IgG and albumin content of cerebrospinal fluid, and its interpretation. Clin. Chem. 20:571, 1974.
13. Tibbling, G., Link, H., and Ohman, S.: Principles of albumin and IgG analysis in neurological disorders. I. Establishment of reference values. Scand. J. Clin. Lab. Invest., 37:385, 1977.
14. Link, H., and Tibbling, G.: Principles of albumin and IgG analysis in neurological disorders. II. Relation of the concentration of the proteins in serum and cerebrospinal fluid. Scand. J. Clin. Lab. Invest., 37:391, 1977.
15. Link, H., and Tibbling, G.: Principles of albumin and IgG analysis in neurological disorders. III. Evaluation of IgG synthesis within the central nervous system in multiple sclerosis. Scand. J. Clin. Lab. Invest., 37:397, 1977.
16. Olsson, T., Kostulas, V., and Link, H.: Improved detection of oligoclonal IgG in cerebrospinal fluid by isoelectric focusing in agarose, double-antibody peroxidase labeling, and avidin-biotin amplification. Clin. Chem., 30:1246, 1984.
17. Strand, T., et al.: Brain and plasma proteins in spinal fluid as markers for brain damage and severity of stroke. Stroke, 15:138, 1984.
18. Al-Kassab, S., Skyhoj Olsen, T., and Bech Skriver, E.: Blood-brain barrier integrity in patients with cerebral infarction investigated by computed tomography and serum-CSF-albumin. Acta Neurol. Scand., 64:438, 1981.
19. Palm, R., Strand, T., and Hallmans, G.: Zinc, total protein, and albumin in CSF of patients with cerebrovascular diseases. Acta Neurol. Scand., 74:308, 1986.
20. Hornig, C.R.: et al.: Changes in CSF blood-brain barrier parameters in ischaemic cerebral infarction. J. Neurol., 229:11, 1983.
21. Wallin, A., et al.: Blood-brain barrier function in vascular dementia. Acta Neurol. Scand., 81:318, 1989.
22. Blennow, K., et al.: Blood-brain barrier disturbances in Alzheimer's disease is related to vascular factors. Acta Neurol. Scand., 81, 323, 1989.
23. Riisoen H.: Reduced prealbumin (transthyretin) in CSF of severely demented patients with Alzheimer's disease. Acta Neurol. Scand., 78:455, 1988.
24. Tourtellotte, W.: On cerebrospinal fluid immunoglobulin-G (IgG) quotients in multiple sclerosis and other diseases. A review and a new formula to estimate the amount of IgG synthesized per day by the central nervous system. J. Neurol. Sci., 10:279, 1970.
25. Tourtellotte, W., and Booe, I.: Multiple sclerosis: The blood-brain-barrier and the measurement of de novo central nervous system IgG synthesis. Neurol., 28:76, 1978.
26. Christenson, R., et al.: Interpretation of cerebrospinal fluid protein assays in various neurologic diseases. Clin. Chem., 29:1028, 1983.
27. Elovaara, I., et al.: Oligoclonal immunoglobulin bands in cerebrospinal fluid of patients with Alzheimer's disease and vascular dementia. Acta Neurol. Scand., 77:397, 1988.
28. Cohen, S.R., et al.: Myelin basic protein in cerebrospinal fluid. Index of active demyelination. In: *Neurobiology of Cerebrospinal Fluid.* 2nd. Ed. (Ed) J.H. Wood. New York, Plenum Press, 1982.
29. Karlsson, B., and Alling, C.: Molecular size of myelin basic protein immunoactivity in spinal fluid. J. Neuroimmunol., 6:141, 1984.
30. Alling, C., Karlsson, B., and Vallfors, B.: Increase in myelin basic protein in CSF after brain surgery. J. Neurol., 223:225, 1980.
31. Whitaker, J.N., et al.: Immunoreactive myelin basic

protein in the cerebrospinal fluid in neurological disorders. Ann. Neuro., 7:58, 1980.

32. Thomson, A.J., et al.: CSF myelin basic protein in multiple sclerosis. Acta Neurol. Scand., 72:577.

33. Cutler, N.R., et al.: Cerebrospinal fluid neuron-specific enolase is reduced in Alzheimer's disease. Arch. Neurol., 43:153, 1986.

34. Lamour, Y., et al.: Serum neuron-specific enolase in senile dementia of the Alzheimer type. Neurosci. Lett., 86:241, 1988.

35. Sulkava, R., et al.: Cerebrospinal fluid neuron-specific enolase is decreased in multi-infarct dementia, but unchanged in Alzheimer's disease. J. Neurol. Neurosurg. Psychiat., 51:549, 1988.

36. Lowenthal, A., et al.: Alfa-Albumin (glial fibrillary acidic protein) in normal and pathological human brain and cerebrospinal fluid. J. Neural., 219:87, 1978.

37. Hyakawa, T., et al.: Levels in stroke patients of CSF astroprotein, an astrocyte-specific cerebroprotein. Stroke, 10:685, 1979.

38. Michetti, F., Massaro, A., and Murazio, M.: The nervous system-specific S-100 antigen in cerebrospinal fluid of multiple sclerosis patients. Neurosci. Lett., 11:171, 1979.

39. Grubb, A., and Lofberg, H.: Human gamma-trace, a basic microprotein: Amino acid sequence and presence in the adenohypophysis. Proc. Natl. Acad. Sci., 79:3024, 1982.

40. Palsdottir, A., et al.: Mutation in cystatin C gene causes hereditary brain hemorrhage. Lancet., Sep., 10:603, 1988.

41. Jensson, O., et al.: Hereditary cystatin C (gamma-trace) amyloid angiopathy of the CNS causing cerebral hemorrhage. Acta Neural. Scand., 76:102, 1987.

42. McRae Degueurce, A., et al.: Antibodies in the CSF of a Parkinson patient recognizes neurons in rat mesencephalic regions. Acta Physiol. Scand., 126:313, 1986.

43. McRae Degueurce, A., et al.: Immunocytochemical investigations on the presence of neuron-specific antibodies in the CSF of Parkinson's disease cases. Neurochem. Res., 13:679, 1988.

44. McRae Degueurce, A., et al.: Antibodies in cerebrospinal fluid of some Alzheimer disease patients recognize cholinergic neurons in the rat central nervous system. Proc. Natl. Acad. Sci., 84:9214, 1987.

45. McRae Degueurce, A., et al.: Antibodies recognizing cholinergic neurons and thyroglobuline are found in the cerebrospinal fluid of a subgroup of patients with Alzheimer's disease. Drug Develop. Res., 15:153, 1988.

46. Foley, P., et al.: Evidence for the presence of antibodies to cholinergic neurons in the serum of patients with Alzheimer's disease. J. Neurol., 235:466, 1988.

47. Wood, J.H.: Neurochemical analysis of cerebrospinal fluid. Neurology, 30:645, 1980.

48. Nordin, C., Siwers, B., Bertilsson, L.: Site of lumbar puncture influences levels of monoamine metabolites. Arch. Gen. Psychiatry, 39:1445, 1982.

49. Bertilsson, L., et al.: Gradients of monoamine metabolites and cortisol in cerebrospinal fluid of psychiatric patients and healthy controls. Psychiat. Res., 6:77, 1982.

50. Bertilsson, L.: 5-Hydroxyindoleacetic acid in cerebrospinal fluid-methodological and clinical aspects. Life Sci., 41:821, 1987.

51. Stanley, M., Traskman-Bendz, L., and Dorovini-Zis, K.: Correlations between aminergic metabolites simultaneously obtained from human CSF and brain. Life Sci., 37:1279, 1985.

52. Gibson, C.J., Logue, M., and Growdon, J.H.: CSF monoamine metabolite levels in Alzheimer's disease and Parkinson's disease. Arch. Neurol., 42:489, 1985.

53. Raskind, M.A., et al.: Norepinephrine and MHPG levels in CSF and plasma in Alzheimer's disease. Arch. Gen. Psych., 41:343, 1984.

54. Risby, E.D., et al.: The effects of antidepressants on the cerebrospinal fluid homovanillic acid/5-hydroxyindoleacetic acid ratio. Clin. Pharmacol. Ther., 42:547, 1987.

55. Seeldrayers, P., et al.: CSF levels of neurotransmitters in Alzheimer-type dementia. Effects of ergoloid mesylate. Acta Neurol. Scand., 71:411, 1985.

56. Kaye, J.A., et al.: Cerebrospinal fluid monoamine markers are decreased in dementia of the Alzheimer type with extrapyramidal features. Neurol, 38:554, 1988.

57. Soininen, H., et al.: Homovanillic acid and 5-h hydroxyindoleacetic acid levels on cerebrospinal fluid of patients with senile dementia of Alzheimer type. Acta Neurol. Scand., 64:101, 1981.

58. Parmetti, L., et al.: Monoamines and their metabolites in cerebrospinal fluid of patients with senile dementia of Alzheimer type using high performance liquid chromatography and gas chromatography-mass spectrometry. Acta Psychiat. Scand., 75:542, 1987.

59. Brane, G., et al.: Monoamine metabolite in CSF and behavioral ratings in patients with early and late onset of Alzheimer dementia. Alzheimer Dis. Assoc. Disord., 3:148, 1989.

60. Wester, P., et al.: Monoamine metabolite concentrations and cholinesterase activities in cerebrospinal fluid of progressive dementia patients: relation to clinical parameters. Acta Neurol. Scand., 77:12, 1988.

61. Soininen, H., Halonen, T., and Riekkinen, P.J.: Acetylcholinesterase activities in cerebrospinal fluid of patients with senile dementia of Alzheimer type. Acta Neurol. Scand., 64:271, 1981.

62. Arendt, T., et al.: Decreased ratio of CSF acetylcholinesterase to butyrylcholinesterase activity in Alzheimer's disease. Lancet, 1:173, 1984.

63. Jolkkonen, J.T., Soininen, M.S., and Riekkinen, P.J.: Cerebrospinal fluid cholinesterase, beta-endorphin and somatostatin in Alzheimer's disease. Acta Univ. Tamperenis, 21:104, 1984.

64. Tune, L.E., et al.: CSF acetylcholinesterase activity in senile dementia of the Alzheimer type. Ann. Neuro., 17:46, 1985.

65. Gomez, S., et al.: Acetylcholinesterase activity and somatostatin-like immunoreactivity in lumbar cerebrospinal fluid of demented patients. In: *Alzheimer's and Parkinson's Disease.* (Ed) Fisher, et al. New York, Plenum Press, 1986.

66. Atack, J.R., et al.: Cerebropsinal fluid colinesterases in aging and in dementia of the Alzheimer type. Ann. Neurol., 23:161.

67. Kaye, J.A., et al.: Cerebrospinal fluid neurochemistry in the myoclonic subtype of Alzheimer's disease. Ann. Neurol., 24:647, 1988.

68. Kumar, V., and Giacobini, E.: CSF choline, and acetylcholinesterase activity in familial vs. non-familial Alzheimer's disease patients. Arch. Gerontol. Geriatr., 7:111, 1988.

69. Black, P.: Neuropeptides in cerebrospinal fluid. Neurosurg., *11*:550, 1982.

70. Sagar, S.M., et al.: Implications of neuropeptides in neurological disease. Peptides, 5:255(1), 1984.

71. Jackson, I.: Neuropeptides in the cerebrospinal fluid. Neuroendocrine Perspectives, 3:121, 1984.

72. Berrettint, W.H., et al.: Neuropeptides in human cerebrospinal fluid. Life Sci., 37:1265.

73. Widerlov, E.: Neuropeptides and psychiatry-basic and clinical aspects. Nordic J. Psch., *39*(11):9, 1985.

74. May, C., et al.: Cerebrospinal fluid (CSF) corticotropin releasing factor (CRF) is reduced in Alzheimer disease (AD). Neurology (N.Y.), *35(1)*:91, 1985.

75. Soininen, H.S.: Reduced cholinesterase activity and somatostatin-like immunoreactivity in the cerebrospinal fluid of patients with dementia of the Alzheimer type. J. Neurol. Sci., *63*:167, 1984.

76. Oram, J.J., Edwardson, J., and Millard, P.H.: Investigation of cerebrospinal fluid neuropeptides in idiopathic senile dementia. Gerontology, 27:216, 1981.

77. Rogers, R.L., et al.: Decreased cerebral blood flow precedes multi-infarct dementia, but follows senile dementia of Alzheimer type. Neurology, 36:1, 1986.

78. Facchinetti, F., et al.: Central ACTH deficit in degenerative and vascular dementia. Life Sci., 35:1691, 1984.

79. Nemeroff, C.B., et al.: Elevated cerebrospinal fluid concentrations of cortico tropin-releasing factor-like immunoreactivity in major depression. Science, *226*:1342, 1984.

80. Ferrero, P., et al.: Diazepam-binding inhibitor-like immunoreactivity (DBI-LI) in human CSF. Correlation with neurological disorders. J. Neurol. Sci., *87*:327, 1988.

81. Ernst, A., et al.: Comparison of DSIP-(delta sleeping-inducing peptide) and P-DSIP-like (phosphorylated) immunoreactivity in cerebrospinal fluid of patients with senile dementia of Alzheimer type, multi-infarct syndrome, communicating hydrocephalus and Parkinson's disease. J. Neurol., *235*:16, 1987.

82. Atack, J.R., et al.: Cerebrospinal fluid somatostatin and neuropeptide Y. Arch. Neuro., 45:269, 1988.

83. Widerlov, E., et al.: Elevated CSF somatostatin concentrations in demented patients parallel improved psychomotor functions induced by integrity-promoting care. Acta Psychiat. Scand., 79:41, 1989.

84. Adams, R.D., and Kubik, C.S.: subacute degeneration of the brain in pernicious anemia. N. Engl. J. Med., *231*:1, 1944.

85. Ferraro, A., Arieti, S., and English, W.H.: Cerebral changes in the course of pernicious anemia and their relationship to psychiatric symptoms. J. Neuropathol. Exp. Neurol., 4:217, 2945.

86. Cole, M.G., and Prchal, J.F.: Low serum vitamin B_{12} in Alzheimer-type dementia. Age Ageing, *13*:101, 1984.

87. Mitsuyama, Y., and Kogoh, H.: Serum and cerebrospinal fluid vitamin B_{12} levels in demented patients with CH_3-B_{12} treatment-Preliminary study. Jpn. J. Psychiat. Neurol., *42*:65, 1988.

88. Regland, B., et al.: Low B_{12} levels related to high activity of platelet MAO in patients with dementia disorders. Acta Psychiat. Scand., *78*:451, 1988.

89. Regland, B., Gottfries, C.G., and Lindstedt, G.: Dementia patients with low cobalamins: Relationship to atrophic gastritis. In press, 1989.

90. Bridge, J.P., et al.: Peripheral catecholamine enzyme function and cognitive impairment of elderly schizophrenics and controls. J. Am. Geriatr. Soc., *32*:259, 1984.

91. Oreland, L., and Gottfries, C.G.: Platelet and brain monoamine oxidase in aging and in dementia of Alzheimer's type. Progr. Neuro-Psychopharmacol. Bio. Psychiat., *10*:533, 1986.

92. Adolfsson, R., et al.: Increased activity of brain and platelet monoamine oxidase in dementia of Alzheimer type. Life Sci., *27*:1029, 1980.

93. Alexopoulos, G., Liebermann, K.W., and Young, R.C.: Platelet MAO activity in primary degenerative dementia. Am. J. Psychiatry, *141*:97, 1984.

94. Agnoli, A., et al.: Prolactin response as an index of dopaminergic receptor function in Parkinson's disease. Correlation with clinical finding and therapeutic response. J. Neural Transm., *51*:123, 1981.

95. Martinez, C., et al.: Thyrotrophine and prolactin responses to thyrotropin-releasing hormone in patients with Parkinson's disease. Acta Endocrinol., *99*:344, 1982.

96. Balldin, J., et al.: Dexamethasone suppression test and serum prolactin in dementia disorders. Br. J. Psychiat., *143*:277, 1983.

97. Balldin, J., et al.: Relationship between DST and the serotonegic system results from treatments with two 5-HT reuptake blockers in dementia disorders. Intl. J. Geriat. Psychiat., *3*:17, 1988.

98. McAllister, T.W., and Hays, L.R.: Thyrotropin-releasing hormone stimulation test and Alzheimer's disease. Biol. Psychiat., *21*:553, 1986.

99. Stahelin, H.G., et al.: Die THR-TSH-Regulation bei Hochbetagten und bei Patienten mit seniler Demenz. Schweiz. Med. Wochenschr., *112*:1784, 1982.

100. Sunderland, T., et al.: TRH stimulation test in dementia of the Alzheimer type and elderly controls. Psychiat. Res., *16*:269, 1985.

101. Peabody, C.A., et al.: Thyrotropin-releasing hormone stimulation test and Alzheimer's disease. Biol. Psychiat., *21*:553, 1986.

102. El Cobky, A., et al.: Anterior pituitary response to thyrotrophin releasing hormone in senile dementia (Alzheimer type) and elderly normals. Acta Psychiat. Scand., *74*:13, 1986.

103. Balldin, J., et al.: The clondine test in patients with dementia disorders: Relation to clinical status and cerbrospinal fluid metabolite levels. Intl. J. Geriat. Psychiat., *3*:15, 1988.

CHAPTER 20

Neuroradiology

O.F. AGEE

As a medical specialty, pathology long antedates the discovery of x-rays. Its first subspecialty with supplemental board examinations (1948) was neuropathology. Clinically, the latter is a consultative service responsive to influences from other disciplines. One such has been neuroradiology, and its impact is likely to increase.

This chapter explores areas of mutual interest, eventually addressing interdisciplinary interchanges in which the neuroradiologist can assist the neuropathologist. It will first introduce neuroimaging and present a portfolio of representative portrayals of neuroradiology's armamentarium. Illustrations have been chosen for their aptness in emphasizing principles rather than as specific histologic studies, although most diseases shown occur in the elderly. Intracranial abnormalities dominate but lesions within the spinal axis are represented. It is ironic at a time that neuroradiology increasingly turns toward function, rather than form, that the emphasis here remains classically anatomic.

HISTORICAL PERSPECTIVE AND OVERVIEW

The world has known of Roentgen's discovery for almost century.[1] Potential medical applications were recognized instantly, but for almost half a century, radiologists mostly exploited "plain-film" radiography. Few invasive procedures existed and use of parenteral contrast (material) was limited. Diagnostic results were astonishingly useful despite methodologic limitations, but they required an imaginative synthesis of subtle observations to indict a specific disease. Conventional radiographs showed only large differences in tissues, such as those between bone and soft tissue. (Of naturally occurring bodily inclusions, plain films recognize five general classes—gas, fat, water density (solid organs, blood, muscle, cerebrospinal fluid (CSF)), bone, and the enamel of teeth.) Unless adjacent structures fell in different categories, they were inseparable on film. Within the central nervous system (CNS), the brain and spinal cord were indistinguishable from CSF. Except for calcifications, aberrant gas, or large fat collections, everything within the skull and bony spinal canal appeared identical.

In 1918, Dandy began to explore the usefulness of introducing gas into the intracranial ventricles; ventriculography, and shortly, pneumoencephalography were born.[2,3] Notwithstanding associated morbidity and specificity limitations (proved a lesion's presence indirectly), "air-studies" remained diagnostic mainstays until gradually usurped by angiography in the 1960s; in refined form, they were sparingly used into the mid-1970s.

Sicard reported his experience with positive contrast material for myelography in 1922.[4] (Negative contrast, or gas myelography, even when combined with tomography, never enjoyed popularity in the United States.) A later iodine-containing, oily compound, iophendylate (Pantopaque, Lafayette Pharmacal, Inc., Lafayette, IN), was synthesized in the early 1940s and in turn replaced earlier materials.[5] Used widely through the 1970s, it allowed better definition of pathologic conditions in the spinal canal than in the head. Unfortunately, the material proved too opaque for optimal visualization of structures and was associated with arachnoiditis. In the late 1970s, water soluble media, offering salubrity and technical advantages,[6,7] replaced it. Myelography is still done, almost always in conjunction with computed tomography (CT), but with the advent of magnetic resonance imaging (MRI), the technique's days are numbered. Even in conjunction with CT, surrounding bone prohibits assessment of the internal character of cordal disease, displaying only a lesion's outline as reflected by surrounding subarachnoid contrast.

Within a month of Roentgen's epochal paper, an eerily prescient radiography was published showing a post mortem angiogram of a hand.[8] Almost 60 years would pass before angiography came into common clinical use. In 1927, Monitz published his experiences in angiography.[9] Struggling independently with primitive equipment and dangerous contrast materials, he suggested the method's potential. Done sporadically until the late 1950s, angiography languished because of the same deficits as in Monitz's time. As contrast media improved, other technical obstacles fell. Powerful generators came into wide use; mechanical film changers and reliable pressure injectors became available; image-intensified fluoroscopy proliferated, allowing intravascular catheters to be maneuvered. With the advent of percutaneous catheter insertion,[10] needle-delivery systems were abandoned. First $4\frac{1}{2}$, then $1\frac{1}{2}$-minute film processors replaced their predecessors and by the early 1960s, angiography flourished. Its acceptance wrought fundamental changes. With detailed vascular depiction, surgical correction of a wide spectrum of vascular lesions became possible. Because angiograms reflected the internal vasculature of a lesion, radiologists began to focus on a lesion's composition as well as its outline. By emphasizing time and flow direction as factors in the evaluation of ischemia, angiography introduced a dynamism to pathologic situations. Finally, the neuroradiologist became the doer and interpreter of interventional studies, rather than only the latter, thus changing his role and reacquainting him with the patient.

By the early 1960s, complementary approaches were developing in nuclear medicine. Improvements in detection hardware and isotopic tracers offered geographic information similar to that of air studies and included data about the internal functioning of a lesion.[11] Radionuclide brain scans became common, and by mid decade spinoffs permitted evaluation of cerebral blood flow,[12] an enterprise that persists.

Important, but largely evolutionary, incremental improvements of conventional techniques continued, but by the early 1970s, progress had plateaued.

In 1973, Ambrose published the first report of CT usage.[13] By applying computer technology to severely collimated x-ray sources in a unique geometry, Hounsfield provided a tool that allowed a revolutionary improvement in safety and diagnostic accuracy.[14] Recognizing the debt that still newer methods owe to CT approaches, one might legitimately divide neuroradiology into pre- and post-CT eras. The number of air studies and radionuclide brain scans done declined to almost zero within months.

CT allowed subdivision of the five plain-film compartments, a refinement crucial in the middle, "water density" group. Intracranial contents no longer appeared homogeneous; brain became distinguishable from blood clot, CSF, edema, and many neoplasms. Still based on tissue x-ray absorption, irrespective of electronic exaggeration, images retained the white/black orientation of conventional filming (bone white, gas black), thereby mitigating initial disaffection with unfamiliar axial images. An early refinement was the use of parenteral iodinated contrast material.[15] Subsequently, inhaled rather than injected contrast would be used to evaluate blood flow.[16] A significant later application proved to be CT stereotactic localization of lesions.[17]

CT has hazards, applying radiation and, frequently, contrast. It is ideally suited for imaging only in the axial plane, although coronals could be made directly and reformatted images in nonaxial planes were sometimes satisfactory. Although there were some technical compromises, CT found many lesions that had previously been missed. It represented a giant step.

CT technology spawned spinoff applications. Surmising that the same strategies might be used with other energy sources, similar approaches were applied to nuclear medicine and ultrasound. The latter, afflicted with unusual complexity, has enjoyed limited success, but nuclear medicine exploited the techniques splendidly—for example, in SPECT scanners. As a result, and in combination with newer tracer materials, nuclear medicine emerged from its nadir and promises much in the investigation of neurologic disease. SPECT and PET scanning, offering access to more functional data, along with MR spectroscopy, seem likely to cause an unprecedented change of emphasis to the physiologic.

Within a short time, CT was extended to other parts of the body, including the spine. Patients with neurologic diseases benefited earlier than those requiring studies of the abdomen or chest. Although artifacts sometimes degraded images of the brain and spine, the scans of other organs were so afflicted that detail failed to match that obtained of the CNS. CT became the standard to which other tests were compared, and the 1980s opened with a mood of optimism, even satisfaction, with the diagnostic armamentarium.

Nuclear magnetic resonance (NMR) spectroscopy has been an entrenched analytical tool since the 1950s.[18,19] Cognizant of CT's techniques, visionaries in that field began to wonder whether MR might support imaging.[20] In September of 1980, the first "clinical" symposium on NMR imaging was held at Vanderbilt University. Attended by almost equal numbers of basic scientists and radiologists, many of the latter concluded that the enterprise might offer promise after years of development, but did not warrant committing resources. At the next year's symposium, held at Bowman-Gray, the change was dramatic. MR imaging was on the threshold of clinical application.

MRI terminology/technology was novel to most physicians. Radiologists resurrected physics texts in an effort to understand even the commonly used measure of magnetic force, the gauss, only to quickly find the preferred terminology changing to the more convenient tesla (T), 10,000 times a gauss. Clinical units operate at field strengths between 0.15 T and 1.5 T. Those between about 0.15 and 0.3 T are spoken of as "low field," while those between 0.3 and 0.8 ± T are termed "mid field," and above that, "high field magnets." (The earth's magnetic field is approximately 0.5 gauss, or about 30,000 times less than that of a 1.5 T unit.) Mid- and high-field units have dominated the market in recent years, partly because of better images, but also because they might support future applications, such as spectroscopy. Reflecting that trend, most images shown are products of either the General Electric Signa (1.5 T) or the Siemens Magnetom S/P scanner (1.0 T). Some illustrations show scans from our earlier Technicare units (0.15 T). CT scans are mostly the products of our GE 9800 units. It is uncertain which magnitude is best, or whether 1.5 T units will be ideal for spectroscopy or in imaging of other elements. It is structurally difficult to preserve a large bore (the aperture in which specimens are studied) in very high-field units, and as a consequence, experimental units in the 10- to 12-T range have quite small apertures (up to about 9 cm diameter), unsuitable for a patient. Such may be moot if very high fields prove hazardous, although experimental whole-body units presently operate at 4.0 T.[21]

The magnets used are bulky, complex, and expensive. They must maintain a uniform magnetic field within the bore and require constant maintenance. Some, mostly in the lower mid-field range, are permanent magnets, and although simpler in construction, cheaper to maintain, and easier to shield (both from and to the environment), they are greatly outnumbered by electromagnets, either resistive (low field) or superconducting. The latter perform at near 0° K and are cooled by coaxial envelopes containing liquid helium and liquid nitrogen.

Although a resistive magnet may be shut off when not in use, a permanent magnet cannot be, and for practical reasons superconductors are not. Even when not in clinical use, most superconductors are powerful attracters of ferromagnetic material. A screwdriver placed near a high-field unit becomes a missile streaking toward the magnet. A metal gurney wheeled too close will slam itself against the unit's surface, attracted so strongly that several persons cannot pry it loose. Watches may be stopped, credit cards erased, etc.

MRI is the modality of choice for the evaluation of most neurologic disease. For clinical purposes, its resolution (about 0.5 millimeter) matches CT, and by further fractionating tissue differences, it permits the recognition of even subtler variations; for example, an exaggerated differentiation of white from gray matter, an accomplishment crudely done with CT. There are other formidable advantages. Unlike CT in which the section plane is dependent on the geometric relationship between patient and machinery (gantry), MRI equipment defines the plane (or volume) electronically; no positional changes of the patient are required. CT images of the spine were always made axially, and with the head, usually. Head images could be made coronally, provided the patient's neck was flexible enough to maintain the contorted, neck hyperextended position required, and for practical purposes, sagittal images were never directly obtained. MRI scans are obtained with the patient in a single, comfortable position—usually supine. Coronal, sagittal, and useful "off plane" images in any axis can be made with the same facility as axials, permitting scrutiny in the most suitable

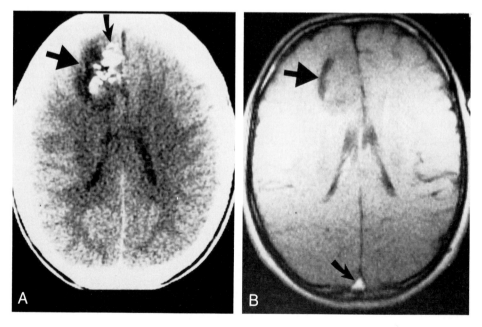

Fig. 20–1. A, Axial CT without contrast. This oligodendroglioma shows dense calcification medially (small arrow) and a crescentic cystic space laterally (large arrow). B, T1 axial image. The cystic space is shown (large arrow) but the bulky calcification is not. Note the high signal of slowly flowing blood in the sigmoid sinus (small arrow).

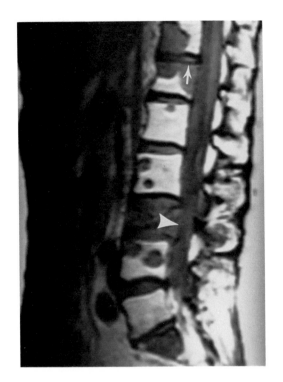

Fig. 20–2. The vertebral end-plates' cortical bone is shown as a thin black line devoid of signal (small arrow). The bone marrow, containing considerable fat, generates a high signal, and when replaced by breast carcinoma metastases, reverts to an easily recognizable lower signal. L3 and S1 are completely replaced by tumor, and the former shows a fragment projecting posteriorly into the thecal space (arrowhead).

view for evaluation. A critical by-product, particularly in the spine with its length orthogonal to the axial plane, is the ability to inspect, in the coronal or sagittal view, many levels simultaneously rather than by integrating a ponderous number of axial slices. Finally, MRI permits numerous acquisition variations, a versatility allowing customized images to portray the pathologic condition expected. CT permits two variations (with and without contrast material); MRI retains those and offers others.

With CT, reliance on abnormal calcification as a diagnostic clue persisted, for example, with neoplasms and aneurysms. Although such deposits, and cortical bone, contain protons (used here as specifically equivalent to the hydrogen nucleus), the latter are bound in a tissue matrix prohibiting an MRI signal and

appear as black voids "seen" vaguely in negative—easily overlooked unless especially large (Figs. 20–1 and 20–2). Thus, when appreciation of cortical detail and/or calcium is crucial, supplementation by CT is necessary, a situation commonly prevailing, for example, within the petrous pyramids. The lack of signal from dense bone is, however, also a boon. It is difficult for CT to image soft tissue within or immediately adjacent to dense bone. With MRI, bone, having no signal, disappears from view, and thus denuded, intraosseous soft tissues are clearly seen (Fig. 20–3).

Shortly after CT's appearance, investigators theorized that conventional, iodine-containing contrast materials could be used in conjunction with it; such media should cause the same x-ray attenuation as seen in conventional filming. Expectations were exceeded because of the increased sensitivity of CT. Not only were vessels discernible with relatively trivial amounts of circulating contrast, but intra/perilesional leakage into interstitial spaces, because of blood-brain barrier (BBB) breakdown, was detectable, adding a new dimension. As MRI evolved, the same thoughts emerged, but with a new problem: what sort of material would furnish a suitable contrast medium for the totally different magnetic resonance imaging? The usual iodine-containing media were worthless; compounds were needed that would affect the magnetic properties of tissues. Theory, and a long familiarity with contaminates in MR spectroscopy suggested answers, and by the mid-1980s clinical trials began on the first of an emerging group of paramagnetic agents, Gd-DTPA.[22] (Gadolinium diethylenetriamine pentaacetic acid, now usually designated gadopentotate dimeglumine [Magnevist, Berlix Laboratories, Inc., Wayne, NJ], the term is frequently shortened to "gadolinium", or in the vernacular, "gad", abbreviations emphasizing the diagnostically active ingredient rather than its carrier molecule. The modifier "Gd" will appear in explanatory legends of illustrations in this chapter if contrast has been used). After extensive testing, the material came into general usage, having been pronounced safe for all but a few patients,[23] generally age group and/or special situation classes in which insufficient data have emerged to prove safety. The material is well

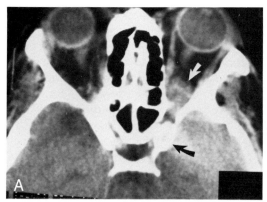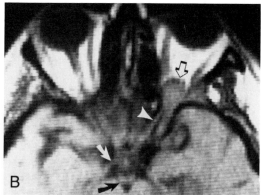

Fig. 20–3. A, Axial CT with contrast. An orbital apex mass (white arrow) extends posteriorly into an enlarged superior orbital fissure, but intracranial extension is obscured by surrounding bone, principally the anterior clinoid (black arrow). B, Axial T1 image. The anterior end of the club-shaped mass (hollow arrow) is still seen, as is its intracranial component. Cortical bone, devoid of signal, has been "removed." The optic nerves can be seen intracranially and the left (arrowhead) is separate from the mass, which proved to be a neurofibroma of the ophthalmic division of the trigeminal nerve. More posteriorly, the anterior portion of the optic tracts can be seen (white arrow) emerging from the chiasm. The faint white dot behind the chiasm is the end-on pituitary stalk and behind it, the mamillary bodies (black arrow) project into the interpeduncular fossa.

tolerated and retains the diagnostic effectiveness of iodinated materials. It is expensive, the usual adult dose exceeding $100.

Other MRI contrast materials will be marketed soon. The next generation also contains gadolinium, varying the carrier's molecular structure to accomplish goals such as a nonionic structure and/or iso-osmolarity,[24] but many other elements known to influence magnetic properties of tissue are potentially usable.[25] Eventual permutations may allow specialized applications far transcending conventional materials.

Gd-DTPA shows the same events as conventional iodine-containing contrast; while circulating in the blood, it may visibly inline vessels, and, in the brain and cord, it accumulates in metabolically active, pathologic tissue. Except with brain and spinal cord, contrast *normally* exits blood vessels and enters surrounding parenchyma. Normal tissues will, therefore, "enhance." An extraneural lesion, depending on its vascularity and avidity for contrast may appear as an abnormal low-signal area, because enhancement within the lesion may not be as great as in the normal. Alternatively, enhancement may be identical to or greater than normal. Meninges and anterior

pituitary react in the same fashion. In the brain and cord, no normal extravascular escape of contrast occurs because of the BBB. Unless pathology is cystic and/or devoid of viable tissue, breakdown of the BBB allows unique enhancement of the lesion. The lack of any normal tissue enhancement increases the conspicuity of lesions, thereby leading to fewer ambiguities, i.e., situations in which a lesion's enhancement matches the organ's. Further, because enhancement depends solely on a BBB breakdown, it is a nonspecific attribute of all pathology. The degree of enhancement is dependent on the timing of scanning following contrast administration, with most scans done immediately following injection.

It is hardly an exaggeration to maintain that MR images effectively match gross observation of the brain at autopsy, notwithstanding the ability of a prosector to discern color or to appreciate textural changes tactily. Even with continuing refinements in histopathology, with the advent of CT and MRI neuroradiology narrowed the gap between neuropathology and itself. As the two disciplines' limits converge, dialog becomes more mutually helpful and problems may begin to show a surprising commonality. In vitro microscopic MRI is done with the use of 4.0 to 12 T laboratory units. The present resolution is at about 4 micrometers (μm),[26] but this is achieved only in small-bore magnets. The practical resolution limit may be about 1 μm, with greater magnification prohibited by the sparcity of signal generated by minute populations of protons (poor signal-to-noise ratio) and the intrinsic motion of protons that produces discernible blur within the time necessary to produce an image.[27] The latter effect, "diffusion," is itself measurable and may well be an important clinical tool in the future.[28] In vivo specimens are even more mobile, and the time required to generate data for microscopic detail may be prohibitive.

Ultimately, the two disciplines will likely become more dependent upon one another.

MAGNETIC RESONANCE IMAGE

Angiograms, myelograms, and even CT exams are shown sparingly in this chapter, with the focus being on MRI. The appearance of images from the first three are well understood but that of MRI is not. This section introduces certain MRI theory, technique, and terminology, illustrating the effects with examples from four general disease categories, namely, neoplasia, edema, hemorrhage, and tissue loss or hypoplasia.

In a strong magnetic field, the nuclei of some elements preferentially align themselves coincident with the field's axis. One such nucleus, that of hydrogen (^{1}H)—a single proton—has, because of its relatively strong magnetic properties and abundance in tissue, proven the most suitable for imaging. Although present in other substances, such as fat, its incorporation into the water molecule and the latter's ubiquity ensure a satisfactory composition for signal production from most tissues. Generally, ^{1}H MRI reflects water concentration. Because the latter is frequently deranged in or around pathology, a pictorial record of that association is useful. Once protons are aligned with the magnetic field, radio pulses at an element-specific frequency excite reorientations of nuclei. When the radiofrequency (RF) pulsing is stopped, nuclei return to their original field orientation, losing energy in the form of an outgoing radio signal that is measurable. Super-

imposing a complex system for geographically locating the origin of such responses, a tissue map is then displayed on a TV screen. A variety of pulses may be imposed, resulting in different-appearing images that may reflect small compositional differences between tissues, or alternatively, optimally portray overall organ configuration. Others accentuate motion, such as with blood flow. The result is a repertoire of pulse sequences designed to elicit different characteristics of the same tissue. Innovative variations surface continuously.

Some sequences, resulting in depiction of proton density (concentration), appear bland and usually are not helpful. Others emphasize one of two characteristic decay patterns (toward ground magnetization state) and the results are spoken of as T1 or T2 images. "T1" and "T2" images are invariably a combination of both, but with one dominant. Hence, proper terminology would designate them T1- or T2-*weighted* images, but in this chapter the "weighted" modifier is deleted. Actual T1 and T2 numerical values may be (rather laboriously) calculated for any given tissue, an enterprise rarely attempted clinically. The values, expressed in milliseconds, are the tissue "relaxation times." Although notable exceptions exist, most CNS pathology has longer relaxation times than normal tissue. On a T1 scan such lesions appear darker than normal (low signal), but on T2, whiter (high signal). It is visually easier to detect abnormal high signal against the dark background normal, this being one reason that T2 images display abnormalities more conspicuously.

Broadly speaking T1/T2 differences are based on variations in the interactions of targeted nuclei with atoms in their immediate environment. The most common sequence of pulses used clinically is a variety termed "spin-echo" and may result, depending on pulse timing, in either a T1 or a T2 image. Several other, lesser used sequences, such as inversion recovery (IR) (Fig. 20–4) exist to generate a T1 image, and most generic sequences are modified further. An increasingly common variation, frequently proprietarily designated, is the gradient-echo sequence, used to diminish scan time, to selectively influence certain tissue signals, or to emphasize flow-related events. The more readings obtained during an acquisition

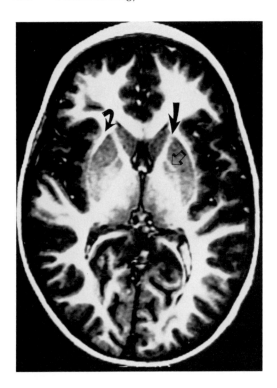

Fig. 20–4. Axial T1 image. The white matter shows a high signal in this 3-year-old's normal scan. The anterior limbs of the internal capsules are well shown (solid arrow on left). The gray matter of the adjacent caudate nuclei heads and lentiform nuclei are shown with a separation between the globus pallidus and putamen (hollow arrow). The right external capsule is indicated by a curved arrow. The inversion recovery sequence is infrequently used, requiring more time than spin-echo variations. On spin-echo T2 images, white matter appears darker than gray.

series, the better the image, assuming no specimen motion. Because patient motion is always a risk, practical acquisition times are compromises; lengthy scan times may allow enough motion to offset theoretical advantages. For clinical usage, a fast but "noisy" set of images may be obtained in less than 1 minute but most acquisitions will require between 4 and 12 minutes. (Lengthening examination time to 1 hour also approaches economic unfeasibility.) "Gating" procedures that synchronize acquisitions with the heart cycle are not now frequently used for CNS imaging. The thickness of sections may be varied, with or without gaps between sections, and with data acquired volumetrically instead of in a planar fashion,

then to be displayed either in "pseudo 3D" or broken into planar images in a conventional way, in any plane the viewer specifies. With planar acquisitions, high-field units provide 2- to 3-mm thick sections as minimum thicknesses and about one-half that if obtained volumetrically. Usually, resultant data are arranged in a planar, grid-like matrix of variable proportion, commonly ranging from 128 × 195 to 512 × 512, which determines pixel size, referring to the smallest, en face (x–y axis) *area* separately distinguishable. The smaller the pixels, the better the spatial resolution. The depth, or z axis, is determined by slice thickness, and when this parameter is added, the unit of indivisibility, now *volume*, is called a voxel. Several views and sequences are used during a single examination and the number of images resulting may be bewildering, commonly up to 80 or more. Hard-copy annotations document much information about acquisition sets, and it is wise to appraise these, because the techniques used influence image type and quality; particularly notable are the TR and TE values, both time measurements in milliseconds. TR is an abbreviation of repetition time and refers to the total time required for a "single" RF excitation, then later decay and measurement of the resulting signal, a process repeated over and over again until the requisite sample is obtained to define necessary detail. (The summed TRs required for a given image set is its acquisition time.) TRs usually range between 500 and 2500 msec. In general, if TR is less than 1 second ("short TR") in spin-echo sequences, resultant images are T1 in type. If TR is in the range of 2000 to 3000 msecs, the result tends toward T2; thus, for the same number of excitations, T2 images require two to three times the acquisition time of a T1 image. TE, an abbreviation of echo-time, varies from about 10 to 25 msec for T1 images accompanying a short TR and up to about 150 msec for the longer TR T2 images. For specialized uses, very short, 100-msec acquisition times suffice for an image.[29] If contrast has been used, annotations so indicate. Images may show a difference in brightness at one edge compared with others; this is usually due to the geometry of surface coils used as RF receiver antennae. The signal is greatest closest to the coil. The size and shape of coils are variable because they are specifically chosen to match the subject's volume of interest. (Most large MRI facilities depend not only on coils supplied by manufacturers, but also on ingenious variations designed by their own engineer/physicists.)

Although images are frequently accompanied by orientative annotations indicating right and left, it is useful to know standard conventions that automatically determine laterality. On axial views, the head or spine is oriented as though one is inspecting it from a caudal direction and with the patient supine. Thus, the ventral aspect of the patient is directed superiorly (nose up), and the patient's right side is on the viewer's left. On coronal views, the images are as though one is looking at the patient from the front. The top of the head is at the top of the film and the patient's right side is on the viewer's left. On sagittal views, the top of the patient's head is at the top of the film and customarily, the patient faces the viewer's left. Anatomic landmarks easily establish the orientation of axial and coronal images but it may be difficult to recognize laterality on sagittal views because the two halves of the brain may appear identical. (Some units give approximate right–left annotations on sagittal series but others do not, and it is advisable to ask about a particular unit's conventions. Most units proceed from the left side of the patient toward the right, an unreliable generalization.) Many studies, especially of the spine, include an image (usually sagittal) with annotation of the planes of accompanying coronal and axial sections, an indispensable aid for orientation.

For imaging, the hydrogen nucleus is an attractive target but other magnetically influenced elements possess properties recommending them as alternatives. A partial list of biologically significant elements includes ^{13}C, ^{15}N, ^{23}Na, and ^{31}P; preliminary investigation of some of these is already occurring.[30] In general, the sparcity of these elements in tissue prohibits the elegant resolution obtained with ^{1}H; but, because several elements directly reflect crucial biochemical processes, scans showing their distribution are of interest. More importantly, some, such as ^{31}P, have potential for in vivo MR spectroscopy,[31] combined with a gross form of localizing imaging. By reflecting

energy transfer mechanisms, such studies should have a major impact on the diagnosis and treatment of ischemia, neoplastic growth, etc.[32,33]

A patient's safety and comfort are paramount considerations in any medical procedure. Many reports attest to the safety of ^{1}H MRI.[34] With the stronger magnetic fields required for nonproton MRI, spectroscopy, and/or microimaging, ultimately a point may be reached at which safety is abridged. Present imaging, without hazard for most patients, is unsuitable for certain individuals. Patients may harbor crucially positioned ferromagnetic materials within their bodies, frequently placed surgically, that, perturbed by the strong magnetic field could cause damage by moving; for example, berry aneurysmal clips.[35] Most institutions have long adopted strategies to screen patients against the possibility of untoward foreign body motion. (A subsidiary industry has developed to convert ferromagnetic medical devices to materials unaffected by magnetic fields and/or RF pulsing. Similarly, appropriately constituted life-support/anesthesia systems are being developed.) Another group adversely affected is that with implanted devices such as pacemakers or spinal cord stimulators.[36] Finally, although the number of patients experiencing claustrophobia in the long tube-like gantry (much more confining than the shorter, doughnut-like CT gantry) has not matched predictions, about 1 patient in 20 cannot tolerate the enclosure. The gantry aperture is confining, and not infrequently, a patient's bulk prevents entry. Once in the unit, a monotonous, metronome-like clicking noise is the patient's chief external stimulus and many go to sleep, an undesirable eventuality in cooperative patients, because movement can no longer be volitionally prevented.

MRI's relatively long scan times, dangers of ferromagnetic materials in or around the patient (such as life-support utensils) and lack of signal from cortical bone conspire to reduce the usefulness in MRI in the acutely traumatized patient, and CT is usually chosen. (Furthermore, fresh hemorrhage is not as easily appreciated on MRI as on CT.)

CT and MR scans are afflicted with image degrading and sometimes confusing artifacts. Only a few examples will be cited. The most

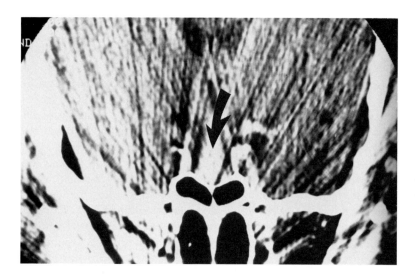

Fig. 20–5. Coronal CT with contrast. The sellar area (arrow) is obscured by linear artifacts generated from dental amalgam, a problem avoided with MRI. Some orthodontic devices create artifacts in the face area on MRI, but do not usually mar brain visualization.

common serious degradation is secondary to patient motion. (Outside the CNS where vascular pulsatility, respiration and/or mobile intestinal gas contribute their own movements, motion is a more extreme problem.) Metallic inclusions affect either type of scan, but in general, MRI enjoys an advantage, if for no other reason than dental amalgam has little adverse effect (Fig. 20–5). Nonetheless, even minute ferrous materials, not dangerous because of position and size, can create substantial distortion (Fig. 20–6). Metal artifacts are usually recognizable and are unlikely to be mistaken for lesions. One common CT artifact, beam "hardening" by bone, has no counterpart in MRI. The result is that MRI does a better job of depicting soft tissue in certain areas, particularly the brain stem (Fig. 20–7) or low temporal lobes. On CT, beam hardening usually results in false-negative impressions, hiding ossified lesions, but may occasionally produce false-positive overcalls, particularly of extracerebral fluid collections. A different limitation geographically related to bone is that of visualization of convexity cortex; bone produces on CT such a dominant whiteness that it is impossible to depict immediately adjacent soft tissue. Meninges, relatively small cortical vessels, and other such tissues are lost in the bone aggregate. With MRI, the inner table has no signal and surface detail is seen, a property increasing the conspicuity of abnormal Gd enhancement nearby and furnishing justification for MRI's dominance in detecting meningeal

disease. All scans potentially suffer from sampling error. Unless planar sections are contiguous, unsampled tissue will intervene between images, a phenomenon most apparent with CT of the spine in which long segments are studied axially, precluding contiguous slices. A potentially serious pitfall (and another reason for CT's difficulty in depicting cortex near the inner table) is "partial volume averaging." Most offensive in the z, or depth plane (slice thickness, usually the longest axis of a voxel), it is the inevitable result of a voxel's finite size. A structure smaller than or only partly included within a voxel contributes only part of the value within the volume that will be represented in the resultant image. It is averaged with other tissue to produce a net value that may not reflect its presence. If an isolated group of voxels has enough of its average contributed by aberrant values from a mostly out-of-plane tissue, the latter's origin may not be recognized and may be erroneously thought to be diseased. The visual effect is rather like viewing the tip of an iceberg from the sky. Just as inspection of the iceberg beneath the water clarifies its character, integration with adjacent scan slices allows recognition. Thin, contiguous sections minimize confusion. Electronic artifacts occur; usually recognizable, they may obscure pathology. One artifact unique to MRI is that of chemical shift.[37] Noticeable at high-field strengths, differential spatial shifts of certain chemical groups create geographic distortion. Most apparent with fat, the phenomenon

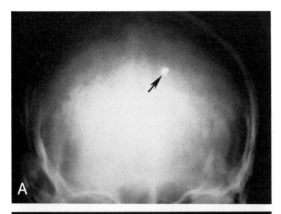

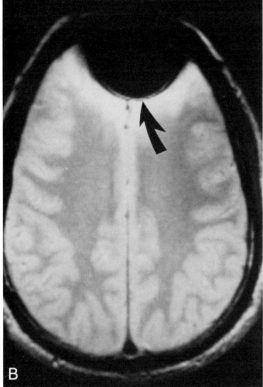

Fig. 20–6. A, PA plain film of skull. Note the small metallic foreign body. Located in the scalp, its presence did not contraindicate MRI. B, Axial proton density image. Although the patient experienced no discomfort during the MR scan and no complications ensued, the foreign body created a disproportionately large artifact.

is recognizable and is even an exploitable trait.[38] Finally, one MRI artifact, truncation,[39] can simulate abnormality, particularly in the spinal cord. Pseudosyrinxes may result. When technical and anatomic factors favor trunca-

tion artifact production, "lesions" must be more stringently proven and extra acquisitions may be necessary for authentication.

Illustrations emphasize the signal characteristics of tissues as shown by MR scans, with only incidental mention of secondary changes in bone, location and multiplicity of lesions, and mass effects. For those requiring a more scrupulously detailed description of MRI theory, a comprehensive reference is provided.[40]

MRI APPEARANCE OF NEOPLASMS

This heterogeneous group shows such diversity that it is useful in the description of all but a few of MRI's repertoire. Gadolinium is usually used. Lesions separate into those primarily from CNS parenchyma, either neural or supporting elements, or extra-axial, arising from bone, meninges, nerve sheaths, etc. Some contain unusual tissues such as fat, blood clot, or melanin, which may reduce differential diagnostic probabilities.

The usual intra-axial tumor generates less signal than does normal brain on T1 images and appears darker (Fig. 20–8A), although the difference may be difficult to appreciate. Secondary perilesional edema has a similar appearance. T2 images also show their version of relaxation time lengthening, but instead of a low signal, a high signal results (white) and is strikingly different from background (Fig. 20–8B). Unfortunately, edema also shows a high signal and may be indistinguishable from a neoplastic nidus. Although differentiation may be possible with improvised pulse sequence acquisitions, separation is usually made by administering contrast and then repeating at least one T1 set. Edema does not ordinarily sequester gadolinium, and hence, viable neoplasm is identified by its then uniquely high signal (Fig. 20–8C); nonaxial views frequently excel in defining a tumor's margin (Fig. 20–8D). Even with contrast, the scan margin of neoplasia is not necessarily indicative of the microscopic extent of tumor but is a reasonable approximation. If the margin is distinctly defined, the neoplasm is likely to be a less aggressive variety, whereas poor definition suggests more substantial infiltration into surrounding tissues and greater atypia. The tumor interior may have cystic and/or necrotic components, and

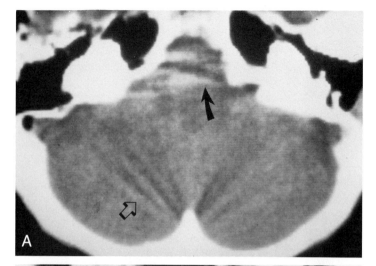

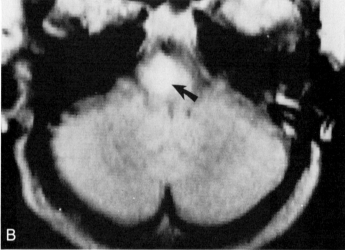

Fig. 20-7. A, Axial CT without contrast. The patient had signs of a brain stem lesion but beam hardening artifact, particularly overlying the brain stem ("Hounsfield artifact"—solid arrow) hides the disease process. The alternating black/white linear radiations from the internal occipital protuberance are also caused by beam hardening. B, Axial T1 image. A high-signal blood clot is discernible in the right lower pons area (arrow). A result of bleeding from an AVM, the lesion owes its signal to contained methemoglobin.

in both, the signal resembles that of CSF, showing the same progression from black toward high-signal white as the T2 effect increases (Fig. 20–9). Necrotic spaces, as in glioblastoma multiforme, tend to have a thicker, more irregular wall than, for example, the sharply defined cysts of benign astrocytomas. If associated with intense hypervascularity, abnormally dilated blood vessels within and surrounding a lesion can be appreciated (Fig. 20–10). Particularly with contrasted studies, spread into nearby subarachnoid spaces is often discernible, a difficult observation on CT.

A tumor containing uncharacteristic intracranial material, such as fat and/or cholesterol (Fig. 20–11), or certain products of hemorrhage is easily discerned by a *shortening* of re-laxation time, best appreciated on T1 images as an aberrant, whitish area of high signal. Calcifications are poorly appreciated but are expected to have no signal (black).

Excluding the pituitary, most primary extra-axial neoplasms arise from the meninges or Schwann cells. Usually internally homogeneous, with T1 and T2 essentially identical to normal brain, without contrast they are recognized by mass effect, rather than an aberrant signal (Fig 20–12A,B). Because BBB is not involved, such lesions enhance spectacularly and are then easily discerned (Fig. 20–12C), sometimes showing a cleft of intervening subarachnoid space between themselves and neural tissue. Even within foramina, the absence of a signal from bone allows identification (Fig.

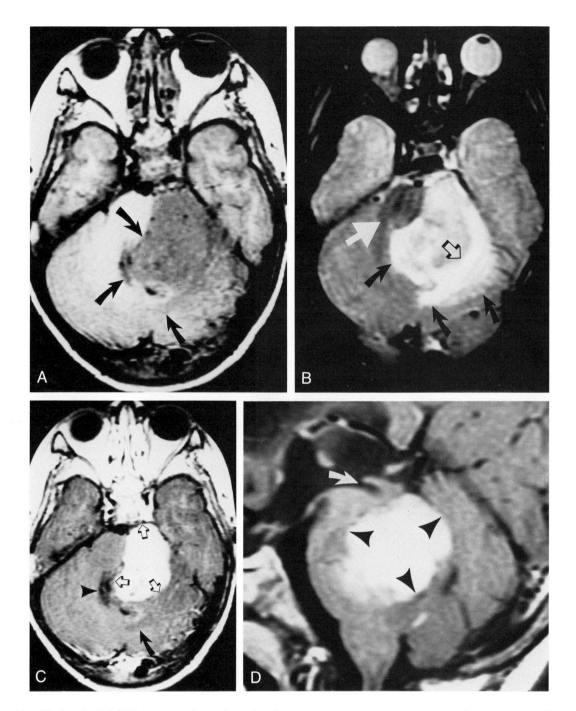

Fig. 20–8. A, Axial T1 image. A large, low-signal mass occupies the anterior 70% of the left cerebellar hemisphere and herniates across the midline toward the right. Its posterolateral margin is poorly defined. B, Axial T2 image. The lesion (black arrows) is better defined on T2 images as a region of increased signal. The signal is inhomogeneous and there is a margin (hollow arrow) between that which will ultimately be shown neoplasm anteromedially, and posterior edema. Without subsequent contrast images, differentiation of neoplasm from edema would have been uncertain. The low-signal brain stem (white arrow) is compressed and distorted as it is pushed toward the right. Incidentally, the patient shows high-signal mucosal swelling in the ethmoid air cells. C, Axial T1 image with Gd. The neoplasm is enhanced (hollow arrows) but the edema is not. Note the posteromedial finger of edema reverting to a T1 low-signal (solid arrow). The distorted fourth ventricle is displaced well to the right of midline (arrowhead). D, Sagittal T1 image with Gd. The ability to view the lesion in multiple projections frequently adds to better appreciation of its geography and the involvement of adjacent structures. This tumor (arrowheads) causes aqueductal obstruction; note the dilated rostral aqueduct (arrow) and third ventricle.

471

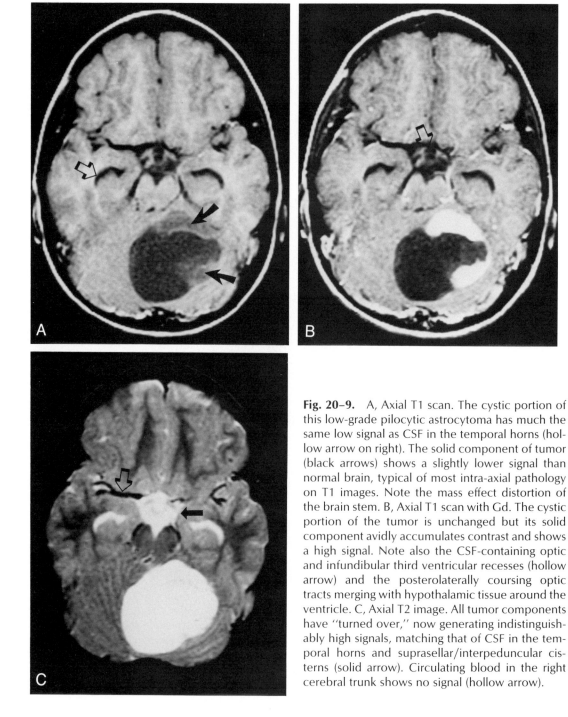

Fig. 20–9. A, Axial T1 scan. The cystic portion of this low-grade pilocytic astrocytoma has much the same low signal as CSF in the temporal horns (hollow arrow on right). The solid component of tumor (black arrows) shows a slightly lower signal than normal brain, typical of most intra-axial pathology on T1 images. Note the mass effect distortion of the brain stem. B, Axial T1 scan with Gd. The cystic portion of the tumor is unchanged but its solid component avidly accumulates contrast and shows a high signal. Note also the CSF-containing optic and infundibular third ventricular recesses (hollow arrow) and the posterolaterally coursing optic tracts merging with hypothalamic tissue around the ventricle. C, Axial T2 image. All tumor components have "turned over," now generating indistinguishably high signals, matching that of CSF in the temporal horns and suprasellar/interpeduncular cisterns (solid arrow). Circulating blood in the right cerebral trunk shows no signal (hollow arrow).

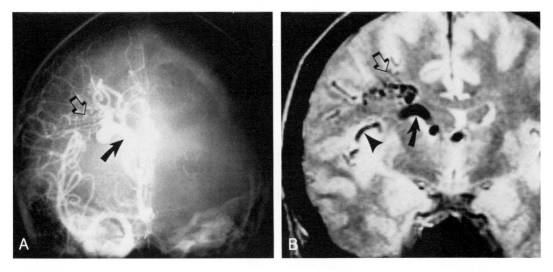

Fig. 20–10.   A, AP right carotid angiogram—arterial phase. The somewhat diffuse nidus of a high parietal AVM (hollow arrow) promptly shunts into dilated veins draining to the deep venous system. Note the similarity of Figure 10B and of the veins lateral to the solid arrow. B, Coronal T2 image. The components of the AVM are shown as signal voids, with the lesion's nidus (hollow arrow) superolateral to enlarged veins. A slightly dilated middle cerebral feeder is seen (arrowhead) over the insular surface. The depiction of the lesion is less complete than on the angiogram because the image is a tomographic section with other components seen in adjacent slices; "3D" images would show the entire lesion.

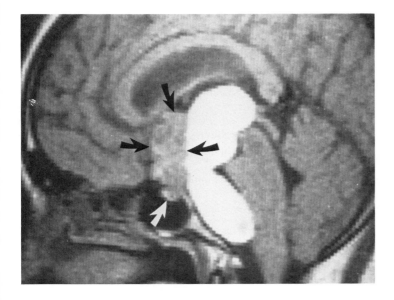

Fig. 20–11.   Sagittal T1 image. Above the normal size sella (white arrow) there is a large trilobular mass. While this craniopharyngioma's anterior component (black arrows) has a nondescript appearance, cholesterol laden material in the posteriorly directed cyst generates a high signal.

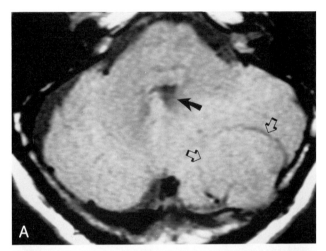

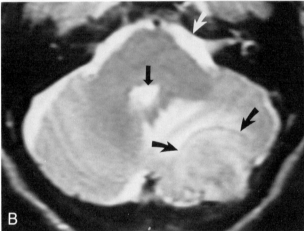

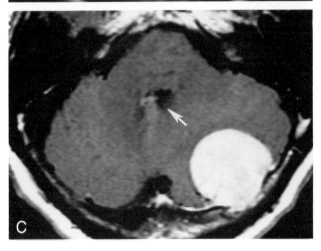

Fig. 20–12. A, Axial T1 image. This large posterior fossa meningioma has a signal identical to normal parenchyma, a feature common in extra-axial neoplasms. Its presence can be deduced from its mass effect (distorting the fourth ventricle—solid arrow) and by a margin of low signal partially outlining its surface (hollow arrows). Edema between the tumor and the fourth ventricle is impossible to appreciate. B, Axial T2 image. The lesion margin retains its low signal (curved black arrows) and is a capsule rather than a CSF cleft. Edema behind the fourth ventricle (straight black arrow) has converted to a high signal like the CSF in the ventricle and pontine/CP angle cisterns (white arrow). Of incidental note is the basilar artery, shown as a circular midline flow void in the pontine cistern, and CSF in the left internal auditory canal. Fluid is seen within the vestibular apparatus posterior to the canal and within the cochlea anteriorly. The meningioma has acquired a slightly higher signal than parenchyma; commonly, extra-axial tumors are identical with normal tissue on T2 images. C, Axial T1 image with Gd. CSF in the fourth ventricle (arrow) and anterior basal cisterns show the usual low T1 signal, but the meningioma shows striking contrast accumulation. Its location and discreteness, as well as its noncontrast signals, are characteristic of an extra-axial origin. The blunting of the posteromedial abutment of tumor with dura and the high-signal "tail" of contrast proceeding medially is a combination of plaque-like tumor spread and contrast within draining veins.

20–13). Without contrast, small tumors may be overlooked. Neoplasms within the spinal cord or adjacent spaces respond similarly (Fig. 20–14).

Although uncommon in the geriatric patient, pituitary tumors merit mention because their signal characteristics re-enforce aforementioned concepts. With no BBB in the anterior pituitary, tissue normally shows enhancement following contrast administration. Most small neoplasms exhibit lesser enhancement and are seen as low-signal areas (Fig. 20–15), a nonspecific characteristic. One MRI advantage, compared with CT, is the exquisite visualization of perisellar structures, such as the optic chiasm and cavernous sinuses, important for the surgeon to evaluate prior to intervention.

Many non-neoplastic lesions also show abnormal enhancement from BBB breakdown, including cerebritis and abscess, the margins of infarctions, and acute demyelinating proc-

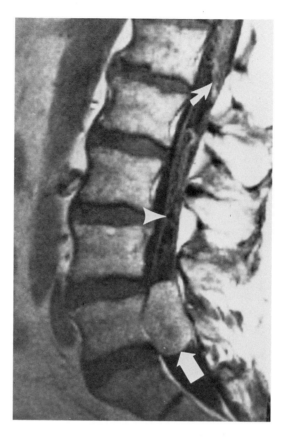

Fig. 20–14. Sagittal T1 image with Gd. Approximately isodense with disc material on noncontrasted T1 images, this large, filum paraganglioma (broad arrow) shows enhancement. Within the thecal space rostrally, one can faintly see serpiginous areas of signal void (arrowhead), indicating dilated vascular channels subsequent to the tumor's internal hypervascularity. The cord can be seen (small arrow) ending at the L1–2 interspace.

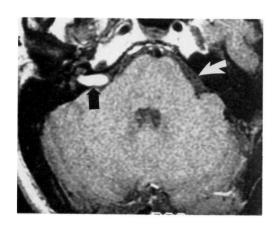

Fig. 20–13. Axial T1 image with Gd. Instead of a low T1 signal as in cisterns (white arrow), the right internal auditory canal is filled with a sausage-shaped enhancing mass (black arrow). The neuroma barely projects into the adjacent CP angle cistern. With nondescript T1 and T2 signals before contrast, it was almost imperceptible. It is common to diagnose acoustic neuromas smaller than this, a formidable challenge with CT because of the competing whiteness of surrounding bone. With CT, intrathecal contrast likely would have been required. The high-signal material anterior to the pontine and CP angle cisterns is fatty marrow within the petrous apices.

esses. More disturbingly, reparative processes, gliosis, and meningeal scarring also enhance (Fig. 20–16),[41] and along with radionecrosis, confound differentiation from neoplasia.

MRI APPEARANCE OF EDEMA

Edema accompanies most intra-axial abnormalities, and therefore, is a nonspecific finding. As an interpretive strategy, edema is characterized as one of three types: vasogenic, cytotoxic, and interstitial.[42] Unless serving an

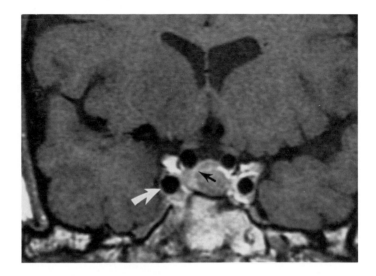

Fig. 20–15.   Coronal T1 image with Gd. This nonenhancing 1-cm prolactinoma (overlaid by black arrow) balloons the sellar diaphragm upward into the supersellar cistern and bows the left sellar floor downward. A rim of residual pituitary tissue is present (black arrow), which, because of its normal enhancement, can be differentiated from tumor. The parasellar higher signal material is circulating, contrast-laden blood in the cavernous sinuses, containing the on-end internal carotid arteries (one loop on right indicated by white arrow). Intracavernous structures such as cranial nerves III, IV, VI, and the ophthalmic division of V are frequently discernible. Curiously, large pituitary tumors with extrasellar spread usually show abnormal contrast enhancement. Although MRI is preferred for sellar investigations, CT performs almost as well and has the advantage of better depiction of bone distortion.

unusual patient mix, most facilities will see mainly vasogenic edema, the type seen surrounding intra-axial neoplasms (Fig. 20–17). Edema also occurs with other types of lesions, such as inflammatory. Characterized by involvement of white matter, it represents fluid seeping into the interaxonal interstices. Its extent, relative to the original inciting lesion, is variable and frequently disproportionately extensive. Without contrast it may be difficult to differentiate reactive edema from tumor.

Cytotoxic edema is seen with infarction (Fig. 20–18). It reflects geographically the vascular territory involved, and if cortically arterial in origin, it has a recognizably triangular configuration with a centrally directed apex and affects both gray and white matter. It is thought to be secondary to an abnormal intracellular accumulation of fluid as a result of a sodium/potassium "pump" malfunction.

Interstitial edema, a somewhat unfortunate appellation, reflects a special situation. Occurring when CSF, under pressure within the ventricular system, leaks transependymally into the periventricular tissues, it creates a halo of edema around mostly the lateral, but sometimes, the third and fourth ventricles (Fig. 20–19). Seen capriciously with hydrocephalus, early anticipation that the finding would become a valuable tool for differentiating atrophy from "normal pressure" hydrocephalus has gone unrealized. Furthermore, normally, a faint rim of periventricular high signal mimics interstitial edema. (True transependymal leakage must also be differentiated from the several demyelinating diseases that occur periventricularly, although the latter are generally more irregularly distributed.)

Recognition of a dominant variety of edema is helpful, but some examples are not purely of one category. The diagnostic usefulness of the pattern is frequently transcended by recognition of the primary lesion. The elegant depiction of edema by MRI probably has been most valuable conceptually by illustrating the impact of edema in the production of mass effect. If delayed images are obtained, edema may show slight enhancement.

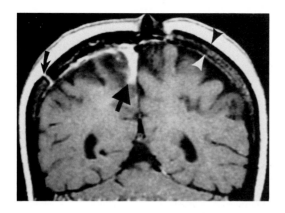

Fig. 20–16. Coronal T1 image with Gd. This patient had a right parietal parafalcine meningioma removed 3 months previously. Precontrast T1 images showed no significant high signal in the area, but this image shows a band of meningeal enhancement (large black arrow). Perhaps this is simply meningeal reaction to surgery, but it is impossible to exclude residual tumor. Although craniotomy margins may be difficult to define on MRI, the inferior margin of this flap is well delineated (small black arrow). Note the opposite parietal bone. The inner and outer tables (arrowheads) are low-signal black structures, with the intermediate signal diploë intervening. Internal to the inner table is a thin intermediate signal structure that is dura, showing slight normal enhancement. External to the outer table is high-signal subcutaneous fat. The dilated sulci over both high convexities indicate atrophy, exaggerated on the right by postoperative encephalomalacia.

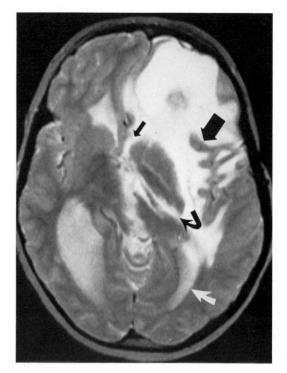

Fig. 20–17. Axial T2 image. Predominantly white matter edema creates a very high signal in the left frontoparietal region. Note the involvement of both internal capsule limbs (small arrows) and sparing of the distorted, adjacent lentiform nucleus and thalamus. Enfolded cortex in the sylvian fissure area (large arrow) retains its normal signal also. The edema's signal is even higher than intraventricular CSF (white arrow). The mass effect of the edema was greater than that of the inciting glioblastoma, above this section plane.

MRI APPEARANCE OF HEMORRHAGE

MRI reveals its dependence on the magnetic properties of tissues most evidently with hemorrhage.[43] With the exception of subarachnoid hemorrhage in which extravasated blood may not easily convert to deoxyhemoglobin because of oxygen in circulating CSF, hemoglobin degradation products show characteristic appearances. Circulating blood, containing considerable oxyhemoglobin, does not give a conspicuous signal.

Consider a fresh parenchymal hemorrhage. Within a few hours, oxyhemoglobin converts to deoxyhemoglobin. The latter, evoking magnetic susceptibility effect, has a nondescript T1 signal, but a shortened T2 relaxation time, and

appears as an abnormally dark, or low-signal area (Fig. 20–20). In about 4 to 6 days, transition to methemoglobin occurs and the signal changes. The change occurs first in the clot's periphery, progressing centrally until all is converted, a process requiring several days, depending on the lesion's size. At this stage, the clot exhibits an unusual, high T1 signal (Fig. 20–21). The shortening of T1 relaxation time is accompanied by a lengthening of T2. T1 shortening is a direct consequence of paramagnetic methemoglobin, an effect also operative in T2 images, but more than offset by fluid within the clot and its immediate environs. The net result is T2 lengthening instead,

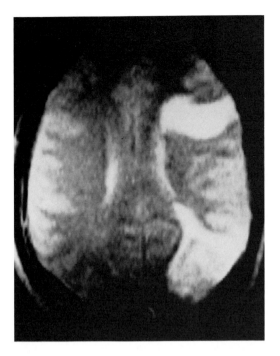

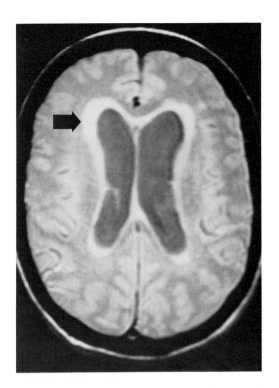

Fig. 20-18. Axial T2 image (blurring patient motion). Two left-sided high-signal areas of cytotoxic edema are present, both in middle cerebral arterial territories. Both extend from the cortex through the white matter to the left lateral ventricle. Despite their size, there is relatively little mass effect. These ischemic infarcts were approximately 48-hours old.

Fig. 20-19. Axial proton density image. A high-signal halo surrounds the slightly dilated lateral ventricles. The patient had acute obstructive hydrocephalus secondary to compression of the fourth ventricle.

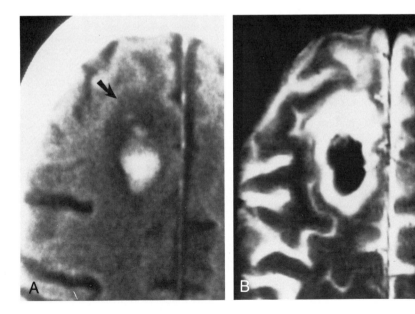

Fig. 20-20. A, Axial CT without contrast. This high right frontal parenchymal hemorrhage shows a broad zone of lucent-appearing edema surrounding a smaller hyperdense hematoma. B, Axial T2 image. The acute hemorrhage, deoxyhemoglobin, is shown as an area of very low signal surrounded by high-signal edema.

478

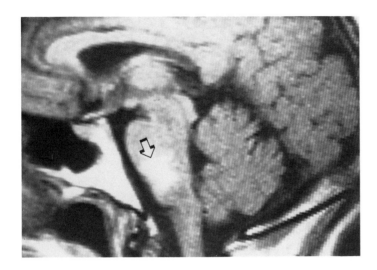

Fig. 20–21. Sagittal T1 image of the same patient as in Figure 20-7. The methemoglobin in this subacute hemorrhage is easily recognized. The versatility of MRI in allowing off-axial views facilitates lesion localization.

thus resulting in the usual high, instead of low signal. Melanin has the same effect (Fig. 20–22).[44] Fat has much the same appearance, but tends to fade with long TEs, and is seldom mistaken for clot or melanin, partly because subcutaneous fat offers a standard for compar-

ison. The methemoglobin signal is retained for several months. As it is degraded, hemosiderin and ferritin appear and are phagocytized, producing images that are the reverse of those of methemoglobin—low signals on both T1 and T2, persisting for years. The end result is an

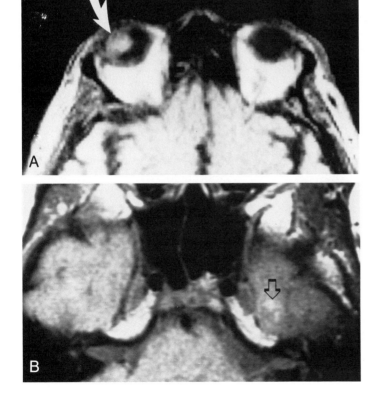

Fig. 20–22. A, Axial T1 image. A melanotic malignant melanoma in the patient's right globe shows a characteristic high signal. B, Axial T1 image. This small mixed neuronal/glial tumor (hollow arrow), similar to a ganglioglioma, was shown better on T2 and T1 Gd images, but its most interesting feature was a high signal on noncontrasted T1s, thought likely to be secondary to past hemorrhage. Histologically, there was none, but many glial cells contained large amounts of melanin.

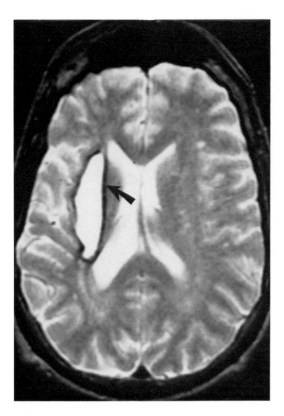

Fig. 20-23. Axial T2 image. A cystic lesion is in the left centrum semiovale; its contents match the high signal of CSF in the ventricular system. The pronouced low-signal (black) margin (arrow) to the cyst is thought to represent hemosiderin. The patient had sustained a hemorrhagic infarct 3 years and 2 weeks previously.

encephalomalacic space with a black peripheral rim of hemosiderin/ferritin (Fig. 20-23).

CT shows simpler time-dependent changes of clot because of different tissue properties.[45] X-ray absorption is dependent on atomic number, and proteins in the hemoglobin molecule cause more attenuation than brain tissue (iron contributes minimally to a clot's radio-opacity), until hemoglobin is broken down, clot appears white (Fig. 20-24). Normal flowing blood on CT has a higher attenuation than does brain tissue, with a faint whitish appearance compared with the latter. (To digress, a seriously anemic patient's blood may contain so little hemoglobin that a clot may appear aberrantly CT lucent. With MRI, such a clot's signal should be qualitatively the usual, al-

though its strength might be reduced.) As clot retraction occurs over the course of a few hours, attenuation increases, but thereafter gradually converges toward normal brain opacity as component molecules become smaller and more diluted. At about 10 to 14 days, clot will resemble normal brain, and is termed "isodense"; it may then be overlooked on scan (Fig. 20-25). By about 3 weeks post-hemorrhage, the clot becomes relatively "lucent" compared with brain and increasingly resembles CSF (Fig. 20-26). At that point, a fluid collection can be appreciated, but its hemorrhagic origin is not apparent. Eventually, the clot may show dystrophic calcification, poorly detectable on MRI but unmistakable on CT. Subacutely, it may show a peripheral ring of abnormal CT and MR contrast enhancement as a result of a disrupted BBB and/or reparative hypervascularity. Temporal differences in the appearance of clots seen on MR and CT scans make the two types of studies complementary (Fig. 20-27). Clot and subarachoid hemorrhage are seen hyperacutely more convincingly by CT (first 3 days), a fortunate circumstance, because other factors also reduce MRI performance in the same period. At about 1 week, either imaging method will conspicuously show clot as an abnormally white lesion. Beyond 10 to 12 days, MRI is superior, continuing to depict blood with a high signal, whereas on CT, the lesion will either be "isodense," or nonspecifically "lucent." Years later, MRI may still indicate prior hemorrhage by hemosiderin/ferritin deposits.

Even at a time of maximal conspicuity on CT, there are sites at which a clot might go unrecognized because of artifact from adjacent bone, notably in the posterior fossa and the spinal cord.

In summary, blood clots can be recognized on both CT and MRI, but the latter is more useful except in the immediate post-hemorrhage period. To exploit MRI, both T1 and T2 images must be obtained, and it is particularly useful in detection of hemorrhage in certain locales. Contrast administration is unnecessary except to exclude underlying pathology. A clot of unknown age may be vintaged up to an age of about 3 weeks, and older clots can be identified.

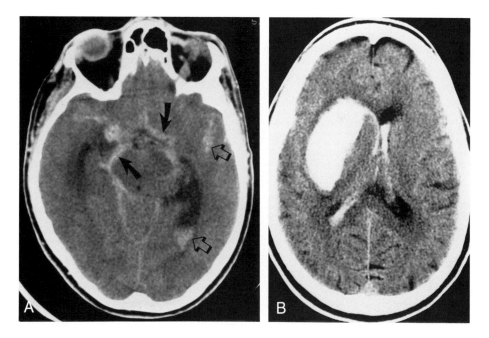

Fig. 20–24. A, Axial CT without contrast. The patient suffered a subarachnoid hemorrhage 24 hours previously. Opaque blood is widely scattered in the ventricular cistern, over the insular surface (both hollow arrows) and in the basal cisterns (solid arrows). A right carotid bifurcation aneurysm had ruptured. B, Axial CT without contrast. A large, day-old frontal hemorrhage is shown dissecting into the frontal horn and spreading throughout the lateral ventricles. Minimal edema surrounds the clot. As an incidental comparison to MRI, note that the calvarium is white and the subcutaneous fat is black, the reverse of that seen on MRI.

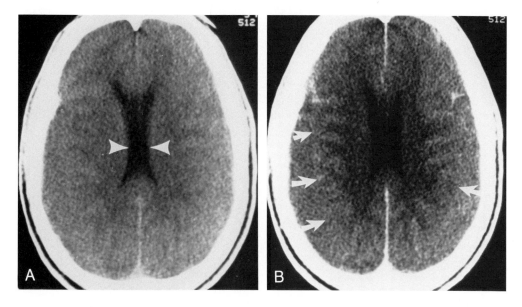

Fig. 20–25. A, Axial CT without contrast. The lateral ventricles have an appearance that suggests bilateral compression, but no specific lesion can be identified. In fact, large symmetrical parietal subdural hematomas are present. B, Axial CT with contrast. Rescanning after administration of IV contrast shows a faintly discernible brain margin displaced well medially (white arrows). The 12-day-old hematomas have neither internal vascularity nor leakage of contrast into them and become detectable. Inward displacement of white matter is also apparent.

481

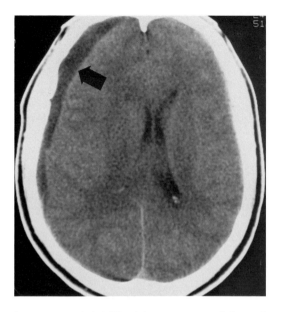

Fig. 20-26. Axial CT without contrast. A 3- to 4-week-old lucent subdural hematoma displaces brain. Mass effect distorts the lateral ventricles.

MRI APPEARANCE OF CNS MALDEVELOPMENT OR TISSUE LOSS

This section emphasizes those processes in which tissue has been lost, focally or diffusely in an atrophic/encephalomalacic fashion, with mention of developmental anomalies. MRI is the best imaging tool for most such processes. Some hypoplasias, such as in the corpus callosum, resulting in rather trivial deficits are not uncommonly incidentally discovered in the elderly and may be easier to appreciate on multidirectional images (Fig. 20–28) than by autopsy sectioning processes. An appreciation of overall organ configuration is paramount and T1 images excel. (They are usually supplemented with T2s in case other pathology exists, or for more pronounced differentiation of gray from white matter.) Focal tissue loss is well shown and may suggest the nature of the original insult (Fig. 20–29). Brain stem and cerebellar degenerations or anomalies are well shown (Fig. 20–30). Because of the large number of patients afflicted, MRI may prove most

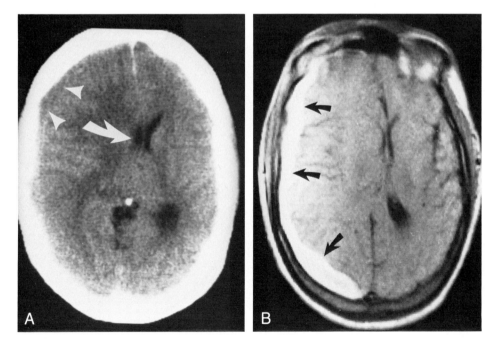

Fig. 20-27. A, Axial CT without contrast. Mass effect from the right frontal area displaces the ventricular system (arrow), but the lesion is unseen. One might make a tenuous case for a small, faintly lucent extracerebral fluid collection (arrowheads). B, Axial T1 image; done within 24 hours of the preceding CT. A large, 2-week-old right convexity subdural hematoma is identified.

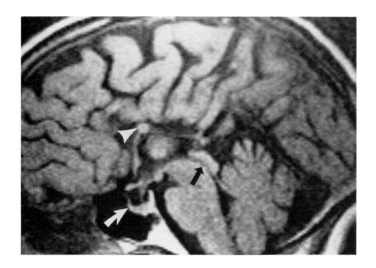

Fig. 20–28. Sagittal T1 image. This 63-year-old patient was incidentally found to have an almost absent corpus callosum, with a small remnant (arrowhead) present near the genu area. The cingulate gyrus is absent. The patient also shows a partly "empty" sella (white arrow) with its superior half filled with CSF. The pituitary stalk passes downward to residual pituitary tissue in the sellar depths. Other normal structures can be identified, including the aqueduct (black arrow), a large mass intermedia, and mamillary bodies.

valuable in assessing regional or diffuse brain loss.

Marginally dilated sulci and ventricles are difficult to distinguish from normal variations, and it is even harder to correlate the degree of atrophy with neurologic malfunction, or with a clinical syndrome or specific dementia (Fig. 20–31).[46] The distinction between mild hydrocephalus and atrophically enlarged ventricles is frequently uncertain, notwithstanding a variety of measurement algorithms;[47] the lack of their widespread adoption is probably a testament both to the laboriousness of calculations and to a lack of specificity. Such categorization problems may yield to computer solutions. "Mapping" software that more or less independently (little human direction) measures such things as the relative volumes of brain tissue and CSF, lobar or basal ganglion symmetry, and white versus gray matter is a realistic prospect. Abnormal symmetry of the temporal lobes may shortly be quantitated in dyslexics,[48] and almost certainly patterns of regional abnormality in the dementias will emerge. It may be possible to document associated cortical thinning. The cortical mantle, infrequently studied by neuroradiologists in the past, is likely to become an unaccustomed object of interest (Fig. 20–32).

The foregoing text and accompanying illustrations should have furnished familiarization with MRI's potentials and image appearances. We shall now consider interdisciplinary impacts.

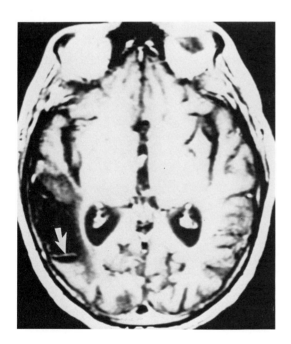

Fig. 20–29. Axial T1 image. A discrete lesion can be seen in the right temporal region; its internal signal matches CSF in the ventricles. It is the encephalomalacic result of infarction. Note surviving string-like vessels bridging the space (arrow).

NEUROPATHOLOGY-NEURORADIOLOGY SYNERGIES

Following appraisal of specimens, the pathologist casts the decisive vote identifying a specific disease process. By furnishing feed-

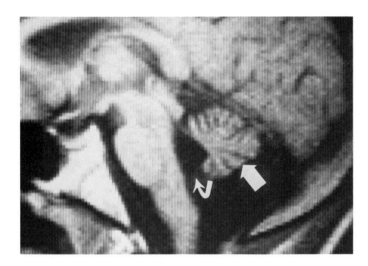

Fig. 20–30. Sagittal T1 image. This patient shows a well formed but diminutive vermis (broad arrow). In more lateral images, both inferior cerebellar hemispheres were also hypoplastic. Note the broad foramen of Magendie (small arrow). The brain stem is normal.

back to other specialties, such as radiology, other disciplines improve their own specificity. The aim of this section is to examine potentially fruitful areas of cooperation. Some clini-

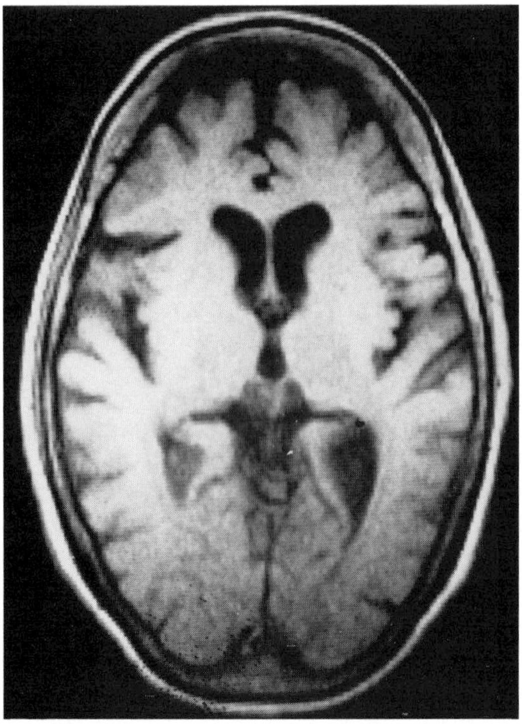

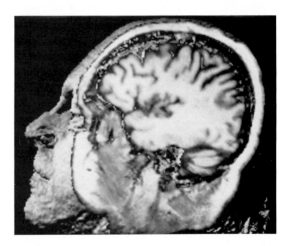

Fig. 20–31. Axial T1 image. Clinically thought to have Pick's disease, this patient shows atrophy in the frontotemporal regions. Note the dilated frontal horns and third ventricle and the almost exclusively enlarged frontal lobe sulci. Yet, a busy neuroradiologist will see many ostensibly similar scans in patients without Pick's.

cal abnormalities, particularly those temporary in nature, such as transient ischemic attacks, are better appreciated clinically than pathologically and are amenable to radiologic demonstration. In addition, there are situations in which neuroradiologic evidence may be of considerable benefit to the neuropathologist. Probably the two most important areas of information flow from radiology lie in appraising the environment of a lesion and in the intro-

Fig. 20–32. Sagittal T1 section from "3D" image. Once a 3D image is constructed, sections in any appropriate deep plane may be extracted. Although the plane chosen may be curved to match the cortical surface, this section is flat, cut in the parasagittal plane, showing the deep sylvian fissure and part of the insular surface. The implications for mapping of brain surface and correlation with external landmarks are obvious. The "ice crystal" effect surrounding the brain is electronic noise.

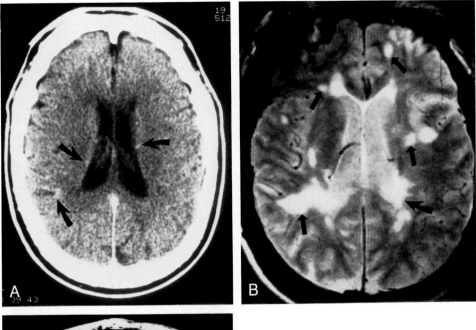

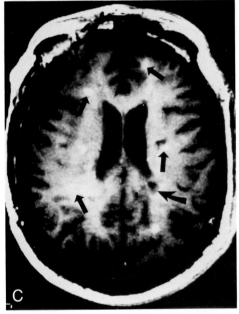

Fig. 20–33. A, Axial CT with contrast. Clinically, this patient was thought to have multiple sclerosis, but the CT was only marginally supportive of that diagnosis. This scan shows only questionable areas of enhancing plaques (arrows). B, Axial T2 image. Almost all T2 sections showed myriad high-signal demyelinations. Some are indicated with arrows. Many lesions merge with the ventricles but others are peripheral. C, Axial T1 image with Gd. About half of the biopsy-proven MS plaques show enhancement. Compare these with the same lesions in B. The lesion marked with a curved arrow appears largely inactive. Many more enhancing lesions are seen on this image made during an exacerbation of disease than on studies done about a year earlier and a year later.

duction of time as a variable, most applicable in fluid (blood or CSF) dynamics.

NEURORADIOLOGIC CONTRIBUTIONS TO THE NEUROPATHOLOGIST

Understanding the Milieu

The basic issue here is that of obtaining a representative sample for histologic analysis. Even at autopsy, with the entire specimen available, isolated tiny lesions might go undetected without the focused attention of the prosector. Although it is likely that most common demyelinating diseases, such as subcortical arteriosclerotic encephalopathy or multiple sclerosis (MS), would be represented on routine brain sections, it is advantageous for the prosector to have advance knowledge of the lesions' distribution. MR scans show MS plaques with considerable accuracy (Fig. 20–33A,B), a property furnishing one of the early

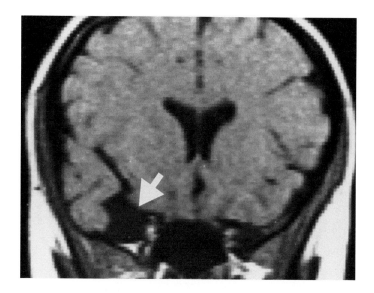

Fig. 20–34. Coronal T1 image. A low-signal CSF collection is producing minimal mass effect in the medial temporal area on the right. It proved to be a subarachnoid cyst.

justifications of the method.[49] Indeed, the combination of contrast scans and the facility of follow-up studies provide objective evidence of the efficacy of treatment, separating new and/or active lesions from malacia of past disease (Fig. 20–33C). Parenthetically, feedback from the pathologist is crucial in differentiating other scan-similar pathology such as subcortical arteriosclerotic encephalopathy (Binswanger's dementia), in specifying the nature of frequently seen leukoaraiotic foci ("UBOs"—unidentified bright objects), and in distinguishing all from normal structures such as Virchow-Robin spaces. Such correlations are in part the justification for routine post mortem MRI of brain specimens at some institutions.

Another neuroradiologic contribution, along with clinical evidence, is to emphasize the need for detailed study of structures not normally examined at routine autopsy. In the main, these lie outside the brain or pituitary, structures routinely sectioned. Dural venous sinuses (particularly the cavernous), the calvarium, and facial sinuses are not routinely sampled. A neoplasm causing substantial cranial nerve involvement within a jugular bulb might go unnoted, and a basisphenoid mass might not be discernible. Finally, there are certain, mainly extra-axial, lesions such as subarachnoid cysts that may be clearly identified on MRI (Fig. 20–34) but are so fragile that

organ removal may distort them enough to escape histologic examination.

In surgical pathology the necessarily selective biopsy accentuates the pathologist's vulnerability. Consider the matter of multiplicity of lesions. A biopsied hamartoma or giant cell astrocytoma may suggest the possibility of tuberous sclerosis, but prior knowledge of numerous periventricular, calcific lesions on CT effectively makes the diagnosis. (Tuberous sclerosis, notwithstanding its characteristic clinical triad of findings, is frequently first diagnosed by scan, with the clinical findings then retrospectively apparent.) Although a thorough prosector, recognizing the likelihood of allied disease processes would sample facial sinusoidal and/or mastoid cells in a case of epidural abscess, direction from prior scans provides a reassuring measure of completeness (Fig. 20–35).

Particularly since the advent of CT stereotactically guided biopsy, sample sites are increasingly selected by neuroradiologic methods. A biopsy obtained from the center of a necrotic area is unlikely to offer definitive information, whereas tissue from the active margin of a diseased area, obtainable with reasonable assurance stereotactically, usually allows an accurate diagnosis (Fig. 20–36). In fact, stereotactic biopsies have affected even the spectrum of disease submitted to the pathologist, since many lesions previously considered

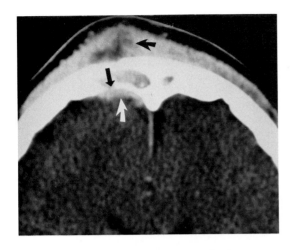

Fig. 20–35. Axial CT with contrast. The low attenuation area in the forehead (curved black arrow) surrounded by edematous tissue is an abscess. The frontal sinus is filled with pus and there is a destructive defect in its posterior wall (straight black arrow) leading to an area of enhancement (white arrow) in the frontopolar extracerebral space—an epidural abscess.

unapproachable are now biopsied. The technique is one of the great breakthroughs of the last few decades.

Certain disease processes impinging on the CNS are poorly appreciated by biopsy; tissue obtained is insufficient, in itself, to clarify the pathologic process, and the sample must be considered in its in vivo setting. Material obtained during repair of dysraphic lesions and disc herniations—normal tissue out of context (Fig. 20–37)—may not reveal the pathophysiology involved. Without surgical observations or radiologic evidence, the pathologist's appraisal of herniated disc fragments is almost meaningless. The same deficit is operative in the histologic examination of a blood clot, inasmuch as the specimen might not reveal causation or its impact on the CNS. A more subtle limitation occurs when the CNS is damaged by an abnormality that is operative only with the patient in certain postures. Neither histologic evidence of post-traumatic myelomalacia or rheumatoid arthritic pannus at the C1–2 area

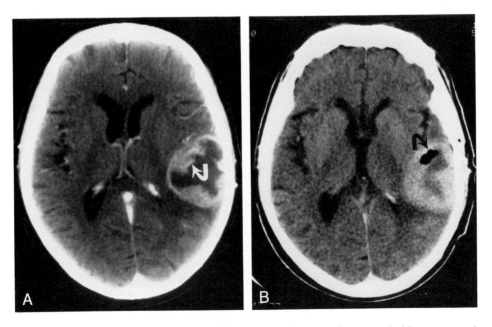

Fig. 20–36. A, Axial CT with contrast. This internally necrotic, ring-enhancing glioblastoma was biopsied with BRW stereotactic technique at the indicated site (curved arrow). B, Axial CT with residual contrast from previous study, done a few minutes after the biopsy. It shows a bubble of gas near the biopsy site in the viable ring of tissue. Contrast has diffused toward the lesion's center and the margins of viable tumor are less well-defined.

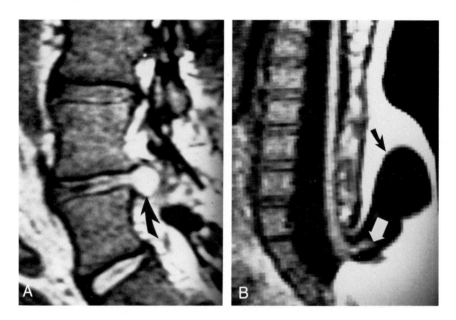

Fig. 20–37. A, Sagittal T1 image, lumbar spine. This patient has a large lateral herniated nucleus pulposus (arrow) at the L4–5 level. Note the continuity of the herniation with the narrowed and abnormally low-signal disc more anteriorly. The low signal, shared with L3–4, indicates desiccation. The horizontal clefts in the discs are normal. B, T1 sagittal image shows a classic meningomyelocele, with neural tissue (white arrow) extending into the sac from the abnormally caudally positioned (tethered) cord. The serrated margin of the meningocele (black arrow) is a result of a relatively large pixel size.

conveys the mechanics of pathophysiology as do sagittal MRI images in the flexed position (Fig. 20–38).

In summary, by showing abnormalities in their environmental contexts, CT and MRI scans amalgamate abnormalities in a fashion that isolated tissue samples can only suggest. For a thorough understanding of the impact of pathologic processes, the neuropathologist might do well to use neuroradiologic images as a consolidating resource.

Time-Related Phenomena—Mostly Fluid Dynamics

Anatomic pathologists inspect tissue at a moment in time, and without uncommonly performed repeated sampling, are ignorant of temporal events, both rapidly and slowly consummated, that contribute to clinical symptoms. Nowhere is this more apparent than in the patterns and flow-rate of blood.

Although it is easy histologically to identify berry or mycotic aneurysms, arteriovenous malformations, and a variety of other angiomatous lesions, the same information is available on angiograms, and increasingly, on flow-emphasizing MR scans. (A more incomplete depiction is afforded on contrast-enhanced CT scans.) Conventional MRI techniques result in flowing blood producing no signal—a "flow void." Protons in moving blood may produce signals upon decay from RF excitation, but not remain in the sample plane long enough to be magnetized and/or release energy within the allotted time of scrutiny. The result is often a reasonable depiction of vascular lumens "in negative," with the caveat that turbulence results in false luminal estimations. Even without measures that improve flow evaluation, abnormal peri/intralesional vascularity can be seen noninvasively. Much effort is being invested in improving the visualization of vessels.[50,51] Intravascular contrast material helps, but activity has been mostly directed to developing specialized pulse sequences that accentuate flow (Fig. 20–39). Combined with pseudo-3D imaging, such techniques will supplant conventional angiography in many clinical situations. CT and MR scanning have relegated angiography mostly to a "road-map-

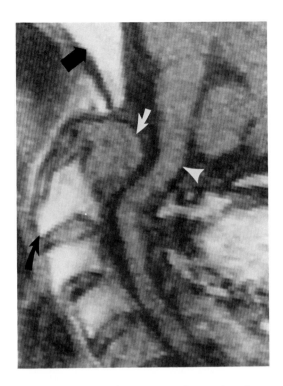

Fig. 20–38. Sagittal T1 image shows the distortions that may result from rheumatoid arthritis. The clivus (thick black arrow) and anteroinferior corner of the body of C2 (small black arrow) are identified. The odontoid process has been replaced by posterosuperiorly directed pannus (white arrow) that increasingly distorted the adjacent upper cervical cord (arrowhead) with flexion.

ping" procedure preparatory to surgery, rather than one for diagnostic purposes.

All forms of angiography depict clinically significant phenomena that are invisible on histologic examination. Intense arterial spasm as a result of subarachnoid hemorrhage, unless it results in infarction and/or sufficient dropout of neuronal elements from ischemia, is unappreciated. Abnormal direction of flow, frequently reversed in collateral channels, goes unnoticed. (MRI is emphasized in this chapter, but other radiologic techniques for the evaluation of flow phenomena, such as Doppler ultrasound, nuclear medicine studies, and xenon CT, contribute to their understanding.)

PET scanning and MR spectroscopy offer special information. If ^{31}P spectroscopy fulfills its promise, even temporarily ischemic tissue not proceeding to infarction will be identifiable. The prospect of timely intervention in pre-stroke situations has enormous implications.

Neuroradiologists have long been interested in the dynamics of CSF production, resorption, and flow, primarily because of applications in hydrocephalus. Recent investigations show the value of a specialized variation of MRI in the depiction of CSF flow. Based on the pulsatile movement of CSF, aberrations in flow patterns appear to be detectable.[52] This direct measure of dynamics, rather than the morphologic end-result as mirrored by ventricular size and configuration, may finally differentiate between hydrocephalus and atrophic ventricular enlargement.

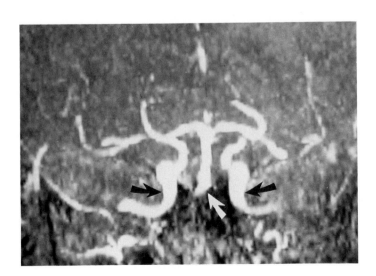

Fig. 20–39. Coronal gradient echo image. Part of an "MR angiogram," this image shows the major vessels of the base of the brain, including the carotids (black arrows), the basilar (white arrow), and their adjacent major branches. Such techniques may obviate the need for invasive angiographic alternatives.

NEUROPATHOLOGY INPUT TO NEURORADIOLOGY

The radiologist is beholden to the pathologist to prove the nature of the abnormalities that are discovered. With sufficient correlation, enough specificity is established to be useful. Needed, for example, is a solution to the difficulty MRI has in distinguishing between a unicameral cystic space and microcystic encephalomalacia. Another problem area is that of postoperative reparative change. With an abnormal signal following contrast, it is difficult to distinguish scar from a recurrence of the original lesion. The same may be said of radiation necrosis. Collaborative effort is needed in assessing the effectiveness of therapeutic embolization materials. Many similar challenges remain.

Some MRI abnormalities sufficient to prompt appropriate (surgical?) therapy are relatively nonspecific. A growth hormone producing pituitary tumor appears identical to a prolactinoma or an ACTH producing tumor. Joint effort is needed to develop contrast material that imitates immunocytochemical staining specificity.

FUTURE "NEURORADIOLOGIC" DIRECTION

Prognostication is an inherently humbling exercise. It is done here with little confidence, but in the hope of enough accuracy to focus thinking on emerging investigative areas of radiology with which neuropathology will likely interface.

Judging by the avalanche of technical refinements to MRI described in the literature, many incremental improvements in image acquisition, detail, and display formats are anticipated. One spinoff will be cine MRI, an undertaking being embarked upon now.[52] Pseudo, or real, 3D images will become commonplace. But fundamentally, such advances do not open new avenues, they "merely" improve existing techniques. Other enterprises are likely to be more revolutionary.

One might anticipate specific cell type, organ-seeking, or disease-specific contrast agents analogous to the immunocytochemical stains used in pathology. Increased reliance on blood or CSF flow/utilization studies will almost certainly emerge, both with MRI and radionuclide techniques. We should see increasing interest in the brain's surface and in peripheral nerves. The most promising new technique is in MR spectroscopy by which malfunction may be identified before permanent damage occurs; conventional pathologic proof of such evanescent "lesions" will be difficult to obtain. The emerging field of micro-MRI might, because of prior histologic expertise, be a matter of pathologic interpretation within an originally radiologic method, offering the advantage of nondestructive observations. Molecular diffusion phenomena also involve analysis of small samples, an enterprise that pathologists might be deeply involved in. The next decade promises to be exciting.

INTERDISCIPLINARY COMMUNICATION

CT, MR, and radionuclide scans provide data in a digital form that is ideal for manipulation and image transmittal. Currently, teleradiography emphasizes intraradiologic and clinical area networks where almost real-time viewing is desirable, such as critical care units; eventually, pathology departments will be included in such liaisons. Coupled with intercoms, timely communication between pathology and radiology departments should improve. The pathologist, as he receives a specimen for examination, will be able to review pertinent radiologic studies at the push of a few buttons.

COST FACTORS

The costs of a unit's initial purchase, maintenance, expendable supplies and personnel make MRI an expensive enterprise. A unit's typical price approaches 2 million dollars. A brain study is likely to cost $800 ±, and depending on their scope, spinal studies may cost more. Third party payers reimburse for scans, but society's limit of affordability, almost irrespective of merit, appears to approach. Progress and usage are predicted on the assumption that a valuable resource will be fully exploited, now a somewhat tenuous axiom. Audits should eventually show a favorable cost/benefit balance, as with CT, but to achieve this, MRI must be used selectively. One of the radiology department's responsibilities will be the education of referring physicians so that costs are justified.

CONCLUSION

More than any other radiologic tool, MRI exposed the myopia of complacency with existing methods. It could be years before medicine fully exploits even present day ^{1}H imaging, and optimization will doubtless be the result of joint efforts by clinicians, radiologists and pathologists, with radiology continuing to furnish a bridge between the patient or clinician and the pathologist. As present subsidiary efforts such as spectroscopy, nonhydrogen imaging, diffusion techniques, and microimaging evolve, it is hard not to foresee closer neuropathology/neuroradiology interdisciplinary symbiosis.

And, what will tomorrow bring?

ACKNOWLEDGMENTS

I am grateful to my colleagues E. Raymond Andrew, Ph.D. (Radiology and Physics) and William E. Ballinger, Jr., M.D. (Neuropathology) for insights into areas beyond my expertise. Thanks also to Ms. Linda Pigott, manuscript preparation specialist.

REFERENCES

1. Roentgen, W.C.: On a new kind of rays. Erste Mitt Sitzber Phys-Med Ges (Wurzburg), *137*:132, 1895.
2. Dandy, W.E.: Ventriculography following the injection of air into the cerebral ventricles. Ann. Surg., *68*:5, 1918.
3. Dandy, W.E.: Röntgenography of the brain after the injection of air into the spinal canal. Ann. Surg. *70*:397, 1919.
4. Sicard, J.A., and Forestier, J.: Methode générale d'exploration radiologique par l'huile iode (Lipiodol). Bull. Mem. Soc. Med. Hop. (Paris), *46*:463, 1922.
5. Ramsey, G.H., French, J.D., and Strain, W.H.: Iodinated organic compounds as contrast media for radiographic diagnosis. Radiology, *43*:236, 1944.
6. Skalpe, I.O., and Amundsen, P.: Lumbar radiculography with metrizamide. Radiology, *115*:91, 1975.
7. Skalpe, I.O., and Amundsen, P.: Thoracic and cervical myelography with metrizamide. Radiology, *116*:101, 1975.
8. Haschek, E., and Lindenthal, O.T.: A contribution to the practical use of the photography according to Röntgen. Wien. Klin. Wochenschr., *9*:63, 1986.
9. Moniz, E.: Arterial encephalography: Its importance in the location of cerebral tumors. Rev. Neurol., *2*:72, 1927.
10. Seldinger, S.I.: Catheter replacement of the needle in percutaneous arteriography. Acta Radiol., *39*:368, 1953.
11. Mealey, J., Dehner, J.R., and Reese, I.C.: Clinical comparison of two agents used in brain scanning. Radioiodinated serum albumin vs. chlormerodrin Hg 203. JAMA, *189*:260, 1964.
12. Ingvar, D.H., Cronqvist, S., Ekberg, R., et al.: Normal values of regional cerebral blood flow in man. Acta Neurol. Scand. Suppl., *14*:1, 1965.
13. Ambrose, J.: Computerized transverse axial scanning (tomography). 2. Clinical application. Br. J. Radiol., *46*:1023, 1973.
14. Hounsfield, G.: Computerized transverse axial scanning (tomography): Part 1. Description of System. Br. J. Radiol., *46*:1016, 1973.
15. Kramer, R.A., Janotos, G.P., and Peristein, G.: An approach to contrast enhancement in computed tomography of the brain. Radiology, *116*:641, 1975.
16. Gur, D., Wolfson, S.K., Yonas, H., et al.: Progress in cerebrovascular disease: Local cerebral blood flow by xenon enhanced CT. Stroke, *13*:750, 1982.
17. Heilbrun, M.P., Roberts, T.S., Apuzzo, M.L.J., et al.: Preliminary experience with Brown-Roberts-Wells (BRW) computerized tomography stereotaxic guidance system. J. Neurosurg., *59*:217, 1983.
18. Purcell, E.M., Torrey, H.C., and Pound, R.F.: Resonance absorption by nuclear magnetic moments in a solid. Physiol. Rev., *69*:37, 1946.
19. Block, F.: Nuclear induction. Physiol. Rev., *70*:460, 1946.
20. Lauterbur, P.: Image formation by induced local interactions: Examples employing nuclear magnetic resonance. Nature, *242*:190, 1973.
21. Schenck, J.F., Dumoulin, C.L., Souza, S.P., et al.: Health and physiological effects of human exposure to whole-body 4 tesla magnetic fields during magnetic resonance scanning. Abstracts, Society of Magnetic Resonance in Medicine, Ninth Annual Scientific Meeting and Exhibition, New York, *1*:277, 1990.
22. Carr, D.H., Brown, J., Bydder, G.M., et al.: Gadolinium-DTPA as a contrast agent in MRI: Initial clinical experience in 20 patients. AJR, *143*:215, 1984.
23. Goldstein, H.A., Kashanian, F.K., Blumetti, R.F., et al.: Safety assessment of gadopentetate dimeglumine in U.S. clinical trials. Radiology, *174*:17, 1990.
24. Van Wagoner, M., O'Toole, M., and Quay, S.C.: Nonionic magnetic resonance imaging contrast agents: Clinical trial experience of safety, tolerance, and efficacy of gadodiamide injection. Invest. Radiol., *25* (Suppl. 1):S39, 1990.
25. Engelstad, B.L., and Wolf, G.L.: Contrast agents. In: *Magnetic Resonance Imaging.* Edited by D.D. Stark and W.G. Bradley, Jr. St. Louis, C.V. Mosby, 1988.
26. Cho, Z.H., Ahn, S.C.J., Lee, H.K., et al.: Nuclear magnetic resonance microscopy with 4-μm resolution: Theoretical study and experimental results. Med. Phys., *15*:815, 1988.
27. Johnson, G.A., Benvenisti, H., Cofer, G.P., et al.: MR microscopy—applications in basic sciences. Abstracts, Society of Magnetic Resonance in Medicine, Ninth Annual Scientific Meeting and Exhibition, New York, *1*:254, 1990.
28. Le Bihan, D., Breton, E., Lallemand, D., et al.: MR imaging of intravoxel incoherent motions: Application to diffusion and perfusion in neurologic disorders. Radiology, *161*:401, 1986.

29. Ordidge, R.J., Howseman, A., Coxon, R., et al.: Snapshot imaging at 0.5 T using echo-planar techniques. Magn. Reson. Med., *10*:227, 1989.

30. Hilal, S., Maudsley, A.A., Ra, J.B., et al.: In vivo imaging of sodium-23 in the human head. J. Comput. Assist. Tomogr., *9*:1, 1985.

31. Bottomley, P.: Human in vivo NMR spectroscopy in diagnostic medicine: Clinical tool or research probe? Radiology, *170*:1, 1989.

32. Brant-Zawadzki, M., Weinstein, P., Bartkowski, H., et al.: MR imaging and spectroscopy in clinical and experimental cerebral ischemia: A review. AJNR, *8*:39, 1987.

33. Evanochko, W.T., Ng, T.C., and Glickson, J.D.: Application of in vivo NMR spectroscopy of cancer. J. Magnet. Reson. Med., *1*:508, 1984.

34. Kanal, E., Shellock, F.G., and Talagala, L.: Safety considerations in MR imaging. Radiology, *176*:593, 1990.

35. New, P.F.J., Rosen, B.R., Brady, T.J., et al.: Potential hazards and artifacts of ferromagnetic and nonferromagnetic surgical and dental materials and devices in nuclear magnetic resonance imaging. Radiology, *147*:139, 1983.

36. Pavlicek, W., Geisinger, M., Castle, L., et al.: The effects of nuclear magnetic resonance on patients with cardiac pacemakers. Radiology, *147*:149, 1983.

37. Smith, A.S., Weinstein, M.A., Hurst, G.C., et al.: Intracranial chemical-shift artifacts on MR images of the brain: Observations and relation to sampling bandwidths. AJR, *154*:1275, 1990.

38. Wismer, G.L., Rosen, B.R., Buxton, R., et al.: Chemical shift imaging of bone marrow: Preliminary experience. AJR, *145*:1031, 1985.

39. Czervionke, L.F., Czervionke, J.M., Daniels, D.L., et al.: Characteristic features of MR truncation artifacts. AJR, *151*:1219, 1988.

40. Wehrli, F.W., Sprawls, P., Fullerton, G.D., et al.: Introduction to MRI (Unit 1). In: *Magnetic Resonance Imaging*. Edited by D.D. Stark and W.G. Bradley, Jr. St. Louis, C.V. Mosby, 1988.

41. Elster, A.D., and DiPersio, D.A.: Cranial postoperative site: Assessment with contrast-enhanced MR imaging. Radiology, *174*:93, 1990.

42. Fishman, R.A.: Brain edema. N. Engl. J. Med. *293*:706, 1975.

43. Gomori, J.M., Grossman, R.I., Yu-Ip, C., et al.: NMR relaxation times of blood: Dependence of field strength, oxidation state and cell integrity. J. Comput. Assist. Tomogr., *11*:684, 1987.

44. Woodruff, W.W., Jr., Djang, W.T., McLendon, R.E., et al.: Intracerebral malignant melanoma: High-field strength MR imaging. Radiology, *165*:209, 1987.

45. New, P.F.J., and Aronow, S.: Attenuation measurements of whole blood and blood fractions in computed tomography. Radiology, *121*:635, 1976.

46. Jack, C.T., Mokri, B., Laws, E.R., Jr., et al.: Findings in normal-pressure hydrocephalus: Significance and comparison with other forms of dementia. J. Comput. Assist. Tomogr., *11*:923, 1987.

47. Guldensted, C., and Kosteljanetz, M.: Measurements of the normal ventricular system with computer tomography of the brain. A preliminary study on 44 adults. Neuroradiology, *10*:205, 1976.

48. Jack, C.R., Gehring, D.G., Sharbrough, F.W., et al.: Temporal lobe volume measurement from MR images: Accuracy and left-right asymmetry in normal persons. J. Comput. Assist. Tomogr., *12*:21, 1988.

49. Young, I.R., Hall, A.S., Pallis, C.A., et al.: Nuclear magnetic resonance imaging of the brain in multiple sclerosis. Lancet, *2*:1063, 1981.

50. Masaryle, T.J., Modic, M.T., Ross, J.S., et al.: Intracranial circulation: Preliminary clinical results with three-dimensional (volume) MR angiography. Radiology, *171*:793, 1989.

51. Pernicone, J.R., Seibert, J.E., Potchen, E.J., et al.: Three-dimensional phase-contrast MR angiography in the head and neck: Preliminary report. AJNR, *11*:457, 1990.

52. Quencer, R.M., Post, M.J.D., and Hinks, R.S.: Cine MR in the evaluation of normal and abnormal CSF flow: Intracranial and intraspinal studies. Neuroradiology, 1990. (In press.)

Index

Page numbers in *italics* indicate figures; numbers followed by "t" indicate tables.